PAEDIATRIC SURGERY:
A COMPREHENSIVE TEXT FOR AFRICA

EDITORS:

EMMANUEL A. AMEH
STEPHEN W. BICKLER
KOKILA LAKHOO
BENEDICT C. NWOMEH
DAN POENARU

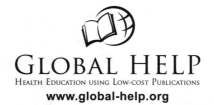

GLOBAL HELP
HEALTH EDUCATION USING LOW-COST PUBLICATIONS
www.global-help.org

Table of Contents: Volume I

TABLE OF CONTENTS: VOLUME II

CONTRIBUTING AUTHORS

Francis A. Abantanga, MD, Cert Paed Surg, PhD, FWACS,
Cert Cardio Surg, FGCS
Associate Professor, Head, Department/Directorate of Surgery
School of Medical Sciences/Komfo Anokye Teaching Hospital
College of Health Sciences
Kwame Nkrumah University of Science and Technology
Kumasi, Ghana

Hesham M. Abdelkader, MD, MRCS, FEBPS
Lecturer of Pediatric Surgery
Division of Pediatric Surgery
Ain Shams University
Cairo, Egypt

Lukman O. Abdur-Rahman, MBBS, MPH, FWACS
Senior Lecturer and Consultant Paediatric Surgeon
Paediatric Surgery Unit, Department of Surgery
College of Health Sciences, University of Ilorin and University of Ilorin
Teaching Hospital
Ilorin, Nigeria

Auwal M Abubakar, MBBS, FWACS, FICS
Associate Professor and Consultant Paediatric Surgeon
Paediatric Surgery Unit, Department of Surgery
College of Medical Sciences, University of Maiduguri and
University of Maiduguri Teaching Hospital
Maiduguri, Borno State, Nigeria

Adesoji O. Ademuyiwa, MBBS, FWACS, FMCS (Nig)
Lecturer and Consultant Paediatric Surgeon
Paediatric Surgery Unit, Department of Surgery
College of Medicine, University of Lagos
Lagos, Nigeria

James O. Adeniran, MBBS (Ib), FRCS (Glasg), FWACS,
Dip Paed Surg (Lond)
Professor of Paediatric Surgery
Paediatric Surgical Unit
University of Ilorin and University of Ilorin Teaching Hospital
Ilorin, Nigeria

Frank Agada, FRCS Ed
Department of ENT, Head and Neck Surgery
York Hospital
York, U.K.

Sunday Olusegun Ajike, BDS, FWACS, PGDPA
Associate Professor and Consultant Maxillofacial Surgeon
Department of Dental Surgery
Ahmadu Bello University and Ahmadu Bello University Teaching Hospital
Zaria, Nigeria

Jennifer H. Aldrink, MD
Assistant Professor of Clinical Surgery
The Ohio State University College of Medicine
Division of Pediatric Surgery
Nationwide Children's Hospital
Columbus, Ohio, U.S.

Christopher C. Amah, MB ChB, FWACS
Senior Lecturer & Consultant Pediatric Surgeon
Department of Pediatric Surgery
University of Nigeria and University of Nigeria Teaching Hospital
Enugu, Nigeria

Emmanuel A. Ameh, MBBS, FWACS, FACS
Professor and Consultant Paediatric Surgeon
Chief, Division of Paediatric Surgery, Department of Surgery
Ahmadu Bello University and Ahmadu Bello University Teaching Hospital
Zaria, Nigeria

Nkeiruka Ameh, MBBS, FWACS
Senior Lecturer and Consultant Obstetrician and Gynecologist
Reproductive Endocrinology & Infertility Unit
Department of Obstetrics & Gynecology
Ahmadu Bello University and Ahmadu Bello University
Teaching Hospital
Zaria, Nigeria

Manali S. Amin, MD, FACS
Instructor, Department of Otology and Laryngology
Harvard Medical School
Associate in Otolaryngology, Department of Otolaryngology
and Communication Disorders
Children's Hospital Boston
Boston, Massachusetts, U.S.

Safwat S. Andrawes, MBChB, MMed Surgery, MSc Urology,
FICS, FCS (ESCA)
Consultant Paediatric Surgeon and Paediatric Urologist
Gertrude's Children Hospital
Nairobi, Kenya

William Appeadu-Mensah, MB, CHB, FWACS, FGCS
Paediatric Surgery Unit, Department of Surgery
University of Ghana Medical School
Korle-Bu Teaching Hospital
Accra, Ghana

Marion Arnold, MBChB, DCH (SA)
Division of Pediatric Surgery
University of Stellenbosch
Tygerberg, South Africa

Johanna R. Askegard-Giesmann, MD
Clinical Research Fellow
Department of Pediatric Surgery
Nationwide Children's Hospital
The Ohio State University
Columbus, Ohio, U.S.

Jane P. Balint, MD
Associate Professor of Clinical Pediatrics
The Ohio State University College of Medicine
Director, Intestinal Support Service
Division of Pediatric Gastroenterology, Hepatology, and Nutrition
Nationwide Children's Hospital
Columbus, Ohio, U.S.

Behrouz Banieghbal, MB, BCh, BAO, FRCSI,
FRC (SA) Paed Surg
Paediatric Surgeon and Senior Lecturer
Division of Paediatric Surgery
Johannesburg General Hospital
University of the Witwatersrand
Johannesburg, South Africa

Nick Bauman, MD, FRCSC
BethanyKids at Kijabe Hospital
Kijabe, Kenya

Peter Beale, FCS (SA); M Med Chir (Pret), FRCS (Edin)
Head of Paediatric Surgery Division
University of the Witwatersrand
Johannesburg, South Africa

Stephen W. Bickler, MD, DTM&H, FACS, FAAP
Professor of Surgery & Pediatrics
University of California, San Diego
Attending Pediatric Surgeon
Children's Hospital of San Diego
San Diego, California, U.S.

Christopher Bode, MBCHB, FWACS, FMCS (Nig)
Associate Professor and Consultant Paediatric Surgeon
Paediatric Surgery Unit, Department of Surgery
Lagos University and Lagos University Teaching Hospital
Lagos, Nigeria

Laura Boomer, MD
Resident in General Surgery
University of Nevada School of Medicine
Las Vegas, Nevada, U.S.

Eric Borgstein, MD, FRCS (Edin), FCS (ECSA)
Professor of Surgery
Consultant Paediatric Surgeon
College of Medicine, University of Malawi
Queen Elizabeth Central Hospital
Blantyre, Malawi

Richard Bransford, MD, FACS
Program Director
BethanyKids at Kijabe Hospital
Kijabe, Kenya

Mairo Adamu Bugaje, MBBS (ABU), FWAC-Paed
Senior Lecturer and Consultant Paediatrician
Head, Department of Paediatrics
Ahmadu Bello University and Ahmadu Bello University Teaching Hospital
Zaria, Nigeria

Brian H. Cameron, MD, FRCSC, FACS
Associate Professor of Pediatric Surgery
McMaster Children's Hospital
Hamilton, Ontario, Canada

Louise Caouette-Laberge, Paediatric Plastic Surgeon
and Professor of Surgery
Hospital Sainte-Justine
Université de Montréal
Montréal, Qubec, Canada

Richard F. Carter, MD
Senior Resident, General Surgery
Department of Surgery
Virginia Commonwealth University School of Medicine
Richmond, Virginia, U.S.

John Chinda, MBBS, FWACS
Lecturer and Consultant Paediatric Surgeon
Paediatric Surgery Unit, Department of Surgery
University of Maiduguri and University of Maiduguri Teaching Hospital
Maiduguri, Nigeria

Lohfa B. Chirdan, MBBS, Dip Paed Surg (Lond), FWACS
Associate Professor and Consultant Paediatric Surgeon
Paediatric Surgery Unit, Department of Surgery
University of Jos and Jos University Teaching Hospital
Jos, Nigeria

Andrew Coatesworth, FRCS (ORL-HNS)
Department of ENT, Head & Neck Surgery
York Hospital
York, U.K.

Oriana D. Cohen, BA
Department of Surgery, Division of Pediatric Surgery
New York University Langone Medical Center
New York, New York, U.S.

Sharon Cox, MBChB, FCS (SA), Cert Paed Surg (SA)
Senior Consultant in Paediatric Surgery
Department of Pediatric Surgery
School of Child and Adolescent Health and Red Cross War Memorial Children's Hospital
University of Cape Town, Rondebosch
Cape Town, South Africa

Olamide O. Dairo, MD
Assistant Professor of Anesthesiology
The Ohio State University
Attending Anesthesiologist
Nationwide Children's Hospital
Columbus, Ohio, U.S.

Osarumwense David Osifo, MBBS, FWACS, FICS
Lecturer/Consultant Paediatric Surgeon
University of Benin Teaching Hospital
Benin City, Nigeria

Miliard Debrew, MD, FRCS (Eng), FCS (ECSA)
Assistant Professor of Paediatric Surgery
Black Lion Hospital, Addis Ababa University
Addis Ababa, Ethiopia

Ashish Desai, FRCS, FEBPS, MCh Paed, DNB Paed Surg
Consultant Paediatric Surgeon
King's College Hospital
London, U.K.

David P. Drake, MA, MB, BChir, FRCS, DCH
Consultant Paediatric Surgeon
Department of Paediatric Surgery
Great Ormond Street Hospital for Children
London, U.K.

Felicitas Eckoldt-Wolke, Professor of Pediatric Surgery
Chair and Chief of Clinic of Paediatric Surgery
Jena University Hospital
Friedrich Schiller University of Jena
Jena, Germany

Stella A. Eguma, MBBS, DA, FWACS
Professor of Anaesthesia
Ahmadu Bello University
Consultant Anaesthetist
Ahmadu Bello University Teaching Hospital
Zaria, Nigeria
Consultant Anaesthetist
John F Kennedy Memorial Hospital
Monrovia, Liberia

Sebastian O. Ekenze, MBBS, FWACS
Senior Lecturer & Consultant Pediatric Surgeon
Department of Pediatric Surgery
University of Nigeria and University of Nigeria Teaching Hospital
Enugu, Nigeria

Khalid A. ElAsmar, MBBCH, MS, MRCS
Division of Pediatric Surgery
Ain Shams University
Cairo, Egypt

Hesham Soliman El Safoury, MD
Professor of Pediatric Surgery
Ain-Shams University
Cairo, Egypt

Charles F.M. Evans, BSc, MBBS, MRCS (Eng), MD
Department of Paediatric Surgery
Oxford Children's Hospital
John Radcliffe Hospital
Oxford, U.K.

Iyekeoretin Evbuomwan
Professor and Consultant Paediatric Surgeon
Department of Surgery
University of Benin and University of Benin Teaching Hospital
Benin, Nigeria

Renata Fabia, MD, PhD, FACS
Assistant Professor of Clinical Surgery
The Ohio State University
Director of Burn Unit
Nationwide Children Hospital
Columbus, Ohio, U.S.

Julia B Finkelstein
New York University Langone School of Medicine
New York, New York, U.S.

Andrew P Freeland, FRCS
Consultant ENT Surgeon
John Radcliffe Hospital
Oxford, U.K.

Howard B Ginsburg, MD
Director
Division of Pediatric Surgery, Department of Surgery
New York University Langone School of Medicine
New York, New York, U.S.

John R. Gosche, MD, PhD
Chief, Division of Pediatric Surgery
Professor of Surgery, Department of Surgery
University of Nevada School of Medicine
Las Vegas, Nevada, U.S.

Hugh W. Grant, BSc, MB ChB, MD, FRCS (Edin), FRCS (Eng)
Consultant Paediatric Surgeon
John Radcliffe Hospital
Oxford, U.K.

Jonathan I. Groner, MD, FACS, FAAP
Professor of Clinical Surgery
The Ohio State University College of Medicine
Interim Chief, Department of Pediatric Surgery
Trauma Medical Director
Nationwide Children's Hospital
Columbus, Ohio, U.S.

Devendra K Gupta, MBBS, MS MCh, FAMS, FRCS,
   DSc (Honoris Causa)
Professor and Head, Department of Pediatric Surgery
All India Institute of Medical Sciences
New Delhi, India

Ahmed T. Hadidi, MB, BCh, MSc, MD, FRCS (Eng, Glasgow),
   FA (Germany), PhD
Professor of Pediatric Surgery
Chairman of Pediatric Surgery Dept. Offenbach Hospital, Offenbach
Chairman of Pediatric Surgery Dept., Emma Hospital, Seligenstadt
Frankfurt, Hessen, Germany

Larry Hadley, MB.CHB.,FRCS (Edin),FCS (SA)
Professor and Head of Department of Paediatric Surgery
Nelson Mandela School of Medicine
University of KwaZulu-Natal
Durban, South Africa

Alaa F. Hamza, MD, FRCS, FAAP (Hon)
Professor of Pediatric Surgery
Head of Liver Transplantation Unit
Division of Pediatric Surgery
Ain Shams University
Cairo, Egypt

Edward Hannon, BSc (Hons), MBChB (Hons), MRCS
Specialist Registrar in Paediatric Surgery
Oxford Children's Hospital
Oxford, U.K.

Sameh Abdel Hay, MD
Professor and Chief, Pediatric Surgery Unit
Ain Shams University
Cairo, Egypt

Hugo A. Heij, MD, PhD
Professor of Paediatric Surgery and Head
Paediatric Surgical Centre of Amsterdam
Emma Children's Hospital AMC and VU University Medical Centre
Amsterdam, The Netherlands

Chris Heinick, Paediatric Surgeon
Klinik für Kinderchirurgie der Friedrich-Schiller Universität
Jena, Germany

Afua A. J. Hesse, MB.ChB FRCS (Ed), FWACS, FGCS,
   Cert,HMPP (Leeds)
Associate Professor and Consultant Paediatric Surgeon
Head, Department of Surgery
Korle-Bu Teaching Hospital and the University of Ghana Medical School
Accra, Ghana

Rowena Hitchcock, MB BCh, MA, MD, FRCS
Consultant Paediatric Urologist
Oxford Children's Hospital
Oxford, U.K.

Piet Hoebeke, MD, PhD
Head of Department of Urology
Paediatric Urology and Urogenital Reconstruction
Ghent University Hospital
Ghent, Belgium

Sarah Howles, MRCS (Eng), MA
Department of Paediatric Surgery
Oxford Children's Hospital
Oxford, U.K.

Amy Hughes-Thomas, BSc (Hons), MBBS, MRCS (Eng)
Specialist Registrar Paediatric Surgery
The Children's Hospital, John Radcliffe NHS Trust
Oxford, England

Akanidomo J. Ibanga, BSc, MSc (Clin Psych)
School of Psychology
University of Birmingham
Birmingham, West Midlands, U.K.

Hannah B. Ibanga, MBBS, FWACP (Paeds), Child Psychology (Dip)
Emergency Department
Birmingham Children's Hospital
Birmingham, West Midlands, U.K.

Rebecca Inglis, BM BCh, MA (Cantab)
Junior Research Fellow
Department of Paediatric Surgery
John Radcliffe Hospital
Oxford, U.K.

Sha-Ron Jackson, IeMD
Pediatric Surgery Research Fellow
Children's Hospital Los Angeles
Keck School of Medicine
University of Southern California
Los Angeles, California, U.S.

Iftikhar Ahmad Jan, MBBS, FCPS, FRCS (Eng + Edin), FACS,
FEBPS
Professor of Pediatric Surgery
The Children's Hospital
PIMS Islamabad and National Institute of Rehabilitation Medicine
Islamabad, Pakistan

Jayaratnam Jayamohan, MBBS, FRCS, BSc
Consultant Paediatric Neurosurgeon
Oxford Children's Hospital
Oxford, U.K.

V. T. Joseph, FRCS, MD
Consultant Paediatric Surgeon
John Radcliffe Hospital
Oxford, U.K.

Jonathan Karpelowsky, MBBCh, FCS (SA), Cert Paed Surg (SA)
Senior Specialist
Department of Paediatric Surgery
Red Cross War Memorial Children's Hospital
Cape Town, South Africa

Brian D. Kenney, MD
Assistant Professor of Clinical Surgery
Department of Pediatric Surgery
Nationwide Children's Hospital
The Ohio State University
Columbus, Ohio, U.S.

John Kimario, MMed
Consultant ENT Surgeon
Muhimbili National Hospital
Dar es Salaam, Tanzania

Sharon Kling, FCPaed (SA), MMed (Paed), M Phil
Tygerberg Children's Hospital and Stellenbosch University
Cape Town, South Africa

Sanjay Krishnaswami, MD, FACS, FAAP
Educational Director, Pediatric Surgical Residency
Assistant Professor, Division of Pediatric Surgery
Oregon Health & Science University
Portland, Oregon, U.S.

Neetu Kumar, MBBS, MRCS
Jenny Lind Children's Department
Norfolk & Norwich University Hospital
Norwich, U.K.

Jean-Martin Laberge, MD, FRCSC, FACS
Paediatric Surgeon and Professor of Surgery
Division of Pediatric General Surgery
The Montreal Children's Hospital of the McGill University
    Health Center
Montreal, Québec, Canada

Kokila Lakhoo, PhD, FRCS (Eng + Edin), FCS (SA),
    MRCPCH (U.K.), MBCHB
Consultant Paediatric Surgeon and Senior Lecturer
Children's Hospital Oxford and University of Oxford
Oxford, U.K.
African Affiliation: KCMC Tanzania

Richa Lal, MS, MCh
Additional Professor and Head
Department. of Pediatric Surgery
Sanjay Gandhi Post Graduate Institute of Medical Sciences
Lucknow, Uttar Pradesh, India

David A. Lanning, MD, PhD
Surgeon-in-Chief, Children's Hospital of Richmond
Associate Professor of Surgery and Attending Pediatric Surgeon
Department of Surgery
Virginia Commonwealth University School of Medicine
Richmond, Virginia, U.S.

Michael Laschat, MD
Consultant, Paediatric Anaesthesia
Children`s Hospital
Cologne, Germany

Mohammed A. Latif Ayad, MD
Consultant of Pediatric Surgery
Division of Pediatric Surgery
Ain Shams University
Cairo, Egypt

John Lazarus, MBChB, FC UROL (SA), MMed (Urology)
Paediatric Urologist
Red Cross War Memorial Children's Hospital
University of Cape Town
Cape Town, South Africa

Jacob N. Legbo, MBBS, FWACS, FMCS (Nig), FRCSEd, FICS
Senior Lecturer and Consultant Plastic and Reconstructive Surgeon
Plastic Surgery Unit, Department of Surgery
Usmanu Danfodiyo University and Usmanu Danfodiyo University
    Teaching Hospital
Sokoto, Nigeria

Katrine Lofberg, MD
Surgical Resident
Oregon Health & Science University
Portland, Oregon, U.S.

Muhammad Raji Mahmud, MBBS, FWACS
Lecturer and Consultant Neurosurgeon
Division of Neurosurgery, Department of Surgery
Ahmadu Bello University and Ahmadu Bello University
    Teaching Hospital
Zaria, Nigeria

Amaani K. Malima, MD (Bulgaria), MMed (Orthop-Tumaini),
    FCS (ECSA)
Head, Department of Surgery
Temeke Municipal Hospital
Dar es Salaam, Tanzania

N. Marathovouniotis, MD
Department of Paediatric Surgery and Paediatric Urology
Childrens Hospital
Town of Cologne, Germany

Franklin C. Margaron, MD
Senior Resident, General Surgery
Department of Surgery
Virginia Commonwealth University School of Medicine
Richmond, Virginia, U.S.

Maurice Mars, MBChB, MD
Department of TeleHealth
Nelson R Mandela School of Medicine
University of Kwa-Zulu Natal
Durban, South Africa

Ruth D. Mayforth, MD, PhD
Consultant Paediatric Surgeon
BethanyKids at Kijabe Hospital
Kijabe, Kenya

Hyacinth N. Mbibu, BSc, MBBS, FWACS
Professor and Consultant Urologist
Division of Urology, Department of Surgery
Ahmadu Bello University and Ahmadu Bello University
    Teaching Hospital
Zaria, Nigeria

Merrill McHoney, MB, BS, FRCS (Paeds), PhD
Academic Clinical Lecturer
Department of Paediatric Surgery
Oxford Radcliffe Hospital
Oxford, U.K.

Vivien M McNamara, BM, BS, FRCS (C/Th), FRCS (Paed Surg)
Department of Paediatric Surgery
Great Ormond Street Hospital for Children
London, U.K.

Alice Mears, MBCHB, FRCS
Paediatric Surgery Specialist Registrar
Oxford Children's Hospital and University of Oxford
Oxford, U.K.

Donald E. Meier, MD, FACS, FWACS
Professor and Endowed Chairman
Division of Pediatric Surgery
Texas Tech University Health Sciences Center, El Paso
El Paso, Texas, U.S.
Consultant Surgeon
Baptist Medical Centre
Ogbomoso, Nigeria
Honorary Professor of Pediatric Surgery
Addis Ababa University
Addis Ababa, Ethiopia

Ronald Merrell, MD
Department of Surgery
Virginia Commonwealth University School of Medicine
Richmond, Virginia, U.S.

Alastair J.W. Millar, FRCS, FRACS (Paed Surg), FCS (SA), DCH
Charles F.M. Saint Professor of Paediatric Surgery
University of Cape Town and Red Cross War Memorial
    Children's Hospital, Rondebosch
Cape Town, South Africa

Ashish Minocha, MBBS, MS, MCh, DNB, MNAMS, FICS
Consultant Paediatric and Neonatal Surgeon
Jenny Lind Children's Department
Norfolk & Norwich University Hospital
Norwich, U.K.

Catherine Mngongo, MMED Surg (KCMC), MBBCH (Tanzania)
Consultant Surgeon
Tumaini University
Kilimanjaro Christian Medical Centre
Kilimanjaro Moshi, Tanzania

Charles N. Mock, ScB, MPH, MD, PhD, FACS
Professor, Department of Surgery, and Professor of Epidemiology
University of Washington, Seattle, Washington, U.S.
Visiting Senior Lecturer
Department of Surgery
School of Medical Sciences/Komfo Anokye Teaching Hospital
College of Health Sciences, Kwame Nkrumah University
    of Science and Technology
Kumasi, Ghana

Sam W. Moore, MBChB, FRCS, Doctor of Medicine (MD)
Division of Pediatric Surgery
Tygerberg Hospital
University of Stellenbosch
Tygerberg, South Africa

Paul J. Moroz, MD, MSc, FRCSC, FAAOS
Assistant Professor
Department of Pediatric Orthopaedic Surgery
University of Ottawa and Children's Hospital of Eastern Ontario
Ontario, Ottawa, Canada
African affiliation: Department of Surgery, Kilimanjaro Christian
    Medical Centre,
Moshi, Tanzania

Philip M Mshelbwala, MBBS, FWACS
Consultant Paediatric Surgeon and Senior Lecturer
Division of Paediatric Surgery, Department of Surgery
Ahmadu Bello University and Ahmadu Bello University
    Teaching Hospital
Zaria, Nigeria

David Msuya, MD, MMED surgery, FCS (ECSA)
Consultant Surgeon
Kilimanjaro Christian Medical Centre and Tumaini University
Moshi, Tanzania

Evan P. Nadler, MD
Co-Director, Children's National Obesity Institute
Children's National Medical Center
Associate Professor of Surgery, Pediatrics, & Integrative
    Systems Biology
The George Washington University School of Medicine
    & Health Sciences
Washington, DC, U.S.

Abdulrasheed A. Nasir, MBBS, FWACS
Consultant Paediatric Surgeon
Division of Paediatric Surgery
University of Ilorin Teaching Hospital
Ilorin, Nigeria

Mark Newton, MD, FAAP
Associate Professor of Pediatric Anesthesiology
Vanderbilt University Medical Center
Nashville, Tennessee, U.S.
Consultant Anesthesiologist and Director of Kenya Registered Nurse
Anaesthetist Program
Kijabe Hospital
Kijabe, Kenya

Phuong D. Nguyen, MD
Department of Surgery, Division of Pediatric Surgery
New York University Langone Medical Center
New York, New York, U.S.

Paul T. Nmadu, FMCS (Nig), FWACS, FICS
Professor and Consultant Paediatric Surgeon
Division of Paediatric Surgery, Department of Surgery
Ahmadu Bello University and Ahmadu Bello University Teaching Hospital
Zaria, Nigeria

Peter M. Nthumba, MBChB, MMed (Surgery), FCS (ECSA)
Plastic, Reconstructive and Hand Surgeon
AIC Kijabe Hospital
Nairobi, Kenya

Alp Numanoglu
Red Cross War Memorial Children's Hospital
Cape Town, South Africa

Benedict C. Nwomeh, MD, MPH, FRCS (Eng, Ed, Glas),
    FACS, FAAP, FWACS
Associate Professor of Clinical Surgery
The Ohio State University
Director of Surgical Education
Department of Paediatric Surgery
Nationwide Children's Hospital
Columbus, Ohio, U.S.

Andrew Gustaf Nyman, MBBCh, MRCPCH
Paediatric Intensive Care Registrar
Oxford Children's Hospital
Oxford, U.K.

Modupe Odelola
Imperial College NHS Trust
St. Mary's Hospital
Praed Street
London

Michael O. Ogirima, FMCS, FWACS, FICS, FAOI
Associate Professor and Chief Consultant
Department of Orthopaedics and Trauma Surgery
Ahmadu Bello University and Ahmadu Bello University
    Teaching Hospital
Zaria, Nigeria

G. Olufemi Ogunrinde, MBBS, FWACP
Senior Lecturer and Consultant Paediatrician
Department of Paediatrics
Ahmadu Bello University and Ahmadu Bello University
    Teaching Hospital
Zaria, Nigeria

Adekunle O. Oguntayo, MBBS, FWACS, FICS
Senior Lecturer and Consultant Obstetrician and Gynecologist
Gynaecologic Oncology Unit
Department of Obstetrics and Gynecology
Ahmadu Bello University Teaching Hospital
Zaria Nigeria

Philemon E. Okoro, MBBS, FWACS
Lecturer and Consultant Paediatric Surgeon
University of Port Harcourt and Port Harcourt University
    Teaching Hospital
Port Harcourt, Nigeria

Peter F. Omonzejele, PhD
Department of Philosophy
University of Benin
Benin-City, Nigeria

Richard Onalo, MBBS, FMCP
Consultant Paediatrician
Department of Paediatrics
Ahmadu Bello University Teaching Hospital
Zaria, Nigeria

G. Ifeyinwa Onimoe, MBBS, FAAP
Clinical Fellow
Department of Hematology/Oncology/Bone Marrow Transplant
Nationwide Children's Hospital
Ohio State University
Columbus, Ohio, U.S.

Iyore A. Otabor, MD, MALD
Clinical Instructor and Research Fellow
Department of Pediatric Surgery
Nationwide Children's Hospital
The Ohio State University
Columbus, Ohio, U.S.

Dakshesh Parikh, MBBS, MS, FRCS (Paed), MD
Consultant Paediatric General and Thoracic Surgeon
Birmingham Children's Hospital NHS Foundation Trust
Birmingham, U.K.

Graeme Pitcher, MBBCh, FCS (SA)
Adjunct Professor
Department of Surgery
University of the Witwatersrand
Head, Paediatric Surgery
Chris Hani Baragwanath Hospital
Johannesburg, South Africa

Dan Poenaru, MD, MHPE, FRCSC, FACS, FCS (ECSA)
Consultant Paediatric Surgeon
BethanyKids at Kijabe Hospital
Kijabe, Kenya
Honorary Professor of Surgery
Aga Khan University
Nairobi, Kenya
Adjunct Professor of Surgery and Paediatrics
Queen's University
Kingston, Ontario, Canada

Jean Heuric Rakotomalala, MD
Paediatric Surgery Fellow (COSECSA)
BethanyKids at Kijabe Hospital
Kijabe, Kenya

Ashley Ridout, BM BCh, MA (Oxon), MRCS (Eng)
Oxford Deanery School of Surgery
Oxford, U.K.

Dorothy V. Rocourt, MD
Chief Fellow in Pediatric Surgery
Nationwide Children's Hospital
The Ohio State University
Columbus, Ohio, U.S.

Bankole S. Rouma, MD
Professor, Pediatric Surgery
University Hospital of Treichville
Abidjan, Côte d'Ivoire

Avraham Schlager, MD
Division of Pediatric Surgery, Department of Surgery
New York University School of Medicine
New York, New York, U.S.

Kant Shah, MBBS MRCS
Research Fellow
Department of Paediatric Surgery
Oxford Children's Hospital
Oxford, U.K.

Shilpa Sharma, MBBS, MS, M.Ch, DNB, Ph.D
Assistant Professor
Department of Pediatric Surgery
Post Graduate Institute of Medical Education and Research
Dr RML Hospital
New Delhi, India

Alison Shefler, MD, FRCP (C)
Consultant in Paediatric Intensive Care
Oxford Children's Hospital
Oxford, U.K.

Bello Bala Shehu, MBBS, FRCS, FACS, FWACS
Professor and Consultant Neurosurgeon
Chief, Regional Centre for Neurosurgery
Usmanu Danfodiyo University Teaching Hospital
Sokoto, Nigeria

Daniel Sidler, MD, M.Phil, FCS (SA)
Associate Professor of Paediatric Surgery and Senior Lecturer
Department of Paediatric Surgery
Tygerberg Children's Hospital, Stellenbosch University
Cape Town, South Africa

Michael Singh, MBBS; FRCS (Paed)
Consultant Paediatric General and Thoracic Surgeon
Birmingham Children's Hospital NHS Foundation Trust
Birmingham, U.K.

Saurabh Sinha, MBBS,FRCS
Fellow in Neurosurgery
Oxford Children's Hospital
Oxford, U.K.

Oludayo Adedapo Sowande, MBChB, FRCSEd, FWACS
Senior Lecturer and Consultant Paediatric Surgeon
Paediatric Surgery Unit, Department of Surgery
Obafemi Awolowo University Teaching Hospital
Ile Ife, Nigeria

Helen Sowerbutts, BA, BABCh Oxon
Speciality Trainee (ST1) in Paediatrics
Northwick Park Hospital
London, U.K.

Emily Stamell
Division of Pediatric Surgery, Department of Surgery
New York University School of Medicine
New York, New York, U.S.

Ronald S. Sutherland, MD, FACS, FAAP
Pediatric Urology
Professor of Surgery & Pediatrics (Clinical)
University of Hawaii, John Burns School of Medicine
Honolulu, Hawaii, U.S.

Atonasio Taela
Department of Surgery
Eduardo Mondlane University
Maputo Central Hospital
Maputo, Mozambique

Erin A. Teeple, MD
Bariatric/Minimally Invasive Surgery Fellow
Department of Pediatric Surgery
Nationwide Children's Hospital
The Ohio State University
Columbus, Ohio, U.S.

Ralf-Bodo Troebs, MD
Professor of Pediatric Surgery
Department of Pediatric Surgery
Catholic Foundation Marienhospital Herne
Ruhr University of Bochum
Herne, Germany

Nyaweleni Tshifularo, MBChB, FCS (SA)
Tygerberg Hospital
University of Stellenbosch
Stellenbosch, South Africa

Francis Aba Uba, MB ChB, FMCS, FWACS
Associate Professor of Surgery and Consultant Paediatric Surgeon
Paediatric Surgery Unit, Department of Surgery
University of Jos and Jos University Teaching Hospital
Jos, Nigeria

Jeffrey S. Upperman, MD, FACS, FAAP
Associate Professor of Surgery
Keck School of Medicine
University of Southern California
Director of Pediatric Trauma
Children's Hospital of Los Angeles
Los Angeles, California, U.S.

Usang E. Usang, FWACS, FMCS (Nig), FICS
Lecturer and Consultant Paediatric Surgeon
University of Calabar and Calabar University Teaching Hospital
Calabar, Nigeria

A.B. (Sebastian) van As, MBChB, MMed, MBA, FCS (SA), PhD
Professor and Head, Trauma Unit
Red Cross War Memorial Children's Hospital
Department of Paediatric Surgery
School of Child and Adolescence Health, University of Cape Town
Cape Town, South Africa

Stefan Wolke
Clinic of Paediatric Surgery
Jena University Hospital
Friedrich Schiller University of Jena
Jena, Germany

George G. Youngson, CBE, PhD, FRCS Ed
Professor and Consultant Paediatric Surgeon
Department of Paediatric Surgery
Royal Aberdeen Children's Hospital
Aberdeen, Scotland
African affiliation: External Examiner, University of Malawi

Nathan R. Zilbert
Division of Pediatric Surgery, Department of Surgery
New York University School of Medicine
New York, New York, U.S.

FOREWORD

Paediatric surgery has come of age with the publication of this landmark textbook directed to the African continent. A comprehensive textbook of this nature is long overdue and undoubtedly will serve as a basic reference tome, practical manual, and stimulus for innovative research for generations to come. Most current textbooks are written with an emphasis on surgical conditions and remedies commonly encountered in the developed world. However, in many developing countries, the aetiology, incidence, pathogenesis, clinical manifestations, investigations, treatment, and outcomes for common diseases, as well as diseases endemic to these regions, are different. Hence the need for a textbook to look beyond current texts and address diseases in a more comprehensive way.

The development of paediatric surgery as a speciality in Africa is relatively recent. In many areas, it is still compromised by a lack of demographic information, infrastructure, and trained surgeons familiar with the special needs of children, as well as limited anaesthetic services and fiscal deficiencies. Life for children on the African continent is therefore not easy. It is a constant battle against poverty, parasitic and other infections and diseases, trauma, debilitating congenital and central nervous system abnormalities, and many other factors impairing their growth and development.

Many of the same surgical diseases seen in the developed world must be diagnosed and treated in Africa under substantially less favourable and often adverse circumstances. The morbidity and mortality rates remain unacceptably high, with wide disparities between countries as well as between urban and rural communities. It is in this setting that this textbook will make a valuable contribution toward expanding knowledge and achieving improved surgical outcomes for all children.

Authorship was wisely chosen: each chapter is written by an acknowledged international expert and an African counterpart who has extensive experience. This daunting task is an affirmation of the specific need to address the often neglected surgical diseases of the region and their special circumstances. This collaboration also recognises the important contributions made by surgeons from Africa. They have a breadth of knowledge and experience to help unlock the doors of ignorance and to contribute to setting a standard of quality care. Many of the authors have earned national and international professional distinction as surgeons, teachers, innovative researchers, and leaders.

People often question the relevance of surgery on a continent where so many other issues are a priority. The estimated accumulative risk for a child to have a condition requiring surgical input is 85% by the age of 15 years, making it a significant public health problem. Obstacles to improve paediatric surgical care include a general lack of interest in surgical conditions affecting children, its poorly defined role, and a lack of political commitment. Surgical training in Africa is also very variable and beset with multiple challenges, which further compound the already suboptimal standard of surgical care. Sick children therefore are found on the doorsteps of health care workers, but the only way they can get their rightful due is to have knowledgeable and skilled surgeons caring for them.

This textbook, as a rich source of information, will consequently contribute significantly to paediatric surgical education in Africa, combining home-grown knowledge on the care of children with surgical conditions. Although this book is directed to the needs of surgeons working in Africa, it may also be of great help to those treating children from Africa somewhere in the developed world. Diseases know no boundaries.

Emeritus Professor Heinz Rode
Red Cross War Memorial Children's Hospital
University of Cape Town, South Africa

A NOTE FROM THE PUBLISHER

We are very pleased to partner with the authors to publish this entirely new and important book: *Paediatric Surgery: A Comprehensive Text For Africa*. This is a major achievement resulting from the contributions of many individuals.

All of the authors contributed their time, experience, and expertise, and for busy clinicians, writing is done at great personal sacrifice. Only by knowing the importance of a project do physicians elect to allocate such time for new material. We acknowledge the special contribution of Dr. Emmanuel Ameh for initiating and coordinating the entire undertaking. Please review the list of the text's contributors and note their diversity and impressive credentials.

Our staff also made this publication a priority. Deborah Cughan organized the project and used her graphic skills to integrate the text and illustrations for publication as well as to design the cover. Sandra Rush edited and indexed the book at a reduced non-profit rate. Additionally, Dean Carlson, our manager and web-master, helped to facilitate all aspects of the project.

Friends of the Global HELP Organization covered the cost of producing this book. Expenses include editing, indexing, formatting, web-site management, CD-Rom Library duplication, and hardcopy printing. Scores of generous people made donations and the major contributors were Henry & Cindy Burgess, George Hamilton, Paul & Suzanne Merriman, and Lana & Lynn Staheli.

We plan to distribute this publication as widely as possible. Along with the printed version, the full text is available on low-cost CD-Roms and may be downloaded in PDF format from our web-site without charge or restrictions.

For any new editions of the publication, please visit our web-site at www.global-help.org.

Lynn Staheli, MD, 2011
Founder and Volunteer Director,
Global HELP Organization
Paediatric Orthopaedist
Professor Emeritus, University of Washington
Seattle, Washington, USA

PREFACE

Paediatric surgery has become an established specialty in many parts of Africa and other developing countries. However, the surgical care of children continues to pose significant challenges in these settings, due partly to the enormous disparity between the large volume of patients and the few available paediatric surgical specialists. In addition, many patients present late, frequently with advanced diseases, and, unfortunately, available medical facilities are often suboptimal.

Although a number of good paediatric surgical textbooks are currently in use worldwide, few address the peculiar needs of surgeons in the developing world. Even though most aspects of paediatric surgical care are standard worldwide, in many cases, the approach, methods, and techniques described in Western textbooks may not be applicable to the African setting. Most existing textbooks are written by surgeons who assume a Western audience in their discussion of incidence rates, demographics, and socioeconomic aspects. Discussion of available treatment options and reference to "standard of care" assume a Western level of technology. Understandably, conditions common in Western countries are treated with greater emphasis while those commonly seen in Africa may not be discussed at all. This book presents a comprehensive overview of paediatric surgery that is most relevant to African children and their surgeons. When used along with the already available textbooks, it will provide a more balanced perspective to anyone interested in paediatric surgery in Africa

The authors of this book are primarily reputable paediatric surgeons with vast experience working in Africa, but also include those from developed countries, whose contributions will add the expertise gained from experience in state-of-the-art facilities. It is hoped that this collaboration will provide the reader with a safe approach to surgical care of children under difficult situations as well as up-to-date information on various aspects of paediatric surgery.

Africa is currently experiencing a severe shortage of paediatric surgical specialists, and a significant proportion of surgery on African children is still performed by general surgeons. Therefore, this book is targeted at trainees in both paediatric surgery and general surgery in Africa and similar settings as well as practising surgeons. Undergraduate medical students, paediatricians, and other paediatric health care practitioners will also find this book a useful reference. The recent increase in the numbers of charitable medical missions from Western countries will continue to bring surgeons from developed countries to Africa. These much-needed doctors will find the book an essential accessory to their work in Africa. Ultimately, we hope the children of Africa will be the final beneficiaries.

The Editors,

E. A. Ameh, Zaria, Nigeria
S. W. Bickler, San Diego, California, USA
K. Lakhoo, Oxford, UK
B. C. Nwomeh, Columbus, Ohio, USA
D. Poenaru, Kijabe, Kenya

Every effort has been made to confirm the accuracy of the presented information. The authors and publisher are not responsible for errors of omission or for any consequences from the application of the information in this book, and make no warranty, expressed or implied, with respect to the currency, completeness, or accuracy of the contents of this publication. Application of this information in a particular situation remains the professional responsibility of the practitioner.

Paediatric Surgery: A Comprehensive Text for Africa is published by the Global HELP Organization.

Seattle, WA, USA

ISBN 978-1-60189-128-0

Basic Principles

CHAPTER 1
PAEDIATRIC SURGERY SPECIALTY AND ITS RELEVANCE TO AFRICA

Philip M. Mshelbwala
Benedict C. Nwomeh

Introduction

In Africa, children constitute more than half of the population,[1] and therefore much effort is devoted to the prevention and treatment of childhood diseases. Emphasis is placed on diseases that cause the greatest morbidity and mortality, such as communicable diseases (especially human immunodeficiency virus/acquired immune deficiency syndrome (HIV/AIDS), malaria, and respiratory infections), maternal and perinatal conditions, and nutritional deficiencies.[2] In many African countries, scarce health care resources have been concentrated on the provision of immunisation, HIV control, malaria eradication, and other public health concerns. As a result, diseases for which surgical intervention offers the only hope for prevention, palliation, or cure usually do not come within the radar of health policy makers. Given that surgical diseases have not been considered significant health care problems in Africa, the paediatric surgical speciality has not received the attention it deserves.[3]

Paediatric surgeons have been described as the only true general surgeons;[4] this is especially the case in Africa, where paediatric subspecialisation is rare in orthopedics, urology, otolaryngology, thoracic surgery, plastic surgery and neurosurgery. The paediatric surgeon in Africa, therefore, provides cost-effective care at a considerable bargain for these impoverished countries. A detailed list of paediatric surgical diagnoses encountered in an urban hospital in Africa is provided in Table 1.1. Unaccounted for in most studies are those children for whom treatment is inaccessible due to distance, cost, or lack of qualified personnel. Bickler et al. analyzed all paediatric visits at the main urban hospital in Banjul, The Gambia, and estimated the incidence of paediatric surgical problems at 543 per 10,000 children aged 0–14 years, of which 46% required surgical procedures. Using age-specific incidences, the authors estimated the cumulative risk for all surgical conditions at 85.4% by age 15 years (Figure 1.1).[5,6]

Despite sparse epidemiologic data, there is increasing recognition of the value of surgery as a component of basic health care and an important means of providing both preventive and curative treatment.[7] As such, it is imperative that paediatric surgical care be integrated into a comprehensive strategy to reduce the burden of disease in Africa.

Table 1.1: Surgical conditions seen among children (n = 1200) treated at elective surgery at Komfo Anokye Teaching Hospital, Kumasi, Ghana.

Disease entity	Number of children	Percentage of total
Inguinal hernia and hydrocele	611	51
Undescended testis	93	8
Umbilical hernia	63	5
Extra digits	58	5
Neoplasms	44	4
Cystic hygroma/hemangioma	36	3
Anorectal malformations	34	3
Uncircumcised penis	28	2
Hirschsprung's disease	27	2
Enlarged lymph nodes	26	2
Rectal polyp	14	1
Thyroglossal and branchial cysts	11	0.9
Oesophageal stricture	10	0.8
Epigastric and incisional hernia	10	0.8
Wilms' tumour	9	0.8
Thyroglossal cysts	9	0.8
Rectovaginal fistulas	8	0.7
Sacrococcygeal teratoma	8	0.7
Spina bifida	5	0.4
Ambiguous genitalia	3	0.3
Anal stenosis	3	0.3
Enterocutaneous fistula	3	0.3
Hypersplenism with splenomegaly	3	0.3
Popliteal cyst	3	0.3
Pyloric stenosis	2	0.2
Patent urachus	2	0.2
Miscellaneous other	74	7

Source: Adapted from: Abantanga FA, Amaning EP. Paediatric elective surgical conditions as seen at a referral hospital in Kumasi, Ghana. ANZ J Surg 2002 72(12):890–892.

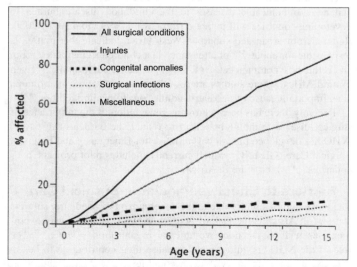

Source: Bickler SW, Rode H. Surgical services for children in developing countries. Bull World Health Organ 2002; 80(10):829–835.

Figure 1.1: Estimated risk of requiring surgical care in a paediatric population living in Banjul, The Gambia. Cumulative risk was estimated by using age-specific incidences.

Historical Background

Modern archaeology has uncovered evidence of surgical operations in Africa that predated the Neolithic age, including children as patients.[8] The first medical school was established in Alexandria, Egypt, by Herophilus in the fourth century B.C.E. and developed further in the third century B.C.E. by Erasistratus.[9] Therefore, the concept of surgery is not alien to the continent, notwithstanding the lack of progress that occurred over many centuries.

The practice of paediatric surgery as a specialty in Africa has its roots in South Africa during the 1920s with paediatric surgeons from the Hospital for Sick Children, Great Ormond Street, London, as pioneers.[10] In the late 1940s and 1950s, the first paediatric surgical unit was established at Groote Schuur Hospital in Cape Town by Jan H. Louw, and since then, the practice of paediatric surgery in Africa has become firmly established. Several national and regional organisations have been formed to promote the practice of paediatric surgery. In 1994, the Pan African Paediatric Surgical Association (PAPSA) was formed, which held its inaugural meeting in Nairobi, Kenya, in March 1995. In 2004, the African Journal of Paediatric Surgery (AJPS) was founded by Francis Uba. This publication has already achieved listing in MEDLINE, thus removing a major obstacle to the growth of the specialty.

In the past five decades, many Africans have trained in paediatric surgery, both overseas and recently in indigenous residency programmes. Paediatric surgery divisions now exist in several departments of surgery, many of which participate in the education of medical students and general surgery residents. In a few centres, subspecialty training in paediatric surgery has been established with a formalised curriculum. Regulation and oversight of paediatric surgery training has been carefully maintained by professional bodies that administer the examination and certification required for credentialing as a subspecialist.

Currently, examination and certification in paediatric surgery have been organised on a regional basis. In South Africa, surgeons who have completed general surgery training and an additional two years of subspecialty training may take the specialty examination in paediatric surgery offered by the College of Medicine of South Africa.[11] In West Africa, surgeons become eligible for examination and certification in paediatric surgery after a minimum of two years of general surgery training and a further 20 months of subspecialty training under the aegis of the West African College of Surgeons.[12]

African surgeons have made significant contributions to the practice of paediatric surgery and have also championed the development of the specialty locally. Many paediatric surgeons with roots in Africa have achieved local and international recognition for their clinical, research, and leadership roles. As a prime example, the dominant hypothesis on the aetiology of intestinal atresia was the outcome of a series of experiments performed by Jan Louw and Chris Barnard at the Red Cross Children's Hospital in Cape Town. This seminal work, published in Lancet in 1955, provided direct evidence for vascular accidents as the likely mechanism in the pathogenesis of intestinal atresia during foetal development. Louw was honoured with the prestigious Sir Denis Browne Gold Medal by the British Association of Paediatric Surgeons (BAPS) in 1980. The 2004 honouree for this award was another South African, Sir Lewis Spitz, who rose to the Nuffield Chair of Paediatric Surgery at the Hospital for Sick Children, Great Ormond Street, London. Recently, Sid Cywes was accorded the honorary fellowship of the American College of Surgeons. Additionally, Donald Nuss, who developed the minimally invasive repair for pectus excavatum, began his training in Africa.

Burden of Surgical Diseases in African Children

With only 11% of the world's population, Africa bears 25% of the global burden of disease. Several well-known factors, including endemic poverty, poor literacy rates, civil conflicts, and corrupt political leadership, contribute to the overwhelming burden of childhood disease in low- and middle-income countries. Although comprehensive data on the incidence of paediatric surgical conditions in Africa is lacking, available information suggests that trauma, congenital anomalies, and surgical infections are common.[13] Yet, the focus on the prevention and treatment of infectious diseases has often led to the neglect of trauma and other surgical disease as important factors in the overall disease burden in children from these regions.[14]

Despite the perceived high costs and limited availability of a trained workforce and equipment, surgery is often an essential and integral part of basic health care, as in cases of treatment of injuries, urinary retention, and inhaled foreign bodies, or preventive, as in the case of elective hernia repair.[5] In fact, Gosselin et al. performed a cost-effectiveness analysis to evaluate the costs and disability-adjusted life years (DALYs) saved by the provision of surgical services to children in a rural hospital in Sierra Leone, and the positive effect was comparable to that of other public health interventions.[15]

Failure to recognise the importance of surgical treatment has led to neglect by both governmental and donor agencies. Of the estimated 234 million major surgical procedures performed worldwide annually,[16] which is 7 times the number of persons infected with HIV, only 3.5% of these are performed in the poorest nations, many of which are in Africa.[17]

The view of surgical disease as being relatively unimportant has been amplified by a lack of accurate epidemiological studies. However, emerging data highlight the need to re-examine conventional thinking. One report from a rural hospital in Malumfashi, Nigeria, and another from a large urban hospital in Banjul, The Gambia, showed that paediatric surgical cases account for 6.6% and 11.3% of all paediatric admissions, respectively.[18,19] In both studies, 80–90% of all paediatric surgical admissions were due to congenital anomalies, surgical infections, and trauma. Determination of the true incidence of congenital anomalies is difficult due to the associated stigma still seen in many native populations. In South Africa, with better surveillance systems and greater awareness among the population, the incidence of congenital anomalies is about 12 per 1,000 live births.[20]

Among surgical diseases, trauma is an important cause of morbidity, mortality, and disability in African children.[21] According to estimates by the World Health Organization (WHO), injuries account for 13% of the childhood disease burden and nearly 1 million deaths per year in developing countries.[22,23] Africa's children are at more risk of dying from motor vehicle crashes than European children.[2] Deen et al.[22] have projected that the relative contributions of injuries and noncommunicable diseases to the childhood disease burden in developing countries will increase from 28% in 1990 to 45% by 2020. Reports from urban and suburban West Africa indicate that trauma is responsible for about 9% of attendance in a children's emergency room and is the most common cause (47%) of paediatric admissions.[19,24] Even in rural Africa, where studies are few, there are indications that trauma is an important cause of paediatric admissions to health facilities.[18,25]

Recently, there has been a growing recognition of the importance of surgical disease in the global effort to reduce the burden of disease.[26] WHO has developed the Global Initiative for Emergency and Essential Surgical Care (GIEESC), which currently includes pilot projects in 17 countries, of which 8 are in Africa.

Barriers to Effective Paediatric Surgical Care

The most significant obstacle to the development of paediatric surgical services in Africa is the lack of interest shown by the various governments as well as the nongovernmental organisations (NGOs).[27] The role of the NGOs is quite crucial because their contribution to health care expenditures in many African countries is substantial and occasionally exceeds the health budget of national governments.[2] These NGOs, especially the UN agencies (World Bank, WHO, and the United Nations Children's Fund (UNICEF)) and private foundations (e.g., The Bill and Melinda Gates Foundation) exert even greater influence because they often set the agenda for health care priorities of many developing countries.

Socioeconomic and Cultural Factors

Africa remains a predominantly illiterate and poor continent, with the majority of the population surviving on less than US$2 daily.[28] Due to the lack of health insurance, out-of-pocket private expenditure on health care is the norm. Therefore, health care is in direct competition with the basic subsistence needs for food, shelter, and clothing. In the few countries where health care is free or subsidised for children, surgical conditions are often excluded. Unfortunately, even families that can afford to pay may be unaware that surgical treatment is feasible or available for a variety of disabling, disfiguring, or life-threatening congenital or acquired conditions.

A persistent cultural attitude toward congenital anomalies continues to hinder access to corrective surgery. Congenital anomalies may be ascribed to supernatural causes or the curse of the gods. Fortunately, egregious behaviour such as the sacrifice of malformed babies has been largely eliminated, although reluctance to seek treatment persists.

Poor Health Care Facilities

Jan H. Louw established the first paediatric surgery unit in southern Africa at the Groote Schuur Hospital in Cape Town in 1948; this became a full department in 1952.[10] Since then, several other centres have emerged in South Africa where medical care in general and paediatric surgery services in particular have advanced to a level comparable with many Western countries. The practice of paediatric surgery as a specialty has now been established in several other African countries, but unfortunately the majority of these are plagued with poor facilities and dysfunctional health care systems. The only dedicated children's hospital in sub-Saharan Africa is the Red Cross War Memorial Hospital, Rondebosch, South Africa. Here, paediatric surgeons enjoy facilities in a major clinical and research paediatric centre recognised both regionally and internationally.[10]

In Nigeria, with a population of 150 million, the government has only recently approved the construction of its first comprehensive children's hospital, expected to open in Zaria in a few years. Currently, most paediatric surgeons in Africa practice in large urban hospitals that principally serve adult patients. Many of these centres are overcrowded, poorly funded, and lack facilities such as a dedicated paediatric ward, paediatric emergency room, neonatal intensive care unit (NICU), paediatric radiology, and paediatric pathology, which are considered basic requirements for a sustainable paediatric surgery practice. Where these facilities exist, they are often poorly equipped and are frequently operated by doctors who have not undergone dedicated paediatric training. The lack of paediatric anaesthesia has caused some surgeons to rely on local anaesthesia or staged procedures for complex cases.[27,29]

Referral and Transport

Poor obstetric services limit the ability to perform prenatal diagnosis and planned delivery for infants with severe congenital anomalies, as is routinely obtained in most developed countries. Many pregnant women do not receive antenatal care, and sometimes the only obstetric service available is delivery by untrained traditional birth attendants (TBAs).[27,30] Untrained TBAs are unable to recognise congenital anomalies for which early surgical treatment is essential to prevent early death. Such conditions include oesophageal atresia, intestinal atresia, and congenital diaphragmatic hernia. Even when referrals to appropriate health care facilities are made, the poor condition of rural roads and inadequate transport facilities often lead to neonatal loss in transit or presentation in a debilitated and decompensated physiological state.

Shortage of Trained Workforce

Despite the increasing number of medical schools in Africa, the number of doctors practicing on the continent remains grossly inadequate. In Ghana, about 1,500 doctors serve the 20 million population, and only

32 specialists work in Malawi, with a population of 10 million.[31,32] In Nigeria, fewer than 40 practicing paediatric surgeons cater to a paediatric population (less than 18 years of age) that exceeds 80 million. This gives a ratio of one paediatric surgeon to about 2 million children (compared to 1:100,000 in North America). The few paediatric surgeons available are often overworked and are largely inaccessible to the overwhelming majority of the populace. The void is filled at best by nonspecialist surgeons or general practitioners and at worst by quacks and traditional healers.

The reasons for the shortage of trained paediatric surgeons are not farfetched. Lack of facilities and supporting personnel has limited the capacity to train paediatric surgeons locally, and opportunities for training overseas have been severely curtailed. To compound this problem, paediatric surgery is not a popular choice of career for aspiring surgeons. This situation has been attributed to the heavy workload, a frustrating lack of facilities, and poor compensation. Under these conditions, it is difficult to attract young surgeons with the promise of a rewarding and satisfying career. The endemic brain drain has also played a role in depleting the number of practicing surgeons, many going overseas for further training but never returning to their home countries. The workforce shortage cuts across the entire spectrum of paediatric care, including nursing, radiology, anaesthesiology, and pathology.

Recommendations

The relevance of paediatric surgery in Africa and other developing regions is no longer in doubt.[33] However, if the impact of the paediatric surgical practice as part of essential health care to children is to be felt, then a major paradigm shift is needed. Some of the ideas presented here have been drawn from the seven-point strategy advocated by Bickler et al., which should be required reading for all paediatric surgeons and health policy makers in Africa (see Table 1.2).[6,13]

Table 1.2: Strategies for improving paediatric surgery care in Africa.

1	Define communities' health needs with input from the communities.
2	Demonstrate the need for paediatric surgical services.
3	Foster community participation.
4	Start with what is available and build on existing services.
5	Integrate preventive and curative services.
6	Facilitate ongoing training.
7	Remain goal-directed within available resources.

Source: Adapted from Bickler SW, Kyambi J, Rode H. Pediatric surgery in sub-Saharan Africa. Pediatr Surg Intl 2001; 17:442–447.

Research

African paediatric surgeons should become more involved in clinical and basic science research in order to improve the care of their patients and generate awareness for their work. The most fundamental task here is to collect, analyze, and publish data reflecting local experience with childhood surgical disease.

Training

Wider exposure of medical students and surgeons-in-training to paediatric surgery would likely generate more interest in the specialty. Trainees could, however, develop an aversion to the specialty if a positive mentoring environment is not provided. The tendency toward exploitative and even brutal treatment of surgical residents is an unfortunate legacy of Halstedian training. Recognition of the deleterious effect of such an abusive environment to surgical education has been the impetus behind the resident work-hour limitations now in force in most Western countries. Unfortunately, the old habits remain the norm in much of Africa, and may be a major obstacle to recruiting bright young talent into the specialty. The quality of paediatric surgery training has been adversely affected by the lack of adequate facilities and limited exposure to current techniques.[34]

Increasing global partnerships provide an opportunity to improve human and material capacity.[17] Such partnerships could involve exchange programmes with colleagues and trainees from developed countries, but also intraregional collaboration that could be incorporated into local residency training programmes.[35] Skills transfer can be achieved by using novel methods, such as telesimulation and telementoring, where mentors or experts in other parts of the world can offer advice or direct real-time surgical procedures being performed in resource-poor hospitals.[36]

Several professional surgical societies have recently developed global surgery initiatives that provide training opportunities for African surgeons, including the American College of Surgeons (ACS),[37] the American Paediatric Surgical Association (APSA),[38] and the Association for Academic Surgery (AAS).[39] Efforts are under way to create a central clearinghouse where all available overseas training opportunities will be made accessible to trainees in developing countries.

Leadership

Although specialty organisations for paediatric surgeons are essential, it is important to be connected to the wider field of surgery. This can be achieved by ensuring that paediatric surgery remains an integral component of the surgery department educational activities as well as morbidity and mortality conferences. Presentation of research work should not be limited to specialty meetings; rather, a strong paediatric surgery presence needs to be maintained in national and regional conferences involving surgeons of different specialties. Furthermore, paediatric surgeons should seek every opportunity to network and collaborate with paediatricians by organising joint educational activities and participating in paediatric meetings. This will give paediatric surgeons visibility among their peers and facilitate public recognition of their vital role in the provision of child health care. The surgical section of the American Academy of Paediatrics is the prototype for such collaboration.[3]

Paediatric surgeons should strive to achieve leadership positions in their surgery departments as well as in umbrella national and regional surgical organisations to ensure that the interests of children and the specialty are well represented. Finally, paediatric surgeons in Africa should maintain strong collaborative relationships with colleagues in other parts of the world at personal, professional, and organisational levels. The quality, reputation, and international recognition of local specialty certification would be enhanced by recruiting examiners from other parts of the world to participate at the various local certification examinations.[3]

Support for Nonsurgical Personnel

Given the dearth of trained paediatric surgeons, it is inevitable that the vast majority of children with paediatric surgical conditions will seek care from adult surgeons, nonsurgeon physicians, and nonphysician health professionals. Many newborn infants die needlessly due to lack of referral for surgical care. Educational programmes that enhance the awareness and diagnostic abilities of health care personnel within the locality of each paediatric surgeon will likely improve early referral, particularly for life-threatening conditions. A pocket manual of common paediatric surgery conditions has been specifically written with such personnel in mind.[40]

Conclusion

The paediatric surgery specialty is now indispensable in the overall effort to relieve the disease burden in Africa and other developing regions. However, for the practice to remain relevant in the coming years, advocacy for funding and public health policies geared towards the needs of children must be intensified and maintained.

Although significant obstacles exist in the infrastructure and workforce, paediatric surgeons must take the lead as advocates for children and in educating the public as well as policy makers on the need to recognize surgical disease in children as a significant health problem. By focusing on clinical excellence, engaging in serious research, and adopting a training model that provides real mentorship, African paediatric surgeons can provide the highest level of care possible to their unique group of patients.

Evidence-Based Research

Table 1.3 presents a study on the costs and DALYs averted by a hospital in Sierra Leone.

Table 1.3: Evidence-based research.

Title	Cost/DALY averted in a small hospital in Sierra Leone: what is the relative contribution of different services?
Authors	Gosselin RA, Thind A, Bellardinelli A
Institution	University of California, Berkeley, California, USA; University of Western Ontario, London, Ontario, Canada; Emergency Hospital, Goderich, Sierra Leone
Reference	World J Surg 2006; 30(4):505–511
Problem	To estimate the cost/disability-adjusted life years (DALYs) averted by health facilities, including surgery in adults and children, thereby providing cost-effectiveness data to guide resource allocation decisions in the developing world.
Intervention	Estimation of the costs and the DALYs averted by an entire hospital in Sierra Leone.
Comparison/ control (quality of evidence)	Cost-effectiveness analysis is a complex undertaking, but the DALYs method is probably the best composite measure.
Outcome/ effect	For the three-month study period, total costs were calculated as $369,774, with an estimate of 11,282 DALYs averted (cost/ DALY averted of $32.78). This compares favourably to other nonsurgical health interventions in developing countries.
Historical significance/ comments	This study suggests that contrary to traditional dogma, surgery in adults and children is a cost-effective public health intervention, particularly in developing countries. If these findings are confirmed by future studies, they provide strong rationale for expanding paediatric surgery care in Africa.

Key Summary Points

1. Childhood surgical disease is an understated cause of morbidity and mortality in Africa.

2. Paediatric surgery saves as many disability-adjusted life years (DALYs) as other public health interventions.

3. African paediatric surgeons have made significant contributions to the specialty.

4. Paediatric surgeons must take the lead as advocates for children among the public and policy makers.

5. Training needs can be partly met by utilising global partnerships.

References

1. UNICEF. State of the world's children, 2007. Available at http://www.unicef.org (accessed: 10 January, 2010).

2. World Health Organization. The World Health Report 2008. Available at http://www.who.int/whr/en/ (accessed: 10 January, 2010).

3. Nwomeh BC, Mshelbwala PM. Paediatric surgery specialty: how relevant to Africa? Afr J Paed Surg 2004; 1(1):36–42.

4. Whalen TV. Presidential address: forgive and remember while punching the clock. Current Surgery 2004; 61(1):116–119.

5. Bickler SW, Rode H. Surgical services for children in developing countries. Bull World Health Organ 2002; 80(10):829–835.

6. Bickler SW, Telfer ML, Sanno-Duanda B. Need for paediatric surgery care in an urban area of The Gambia. Trop Doct 2003; 33(2):91–94.

7. Debas HT, Thind A, Gosselin RA, McCord C. Surgery. In: Jamison DT, Brennan JG, Measham AR, et al., eds. Disease Control Priorities in Developing Countries, 2nd ed. Oxford University Press, 2006, Pp 981–993.

8. Alt KW, Jeunesse C, Buitrago-Tellez CH, Wachter R, Boes E, Pichler SL. Evidence for stone age cranial surgery. Nature 1997; 387(6631):360.

9. Badoe EA, Archampong EQ, da Rocha-Afodu JT. A brief history of surgery. In: Badoe EA, Archampong EQ, eds. Principles and Practice of Surgery Including Pathology in the Tropics. Ghana Publishing Corporation, 2000, Pp 1 –10.

10. Cywes S, Millar A, Rode H. From a "Louw" beginning...paediatric surgery in South Africa. J Pediatr Surg 2003; 38(7 Suppl):44–47.

11. The Colleges of Medicine of South Africa. Regulations for admission to the examination for the post-specialisation certificate in the subspecialty of paediatric surgery. Available at: http://www.collegemedsa.ac.za/index.html (accessed: 10 January, 2010).

12. West African College of Surgeons. Regulations for fellowship examinations. Available at http://www.wacs-coac.org/facult.htm (accessed: 10 January, 2010).

13. Bickler SW, Kyambi J, Rode H. Pediatric surgery in sub-Saharan Africa. Pediatric Surgery International 2001; 17(5–6):442–447.

14. Loefler IJP. Surgery in the third world. In: Watters DAK, ed. Surgery in the Tropics. Baillières Clin Trop Med Commun Dis 1988; 3:173–189.

15. Gosselin RA, Thind A, Bellardinelli A. Cost/DALY averted in a small hospital in Sierra Leone: what is the relative contribution of different services? World J Surg 2006; 30(4):505–511.

16. Weiser TG, Regenbogen SE, Thompson KD, et al. An estimation of the global volume of surgery: a modelling strategy based on available data. Lancet 2008; 372(9633):139–144.

17. Azzie G, Bickler S, Farmer D, Beasley S. Partnerships for developing pediatric surgical care in low-income countries. J Pediatr Surg 2008; 43(12):2273–2274.

18. Ameh EA, Chirdan LB. Paediatric surgery in the rural setting: prospect and feasibility. West Afr J Med 2001; 20(1):52–55.

19. Bickler SW, Sanno-Duanda B. Epidemiology of paediatric surgical admissions to a government referral hospital in The Gambia. Bull World Health Organ 2000; 78(11):1330–1336.

20. Delport SD, Christianson AL, van den Berg HJ, Wolmarans L, Gericke GS. Congenital anomalies in black South African liveborn neonates at an urban academic hospital. S Afr Med J 1995; 85(1):11–15.

21. Nwomeh BC, Ameh EA. Pediatric trauma in Africa. African J Trauma 2003; 1(1):7–13.

22. Deen JL, Vos T, Huttly SR, Tulloch J. Injuries and noncommunicable diseases: emerging health problems of children in developing countries. Bull World Health Organ 1999; 77(6):518–524.

23. Murray CJ, Lopez AD. Global and regional cause-of-death patterns in 1990. Bull World Health Organ 1994; 72(3):447–480.

24. Adesunkanmi AR, Oginni LM, Oyelami AO, Badru OS. Epidemiology of childhood injury. J Trauma 1998; 44(3):506–512.

25. Gedlu E. Accidental injuries among children in north-west Ethiopia. East Afr Med J 1994; 71(12):807–810.

26. Taira BR, McQueen KA, Burkle FM Jr. Burden of surgical disease: does the literature reflect the scope of the international crisis? World J Surg 2009; 33(5):893–898.

27. Ameh EA, Ameh N. Providing safe surgery for neonates in sub-Saharan Africa. Trop Doct 2003; 33(3):145–147.

28. Population Reference Bureau. 2009 World Population Data Sheet. Available at http://www.prb.org. (accessed: 10 January, 2010).

29. Adeyemi SD. Newborn surgery under local anaesthesia. Prog Pediatr Surg 1982; 15:13–23.

30. Tumwine JK. Experience with training of traditional midwives on the prevention and management of birth asphyxia in a rural district in Zimbabwe. J Obstet Gynaecol East Cent Africa 1991; 9(1):11–15.

31. Broaded RL, Muula AS. The challenges facing postgraduate medical training development in Malawi. Africa Health 2004; 26(2):13–15.

32. Peason B. The brain: a force for good? Africa Health 2004; 26(2):10–12.

33. Ameh EA, Adejuyigbe O, Nmadu PT. Pediatric surgery in Nigeria. J Pediatr Surg 2006; 41(3):542–546.

34. Harouchi A. Have the advances of modern pediatric surgery reached the African children? Chir Pediatr 1990; 31(4–5):284–286.

35. Ozgediz D, Wang J, Jayaraman S, et al. Surgical training and global health: initial results of a 5-year partnership with a surgical training program in a low-income country. Arch Surg 2008; 143(9):860–865; discussion 865.

36. Okrainec A, Henao O, Azzie G. Telesimulation: an effective method for teaching the fundamentals of laparoscopic surgery in resource-restricted countries. Surg Endosc 2010; 24(2):417–422.

37. Perkins RS, Casey KM, McQueen KA. Addressing the global burden of surgical disease. In: Proceedings from the 2nd Annual Symposium at the American College of Surgeons. World J Surg, 30 December 2009.

38. Coran AG. Presidential address. Da Vinci and the Penrose drain. J Pediatr Surg 2003; 38(3):267–274.

39. Nadler EP, Nwomeh BC, Frederick WA, et al. Academic needs in developing countries: a survey of the West African College of Surgeons. J Surg Res 2009 (PubMed PMID: 19766242).

40. Bickler SW, Rode H. Paediatric Surgery for the District Hospital. MacMillan, 2010, in press.

CHAPTER 2
NEONATAL PHYSIOLOGY AND TRANSPORT

Larry Hadley

Kokila Lakhoo

Introduction

It is perhaps trite to emphasize that the child is not merely a small adult, but nowhere is this distinction more apparent than in the neonate.

The transition from intrauterine to extrauterine life requires fundamental changes in the circulatory, respiratory, metabolic, and immune functions of the newborn. When a surgical pathology is added to the mix, these essential adaptations can be compromised, leading to organ dysfunction. Single organ dysfunction is frequently the start of a cascade that rapidly results in failure of the entire organism. Thus, the emphasis in neonatal care is on the prevention of problems rather than on the management of disasters once they have occurred. In order to prevent dysfunction, it is important to recognise patients at particular risk but also to have in place general principles of care and to train nursing staff and paramedical personnel in their application. Neonatal care is a team effort. Whenever possible, the team should include the mother and other family members, if culturally appropriate.[1]

Neonatal physiology is not defined by geography or politics, but our ability to recognise and respond to system dysfunction is a factor of the human and material resources available. In a developing country where scarce resources must be utilised for the maximum benefit of numerous constituencies, imaginative alternatives to standard Western care are required. It is in just this environment that maternal ill health and deficient antenatal care add to the considerable difficulties faced by neonates during the perinatal period.

Many of the neonate's survival mechanisms are installed during the third trimester of pregnancy, and preterm delivery can additionally challenge the successful transition to independent life, the difficulties being directly proportional to the degree of prematurity.

Occasionally, the uterus proves to be a hostile environment for the developing foetus and, in conjunction with obstetric colleagues, pregnancy management will need to take account of the interests of both the foetus and the mother. Certainly, the antenatal recognition of surgical disease calls for skilled management of the pregnancy and delivery and provides the surgeon with an unborn patient for whom diagnosis, prognosis, investigation, and management are difficult.

A few specific anomalies can be ascribed to genetic, teratogenic, or infectious causes, but the pathogenesis of most congenital malformations remains unknown. It is improbable, however, that any insult that results in a congenital abnormality will affect a single system or structure without affecting other structures that are developing at the same time. Thus, multiple abnormalities should be suspected and sought in every neonate presenting for surgery.

Neonatal Classification

Neonates come in a variety of sizes and degrees of maturity. It is important to recognise risk factors in any patient presenting for surgery, but particularly so in the neonate, in whom body weight and prematurity are easily assessed and critical to defining the likely co-morbidities and risk factors and help to determine appropriate management (Figure 2.1).

Many "surgical" babies are born before term; in addition, they are often small for their gestational age (SGA). Causative factors include

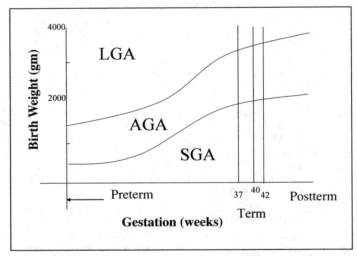

Figure 2.1: Neonatal classification (LGA = large for gestational age; AGA = appropriate for gestational age; SGA = small for gestational age).

maternal infections and poor nutrition, placental insufficiency, maternal cigarette smoking, and maternal substance abuse such as drugs and alcohol. Frequently, polyhydramnios complicates a pregnancy in which the foetus has an intestinal abnormality due to the inability to ingest and recycle amniotic fluid, stimulating early labour. Such babies are therefore exposed to the risks of prematurity and its associated problems as well as the morbidity of a surgical pathology. Recognition of a neonate's status allows prediction of potential clinical problems, thus allowing preventive steps to be taken. Table 2.1 outlines the traditional risks faced by SGA and preterm infants.

The risks associated with prematurity are reflected in the mortality of preterm babies without surgical disease and depend upon the degree of prematurity and body weight (Figure 2.2). This risk of mortality must be weighed against the available resources and the nature of the surgical problem before a decision on management can be taken. Such considerations are particularly germane to the practice of neonatal surgery in a developing country where both human and material resource limitations may be extreme.

Temperature Control

The neonate is designed as a radiator with a large surface area relative to its mass. Heat is lost through convection, conduction, radiation, and the latent heat of evaporation of transdermal fluid loss. In the term neonate, heat loss is reduced by a layer of insulating subcutaneous fat and a thick skin that reduces transdermal fluid loss. Heat production comes from hepatic glycogenolysis and the metabolism of brown fat, a metabolic response termed "nonshivering thermogenesis".[2] All of these defences against heat loss are weakened in the preterm infant, who has a thin skin, increased transdermal water loss, no subcutaneous fat,[3] and who has been born before having the opportunity to lay down any brown

Table 2.1: Predictable problems in small for gestational age (SGA) and preterm average for gestational age (AGA) babies.

	SGA	Pretterm AGA
Lung	Pulmonary haemorrhage	Hyaline membrane disease
Apnoea	+	+++
Hypoglycaemia	+++	+
Hypeglycaemia	+	+++
Jaundice	+	+++
Haemoglobin	Polycythaemia	Normal
Feeding capacity	Normal	Reduced
Congenital malformations	+++	+
Mortality	+++	Depends upon gestational age

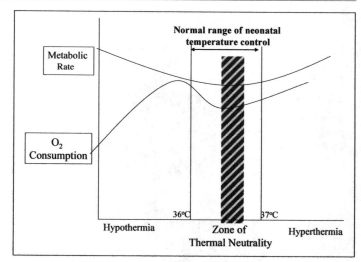

Figure 2.3: Metabolic rates, temperature, and oxygen consumption.

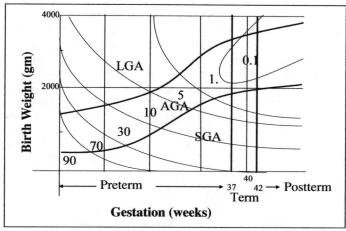

Figure 2.2: Neonatal classification and mortality risk (LGA = large for gestational age; AGA = appropriate for gestational age; SGA = small for gestational age).

fat.[2] In premature babies, insensible water loss can amount to 3 ml/kg per hour, and even in term babies it is around 1 ml/kg per hour. These losses can be minimised by nursing the baby in a humid environment, but this is rarely practicable. Heat loss through convection and conduction can be reduced by nursing the neonate in a warm environment.

In surgically ill neonates, further heat loss occurs in vomitus, tachypnoea, and, of course, during the massive increase in surface area that occurs when the baby's abdomen is opened by the surgeon, or where there is evisceration at birth, as occurs in babies with gastroschisis or ruptured exomphalos.

Babies who become cold must try to maintain temperature by using their scarce energy stores, but these are rapidly exhausted. The well child can replenish these energy stores by feeding. The surgically ill baby cannot. Cold then leads to further depletion of energy stores, protein breakdown, acidosis, sclerema, increased oxygen consumption, sepsis, and death. It is clear from Figure 2.3 that keeping the baby warm minimises the metabolic rate and oxygen consumption, but the zone of thermal neutrality is narrow. Hypothermia is formally defined as a core temperature lower than 36°C.

Prevention is much better than cure. Keeping a baby warm requires strategies different to those required to warm up a cold baby. A baby can be kept warm by enveloping him, and his head, in an insulating material such as a blanket or aluminium foil, obviously ensuring that the airway is not obstructed; doing this to a cold baby will simply keep him cold. The mother's body is an excellent heat source and so-called "kangaroo" care[4] also aids in maternal bonding.[5] It would appear that, at least in the short term, fathers are capable substitutes.[6]

Ideally, surgically ill babies should be kept warm in incubators when these are available. Most babies can be accommodated in incubator temperatures of 32–33°C. Babies in incubators still lose heat by radiating it into space. In a perfect world, double-lined incubators would be standard, but radiation losses can also be reduced by covering the baby with a sheet of paper.

Making a cold baby warm requires an external heat source, and warming should take place slowly[7]; attempting to rapidly warm a baby with an electrical heater inevitably results in dermal burns. During rewarming, it is wise to check the baby's blood sugar level.

Cardiovascular Adaptation

Before birth, the baby's circulation is based upon the placenta, which acts as lung, kidney, and nutrient supply. Thus, the umbilical vessels are of paramount importance. Blood arriving at the foetus from the umbilical vein is shunted across the liver through the ductus venosus and away from the lung through the foramen ovale. The foramen ovale is simply a flap "gate" that is held open because the pressure in the right atrium is higher than the left atrial pressure. Because the lungs require little blood flow before birth, blood is also shunted from the right ventricular outflow into the aorta through the ductus arteriosus before returning to the placenta through the umbilical arteries (Figure 2.4).

When the obstetrician clamps the cord, flow to the right atrium is reduced and the right atrial pressure falls. There is a simultaneous increase in left atrial pressure in response to increased pulmonary blood flow that follows the decreased pulmonary vascular resistance caused by lung expansion with the first breath. This allows the "gate" to close the foramen ovale. With the onset of breathing, there is an increase in peripheral oxygen concentration that stimulates the ductus arteriosus to close, a muscular contraction probably mediated through prostaglandin. The closure of both the foramen ovale and the ductus arteriosus are temporary. They can be reopened by anything that increases right atrial pressure relative to the pressure in the left atrium or that decreases peripheral oxygen concentration. Permanent closure is not achieved in the neonatal period.

Reopening these temporarily closed shunts restores the infant to the foetal circulatory pattern, but there is no longer a placenta that can act as lung or kidney, and unless the adult circulatory pattern can be rapidly re-established, the infant will die. Pulmonary hypertension, seen, for example, in neonates with diaphragmatic hernia, will cause an increase in pressure on the right side of the heart, a right atrial pressure that will exceed left atrial pressure, reopening of the foramen ovale, and ultimately reduction in peripheral arterial oxygen concentration and reversal of ductal closure. Without a placenta, this circulatory pattern

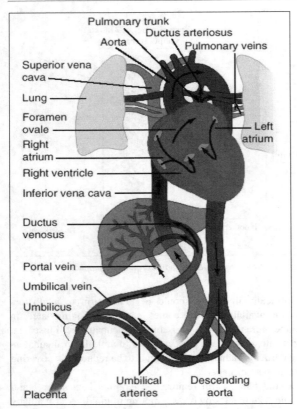

Figure 2.4: Schematic diagram of foetal circulation, with red indicating arterial blood, blue indicating venous blood, and purple indicating admixed blood.

is unsustainable. Pulmonary vascular resistance can be increased, and the foetal circulation reproduced, by hypoxia, acidosis, catecholamine secretion, hypothermia, or hypoglycaemia, as well as conditions that primarily cause pulmonary hypertension.

The circulating blood volume of a term neonate is in the order of 80 ml/kg body weight.[8] This small volume means that precision is essential in the prescription of intravenous fluids, as an apparently trivial error of 1 ml/kg per hour in a 3-kg baby will result in an error of 10% of the circulating blood volume by the end of the day. Similarly, all losses should be carefully measured and replaced.

Respiratory Adaptation

During normal delivery, the fluid that has filled the lungs during foetal life is expelled and the lungs are expanded with air during the first breath. Along with lung expansion, there is a reduction in pulmonary vascular resistance and a redirection of blood flow to allow gas exchange.

Neonates are obligatory nasal breathers and obligatory diaphragmatic breathers. Resistance to air flow is increased by nasogastric intubation, and for this reason—as well as the danger of perforation of the cribriform plate during insertion[9]—orogastric intubation is preferred in this group of patients.

Abdominal distention of any cause will impair diaphragmatic mobility and therefore impede breathing. The number of alveoli in the neonatal lung is less than 10% of the adult quota, but new alveoli are continually added up to 8 years of age. Despite this paucity of alveoli, the resting neonate requires more oxygen per kilogram body weight than an adult, so the neonate is at risk if oxygen requirements are increased or if any pathology diminishes the surface available for gas exchange.

Alveolar stability is maintained by surfactant, a phospholipid wetting agent produced by the type II pneumocyte, which reduces the surface tension in the fluid lining the alveoli. Adequate levels of surfactant are achieved around 35 weeks of gestation. Babies born before this are at risk of developing hyaline membrane disease. It is

possible to predict lung maturity antenatally by measuring amniotic fluid phospholipid concentrations.

Air flow is proportional to the fourth power of the radius of the airway, and a small reduction in calibre (for example, by mucosal oedema) can have a major effect on resistance to air flow and therefore on the work of breathing. Decreased ventilation will result in alveoli being perfused but not aerated, creating an intrapulmonary shunt, with a fall in peripheral oxygen saturation and an increase in the partial pressure of carbon dioxide in the arterial blood ($paCO_2$).

Aspiration of vomitus is common in surgical babies at all phases of their management and is a leading cause of airway oedema, lung contamination, and death.[10] It can be prevented simply by never allowing a surgically ill baby to be nursed supine. A neonate cannot turn over to protect his airway, and vomiting in a supine position inevitably leads to aspiration. Babies are perfectly happy on their sides or prone, and the culture of nursing babies supine has little merit.[11] The canard that it reduces the risk of sudden infant death syndrome (SIDS) is vastly outweighed by the numbers lost each year to aspiration pneumonia.

Similarly, analgesia is important for postoperative respiratory care, as a baby in pain will not breathe deeply, or cry, and will have diminished respiratory excursion, leading to atelectasis, intrapulmonary shunting, and ultimately infection.[12] After thoracic or upper abdominal surgery, adequate analgesia may obviate the need for postoperative ventilation.[13]

Immaturity of the respiratory centre is held to be the cause of apnoea in prematurity. This usually responds to tactile stimulation but may require treatment with theophylline. The risk of apnoea following a general anaesthetic remains for up to a year postnatally in formerly premature babies. All such babies undergoing an anaesthetic for whatever reason should be kept under observation, with apnoea monitoring, for 24 hours after surgery.

Clinical Evaluation

Because babies cannot vary their tidal volume, their initial response to inadequate ventilation is to increase the rate of breathing. Due to the flexible cartilaginous nature of the chest wall, any increase in the work of breathing is manifest by intercostal, sternal, and subcostal recession as well as alar flaring. As the neonate tries to increase positive end expiratory pressure (PEEP) to maintain alveolar patency, grunting may occur. The increased work of breathing will eventually tire the baby, who will be unable to sustain these compensatory tactics and will go into respiratory failure.

Babies with clinical signs of respiratory insufficiency should receive supplementary oxygen pending investigation with a chest x-ray and blood gas analysis, if available. Any increased work of breathing associated with abdominal distention can often be ameliorated by the passage of an orogastric tube and maintenance of gastrointestinal decompression. Viscid tracheal secretions can sometimes be suctioned following humidification, best effected by nebulisation with saline.

Nutrition

The provision of energy as well as the substrate for growth and development is critical to the neonate, and the provision of adequate nutrition is particularly important for the developing brain. Perinatal deficiencies may have lifelong consequences for the patient, particularly with regard to brain growth and development.[14] Nutrition is also pivotal to wound healing, temperature maintenance, and immune function.

Babies who start life with the handicap of intrauterine growth retardation, and those with surgical disorders that are not promptly recognised, are at particular risk of neonatal malnutrition. Whereas normal babies can be fed through the alimentary tract, the surgically ill neonate is frequently unable to tolerate feeding.

In the developed world, this conundrum is resolved by using total parenteral nutrition (TPN), but in many developing countries this is unavailable. The standard of care in the developed world has evolved on the back of the availability of TPN and is often inappropriate care when TPN is unavailable. As getting energy and substrate into the patient is a priority, there may be no alternative to adjusting surgical strategy to allow early use of the alimentary tract. This may involve placing feeding tubes distal to, or through, an anastamosis or creating a stoma above, or instead of, an anastamosis. An extracorporeal gastrointestinal bypass can be created by aspirating bile-containing fluid from above an obstruction and returning it with a feed either via a stoma or via a trans-anastamotic tube, distal to the obstruction. Even when full feeds are not tolerated, there is merit in providing "trophic" or "trickle" feeds that maintain the integrity of the intestinal mucosa.[15]

The advent of the human immunodeficiency virus (HIV), particularly the recognition of the seroconversion of breast-fed babies, has added a further confounding variable.[16] Breast milk is the best, cheapest, and generally most readily available feed for babies, and it is ideal for the surgical patient. These advantages must be weighed against the risk of transmission of HIV and the economic circumstances of the family.[17] It should be remembered that breast milk contains lactose and that many gastrointestinal disorders result in temporary lactose intolerance with resulting diarrhoea.[18]

The term neonate requires about 120 kCal/kg per day to maintain health. The surgical neonate, after a very brief postoperative increase in metabolic rate that lasts only four to six hours,[19] may require fewer calories than normal due to immobility and growth inhibition as well as reduced thermogenesis.[20] Providing too many calories (overfeeding) may increase CO_2 production from lipogenesis.

The premature baby has an increased caloric requirement, up to 130 kCal/kg per day.[21]

Hypoglycaemia

SGA infants, those with diabetic mothers or who have specific conditions such as Beckwith-Wiedemann syndrome are at risk of hypoglycaemia in the first few hours of life. Failure to recognise hypoglycaemia will result in unnecessary neurological morbidity. Clinical signs include apnoea, the tremors or jitteriness, followed by convulsions. The blood sugar should be kept above 2.2 mmol/l by infusion of 10% dextrose if necessary. The blood sugar level should be monitored in all at-risk babies.

Hyperglycaemia

The stress response results in hyperglycaemia in many neonates with emergency surgical conditions, and is common after surgery.[22] Premature babies appear to have a higher normal blood sugar, and moderate degrees of hyperglycaemia (blood glucose < 15 mmol/l) can be tolerated. Glycosuria with a resultant osmotic diuresis occurs only with glucose levels around 12 mmol/l due to greater renal retention in the premature infant.

Immune Function

The normal intrauterine environment is sterile, and the neonate has limited exposure to antigens before birth. Both the B-cell and T-cell populations are naïve, and the neonate depends primarily on the "innate" or nonspecific functions of the immune system.

Circulating neutrophils have a half-life of around 8 hours and must be constantly replenished to effectively combat infection. However, the neonate has a low bone marrow storage pool of neutrophils, and although they are functionally competent, they respond poorly to chemotactic stimuli and are rapidly consumed. The neonate also has deficiencies in the complement system.[23] Almost all immunoglobulin at birth is maternally derived immunoglobulin G (IgG). This immunoglobulin has a half-life of around 3 weeks. Immunoglobulin M (IgM) production is very limited. Immunoglobulin A (IgA), the mucosal surface immunoglobulin, is acquired from breast-feeding.[24] The naïve T-cell population exposes the neonate to the risks of viral and fungal infections, and the "lazy" leukocyte population means that infections are poorly localised and septicaemia is frequent.

Thus, the neonate is immunodeficient when compared to adults. This deficiency becomes more apparent when the nonspecific defences against infection are breached, usually by a well-intentioned physician. Thus, intravenous cannula placement, urinary catheter insertion, endotracheal intubation, and orogastric intubation all bypass important defence structures. Thought must be given to the necessity of these interventions because each has an inherent risk. When deemed essential, all interventions must be performed aseptically. Tubes and catheters should be removed as soon as practicable. It is not possible to make up for deficiencies of hygiene by prescribing antibiotics.

Clearly, antibiotics do have a place in the management of infection but the importance of fungal and viral sepsis must be remembered. The more premature the patient, and the longer the intensive care unit (ICU) stay, the greater must be the clinical suspicion of fungal sepsis, even when cultures are not possible.

Neonatal Transport

The centralisation of neonatal surgical services has made neonatal transportation[25,26] inevitable. From the outset it must be recognised that transportation is not good for babies; it adds to their stress and represents a break in the continuum of care. Neonatal transportation is an exercise that demands the highest professionalism and planning and should only be undertaken in close cooperation with the unit receiving the infant. Formal training in transportation skills is provided in most US paediatric training programmes, but forms only a small part of the undergraduate or postgraduate training in most African schools.

In the Third World, conflicting health care agendas transpire to limit the human and material resources allocated to interhospital transport. This is something of a false economy, as the inexpert transport of a baby results in either a death on arrival (DOA) or delivers a patient in whom resuscitation and avoidable morbidity adds to the cost of management.

Care in transport is also compromised by the infrequency with which any individual medical officer is required to effect transfer, and the small proportion of his practice that this involves. This lack of familiarity often leads to unseemly haste in attempting to get a baby to a tertiary centre. Speed is never an issue; care is.

In an ideal world, the baby would be stabilised in the ICU at the referring hospital, and transported by dedicated medical and paramedical staff in a mobile ICU to the welcoming staff of the ICU at the referral hospital. It is, however, not an ideal world.

Fortunately, most surgically ill babies require minimal technological support during transport, and there is much that can be done without recourse to mobile ICUs and high technology. Most transferred babies have some form of intestinal obstruction and require little other than gastric decompression, intravenous fluid, and temperature maintenance.

Incubators and other devices that rely on electricity or batteries, which always seem to be flat when needed, are not essential. Heat and fluid loss can be minimised by wrapping exposed viscera in clear plastic sheeting such as can be found in most kitchens, or, when necessary, a plastic shopping bag. A warm baby can be kept warm by enveloping him in an insulating blanket of aluminium foil, another kitchen accessory. It is important to include the head, which represents a large proportion of the surface area and contributes significantly to heat loss, but not the face.

Denim bags containing mung beans or any grain, heated for 1 minute in a microwave oven, can provide sufficient heat to keep a neonate warm for two hours during transport, or, more traditionally, hot water bottles (held remote from the skin to prevent burns) can be used. Portable incubators that have hot water bottles as their source of heat were the standard of care when New York City introduced a transport service for premature babies in 1948. That principle is still sound.

An incubator is just a transparent box designed to keep a baby warm. The heat it provides is no better than the heat provided by mung beans or hot water, and it is certainly more expensive. We re-emphasize that there is a difference between keeping a warm baby warm, which is what is required during transport, and making a cold baby warm, which is something that must be done as part of stabilisation before transport. The critical importance of temperature maintenance is demonstrated in the higher mortality of babies who are hypothermic on arrival at a tertiary centre.

Gastric decompression is a vital intervention. By keeping the stomach empty, the risk of vomiting and aspiration is reduced. It can be reduced still further by nursing the baby in the lateral position, or prone, during transport. Gastric decompression also relieves pressure on the diaphragm, reducing the work of breathing. It reduces the diameter of the bowel, thus reducing tension in the bowel wall and allowing greater mucosal blood flow. All of these effects are beneficial, but can be assured only if the nasogastric or orogastric tube is supervised and regularly checked for blockage. None of the benefits of gastric decompression are achieved if the nasogastric tube becomes blocked or displaced.

Pretransport stabilisation should ensure that the baby does not start on a journey with a fluid deficit. Nonetheless, fluid replacement during transport remains essential to replace ongoing losses, particularly nasogastric losses, and to provide maintenance fluid for the duration of the journey. Isotonic fluid losses should be replaced with isotonic fluid, not paediatric maintenance fluids. Modified Ringer's lactate is a reasonable choice. It is overly optimistic to expect a needle to remain in a vein during transport, and fluid will inevitably extravasate if this is attempted. An intravenous cannula should be placed at a site that is accessible for checking during transport.

The amount of fluid required to correct a preexisting deficit can be answered simply. Give enough! "Enough" means that the baby has well-perfused peripheries, adequate urine output (at least 1 ml/kg per hour) signifying adequate renal perfusion, and appropriate cerebral function. If this has not been achieved, "enough" has not been given. Resuscitation is best achieved by aliquots of 10 ml/kg of Ringer's lactate repeated until the desired clinical parameters have been met. Additionally, patients will require maintenance fluids determined by their age and degree of prematurity.

Oxygen administration by mask or by head box supports the baby through any respiratory embarrassment and improves oxygen delivery, particularly to the bowel. Along with the increased mucosal flow following gastric decompression, oxygen administration may play a role in reducing bacterial translocation through a compromised mucosa.

Stabilisation is the sine qua non of transportation. If a baby cannot be resuscitated in a primary care facility, it is unlikely that this can be achieved in a moving vehicle. Stabilisation includes restoration of circulating blood volume with an appropriate fluid, ensuring that there is a clear and sustainable airway, treating hypoglycaemia, and ensuring that the patient is warm.

Whenever possible, the child should be escorted by the most experienced staff available. Successfully supervising the care of a surgically ill neonate during transport is the pinnacle of nursing achievement, and should be recognised as such by medical staff and nurse administrators. To maintain high standards of professionalism in the cramped conditions of a vehicle with a patient who, in the best of circumstances, is a nursing challenge deserves the plaudits of the entire team. Unfortunately, escorting ill babies is often left to the most junior and inexperienced staff member because this impacts the least on the functioning of the referring institution. The mother alone is never a suitable escort. Rarely do mothers have intensive care nursing experience, and the emotional turmoil of giving birth precludes the required precision and objectivity.

Documentation, including a letter of referral outlining the pre-referral progress of the patient and management provided at the primary care facility, must accompany all transported babies. This should augment the telephone discussions with the referral hospital that preceded the decision to transfer the baby. Likewise, any x-rays taken to support the diagnosis should be included with the documentation, or patients will have to endure a repeated radiological examination on arrival, which is a waste of time and money.

Mothers should accompany their babies whenever they are fit enough to do so. If they are unable to do so, it helps if a clotted specimen of the mother's blood is made available to allow a safe matching of blood in case a transfusion becomes necessary.

The principles involved in safe neonatal transfer are outlined in Table 2.2, which presents the mnemonic TWO SIDES as a memory aid for those whose exposure to neonatal transfers is limited.

Table 2.2: Checklist for neonatal transfer.

Tube	Orogastric, maintain gastric decompression; prevent aspiration; improve diaphragmatic excursion; maximise bowel perfusion
Warmth	Conserve energy stores by reducing energy required for thermogenesis
Oxygen	Maximise O_2 delivery to the bowel, brain, myocardium
Sabilisation	Fluid volume restored, rewarmed, before transfer
Intravenous fluids	Ringer's lactate through cannula
Documentation	Referral letter including pre-referral history and progress
Escort	The most skilled nurse or paramedic available
Specimens	X-Rays, mother's clotted blood

Evidence-Based Research

Table 2.3 presents a study on postnatal transfer of preterm infants between hospitals.

Table 2.3: Evidence-based research.

Title	Moving the preterm infant
Authors	Fowlie PW, Booth P, Skeoch CH
Institution	Aberdeen Maternity Hospital, Aberdeen, UK; Princess Royal Maternity Hospital, Glasgow, UK
Reference	BMJ 2004; 329(7471):904–906
Problem	Newborn infants and pregnant mothers may have to move between hospitals for appropriate care because of prematurity or the threat of preterm delivery. Sometimes this move means that the infant and family have to travel hundreds of miles.
Intervention	This article focuses on the postnatal transfer of preterm infants between hospitals.
Comparison/ control (quality of evidence)	When no regional transport service is available, medical and nursing staff from either referring or receiving units undertake the transport on an ad hoc basis. The staff will have variable experience in neonatal transport and the equipment used, and the vehicle may not be dedicated for neonatal use. Running these ad hoc teams often puts resources under strain because there will be fewer staff on site in the unit that carries out the transport.
Outcome/ effect	Anticipating the need for transfer early, appropriate preparation for transfer, and ongoing high-quality care during transfer are the cornerstones of good neonatal transport. To achieve this, staff need to be trained appropriately, all equipment and vehicles must be fitted out for the purpose, and lines of communication must be well established.
Historical significance/ comments	Some newborn infants will always need to be moved between hospitals. Neonatal transport services must be well organised and should aim to provide clinical care to a high standard. The service should be staffed by professionals trained in neonatal transport medicine and in using appropriate equipment.

Key Summary Points

1. A congenital surgical anomaly is usually associated with other system involvement.

2. Birth weight and gestational age affect outcomes.

3. Temperature control is pivotal.

4. Cardiovascular adaptation may be reversed during a surgical insult.

5. Neonates are obligatory nasal breathers and obligatory diaphragmatic breathers.

6. In the absence of TPN, innovative use of tubes and stomas may be necessary to provide nutrition.

7. Unrecognised hypoglycaemia will result in unnecessary neurological morbidity.

8. The neonate is immunodeficient when compared to adults.

9. All interventions must be performed aseptically. Antibiotic prescription will not make up for less than aseptic technique.

10. The principles involved in safe neonatal transfer are present in the mnemonic TWO SIDES.

References

1. Marsh DR, Darmstadt GL, Moore J, Daly P, Oot D, Tinker A. Advancing newborn health and survival in developing countries: a conceptual framework. J Perinatology 2002; 22(7):572–576.

2. Cannon B, Nedergaard J. Brown adipose tissue: function and physiological significance. Physiol Rev 2004; 84:277–359.

3. Rutter N. The immature skin. Euro J Pediatr 1996; 155(S2):S18–S20.

4. Ludington-Hoe SM, Nguyen N, Swinth JY, Satyshur É. Kangaroo care compared to incubators in maintaining body warmth in preterm infants. Biologic Res Nurs 2000; 2(1):60–73.

5. Christensson K, Siles C, Moreno L, Belaustequi A, De La Fuente P, Lagercrantz H, et al. Temperature, metabolic adaptation and crying in healthy full-term newborns cared for by skin-to-skin or in a cot. Acta Pediatrica 1992; 81(6–7):488–493.

6. Erlandsson K, Dsilma A, Fagerberg I, Christensson K. Skin-to-skin care with the father after caesarean birth and its effect on newborn crying and prefeeding behaviour. Birth 2007; 34(2):105–114.

7. Mathur NB, Krishnamurthy S, Mishra TK. Estimation of rewarming time in transported extramural hypothermic neonates. Ind J Pediatr 2006; 73(5):395–399.

8. Aladangady N, McHugh S, Aitchison TC, Wardrop CAJ, Holland BM. Infants' blood volume in a controlled trial of placental transfusion at preterm delivery. Pediatr 2006; 117(1):93–98.

9. Elliot M, Jones L. Inadvertent intracranial insertion of nasogastric tubes: an overview and nursing implications. Austral Emerg Nurs J 2003; 6(1):10–14.

10. Valat C, Demont F, Pegat MA, Saliba E, Bloc D, Besnard JC, et al. Radionuclide study of bronchial aspiration in intensive care newborn children. Nucl Med Commun 1986; 7(8):593–598.

11. Ewer AK, James ME, Tobin JM. Prone and left lateral positioning reduce gastro-oesophageal reflux in preterm infants. Arch Dis Childhood, Fetal and Neonatal Edition 1999; 81(3):F201–F204.

12. Stevens B, Gibbins S, Franck LS. Treatment of pain in the neonatal intensive care unit. Pediatr Clin North Amer 2000; 47(3):633–650.

13. Bösenberg AT, Hadley GP, Wiersma R. Oesophageal atresia: caudo-thoracic epidural anaesthesia reduces the need for postoperative ventilation. Pediatr Surg Intl 1992; 7:289–291.

14. Oyedeji GA, Olamijulo SK, Osinaike AI, Esimai VC, Odunusi ES, Aladekomo TA. Head circumference of rural Nigerian children—the effect of malnutrition on brain growth. Cent Afr J Med 1997; 43(9):264–268.

15. McClure RJ, Newell SJ. Randomised controlled study of clinical outcome following trophic feeding. Arch Dis Childhood, Fetal and Neonatal Edition 2000; 82(1):F29–F33.

16. Miotti PG, Taha ET, Kumwendra NI, Broadhead RB, Mtimavakye LA, van der Hoeven L, et al. HIV transmission through breastfeeding. JAMA 1999; 282(8):744–749.

17. Ogundele MO, Coulter JBS. HIV transmission through breastfeeding: problems and prevention, Annals of Trop Paediatr 2003; 23(2):91–106.

18. Thapa BR, Jagirdhar S. Nutrition support in a surgical patient. Ind J Pediatr 2002; 69(5):411–415.

19. Pierro A. Metabolism and nutritional support in the surgical neonate. J Pediatr Surg 2002; 37(6):811–822.

20. Letton RW, Chwals WJ, Jamie A, Charles B. Early postoperative alterations in energy use increase the risk of overfeeding. J Pediatr Surg 1995; 30(7):988–992.

21. Denne C. Protein and energy requirements in preterm infants. Semin Neonat 2001; 6(5):377–382.

22. Srinivasan G, Jain R, Pildes RS, Kannan CR. Glucose homeostasis during anaesthesia and surgery in infants. J Pediatr Surg 1986; 21:718–721.

23. Schelonka RL, Infante AJ. Neonatal Immunology. Sem Perinatol 1998; 22(1):2–14.

24. Hanson LA, Korotkova M. The role of breastfeeding in prevention of neonatal infections. Sem Neonatol 2002; 7(4):275–281.

25. Hadley GP, Mars M. Improving neonatal transport in the Third World—technology or teaching? South Afr J Surg 2001; 29(4):122–124.

26. Hadley GP. Neonatal transport. Trauma Emerg Med 1998; 15(4):40–44.

CHAPTER 3
RESPIRATORY PHYSIOLOGY AND SUPPORT

John R. Gosche

Mark W. Newton

Laura Boomer

Introduction

The primary function of the lung is to exchange gases between the bloodstream and the environment. The anatomy and physiologic control mechanisms of the lung and its associated pulmonary circulation allow for optimal efficiency of gas exchange. Due to a need for brevity, this chapter addresses only the features of lung development and pulmonary physiology that may impact the care of infants and children. The publications listed in the Suggested Reading at the end of this chapter present a more in-depth understanding of pulmonary physiology,

Pulmonary Physiology in the Neonate

Several unique aspects of neonatal pulmonary physiology related to lung maturation and growth as well as the transition from intrauterine to extrauterine life may significantly complicate management of the surgical neonate.

The structure of the bronchial tree is established by the 16th week of gestation, but alveolar maturation and growth continues throughout foetal life and into adulthood. Prenatal lung development is divided into four phases:

1. *embryonic phase* (3rd through 6th weeks of gestation), during which the primitive lung bud forms;

2. *pseudoglandular phase* (7th through 16th weeks of gestation), during which the bronchial airways are established;

3. *canalicular phase* (16th through 24th weeks of gestation), during which the structure of the distal airways and early vascularisation is established; and

4. *terminal saccular phase* (24th week of gestation to term), during which primitive alveoli are formed and surfactant production begins.

Throughout the period of prenatal lung development, interstitial tissue gradually decreases, resulting in thinning of the walls of the future alveoli. Even at birth, however, the lung does not contain mature alveoli; instead, it has approximately 20 million primitive terminal sacs. Postnatally, the relatively shallow, cup-like terminal saccules of the newborn lung gradually assume the more spherical, thin-walled structure of mature alveoli. In addition, new alveoli continue to develop up to 8 years of age. at which time approximately 300 million alveoli are present. After 8 years of age, lung growth is associated with increases in alveolar size but not number.

Lung hypoplasia is frequently associated with congenital surgical anomalies such as congenital diaphragmatic hernia or congenital cystic adenomatoid malformation that limit lung growth due to compression of the developing lung. Furthermore, because late foetal lung growth is stimulated by rhythmic lung expansion associated with foetal breathing, lung hypoplasia may also be associated with conditions that limit amniotic fluid volume (e.g., renal agenesis) and in patients with severe neurologic abnormalities (e.g., anencephaly). New bronchial development does not occur after the 18th week of gestation, so infants who experienced early inhibition of lung development will not develop completely normal lungs. Lung growth continues well after birth, however, so infants with adequate initial lung parenchyma to support extrauterine life may ultimately be left with little or no functional impairment.

Surfactant production in the foetal lung begins at about 20 weeks of gestation, but is not secreted by the lung until about 30 weeks gestation. Surfactant consists of about 90% glycerophospholipids, of which dipalmitoylphosphatidyl choline (DPPC) is the most important. During late gestation, the ratio of phosphatidyl choline (PC, or lecithin) to other lipid components (phosphatidylglycerol, sphingomyelin) changes, and thus the ratio of the different lipid components of surfactant in the amniotic fluid can be used as an index of lung maturity; that is, a lecithin/sphingomyelin (L/S) ratio >2.0, which normally occurs around 35 weeks gestation and is associated with a low risk of respiratory distress syndrome (RDS). Infants born prior to the age of lung maturity are prone to atelectasis and pulmonary oedema due to a relative lack of surfactant, which can result in the development of hyaline membrane disease.

Foetal lung maturation and surfactant production can also be affected by hormonal influences. Foetal stress associated with uteroplacental insufficiency accelerates lung maturation, probably as a result of the influence of elevated glucocorticoids and catecholamine levels, resulting in a relatively low incidence of RDS in these infants. Elevated insulin levels, however, inhibit surfactant production. Thus, even term infants of diabetic mothers may be prone to the development of RDS.

Due to the relatively greater tissue thickness in the normal newborn lung, lung compliance in the neonate is approximately equal to that of the adult. The chest wall of the newborn, however, is more compliant. Thus, the intrapleural pressure in the newborn is less negative (i.e., only slightly less than atmospheric pressure) than in adults. Given this relationship, one would expect the functional residual capacity (FRC) to be lower in the neonate than in the adult. However, the newborn infant augments FRC by maintaining inspiratory muscle activity throughout expiration thereby splinting the chest wall, and by increasing airway resistance via glottic narrowing during expiration. As a result, the percent FRC of the neonate is similar to that of adults.

Lung expansion and intrapleural pressures affect airway diameters and thus airway resistance. With forceful expiration, increased intrapleural pressure compresses the airways, thus restricting air flow and potentially causing air trapping. In the lung of the adult and older child, cartilaginous support of the airways prevents complete airway collapse. Less cartilaginous support of the central airways in premature infants, however, may result in air trapping during periods of increased respiratory effort.

Haemoglobin in the foetus has a higher oxygen affinity than the haemoglobin found in the normal older child and adult. The increased oxygen affinity of foetal haemoglobin appears to be primarily due to a decreased affinity for 2,3-DPG. This increased oxygen affinity allows for greater uptake of oxygen from the placenta at the lower oxygen tensions normally observed in the foetus. Greater oxygen uptake also reflects higher foetal haemoglobin concentrations. Postnatally, however, the increased oxygen affinity of foetal haemoglobin may limit the delivery of oxygen during periods of hypoxaemia. In the newborn infant, the oxygen-haemoglobin dissociation curve gradually shifts to the right (toward decreased affinity), as adult haemoglobin levels increase and 2,3-DPG levels rise. Thus, by the time the child is 4 to 6 months of age, the oxygen affinity usually approximates that of an adult.

Haemoglobin concentrations also change during the first weeks after birth. The normal haemoglobin concentration of newborn infants varies between 16.7 and 17.9 g/dl. Postnatally, haemoglobin concentrations transiently increase initially, but then gradually fall to reach minimum levels at 8 to 12 weeks of age. The primary explanation for the postnatal decrease in haemoglobin concentration is believed to be the decreased stimulus for haemoglobin synthesis associated with markedly decreased erythropoietin levels in response to the higher oxygen environment of the neonate.

During intrauterine life, the placenta functions as the organ for gas exchange. In the foetus only about 12% of right ventricular output circulates through the pulmonary circulation. The remaining right ventricular output is shunted to the systemic circulation through the ductus arteriosus and foramen ovale. Blood is shunted away from the lung due to the high resistance to flow in the foetal pulmonary vasculature, likely due the combined effects of hypoxic pulmonary vasoconstriction, the local release of vasoconstrictor leukotrienes and anatomic compression of the pulmonary vasculature by the surrounding liquid-filled lung.

At birth, the lung must immediately assume the role of gas exchange. This remarkable transition depends upon the completion of several simultaneous events. First, the collapsed, fluid-filled alveoli of the prenatal lung must be expanded with air, which begins with the first breath. At birth, more than 25 mm Hg of negative pressure is required to overcome the surface tension and open the alveoli for the first time. To accomplish this, the initial inspiratory efforts of the newborn infant are extremely powerful, generating negative pressures of up to 60 mm Hg. In addition, as the newborn's lung fills with oxygen, blood flow must be redirected such that poorly oxygenated blood returning to the right atrium preferentially flows through the pulmonary circulation. The redistribution of blood flow in the newborn occurs as a result of the combined effects of an increase in systemic vascular resistance and an eightfold decrease in pulmonary vascular resistance. The former is due to loss of the low-resistance placental circulation. The latter is due to expansion of the pulmonary vasculature as the lung expands and the pulmonary vessels are no longer compressed by the fluid-filled lung, and due to vasorelaxation in response to increased alveolar oxygen tension. As a result of these adjustments, systemic pressure and left atrial pressure increase while right atrial and pulmonary artery pressure decrease, resulting first in functional closure and then anatomic closure of the foetal shunts (foramen ovale, ductus arteriosus).

Newborn infants with significant impairments in lung function (e.g., RDS, pulmonary hypoplasia) that result in hypoxaemia are prone to persistent pulmonary hypertension of the newborn (PPHN) due to hypoxic pulmonary vasoconstriction. In addition, abnormalities of lung structure are frequently associated with abnormalities of the pulmonary vasculature (i.e., pulmonary vascular hypoplasia), which may also contribute to pulmonary hypertension. As pulmonary blood pressure exceeds systemic blood pressure, blood flow will be shunted again through the anatomic foetal shunts (foramen ovale and ductus arteriosus), resulting in a condition referred to as persistent foetal circulation (PFC). The development of PFC further exacerbates hypoxaemia as unoxygenated blood is shunted away from the pulmonary circulation to the systemic circulation (right-to-left shunt). Occasionally, PFC will respond to measures that increase systemic blood pressure or decrease pulmonary vascular resistance, such as inhaled nitric oxide or oxygen. However, if a significant shunt already exists, these interventions are less unlikely to be successful. Therefore, the optimal strategy is to recognise and treat alveolar hypoxia before pulmonary hypertension develops.

Clinical Correlations

The following scenarios present typical situations and suggested treatments for paediatric respiratory problems.

Case Scenario #1

Presentation

You are seeing a newborn infant at 36 weeks gestational age. The child was born to a nulligravid 18-year-old mother who presented with preterm labor. The child was born after a prolonged labor and difficult assisted vaginal delivery. At the time of rupture of the amniotic membranes, meconium-stained amniotic fluid returned. Examination of the placenta revealed evidence of a partial abruption. The infant's Apgar scores were 7 at 1 minute and 8 at 5 minutes. Upon oropharyngeal suctioning in the delivery room, meconium-stained secretions were noted. The patient is tachypneic and has peripheral cyanosis. Auscultation reveals coarse bilateral breath sounds.

1. What is the likely cause of this patient's respiratory distress?

2. What are the options for supporting this patient?

Treatment

The newborn patient has respiratory distress syndrome. Given the difficult delivery and observed meconium staining of the amniotic fluid, it is likely this patient's respiratory distress is due to meconium aspiration syndrome. The management of patients with meconium aspiration syndrome is primarily supportive. Pulmonary physical therapy and frequent suctioning should be instituted to assist with clearance of the airways. Oxygen therapy with continuous positive airway pressures may improve the patient's cyanosis and decrease the atelectasis associated with disruption of surfactant function.

In many settings in Africa, the use of bubble continuous positive airway pressure, known as "bubble CPAP", may be an option in these types of cases. Bubble CPAP implies placing a short binasal pronged nasal cannulae into the nasal passages of newborns who need some extra airway pressure while their pathology improves and oxygenation increases. The nasal cannulae is attached to the oxygen wall outlet at 8–14 l/min in an effort to maintain pharyngeal pressure with a Y-connector so that an expiratory limb is produced. The expiratory limb can then be placed in 8 cm water pressure; bubbling that stops indicates an excessive loss of airway pressure and the need to confirm for leaks. The water pressure provides for continuous airway pressure, which could allow for these types of patients to improve without the need for intubation.

Steroid therapy may help to decrease airway inflammation, although corticosteroid therapy has not been shown to improve the course or outcome associated with this disease. In addition, antibiotic therapy should be instituted to prevent the frequent complication of secondary bacterial pneumonia, especially if steroids are used.

Case Scenario #2

Presentation

A 7-year-old boy is brought in after being rescued from a burning building. He was sleeping in his home when it caught fire. He was rescued by a neighbor who heard the child screaming for help and coughing. On examination, the child has soot around the nares and in the posterior pharynx, although there are no obvious facial burns. He is anxious and tachypneic, and his skin color is cherry-red.

1. What is the likely cause of this patient's anxiety and tachypnea?

2. What would be your initial treatment?

Treatment

This patient was exposed to a fire in an enclosed environment—a history that raises concern for an inhalation injury. Other findings including soot in the oropharynx and around the nares support the likelihood of inhalation injury, whereas the findings of the cherry-red skin and anxiety are consistent with carbon monoxide poisoning.

Carbon monoxide is a by-product of combustion. Inhaled carbon monoxide is rapidly transported across the alveolar membrane and preferentially binds to the haemoglobin molecule in place of oxygen. Binding of carbon monoxide to haemoglobin (carboxyhaemoglobin) impairs unloading of O_2. Carboxyhaemoglobin is bright red, which explains the cherry-red skin color, and the tachypnea and anxiety suggest tissue (central nervous system) hypoxia.

The most important first step in treating this patient is to provide supplemental oxygen in high concentrations. High oxygen concentration accomplishes two goals: (1) it optimises oxygen delivery to ameliorate tissue hypoxia, and (2) it accelerates unloading of carbon monoxide from the haemoglobin molecule (the half-life of carboxyhaemoglobin is about 90 minutes in 21% oxygen but decreases to 20–30 minutes in 100% oxygen).

An inhalation injury is not commonly due to direct thermal injury to the airways, but these injuries are associated with inhalation of toxic by-products of combustion, which can result in airway oedema due to inflammation. Therefore, fluid resuscitation should be judicious and the patient should have a bladder catheter placed to monitor urine output as an indicator of adequacy of hydration. Care should be taken, however, to avoid overhydration. At times, after fluid resuscitation, the airway can become oedematous, and one needs to monitor for airway obstruction, which may make a definitive airway more difficult. Steroids have been used frequently in the past to attempt to decrease airway swelling. Their use, however, has not been shown to decrease the morbidity or mortality in patients with inhalation injury, and they may increase the risk of infections. Similarly, prophylactic antibiotics have also not been shown to decrease pulmonary complications or mortality in patients with inhalation injuries.

Key Summary Points

1. The primary role of the lungs is to allow for exchange of respiratory gases (intake of oxygen and elimination of carbon dioxide).

2. Pulmonary function requires a balance of ventilation, gas transport, and blood flow.

3. Surgical diseases can negatively impact gas exchange by altering any or all of these factors.

4. Severe derangements may overcome compensatory mechanisms, resulting in hypoxia and acidosis.

5. Due to differences in lung maturation and respiratory mechanics, neonates may be at increased risk of altered gas exchange.

6. Recognition and treatment of causes of dysfunction are key to improving patient outcomes.

Suggested Reading

Cilley RE. Respiratory physiology and extracorporeal life support. In: Oldham KT, Colombani PM, Foglia RP, Skinner M, eds. Principles and Practice of Pediatric Surgery. Lippincott Williams & Wilkins, 2005, Pp 179–221.

Guyton AC, Hall JE. Respiration. In: Guyton AC, Hall JE, eds. Textbook of Medical Physiology, 10th ed. WB Saunders, 2000, Pp 432–492.

Piiper J, Respiratory gas transport and acid-base equlibrium in blood. In: Gregor R, Windhorst U, eds. Comprehensive Human Physiology, from Cellular Mechanisms to Integration. Springer-Verlag, 1996, Pp 2051–2062.

Piiper J. Pulmonary gas exchange In: Gregor R, Windhorst U, eds. Comprehensive Human Physiology, from Cellular Mechanisms to Integration. Springer-Verlag, 1996, Pp 2037–2049.

Staub NC, Dawson CA, Pulmonary and bronchial circulation. In: Gregor R, Windhorst U, eds. Comprehensive Human Physiology, from Cellular Mechanisms to Integration. Springer-Verlag, 1996, Pp 2071–2078.

West JB. Respiration. In: West JB, ed. Best and Taylor's Physiological Basis of Medical Practice, 11th ed. Williams and Wilkins, 1985, Pp 546–613.

Whipp BJ. Pulmonary Ventilation. In: Gregor R, Windhorst U, eds. Comprehensive Human Physiology, from Cellular Mechanisms to Integration. Springer-Verlag, 1996, Pp 2015–2036.

Wilson JW, DiFiore JW. Respiratory physiology and care. In: Grosfeld JL, O'Neill JA, Coran AG, Fonkalsrud EW, eds. Pediatric Surgery, 6th ed. Mosby Elsevier, 2006, Pp 114–133.

CHAPTER 4
CARDIOVASCULAR PHYSIOLOGY AND SUPPORT

Mark W. Newton
John R. Gosche
Laura Boomer

Introduction

Failure of the circulatory system leads to organ dysfunction and ultimately to death. A basic understanding of the physiologic principles of cardiovascular control is essential for early recognition and appropriate treatment of cardiovascular dysfunction.

Cardiac Structure and Function

The force required to pump blood throughout the circulatory system is generated by the heart. The arrangement of the four chambers of the human heart results in two parallel pumping mechanisms (an atrium plus a ventricle, each supplying a separate circulation) that are arranged in series. Due to this series arrangement, failure of one side of the heart usually ultimately results in dysfunction of the other. The force required to pump blood is provided by the contraction of the cardiac muscle, and the valves between the cardiac chambers and at the outflow of the ventricles assure that blood flows in the proper direction. Thus, failure of any of the cardiac valves due to either acquired or congenital defects can severely impair cardiac function.

Cardiac output is the quantity of blood pumped by the heart per unit of time. Cardiac output varies with body size and is proportional to body surface area. Thus cardiac output is frequently normalised to body surface area, which is referred to as the cardiac index. The normal cardiac index per square meter of body surface area for the adult is approximately 3.0 l/min. Normal cardiac index in the newborn infant is approximately 2.5 l/min. This value rapidly increases during early childhood to about 4 l/min by 10 years of age.

Cardiac output is the product of heart rate (contractions per minute) and average stroke volume (ml per contraction) over a time period. Stroke volume, in turn, is affected by changes in preload, afterload, and contractility. During periods of inadequate cardiac output, alterations in all of these variables should be sought and addressed to optimise cardiac function.

Preload is the amount of blood in the ventricle at the end of diastole and reflects the venous return to the heart. Under normal circumstances, the heart pumps whatever amount of blood enters the right atrium without a backup of blood in the atria. This physiologic ability to increase cardiac output is referred to as the Frank-Starling relationship and reflects improved interdigitation of actin and myosin filaments, resulting in optimal force generation during contraction. This ability to increase contractile force even occurs in the weakened heart. Thus, increasing blood volume by giving a fluid bolus or transfusion may improve cardiac output and perfusion even in patients with known cardiac dysfunction.

Of course, there are physiologic limits beyond which increasing end diastolic volume results in excessive stretch of the myocardial fibres and decreases contractile force. This circumstance is seldom observed in patients with normal cardiac function, but may develop in patients with cardiac failure due to ischaemia, valvular disease, myocarditis, or congenital cardiac anomalies. In the absence of valvular disease and pericardial disease, end diastolic right ventricular filling pressure in the right ventricle is equivalent to diastolic atrial pressure and is reflected by central venous pressure. In practice, unfortunately, direct measurements of venous pressure may not always be available. Then indirect indicators such as jugular venous distention and changes in blood pressure with changes in patient position (i.e., orthostatic hypotension) should be looked for, as they may reflect increased or decreased central venous pressures affecting preload.

Afterload is the pressure against which the ventricles must contract to eject blood from the heart. Thus, the afterload on the ventricles is the pressure in the aorta for the left ventricle (or pulmonary main for the right ventricle) throughout systole. In the normal heart, changes in systolic pressure over the physiologic range do not significantly affect cardiac output. Only at extremes of pressure does afterload impair cardiac output in the normally functioning heart. However, congenital anomalies that result in obstruction of blood flow (e.g., coarctation of the aorta, pulmonic stenosis) may create excessive afterload on the heart and impair cardiac output, resulting in heart failure. Furthermore, in patients with poor cardiac function (e.g., myocarditis or valvular heart disease), the judicious use of vasodilators to decrease afterload may significantly increase cardiac output.

Contractility refers to the strength of cardiac muscle contraction and is measured as the change in ventricular pressure generated per unit of time. As noted previously, cardiac contractility is affected by preload due to the Frank-Starling relationship. Cardiac contractility is also influenced, however, by the autonomic nervous system. Specifically, increased sympathetic activity results in increased cardiac contractility, whereas increased parasympathetic activity decreases contractility. Stimuli that increase cardiac contractility are said to have a positive inotropic effect, and those that decrease contractility are said to be negative inotropes. Sympathetic stimulation increases contractility by increasing calcium release during contractions and by increasing the sensitivity of myofilaments to calcium. The negative inotropic effect of parasympathetic activity likely primarily results from loss of normal tonic sympathetic activity. Unfortunately, contractility is a difficult variable to measure in clinical practice. One option for assessing contractile function is to measure ejection fraction by echocardiography.

The final variable that impacts cardiac output is heart rate. Changes in heart rate primarily reflect changes in autonomic nervous activity, with sympathetic stimulation increasing heart rate (i.e., positive chronotrope) and parasympathetic stimulation decreasing heart rate (i.e., negative chronotrope). Heart rate is also affected by intrinsic mechanisms, however. For instance, stretch of the right atrial wall during increases in venous return causes an increase in the heart rate by as much as 10–30%. Increases in heart rate generally correlate with increases in cardiac output, but beyond critical levels, further changes in heart rate may have the opposite effect on cardiac output. As an example, at very high rates above a critical level, stroke volume decreases, thereby limiting cardiac output. Decreased stroke volume at high heart rates results from limited availability of metabolic substrates to support myocardial contraction and a decreased ventricular preload. Conversely, a low heart rate is usually associated with an increase in stroke volume due to increased ventricular preload.

Cardiac output is affected by the above-noted variables in patients of all ages, but neonates are somewhat unique in that they have a limited ability to increase stroke volume. The difference reflects a relatively lower compliance of the neonatal myocardium, thereby limiting increases in cardiac output associated with increases in preload. Also, the neonatal myocardial contractility is less responsive to sympathetic stimulation due to differences in calcium transits. Therefore, the neonate is much more dependent upon changes in heart rate to increase cardiac output in times of need.

Anatomy and Physiology of the Circulation

The body has two circulatory systems: the pulmonary circulation and the systemic circulation. Normally, the two circulations are separate. Structurally, both circulations are similar in that they start with a single large vessel that, through sequential branchings, distributes blood to arteries of decreasing diameter but increasing number. Ultimately the small arteries (arterioles) empty blood into a series of capillaries, which are the primary site of exchange of solutes between the intravascular and extravascular compartments. From the capillaries, blood enters a large number of small veins (venules), which, through a series of junctions with other venous structures of similar calibre, coalesce into several large venous structures that return blood to the atria.

An important concept to remember is that blood always flows down a pressure gradient and will always take the path of least resistance. As a result, points of increased resistance in the circulatory system will result in an increase in pressure proximal to the point of the obstruction until either the pressure is adequate to overcome the cause of the resistance or blood flow is diverted through an alternate pathway. The pulmonary and systemic circulations differ in that the pulmonary circulation is a high-flow, low-resistance, and thus low-pressure system, whereas the systemic circulation has much higher overall resistance and as a result has higher intraluminal pressures. Reflecting these differences in pressures, the relative stiffness and thickness of the arteries are greater in the systemic circulation than in the pulmonary circulation. However, in patients with abnormal connections between the pulmonary and systemic circulations (e.g., patent ductus arteriosus), the pulmonary arteries will ultimately hypertrophy in response to the higher pressures experienced by the pulmonary vessels. The following section primarily addresses the mechanisms that control pressure and blood flow within the systemic circulation.

Control of pressure and blood flow in the systemic circulation occurs both globally and locally. Table 4.1 lists ranges for average blood pressure based upon age, with the mean pressure ±20% at the 95% confidence limit. Values for females are approximately 5% lower than for males. These paediatric blood pressure references may help guide diagnosis and management during times when the patient is demonstrating signs of shock.

The central nervous system (CNS) and the kidneys are the primary organs responsible for global blood pressure control. The CNS affects systemic blood pressure both directly via the autonomic nervous system and indirectly by inducing release of humoral factors. Increased sympathetic nervous system (SNS) activity increases blood pressure by increasing cardiac contractility (as described previously) and by causing vasoconstriction through release of norepinephrine from nerve endings that innervate the vasculature. The latter effect increases arterial resistance, thus increasing proximal pressures, and also increases venous return to the heart—and thus cardiac output—by increasing venous tone and decreasing the capacitance of the venous system. SNS activation also increases blood pressure by stimulating release of the vasoconstrictors, epinephrine, and norepinephrine from

Table 4.1: Age and average blood pressures.

Age	Average blood pressure (mm Hg)
Premature	Systolic 40–60
Full term	75/50
1–6 months	80/50
6–12 months	90/65
12–24 months	95/65
2–6 years	100/60
6–12 years	110/60
12–16 years	110/65
16–18 years	120/65
Adult	125/75

Source: Modified from Zuckerberg AL, Wetzel RC, Shock, fluid resuscitation, and coagulation disorders. In Nichols DG, Yaster M, Lappe DG, Buck JR (eds). Golden Hour: The Handbook of Advanced Pediatric Life Support. Mosby-Year Book, 1991.

the adrenal medullae. Finally, the CNS also affects blood pressure over the long term by releasing vasopression (antidiuretic hormone) from the posterior pituitary, which primarily has an effect by increasing water reabsorption by the renal tubules and increasing intravascular volume. Vasopressin is also a potent vasoconstrictor; however, under normal conditions, the circulating concentration of this hormone is too low to have a direct effect on vascular control.

Given the potent effects of the CNS on blood pressure regulation, it is not surprising that there are multiple mechanisms for controlling the vasomotor centres in the brain. These vasomotor centres are located in the medulla and pons and include both a vasoconstrictor area and a vasodilator area. The vasoconstrictor area causes excitation of vasoconstrictor neurons in the SNS, whereas the vasodilator centre primarily functions to cause inhibition of neurons in the vasoconstrictor area. The activities of these two vasomotor centres are affected by afferent impulses (1) from stretch receptors (baroreceptors) located in the carotid sinus and the wall of the aortic arch, which respond to short-term changes in pressure in these arteries; (2) from low pressure receptors in the atria and pulmonary arteries that reflect changes in blood volume; and (3) from higher brain centres that respond to stressful stimuli (e.g., pain, alarm) and CNS ischaemia. Under normal conditions, the vasoconstrictor centre of the brain stem is continuously active, causing partial contraction of the blood vessels and maintaining baseline vasomotor tone. This explains why rapid loss of SNS activity (such as following a cervical spinal cord injury) often results in hypotension.

The other organ that has important global effects on blood pressure is the kidney. In the kidney, the juxtaglomerular cells located in the proximal arterioles release renin into the bloodstream in response to a decrease in perfusion. Renin is an enzyme that cleaves circulating plasma angiotensinogen, resulting in release of angiotensin I. Angiotensin I is subsequently metabolised to angiotensin II by converting enzyme, which is primarily located in the walls of small vessels in the lung. Angiotensin II has several effects, including vasoconstriction of both arterioles and veins, resulting in an increase in vascular resistance and venous return. It also decreases salt and water loss by the kidney (both by a direct effect on the kidney and by stimulating secretion of aldosterone by the adrenal cortex), resulting in expansion of the circulating blood volume. Ultimately, these effects cause an increase in blood pressure and renal perfusion, resulting in a negative feedback on renin release.

The global mechanisms for affecting blood flow are primarily involved in maintaining adequate central systemic blood pressure and thus assuring adequate perfusion to organs with high metabolic needs, including the heart and CNS. The vasoconstricting effects of sympathetic nervous activity and circulating humoral agents result in a decrease in vascular compliance (the same as an increase in vascular resistance). The cumulative effect of increasing vascular tone contributes to the body's total vascular resistance. The total vascular resistance is one factor that affects pulse pressure, or the difference between systolic and diastolic blood pressures. The other factor is the stroke volume output of the heart. Increases in vascular resistance primarily are reflected by increases in diastolic pressure, whereas increases in cardiac output typically result in an increase in both the systolic and the diastolic pressure. Typically, the diastolic pressure is two-thirds to three-fourths of the systolic pressure. Changes in pulse pressure can be a valuable indicator of circulatory derangements.

Whereas the globally active mechanisms primarily affect systemic blood pressure, local control mechanisms are primarily involved in controlling blood flow to individual organs and tissues. Both metabolic and myogenic mechanisms may be involved in local control of blood flow. Myogenic control reflects the ability of the vascular smooth muscle to constrict in response to increased wall stretch. The myogenic mechanism allows local autoregulation of blood flow that is somewhat independent of upstream pressures. The physiologic importance of the myogenic response is debatable, but it may provide a means for preventing local hyperperfusion and tissue oedema during periods of elevated systemic blood pressure. Likely, the more important control mechanism is metabolic control, which enables the local vasculature to respond to changes in local tissue demand.

Two theories have been proposed to explain how increases in tissue metabolic demand can affect blood flow. The first theory is that a vasodilator substance (e.g., adenosine, carbon dioxide, histamine, or similar) is produced by tissues in response to local decreases in the availability of oxygen or another metabolite. Of the proposed substances, adenosine is a likely candidate. Once released, the vasodilator agent is believed to diffuse locally and induce dilatation of upstream arterioles. The resultant increase in local blood flow would increase the local supply of oxygen and other metabolites to the tissues, thus creating a negative feedback mechanism. The other theory is that local decreases in oxygen tension are directly responsible for causing local vasodilation. This response is based upon the requirement of vascular smooth muscle for oxygen to maintain active contraction. Thus, in response to local decreases in oxygen tension, the vascular smooth muscle of the local upstream arterioles would relax, resulting in an increase in blood flow and oxygen delivery to the tissues in need.

Of course, local vasodilation of downstream blood vessels is of no use if perfusion is limited due to vasoconstriction of more proximal arteries. Local activation of vasodilator responses cannot affect the tone of proximal arterioles. However, as downstream vessels dilate, blood flow velocity in the upstream vessels is increased. The endothelial cells lining arterioles have the ability to sense increases in flow velocity as shear stress. As shear stress increases, endothelial cells release vasodilator substances locally, thereby resulting in relaxation of the adjacent vascular smooth muscle. The most important of these vasodilator agents is the endothelial-derived relaxing factor, nitric oxide. Thus, in response to increases in tissue metabolic need, both local and upstream vessels dilate, resulting in increasing blood flow to meet metabolic demands.

Shock and Clinical Implications in the Paediatric Surgical Patient

Shock is defined as a severe pathophysiological alteration in the normal homoeostatic processes of oxygen delivery and cellular metabolism that, if untreated and prolonged, can lead to major changes in these processes and cellular death. The traditional classifications of shock in the paediatric population include: hypovolaemic, septic, cardiogenic,

and neurogenic. Each of these forms of shock can be present in the paediatric perioperative surgical patient, and it is imperative that each type of shock be adequately treated prior to an elective procedure. One may encounter those occasions when the shock may not be completely resolved, however, and surgery becomes unavoidable or emergency surgery is required. During these types of patient presentations, the understanding of each form of shock needs to be understood and, if possible, treated before surgery ensues and further complications arise.

Hypovolaemic Shock

Hypovolaemic shock is the most common form of shock in the paediatric population and results primarily from a decreased intravascular volume, causing a diminishing venous return and consequently, a decreased preload. Neonates and young infants have a relatively set stroke volume due to the immaturity of their cardiac muscle, which results in the compensation mechanism of an increased heart rate when the preload decreases.

In the typical African clinic, it would be common to see a paediatric patient who has a 2- or 3-day history of diarrhoea or vomiting and presents in hypovolaemic shock with cool, pale extremities; decreased peripheral perfusion (>4 seconds); and decreased urine output. In general, the blood pressure decrease seen in adult patients who have lost 15–25% of their intravascular volume does not occur in the paediatric population, and blood pressure alone is an insensitive indicator of dehydration in children due to their ability to increase their heart rate (Table 4.2). The SNS discharge attempts to compensate for the loss in intravascular volume, but when the acidosis persists and overcomes the vasoconstriction, capillary leak may occur as well.

The paediatric patient may develop tachypnea in an effort to decrease the acidosis that is produced due to the low tissue perfusion occurring during the shock phase. Lethargy and decreased responsiveness to pain occur secondary to decreased cerebral perfusion and low oxygen delivery. These findings associated with a drop in heart rate and blood pressure are ominous signs, and immediate action needs to be quickly pursued. The aetiology of the shock needs to be determined. The most common causes of hypovolaemic paediatric shock include trauma, burns, peritonitis, severe vomiting, and diarrhoea, and in some cases, hyperthermia with decreased intake, which is common with malaria.

Table 4.2: Clinical effects of dehydration based upon percentage of body weight decrease.

Dehydration (% body weight)	Clinical observation
5%	• Increase in heart rate (10–15% above baseline) • Dry mucous membranes • Concentration of the urine • Poor tear formation
10%	• Decrease in skin turgor • Oliguria • Soft, sunken eyes • Sunken anterior fontanelle
15%	• Decrease in blood pressure, tachycardia, tachypnoea • Poor tissue perfusion and acidosis • Delayed capillary refill

Source: Modified from Zuckerberg AL, Wetzel, RC. Shock, fluid resuscitation, and coagulation disorders. In Nichols DG, Yaster M, Lappe DG, Buck JR (eds). Golden Hour: The Handbook of Advanced Pediatric Life Support. Mosby-Year Book, 1991.

Initial management would include the management of the airway, and every patient in shock should receive 100% oxygen by a face mask until the shock resolves. If the airway needs a more definitive measure, then endotracheal intubation needs to be performed because the combination of shock and respiratory problems has a very high mortality rate.

It is always important to remember that shock is a very dynamic process, and changes occur rapidly—this is especially true in the paediatric population, which requires adjustments that are ongoing in the management plan.

Fluid resuscitation in the hypovolaemic patient with a large-bore intravenous cannulae is required, and locations such as the saphenous, femoral, external jugular, and intraossaeous may need to be used. The goal is to replace the intravascular volume as quickly as possible with a crystalloid solution, such as normal saline and not dextrose in water. Normal saline is readily available in most areas of Africa. The expansion effect in the extracellular compartment is greatest, and the cost of the fluid is inexpensive compared to other fluids. At Kijabe Hospital in Kenya, we do not use Ringer's lactate with paediatric patients due to the presence of potassium in Ringer's lactate and its effects on a patient with potentially poor renal function. Figure 4.1 presents an algorithm for treatment of hypovolaemic shock in children. Although this algorithm may need to be adjusted for each specific clinical dilemma, the figure will provide a guide for taking the necessary steps needed to prepare the paediatric shock patient for emergency surgery.

In situations whereby the hypovolaemic shock is due to acute blood loss, the resuscitation team needs to be prepared to infuse appropriate volumes of blood in an attempt to maximise the oxygen-carrying capacity of the intravascular volume. The patient's blood pressure, heart rate, respiratory rate, urine output, and mental status need to be monitored to help determine the appropriate volume to be infused. Most who work in Africa will not have access to central venous monitoring devices; therefore, these indirect measurements of intravascular volume need to act as guides for adequacy of replacement. O-negative or merely type-specific blood can be infused rapidly in the paediatric patient who needs blood urgently to survive due to the shock. If the patient fails to respond to the fluid resuscitation measures, before considering an inotropic agent such as dopamine, look for an additional cause of bleeding or decreased cardiac output, such as tension pneumothorax.

Septic Shock

Septic shock is associated with microorganisms in the blood and the effects of toxic products with an associated inadequate delivery of oxygen to the tissues. Initially, the oxygen delivery can be high, with warm and well-perfused tissues, but this can change if lactic acidosis overcomes the compensatory mechanisms of the paediatric patient due to excessive demand for oxygen. Although gram-negative and gram-positive organisms are a common cause of sepsis, tuberculosis, herpes, and malaria are forms of sepsis seen more often in the African environment. In an environment where the patients arrive late in their course of distress, septic shock can be severe and the mortality very high in the paediatric population.

The factors that indicate septic shock syndrome are as follows:
• clinical suspicion or evidence of infection;

• temperature instability (fever or hypothermia);

• tachycardia/tachypnea; and

• impaired organ system function:

- peripheral hypoperfusion;

- altered level of consciousness;

- oliguria;

- hypoxaemia;

- acidosis; and/or

- pulmonary oedema.

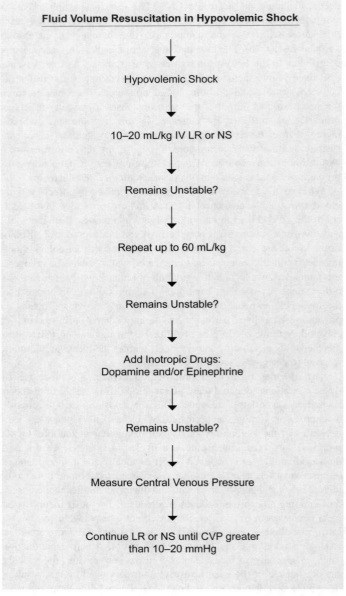

Source: Modified from Litman, RS. Pediatric critical care. In; Litman RS. Pediatric Anesthesia: The Requisites in Anesthesiology. Mosby, Inc., 2004, P 331.

Figure 4.1: Algorithm for treatment of hypovolaemic shock.

The cardiovascular effects that implicate septic shock include lower systemic vascular resistance, increased capillary leak, and increased venous capacitance, which will directly decrease preload and therefore cardiac output. In patients for whom direct myocardial contractility is affected, the inability to provide sufficient oxygen supply for the high demand results in rapid deterioration. The patient who presents early with "warm shock" will demonstrate a significantly different picture than the delayed presenter who is hypovolaemic with "cold shock".

The management of septic shock is similar to hypovolaemic shock in relation to the need for oxygen and fluids, but these patients need to have the aetiology of the septic shock discovered rapidly so that the toxic effect can be diminished and eventually removed from the system. Antibiotics, antituberculosis, or antimalarial drugs need to be administered early and in appropriate doses so that the cause of the sepsis can be resolved. Disseminated intravascular coagulation (DIC), renal failure, acute respiratory failure, and even liver failure can be caused by sepsis.

Cardiogenic Shock

Cardiogenic shock is defined as shock due to cardiac failure, which can be due to infections, trauma, drug overdose, cardiomyopathies, and congenital heart disease. Although cardiac failure may be present in other forms of shock, this form is directly due to the cardiac function. In the newborn period, cardiogenic shock can be caused by a hypoplastic left heart, which is difficult to manage in any environment.

The management of cardiogenic shock depends on the aetiology of the hypotension, but the use of vasopressors such as dopamine and epinephrine with the addition of 5–10 ml/kg boluses of fluids while monitoring cardiac volume indirectly may help temporarily. Arrhythmias may occur more commonly in this form of shock, and the identification of the type of electrocardiogram (ECG) abnormality will help as treatment options are considered.

Cardiogenic shock carries a high mortality rate, and invasive monitoring with mechanical circulatory assistance is sometimes difficult to obtain in resource-poor settings. Without surgical correction of the correctable cardiac paediatric lesions, at times only palliative care can be provided for these patients.

Neurogenic Shock

Cervical spinal cord injury is associated with dysfunction of the sympathetic nervous system, resulting in such cardiovascular changes as severe bradycardia, asystole, and loss of peripheral vascular tone. Cardiovascular problems known to arise from SNS dysfunction include low resting blood pressure, orthostatic hypotension, autonomic dysreflexia, reflex bradycardia, cardiac arrest, limited cardiovascular response to exercise, and alterations in skin microcirculation.

Patients in neurogenic shock initially have warm extremities and low diastolic pressure, which may eventually develop into a situation of acidosis and a decrease in perfusion pressure. With the sudden loss of sympathetic tone, especially if the lesion is above T6, the patient may demonstrate signs of bradycardia and other arrhythmias due to the effect of the cardioaccelerator fibers. Pulmonary oedema may develop due to fluid resuscitation when the loss of sympathetic tone results in peripheral vasodilatation. The management of neurogenic shock depends upon the level of injury and the involvement of the levels for ventilation. If the level is below C8, then the diaphragm is intact and providing the necessary muscles of inspiration needed to maintain oxygenation. Fluid resuscitation and monitoring for bradycardia may prompt the use of intravenous atropine and even vasopressors to maintain the appropriate blood pressure.

Management of Shock

All forms of shock—hypovolaemic, septic, cardiogenic, and neurogenic—can have similar effects on the paediatric patient, and therefore have similar management plans. The foundation of oxygen delivery to compensate for oxygen utilisation allows medical care providers a target to aim toward as they seek to resolve the hypovolaemia, identify the organism in sepsis, search for the cardiac resolution of the shock, or treat the acute spinal cord injury and associated implications of the physiological implications of no sympathetic nervous system. Table 4.3 lists some common cardiovascular medications used in shock management.

Clinical Correlations

The following scenarios illustrate the clinical impact of alterations in cardiovascular function and provide recommendations for management.

Case Scenario #1

Presentation

You are planning a posterior sagittal anorectoplasty (PSARP) on an 8-month-old male with high imperforate anus and unrepaired tetralogy of Fallot (TOF). The patient had a colostomy at one month of age and since that time has had approximately two episodes of central cyanosis, which resolve spontaneously per day. The patient is not on any medications except for iron supplement, and the room air oxygen saturation is 90%. His preoperative haemoglobin level is 8.1. He is small for his age, at 5.1 kg, and has no known respiratory issues.

1. What is the likely aetiology of his cyanotic episodes?

2. How should this patient be managed intraoperatively?

Treatment

This patient has documented tetralogy of Fallot, a cardiac anomaly characterised by right ventricular outflow obstruction associated with a ventricular septal defect (VSD), overriding aorta, and right ventricular hypertrophy. Due to the obstruction of right ventricular outflow, blood flow through the pulmonary circulation in most patients occurs through persistence of the foetal connection between pulmonary and systemic circulations, the ductus arteriosus. Therefore, in these patients, oxygenated blood returning from the lungs and unoxygenated blood returning from the peripheral tissues are mixed in the ventricles through the VSD. The percentage of cardiac output passing through the pulmonary circulation determines the severity of cyanosis.

Patients with TOF frequently experience episodes of worsening cyanosis ("tet" spells) associated with decreased pulmonary perfusion in response to stimuli that increase pulmonary outflow obstruction or decrease systemic vascular resistance. Options for treating cyanotic episodes include IV fluid boluses, pressure on the abdominal aorta, liver compression, morphine 0.1 mg/kg IV, or intravenous sodium bicarbonate. Oxygen is seldom helpful during a "tet" spell due to decreased pulmonary perfusion. During an anaesthetic, it is important to avoid a drop in systemic blood pressure, as this will worsen right-

Table 4.3: Common cardiovascular medications.

Drug	Paediatric dosing	Uses	Classification	Mechanism of action
Dopamine	5–20 mcg/kg per min IV	Shock	Inotropes/ vasopressors	Alpha- and beta1- agonist; stimulates dopaminergic receptors
Epinephrine (Adrenalin)	0.01 mg/kg IV q 3–5 min prn for arrhythmia; SC/IM q 20 min–4 hr for anaphylaxis or asthma	Asystole, VF, pulseless VT, bradycardia, asthma, anaphylaxis	Inotropes/ vasopressors; anti-arrhythmics; anaphylaxis	Sympathomimetic stimulation of alpha- and beta- adrenergic receptors
Phenylephrine (Neo-Synephrine)	5–20 mcg/kg IV bolus, then 0.1–0.5 mcg/kg/min IV; or 0.1 mg/kg SC/IM q 1–2 hr for mild hypotension; or 5–10 mcg/kg IV x 1 for paroxysmal supraventricular tachycardia (PSVT) conversion	Shock, hypotension, PSVT conversion	Inotropes/ Vasopressors	Smooth muscle alpha-agonist (vasoconstrictor)
Ephedrine	10- 50 mg IV (adults) prn hypotension titrated to effect	Hypotension	Inotropes/ Vasopressors; Decongestants	Smooth muscle alpha-agonist (vasoconstrictor)

to-left shunting. Patients may respond to an IV fluid bolus, decreasing inhalation anaesthetic, and vasoconstrictor drugs such as phenylephrine (alpha agonist) to increase systemic vascular resistance. Most cyanotic patients are polycythemic, which improves oxygen delivery. Therefore, consideration should be given to transfusing this patient prior to surgery. Ketamine is a good choice for induction because it tends to maintain systemic blood pressure. Narcotics and low-dose halothane are good choices for this particular surgery, which must be completed without muscle relaxants to allow nerve stimulation during surgery. The goal should be to extubate the patient in the immediate postoperative period to minimise airway stimulation, which can induce a "tet" spell.

Case Scenario #2

Presentation

You are called to see an 8-year-old, previously healthy boy with a 2-day history of abdominal pain and vomiting. On examination, the patient is moderately distended and has diffuse abdominal tenderness with involuntary guarding. The patient seems somewhat anxious, he is tachypneic, his temperature is 39.5°C, his heart rate is 140, and his blood pressure is 90 over 45. His extremities are cool to the touch.

1. What is the likely aetiology of this patient's altered vital signs?

2. What should you do to prepare this patient for surgery?

Treatment

This patient presents with an acute abdomen of two days duration. Based upon the findings on clinical examination, he has diffuse perito-

nitis. His tachycardia, low blood pressure, anxiety, and poor peripheral perfusion are consistent with circulatory shock. He is febrile and has a wide pulse pressure, which would suggest that shock may be due to sepsis. However, patients with peritonitis lose a large amount of intravascular volume due to transudative and exudative losses into the peritoneal cavity. Therefore, this patient likely also has a component of hypovolaemia contributing to his shock state.

The first and most important step in the management of this patient is to recognise that he is in shock. Due to the cardiodepressive effects of most anaesthetic agents, worsening hypotension and organ dysfunction would likely result if this patient were taken directly to the operating room without prior resuscitation. Therefore, an effort should be made to optimise his haemodynamics prior to the induction of anaesthesia. Because both septic shock and hypovolaemic shock respond initially to expansion of the intravascular blood volume, a large-bore IV should be started and the patient should receive one or more boluses of a crystalloid solution. During the period of preoperative resuscitation, vital signs should be monitored frequently, and a bladder catheter should be inserted to monitor urine output as a measure of adequacy of end organ (renal) perfusion. In addition, because sepsis is suspected, the patient should be started on a broad-spectrum antibiotic. It is likely that the ultimate treatment for the cause of this patient's shock will require surgical intervention; therefore, resuscitation should occur as expeditiously as possible.

Key Summary Points

1. Alterations in venous return (preload), vascular resistance (afterload), heart rate, and contractility all impact cardiovascular function.

2. In the healthy patient, compensatory mechanisms allow maintenance of adequate cardiac output and organ blood flow in the face of limited changes in these variables.

3. Neonates have a limited ability to increase cardiac output by increasing contractility and stroke volume, and thus are dependent upon heart rate to maintain cardiac output.

4. Shock is the result when pathologic conditions severely alter one or more factors and overwhelm compensatory responses, resulting in cellular ischaemia due to inadequate cardiac output or a maldistribution of blood flow.

5. Recognition and treatment of the cause of shock is central to optimising patient outcome.

Suggested Reading

Antoni H. Functional properties of the heart. In: Gregor R, Windhorst U, eds. Comprehensive Human Physiology, from Cellular Mechanisms to Integration, Springer-Verlag, 1996, Pp 1801–1823.

Guyton AC, Hall JE. Cardiac output, venous return and their regulation. In: Guyton AC, Hall JE, eds. Textbook of Medical Physiology, 10th ed. WB Saunders, 2000; Pp 210–222.

Guyton AC, Hall JE. Heart muscle: the heart as a pump. In: Guyton AC, Hall JE, eds. Textbook of Medical Physiology, 10th ed. WB Saunders, 2000; Pp 96–106.

Guyton AC, Hall JE. Local control of blood flow by the tissues, and humoral regulation. In: Guyton AC, Hall JE, eds. Textbook of Medical Physiology, 10th ed. WB Saunders, 2000; Pp 175–183.

Hirschl RB, Heiss KF, Cardiopulmonary critical care and shock. In: Oldham KT, Colombani PM, Foglia RP, Skinner M, eds. Principles and Practice of Pediatric Surgery. Lippincott Williams & Wilkins, 2005; Pp 139–178.

Holtz J, Peripheral circulation: fundamental concepts, comparative aspects of control in specific sections and lymph flow. In: Gregor R, Windhorst U, eds. Comprehensive Human Physiology, from Cellular Mechanisms to Integration. Springer-Verlag, 1996, Pp 1865–1915.

Nichols DG, Yaster M, Lappe DG, Buck JR, eds. Golden Hour: The Handbook of Advanced Pediatric Life Support. Mosby-Year Book, 1991.

Ross J, Cardiovascular system. In: West JB, ed. Best and Taylor's Physiological Basis of Medical Practice, 11th ed. Williams and Wilkins, 1985, Pp 108–332.

Teasell RW, Arnold JM, et al. Cardiovascular consequences of loss of supraspinal control of the sympathetic nervous system after spinal cord injury. Arch Phys Med Rehabil 2000; 81:506–516.

CHAPTER 5
FLUIDS AND ELECTROLYTE THERAPY IN THE PAEDIATRIC SURGICAL PATIENT

Mark W. Newton

Berouz Banieghbal

Kokila Lakhoo

Introduction

Perioperative fluid and electrolyte management for infants and children can be confusing due the numerous opinions, formulas, and clinical applications, which can result in a picture that is not practical and often misleading. The basic principles of fluid and electrolyte management are similar in the neonate and the paediatric patient if one considers the exceptions, which include renal maturity, body composition, physiological losses, delivery issues, and autonomic nervous system differences. Understanding the ability of the neonate and older paediatric patient to compensate for fluid and electrolyte alterations due to the surgical pathology is addressed here after an overview of normal fluid and electrolyte metabolism.

Perioperative fluid and electrolyte management addresses dehydration, fasting status, intraoperative fluid management, postoperative issues, and transfusion therapy. When practicing in a resource-limited medical practice setting, one needs to be able to manage extremes of fluid and electrolyte issues with less laboratory and investigative infrastructure in patients who may have delayed presentation after their surgical pathology presented itself. The physician who cares for the surgical needs of the neonate and paediatric patient population must be keenly aware of the perioperative needs regarding fluid and electrolyte metabolism requirements. This understanding will increase the goal of a successful and safe surgical course for both the paediatric patient and the patient's parents.

Renal Function

Physiology of the Newborn

The neonatal renal function is not at adult levels until after the age of 1–2 years due to many factors. The renal blood flow (RBF) reaches adult levels (20% of cardiac output (CO)) around the age of 2 years, whereas the glomerular filtration rate (GFR) shows the effects of increasing in size,

not number, of the glomeruli after the age of 1 year (Table 5.1). Although the neonate is able to cope with routine fluid and electrolyte requirements, it is during times of dehydration, acidosis, trauma, excessive fluid, and solute load that the neonate demonstrates immaturity in renal function. This immaturity in renal function is even more evident in patients who are less than 34 weeks gestational age at birth; studies demonstrate that when a newborn is between 25 and 28 weeks gestational age, it takes 8 weeks for their GFR to reach that of term infants.[1]

The term and preterm neonate will not have a complete diuretic response to a water load until after 5 days of age, and the preterm will have an even slower response when compared to an adult response. Newborns may have an altered ability to concentrate urine, tend to have lower thresholds for glucose excretion, have unnecessary excretions of sodium, and have poor tolerances for fluid loads, all of which are amplified in the preterm infant. By 1 month of age, the full-term infant's kidney is about 70–80% mature in comparison to that of a healthy adult patient. One of the primary homeostatic functions of the kidney is to maintain proper sodium levels in the body.

Term infants in nonphysiological stressful situations can maintain normal sodium levels, but preterm infants less than 32 weeks gestational age would be considered "salt losers". Their ability to conserve sodium is even further altered by hyperbilirubinaemia, hypoxia, and increased intraperitoneal pressure, which may decrease RBF and thus produce a state of hyponatraemia. In the desire to replace the sodium that may be lost in the gastric, due to intestinal obstructional loss, or by diarrhoea, the physician may give the neonate an excessive load of sodium, which may override the tubular functions of the immature renal system and even produce a state of hypernatraemia. Complications, including reopening of the ductus arteriosus and cerebral bleed, can be caused by hypertonicity due to the elevated sodium load.

Table 5.1: Glomerular filtration rate.

	GFR by postnatal age (mean ± SD)		
Gestational age	1 week	2–8 weeks	>8 weeks
Normal GFR (ml/min/1.73 m²)	11.0 ± 5.4[a]	15.5 ± 6.2[a]	47.4 ± 21.5[a,b]
25–28 weeks	10	26	9
No. of subjects	6	9	26
Mean – 1 SD[c]	15.3 ± 5.6[a]	28.7 ± 13.8[a,b]	51.4
29–34 weeks	27	27	1
No. of subjects	10	15	
Mean – 1 SD	40.6 ± 14.8	65.8 ± 24.8[b]	95.7 ± 21.7[b]
38–42 weeks	26	20	28
No. of subjects			
Absolute GFR (ml/min)	0.64 ± 0.33[a]	0.88 ± 0.42[a]	5.90 ± 5.92[a]
25–28 weeks	1.22 ± 0.45[a]	2.43 ± 1.27[a,b]	10.83
29–34 weeks	5.32 ± 1.99	11.15 ± 5.21[b]	20.95 ± 6.40[b]
38–42 weeks			

[a] Significantly less than corresponding value in full-term infants.
[b] Significant increase compared with previous age group.
[c] Mean – 1 SD represents lower cutoff value.

Table 5.2: Clinical significance of newborns' physiological presentations.

Physiology	Clinical significance

Low glomerular filtration due to
    Low perfusion pressure
    High renal vascular resistance
	Poor tolerance volume load
	Poor tolerance sodium level

Only juxtamedullary glomeruli are functional
    Fewer and smaller glomeruli
    Smaller glomerular pore size	

Diminished proximal tubular function
    Low blood flow to juxtamedullary nephron tubules
    Less tubular mass per nephron
    Glomerular-tubular imbalance
	Tendency to excrete filtered sodium
	Low threshold for glucose excretion

Diminished proximal tubular function
    Low blood flow to juxtamedullary nephron tubules
    Less tubular mass per nephron
    Glomerular-tubular imbalance
	Inability to concentrate urine

Potassium balance in the preterm infant can be an issue if the excretion of potassium and the extracellular movement of potassium occur after acidosis. This situation can easily be seen in many situations that would prompt the need for surgical intervention, especially if the presentation to a health care facility is delayed. Usually the newborn can manage with a potassium level of approximately 6 mmol/l, and the technique of taking the blood sample needs to be determined due the common occurrence of haemolysed blood cells and a falsely elevated potassium level.

Additional factors that may influence the renal function include maternal oligohydramnios, maternal drug use (indomethacin), polycystic disease in the family, and some forms of urinary obstruction. Any situation whereby the infant has hypoxia, hypotension, or haemorrhage may lead to a decreased RBF and a subsequent drop in the normal urine output. All of these factors point toward the reminder that infants (especially preterm) must have their fluid status closely monitored so that homeostasis is maintained, or approached, in the circumstance surrounding the need for surgical intervention. The lack of urine pH monitoring and more extensive laboratory testing abilities should not determine the impact that a detailed history and basic renal function monitoring can have on the improvement of surgical outcome, which involves renal function immaturity.

Table 5.2 presents the clinical significance of newborns' physiological presentations.

Clinical Evaluation of Renal Function

The physical characteristics of the newborn may give the examiner a clue as to a possible renal dysfunction. Low-set ears, flattened nose, and VATER (Vertebrae, Anus, Trachea, Esophagus, and Renal) or VACTERAL (Vertebral and spinal cord, Anorectal, Cardiac, TracheoEsophageal, Renal and other urinary tract, Limb) syndrome may heighten the suspicion of renal function issues. The occurrence of an elevated systolic blood pressure, or systolic blood pressure greater than 90 mm Hg in the term infant, may indicate renal insufficiency, but usually these findings are associated not with renal problems but with other issues such as pain or hunger. An accurate measurement of blood pressure is sometimes difficult, but equally necessary, so that the more subtle findings can be helpful in the diagnosis of renal disease.

The absence of abdominal wall musculature can indicate prune belly syndrome, and the evidence of one umbilical artery connecting to the placenta correlates with an increased incidence of cardiac and renal malformations. The examination of the placenta is an easy task that could benefit the care of the newborn surgical or nonsurgical patient when renal function is in question. Oedema in the newborn, which is abnormal in the term child, can also indicate renal disease related to an underlying cardiac problem, hypoxia due to respiratory insufficiency, or low albumin levels, among the list of causes that may include renal dysfunction. The infant with liver failure may present with signs of oedema that are unrelated to any renal problems. A history of asphyxia commonly leads to a marked decrease in urine output. Sepsis is the other common cause of acute renal failure in the neonate. A syndrome of inappropriate antidiuretic hormone (ADH) may accompany asphyxia, which may lead to fluid and electrolyte abnormalities. Once hypotension and oxygen needs are addressed, fluids may need to be restricted until diuresis occurs with fluids.

The perioperative patient who arrives late in the progression of a surgical disease may present with signs of severe dehydration, and it often is difficult to get a detailed history regarding urine output in the neonate. The clinical evaluation of the neonate, which would include alertness, skin turgor, anterior fontanelle size or dimensions, heart rate, blood pressure, and presence or lack of urine, would assist in the determination of renal function and fluid status. Routinely, if the urine output history is questionable, the placement of gauze near the urethra opening could be weighed to assist in obtaining the objective information needed to determine urine output preoperatively.

Laboratory Evaluation of Renal Function

Obtaining the serum creatinine level, which is available in most hospital settings, is the simplest method of determining the glomerular function in the infant. Initially, the creatinine and even sodium level in the newborn is a representation of the maternal electrolyte balance and renal function. A number of factors determine newborn creatinine levels such as maternal levels, gestational age, muscle mass, and fluid balance. Increasing creatinine levels over the first few days of life indicates some form of renal dysfunction. If an infant is born at a gestational age of 25–28 weeks, it will take approximately 8 weeks before the GFR, and thus serum creatinine levels, approach the levels of a term infant.[1]

On a clinical note, the use of gentamicin in the perioperative surgical newborn, if the levels of gentamicin are not measured due to resource constraints, can potentially increase the amount of renal dysfunction in this patient population. In a recent study in India, dosing of gentamicin with the following neonate weights was considered safe:[2]

- 10 mg every 48 hours for the neonate weighing less than 2000 grams

- 10 mg every 24 hours in the neonate weighing 2000–2249 grams

- 13.5 mg every 24 hours for the neonate weighing more than 2500 grams

Gentamicin interval errors are the most common drug error reported in a recent neonatal intensive care unit (NICU) study from the United States, and certainly the effect on renal function is amplified in a setting where drug levels cannot be measured.[3] Gentamicin and ampicillin are the two most commonly prescribed antibiotics in the NICU environment, and inappropriate dosing can cause clinically significant renal damage.

Sodium excretion, which is directly correlated to GFR and indirectly to gestational age, becomes an issue in situations where there is sodium load or the need to retain sodium arises. The kidney's ability to retain sodium in preterm infants will not reach the term infant's level until they reach the gestational age of a term infant. Clinically, this can produce situations of appropriate release of ADH and reabsorption of water in a setting where the patient is getting a volume of hypotonic fluid, such as 0.25% saline in 5% dextrose. If the sodium level goes below 120 mEq/l, then the patient could show signs of neurologic injury, which can be nonreversible.

A urinalysis that shows colour (concentration, presence of bilirubin), red blood cells, white blood cells, protein, and glucose can help to diagnose some renal problems. The observation of protein in the urine can be normal in the first few days of life and then can become expected in cases of hypoxia, congenital cardiac problems, and dehydration. Small amounts of glycosuria can be detected secondary to a low tubular reabsorption with a glucose load, and the glucose load can even result in an osmotic diuresis and dehydration. Glucose in the urine may be an early sign of sepsis, especially in the presence of other factors.

Normal Fluid and Electrolyte Metabolism

Total Body Water

At birth, the infant is suddenly separated from the source of water found in the in utero environment, and now is in an environment with significant water loss from the skin and respiratory tract, thus promoting a potential for early dehydration. During this period of transition, water intake and renal conservation of fluids needs to maintain a homeostatic state to survive.

Total body water compromises intracellular water (ICW) and extracellular water (ECW), with the ECW having an intravascular and interstitial component. With advancing gestational age, the amount of total body water declines from 94% of body weight in the third trimester to approximately 78% at term. In the immediate postnatal period, the amount of extracellular fluid decreases and the percentage of intracellular fluid increases, although the newborn has a large interstitial reserve volume during times of decreased fluid intake. The term infant can compensate more than the preterm infant, but newborns with a large surface-to-weight ratio, higher total water content, limited renal ability to concentrate, greater insensible water loss from thin skin, and high blood flow all can become clinically dehydrated in a very short period of time. The added water loss associated with radiant warmers, which are commonly found in the treatment of the newborn and especially preterm infants, can result in a rapid and progressive level of dehydration without close observation and appropriate fluid

intake adjustments.[1]

Fluid Requirements

Fluid requirements in the newborn or older child depend upon multiple factors, but the majority are determined by the insensible water loss and the newborn's metabolic rate. The evaporation of water from the skin and the respiratory tract has environmental factors, such as air and incubator temperature, humidity, and air flow across the child's body, as well as infant factors, such as patient position, metabolic rate, and elevation in temperature.

Many studies have indicated that water loss from the premature infant is significantly greater than from the term infant, possibly due to decreased subcutaneous fat and increased permeability through the skin. The combination of increased water loss in the premature infant and the use of radiant warmers without humidity, which occurs in many settings, can result in a severely dehydrated premature infant who may need resuscitation. The insensible water loss can increase 50–200% with the use of radiant warmers in the preterm infant. This can have an significant impact on the intraoperative course, as the patient may arrive in the operating theatre dehydrated even though receiving maintenance fluids in the immediate preoperative period. The low-tech approach to humidity can be achieved merely by keeping an open container of water near the newborn while under warming lights. Fluid chambers need to be cleaned and changed routinely in an effort to decrease infection in the nursery unit, and the fluid level of radiant warmers, which may vary depending upon the manufacturer, needs to be monitored.

Many formulas exist to determine the maintenance fluid levels for the neonate or small child. The formula of the "4-2-1 rule" works well for determining the maintenance fluids for weight groups that are less than 30 kg. In this formula, the first 10 kg of body weight is multiplied by 4 ml/hr; the second 10 kg is multiplied by 2 ml/hr; and any additional kilograms of weight are multiplied by 1 ml/hr.[4] Table 5.3 provides examples that apply to newborns and older children to determine maintenance fluids. Intraoperative fluid management is discussed in a later section of this chapter that describes translocated fluid and blood loss. Typically, if one has a 1-ml blood loss, then this 1 ml is replaced by 3 ml of crystalloid, which could be normal saline or Ringer's lactate solution. This amount of replacement allows for the intravascular volume to be maintained, even during times of decreasing intravascular volume, which could be surgery.

Table 5.3: Sample 4-2-1 rule for maintenance fluids for newborns and older children.

Child's body weight	Volume
9 kg	$4 \times 9 = 36$
	$2 \times 0 = 0$
	$1 \times 0 = \underline{0}$
	36 cc/hr
15 kg	$4 \times 10 = 40$
	$2 \times 5 = 10$
	$1 \times 0 = \underline{0}$
	50 cc/hr
26 kg	$4 \times 10 = 40$
	$2 \times 10 = 20$
	$1 \times 6 = \underline{6}$
	66 cc/hr

Table 5.4: Signs and symptoms of dehydration.

Percent of body weight	Signs and symptoms of dehydration
1–5% (mild)	• History of 12–24 hours of vomiting and diarrhoea • Dry mouth • Decreased urination
6–10% (moderate)	• Tenting skin • Sunken eyes, fontanelle • Oliguria • Lethargy
11–15% (severe)	• Cardiovascular instability: mottling, hypotension, tachycardia • Anuria • Sensorium change
20%	• Coma • Shock

Glucose Requirements

Carbohydrate reserves are relatively low in the newborn and certainly will drop to low levels during the prolonged labour course often seen in some areas of Africa. Thirty percent of the glucose reserves are stored as glycogen in the liver, but this cushion is less evident in the low-birth-weight or preterm infant. Within the first four hours of life, the newborn must be given some form of glucose. With prematurity and a gestational age of less than 34 weeks, the ability to swallow is low, so the patient may need an intravenous (IV) line or a feeding tube. Adequate and frequent measurement of the glucose levels of the newborn, especially the newborn pending surgery, is cost effective and will help manage the hypoglycaemia and hyperglycaemia episodes that may harm the infant.

Children who are small for gestational age (SGA), have chronic illnesses, had a prolonged NPO (nothing by mouth) period, premature infants, and infants of diabetic mothers are all at risk for hypoglycaemia during their hospital course. In SGA infants, hypoglycaemia usually occurs 24–72 hours after birth, when the glycogen stores are depleted and the breast milk production may not yet meet demand. In Kenya, we use D 10 (80 ml) mixed with normal saline (NS; 20 ml) in a buretrol of 100 ml and then begin our maintenance fluids and monitor blood glucose levels. The 60 drops per ml buretrols allow us to give the appropriate volume of fluids, which will prevent volume overload (never place more than the volume for 4 hours of maintenance fluids in the buretrol) while adapting the amounts of dextrose and normal saline based upon basic lab values.

Glucose level instability is commonly seen in those patients who are septic or have had a period of hypotension or asphyxia. These patients need close monitoring every hour in the operating theatre to adjust glucose levels; they all need glucose in their operative fluids to prevent the severe complications associated with hypoglycaemia. Intraoperative glucose administration is controversial but, in general, 5% dextrose is adequate because the metabolic stress response to surgery will avoid the patient becoming hypoglycaemic. Neurosurgical cases need very close glucose control due to cerebral ischaemia issues and hyperglycaemia.

Perioperative Fluid and Electrolyte Management

Dehydration

The severity of dehydration should be estimated based upon the history and clinical findings. There are no unique lab values that can accurately determine the severity of dehydration, but certainly an experienced medical care provider becomes adept at the estimation of dehydration in the paediatric population. Oliguria, lethargy, and cardiovascular instability are all symptoms commonly seen when a paediatric patient has severe dehydration.[4] Some common surgical paediatric issues that can cause severe dehydration include bowel obstruction, acute burns, intestinal perforation, myelomeningocele (open), and trauma. Table 5.4 presents signs and symptoms of dehydration by percentage of body weight.[5]

The compensatory mechanisms for dehydration that are seen in the adult population are less well defined in the term infant and even less so in the preterm infant. The body's primary mechanism for compensation is the renin-angiotensin-aldosterone system, which attempts to absorb sodium and water. Renin is released from the kidneys, which then prompts the release of aldosterone and ADH, which then allows for the water and sodium to be reabsorbed. The newborn is able to allocate some of the extracellular fluid to the plasma volume, but this compensation is limited and will result in the loss of skin turgor. The newborn's cardiac output is determined by the heart rate because the intrinsic heart muscle is noncompliant, therefore making the adjustment in preload volume very difficult. If a patient arrives in a state of severe dehydration and shock, then the infusion of 20–30 ml/kg of normal saline must be started while others monitor for the improvement in fluid status. Urine output and concentration (appearance) will be the most accurate and cost-effective measurements that will allow for the monitoring of the overall fluid status. The placement of an intraossaeous line is now preferred if a peripheral intravenous line cannot be placed quickly during the resuscitation time in a severely dehydrated child. Studies have shown that normal saline is as good a volume resuscitator as any fluid available (Table 5.5), and it certainly is cost effective; therefore, there is no need to use the more expensive colloids during fluid resuscitation.

NPO Period in the Paediatric Population

There has been considerable debate about NPO status in children, and NPO guidelines have undergone adjustment. At this time, we no longer use the former prolonged times that once produced surgical patients who were relatively volume depleted upon the start of surgery. It has been shown that clear liquids given 3 hours before surgery results in a lower gastric volume and no change in gastric acidity. A clear liquid is one that has no particulate matter, which means that you can see through the fluid if held up to the light without obstruction.

Infants who are on formula need 6 hours, and breast-feeding infants need 4 hours, at our institution in Kenya, but at some hospitals this would be considered a "clear" liquid and only 3 hours are required for NPO. These modifications have allowed for situations in which the children's veins are more distended and, hopefully, children and parents who are happier during the preoperative period. The type of surgery and reason for the surgical intervention will also dictate the ability to take fluids by mouth. Many neonates who need emergency surgery have never been on any fluids, and NPO is not an issue, but if the patient has a bowel obstruction, for example, then the need for a rapid sequence induction (anaesthesia) may override any NPO concerns.

Intraoperative Fluids

The calculation of intraoperative fluid requirements can be allocated into the following sections: maintenance fluids, preoperative fluid deficit, insensible losses, and estimated blood loss (Table 5.6). Maintenance fluids per hour required based upon a patient's weight was discussed earlier; typically, normal saline or Ringer's lactate are the fluids of choice, as they most closely represent the plasma components. The preoperative deficit will be the patient's weight in kilograms multiplied by the number of hours without any fluids. The insensible losses depend upon many factors, but primarily will be based upon the size of the incision and whether exposure of the bowel or viscus is involved, as this will increase fluid loss (see Table 5.6). The estimated blood loss needs to be replaced as well, with a ratio of 3 ml of normal saline for every 1 ml of blood loss.

Table 5.5: Composition of intravenous crystalloid solutions.

Solution	Glucose (g/l)	Na⁺ (mEq/l)	K⁺ (mEq/l)	Cl⁻ (mEq/l)	Lactate (mEq/l)	Ca⁺² (mEq/l)	pH	Osm
5% dextrose	50	–	–	–	–	–	4.5	253
Ringer's	–	147	4	155	–	4	6.0	309
Lactated Ringer's	–	130	4	109	28	3	6.3	273
D₅ lactated Ringer's	50	130	4	109	28	3	4.9	525
D₅ 0.22% NSS*	50	38.5	–	38.5	–	–	4.4	330
D₅ 0.45% NSS*	50	77	–	77	–	–	4.4	407
0.9% NSS*	–	154	–	154	–	–	5.6	308

Note: NSS = normal saline solution

Table 5.6: Intraoperative fluid requirements.

1. Estimated fluid requirement (EFR) per hour (maintenance fluids)	0–10 kg = 4 ml/kg/hr + 10–20 kg = 2 ml/kg/hr + >20 kg = 1 ml/kg/hr (e.g., 23-kg child = 40 ml + 20 ml + 3 ml, so EFR= 63 ml/hr)
2. Estimated preoperative fluid deficit (EFD)	EFD = Number of hours NPO × weight (in kg) (e.g., 23-kg child NPO for 8 hours EFD = 8 × 23 = 184 ml) 1st hour = ½ EFD + EFR 2nd hour = ¼ EFD + EFR 3rd hour = ¼ EFD + EFR
3. Insensible losses (IL): (add EFR and EFD)	Minimal incision = 3–5 ml/kg/hr Moderate incision with viscus exposure = 5–10 ml/kg/hr Large incision with bowel exposure = 8–20 ml/kg/hr
4. Estimated blood loss	Replace maximum allowable blood loss (ABL) with crystalloid 3:1

The estimated blood loss is extremely difficult to determine in the newborn surgical patient, and the anaesthesia care provider needs to calculate the estimated blood volume and allowable blood loss for every patient before surgery. The surgery team must closely monitor blood loss and, with sponge observation, determine the blood loss at many points during the surgical procedure. Invasive monitoring, even in large surgical procedures, is rare in most areas of Africa, so the use of noninvasive blood pressure, urine output, elevations in heart rate, and capillary perfusion need to provide clues to the overall fluid status of the patient during a surgical procedure. If a pulse oximeter is available, then the waveform changes can help with the perfusion pulse pressure, which may indicate a change in blood volume, cardiac output, or temperature.

If the blood loss is above the allowable blood loss based upon the starting haemoglobin, then fresh whole blood is the most commonly transfused component in Africa. The development of a "walking blood bank" should be an aspect of each hospital involved in operative procedures. This would entail a group of donors known by the hospital lab who can donate blood for emergencies; the opportunity to use warm, fresh (nonstored) blood in the paediatric surgical patient can be life-saving. The inability to adequately warm stored blood is always an issue when a neonate is requiring blood in surgery. If stored (cold) blood is required, a warm bath of water with the tubing within the bath is often useful to help warm the fluids. Hypothermia in a paediatric patient can result in slow awakening and, in the extreme case, cardiac arrhythmias. The use of the buretrol and a three-way stopcock is the most useful manner to give blood in a newborn or very small paediatric patient. A 10- or 20-ml syringe is applied to the stopcock, and the exact amount of blood or volume of other fluid can be given, with this amount accurately recorded. Blood products should be initially given in 10 ml/kg increments and as needed based upon heart rate and blood pressure; more should be added to maintain a normal intravascular blood volume.

The estimated blood volume in the paediatric patient is as follows:

Premature infant	90–100ml/kg
Full-term infant	80–90 ml/kg
3 months–1 year	75–80 ml/kg
>1 year	70–75 ml/kg

Complications that can occur in the surgical neonate or paediatric patient in regard to fluids and electrolytes intraoperatively include fluid overload and pulmonary oedema; hypocalcaemia with large amounts of blood transfusions; elevated potassium levels; hypothermia due to the infusion of cold fluids; hypotension secondary to hypovolaemia; and low sodium levels if D 10 is infused without the addition of any electrolytes. It should be noted that at any sign of bradycardia in the surgical neonate, one must first verify the condition of the respiratory system because bradycardia is one of the first signs of poor oxygenation. Principles for therapy for fluid overload in the paediatric patient include fluid restriction, salt restriction, diuresis or even dialysis, and albumin that is salt poor to help with the fluid status.[4]

Postoperative Fluid Management

In the neonate, postoperative hypothermia is frequently an issue that will affect the recovery time as well as the ability to use fluids that are not warm because this may further decrease the body temperature. *A clinical note:* The cold betadine that is used for surgical procedures can prompt hypothermia because the patient can be soaking in the fluid left over from the initial prep during the length of the procedure. If this sterilisation agent is not removed from the skin of a newborn after the surgery, the patient can develop a chemical burn that can add to the patient's perioperative morbidity.

Electrolytes, glucose, and haemoglobin levels, as well as the documentation of good urine output should be determined within the first few hours after surgery. The normal urine output of >0.5 ml/kg/hr should be measured to help guide the fluid status; at times, a small feeding tube placed in the bladder may be the only method available to measure urine output accurately. The immaturity of the renal system needs to be considered with the intraoperative fluid shifts, which may not promote a diuresis, as expected in older patients. The use of radiant warmers will help with the hypothermia but also add to insensible fluid losses; therefore, removal of these warmers will need to be considered once the temperature returns to a more normal level.

Nausea and vomiting can be seen in the paediatric postoperative patient, but usually this is not an issue in a newborn. Third spacing from the surgical procedure (i.e., loss of fluid from an open abdomen during surgery) is an ongoing issue in the immediate postoperative period, which may influence the overall fluid replacement in this period. The opportunity for the newborn to resume breast milk intake will be dictated by the surgical procedure and the surgeon's preference. Successful surgery in the newborn period is one in which the patient is reunited with the parents so that normal bonding can resume and the patient can quickly return to the family home or village.

Summary of Fluid and Electrolyte Balance

Fluid Balance
- Normal maintenance fluid: Ringer's lactate at rates shown in Table 5.3.
- Resuscitation fluid: 20–30ml/kg bolus using normal saline.
- Preoperative dehydration caused by: vomiting, bowel obstruction, overheating, acute burns, intestinal perforation, myelomeningocele (open), open wounds, abdominal wall defects, and trauma.
- Overhydration: may be iatrogenic.
- Fluid imbalance assessment: see Table 5.6.

Sodium Balance
- Normal sodium requirement: 2–4 mmol/kg per day.
- Normal serum sodium: 135–140 mmol/l.
- Causes of hyponatraemia: iatrogenic with hypotonic solutions, laboratory error, polyuric renal failure, diuretic treatment, congestive cardiac failure, Addison's disease, and maternal hyponatraemia.
- Signs of hyponatraemia: failure to thrive, seizures, and cerebral oedema.
- Causes of hypernatraemia: iatrogenic infusion, laboratory error, dehydration, and maternal hypernatraemia.
- Signs of hypernatraemia: dehydration and seizures.
- Treatment of sodium imbalance: by appropriate usage and adjustment of fluid therapy.

Potassium Balance
- An intracellular ion with a normal requirement of 1–3 mmol/kg per day.
- Normal serum potassium: 3.5–5.5 mml/l.

Hyperkalaemia
- Causes: bruising, haemolysis, renal failure, hypoglycaemia, tissue hypoxia and poor peripheral perfusion, haemolysed blood sample, and inappropriate potassium supplementation.
- Exacerbating factors: hypocalcaemia, hyponatraimia, and acidosis.
- Treatment required for serum potassium levels >7.0 mmol/l:
  - 7.0–8.0 mmol/l without ECG changes: remove potassium source and give calcium resonium 0.5–1 g/kg in divided doses per rectum or orally.
  - >8.0 mmol/l and/or ECG changes (depressed P waves, peaked T waves, wide QRS complexes): emergency treatment required.
  - Emergency treatment for hyperkalaemia:
    1. Remove source of potassium.
    2. 10% calcium gluconate: 1.0 ml/kg IV (dilute 50:50, give over at least 2 minutes). This has a transient effect on electrocardiogram (ECG), not on K+ concentration.
    3. Salbutamol: 4 µg/kg over 10 minutes.
    4. $NaHCO_3$: can be tried, especially if acidotic. Dose is 2 mmol/kg (= 4 ml/kg 4.2% NaHCO3) at 1–2 mmol per minute.
    5. Glucose: 0.5 g/kg per dose: 5 ml/kg of 10% dextrose or 2 ml/kg of 25% dextrose or 1 ml/kg of 50% dextrose, over 15–30 minutes.
    6. Insulin: 0.2 unit per gram of glucose, 1.0 unit/kg insulin with 4ml/kg 25% dextrose over 30 minutes.

Hypokalaemia
- Serum potassium: <3.0 mmol/l.
- Causes: inadequate intake, intestinal obstruction, vomiting, diarrhoea, diuretics, polyuric renal failure, and alkalosis.
- Presentation: cardiac arrythmias, paralytic ileus, urinary retention, and respiratory distress.
- Treatment: by supplementation.

Acid–Base Balance
- Normal: pH is 7.4 and bicarbonate is 25 mmol/l.
- Metabolic acidosis causes: asphyxia, tissue ischaemia, acute renal failure, diarrhoea, dehydration, and stoma losses. Treat cause and bicarbonate infusion is rarely used.
- Metabolic alkalosis causes: vomiting, pyloric stenosis, and upper gastrointestinal obstruction. Correction by fluid, sodium, and potassium replacement.

Glucose Balance
- Normal serum levels: 2.5–7.0 mmol/l.
- Hypoglycaemia: <2–2.5 mmol/l.
- Hypoglycaemia presents with: apnoea, lethargy, seizures, and coma.
- Hypoglycaemia is caused by: poor intake, vomiting, hypothermia, sepsis, and Beckwith-Wiedemann syndrome associated with exomphalos.
- Hypoglycaemia treatment includes: feeding or bolus of 10% dextrose by intravenous infusion (IVI).
- Hyperglycaemia: >14mmol/l.
- Hyperglycaemia is caused by: excess infusion, and should be lowered with less concentrated dextrose solution (5%).

Calcium Balance

- Normal serum values: 2.5 mmol/l.

- Hypocalcaemia may present with: seizures, jitters, and ECG changes of long Q-T interval.

- Treatment includes: calcium supplement orally or calcium gluconate infusion.

Evidence-Based Research

Table 5.7 comments on a paper on the maintenance need for water in parenteral fluid therapy.

Table 5.7: Evidence-based research.

Title	The maintenance need for water in parenteral fluid therapy.
Authors	Holliday MA, Segar WE
Institution	Department of Pediatrics, University of California, San Francisco, California, USA
Reference	Pediatrics 1957; 19:823–832
Problem	Fluid and electrolytes in children.
Historical significance/ comments	Classic paper describing the use of intravenous fluids in the paediatric population involving the perioperative setting to some degree.

Key Summary Points

1. Fluid management in the paediatric surgical population can be a real challenge, especially in the preterm infant with an immature physiological state.

2. With the small circulating blood volume in the paediatric patient, fluid management is a critical aspect of each patient who presents for surgery, and vigilance is critical.

3. Many paediatric patients who present for surgery in Africa have a delayed presentation and need a normal saline (NS) fluid bolus with glucose measurement prior to the onset of surgery.

4. Bowel obstruction in the paediatric patient commonly presents with metabolic acidosis due to delayed presentation.

5. A surgeon preparing the paediatric patient for surgery must determine whether sodium or potassium levels are abnormal and attempt correction prior to surgical management because these abnormalities are much more common than in the adult population.

6. Fluid overload in the paediatric surgical patient is not uncommon, and strict observation of maintenance and third space fluids are essential to avoid this problem.

References

1. Gregory GA, ed. Pediatric Anesthesia, 2nd ed. Churchill Livingstone, 1989.

2. Darmstadt GL. Determination of extended-interval gentamicin dosing for neonatal patients in developing countries. Pediatr Infect Disease J, 2007; 26(6):502–507.

3. Stavroudis TA, Miller MR, Lehmann CU. Medication errors in neonates. Clinics in Perinatology 2008; 35(1):141–161.

4. Cote C, Lerman J, Todres I, eds. A Practice of Anesthesia for Infants and Children, 4th ed. Saunders, 2008.

5. Graef J. Manual of Pediatric Therapeutics, 6th ed. Lippincott-Raven, 1997.

CHAPTER 6
NUTRITIONAL SUPPORT

Afua A.J. Hesse

Jane P. Balint

Introduction

Nutritional support is indicated in paediatric surgical patients for a variety of reasons. Invariably, it is indicated for patients who, for one reason or another, are unable to get enough calories to meet the requirements for daily function and to maintain lean body mass. Preoperatively, most of our patients in Ghana are frankly malnourished or very close to this, which has implications for postoperative outcomes, resulting in varying degrees of poor wound healing. A 2006 World Bank report on nutrition suggests that 24% of children in Africa are underweight and 35% are stunted.[1] This situation puts those children who then go on to develop problems requiring surgery at a distinct disadvantage in relation to their peers in developed countries. Surgical site infections of varying degrees or wound dehiscence are common manifestations of this poor nutrition.

Patients undergoing surgery who are at risk for long periods of ileus postoperatively will require careful planning for nutritional support. Patients with high metabolic requirements postoperatively will also require nutritional support. If surgery is elective, it is better to improve on nutritional status preoperatively. This is the best opportunity to maximise postoperative outcomes. If surgery is emergent, then supplemental nutrition should be offered as soon as possible following surgery. Oral and enteral feeding is always preferred, offering fewer complications than parenteral nutrition. In our environment, and for most centres, full parenteral nutrition is not always available, and other options must be explored.

Nutritional Support Needs

Preoperatively, oral and enteral feeding are the best ways to provide needed calories. The advantages of oral and enteral feeding include promoting the natural flora of the intestine, maintaining the integrity of the intestinal mucosa, and preventing the translocation of bacteria from the gut.[2] These feedings can promote immune function. If the intestinal tract is functional, a large amount of calories can be given by the oral or enteral route. Evidence shows that adequate nutrition can be provided, even to patients with short gut who have only 2 feet of viable bowel, in the absence of parenteral nutrition, by overnight tube feeding with a slow infusion, which also serves to correct fluid and electrolyte imbalance.[3,4] In addition to resulting in fewer complications, enteral feeding is also lower in cost than parenteral feeding.[5]

Generally, in the first year of life, caloric requirements are estimated at 90–150 kcal/kg, gradually decreasing to 40–60 kcal/kg by adolescence.

The Institute of Medicine (IOM) recommendations for children in the United States are shown in Table 6.1. There are no comparative figures currently available for African children.

If parenteral nutrition is necessary, the general guidelines for the distribution of calories (although these are fairly broad) are specifically: not more than 50% of the calories as fat (usually 20–40%), 40–60% of the calories as carbohydrate (specifically dextrose), and 10–20% of the calories as protein. Protein requirements vary by age, as seen in Table 6.2.

The daily trace metals requirements for children are given in Table 6.3.[6] In addition, selenium at 2 µg/kg per day and vitamins should be added to the parenteral nutrition. Fluid and electrolyte needs will vary with the patient's underlying condition and losses, and will need to be monitored for adequacy of supplementation. Routine fluid requirements in children are given in Table 6.4.

Table 6.1: Caloric recommendations for children.

Age	Caloric recommendations
2–3 years	1000–1400 calories
4–8 years	1400–1600 calories
9–13 years	girls: 1600–2000 calories boys: 1800–2200 calories
14–18 years	girls: 2000 calories boys: 2200–2400 calories

Table 6.2: Protein requirements.

Age	Protein requirement
Low birth weight neonate	3.5–4 gm/kg per day
Infant	2.5 gm/kg per day
2- to 13-year-old child	1.5–2 gm/kg per day
Adolescents	1–1.5 gm/kg per day

Table 6.3: Trace minerals requirements.

Trace mineral	Recommended requirements
Zinc	100 µg/kg*
Copper	20 µg/kg
Chromium	0.14–0.2 µg/kg
Manganese	2–10 µg/kg

*There may be increased needs with diarrhoea or losses via an ostomy.
Source: Adapted from Skipper A. Dietitian's Handbook of Enteral and Parenteral Nutrition, 2nd ed. Aspen Publishers, 1998, Pp 80–108.

Table 6.4: Fluid guidelines.

Weight of patient	Basic amount	Additions
<10 kg	100 ml/kg per 24 hours	
11–20 kg	1,000ml	50 ml/kg for each kg >10 kg per 24 hours
21–40 kg	1,500ml	20 ml for each kg >20 kg per 24 hours
>40 kg	1,500ml/m2 per 24 hours	

Source: Adapted from Kerner JA. Manual of Pediatric Nutrition. John Wiley & Sons, 1983.

Pathophysiology of Malnutrition

Paediatric surgical patients who require nutritional support include those who normally would fall within the 50th centile on their weight charts but who, for one reason or another, have not been able to feed orally for more than 5 days; those who, as a result of their surgical problems, have a poor absorptive capacity; those who have high nutrient losses, such as would occur with small bowel enterostomies and

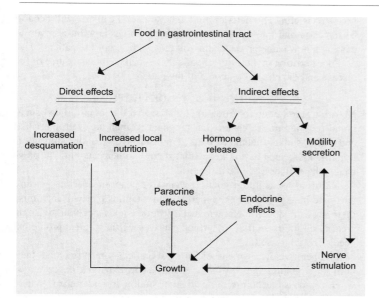

Source: Courtesy of European Society for Clinical Nutrition and Metabolism (ESPEN), Guidelines on Enteral Nutrition.

Figure 6.1: Normal intestinal function.

fistulas; and those with surgical conditions that result in an increase in nutritional needs from increased catabolism, such as occurs in burns and conditions of prolonged sepsis (e.g., peritonitis due to bowel perforation in complicated enteric fever).[7]

Food in the intestinal tract has both direct and indirect beneficial effects, as indicated in Figure 6.1.

Prolonged chronic illnesses that result in overall reduction in total caloric intake will result in poor nutritional state. In addition, any condition in which there is injury to the intestinal mucosa or reduction in total absorptive surface area of the bowel, either from local or systemic disease or any condition in which there is a reduction in overall length of bowel, may result in quantitative nutritional deficiencies and a need for nutritional support. These conditions include, but are not limited to, the following:

• the neonate with an ileostomy;

• antenatal rupture of exomphalos or gastroschisis;

• extensive intestinal resection with short gut and decreased transit time;

• necrotising enterocolitis;

• intestinal atresia ;

• midgut volvulus where there is extensive mucosal damage;

• massive injury, especially to the gastrointestinal tract, in conflict and various situations of violence, where enteral feeding is not feasible;

• inflammatory bowel disease;

• paediatric burns;

• complicated bowel perforations in enteric fever;

• oesophageal strictures from ingestion of corrosives; and

• achalasia of the cardia.

Clinical Evaluation

History

Generally, most communities in Africa place more value on boys than girls. After birth and until babies are weaned, there is usually no difference in nutritional status between girls and boys if the mother is generally well nourished herself. On weaning, however, gender differences in nutritional status in most communities in Africa are more likely to develop, with the boys being favoured.

A history of nutritional intake will be essential. A detail of the composition of the diet for a typical day will give a good indication of the type of nutritional deficiency that may exist. A history of the source of water may help to identify potential micronutrient deficiencies. If these are found to be present, they should then be added to the diet. Teenage and unmarried mothers are more likely to have undernourished or malnourished children because they generally belong to the lower socioeconomic classes and thus may not be able to obtain adequate food. The specific disease conditions listed in the previous section may be indications for additional nutritional support.

Physical Examination of the Child

Physical examination of the child will help to determine the degree of nutritional deprivation. The traditional parameters to measure include the weight and height, which can be compared with standard age, weight, and height charts, and the triceps skinfold thickness or midarm circumference determination. Among the various indices that help in determining nutritional status in children are anthropometric indicators, specifically weight-for-age, height-for-age, weight-for-height, weight/height index, upper arm anthropometry, and head circumference.[8] For preterm infants, crown-heel length and weight gain are the most sensitive indices of the adequacy of intake of nutrients.[6,8,9]

Investigations

Basic investigations required to confirm the proposed clinical diagnosis will be covered in the relevant chapters of this book. The discussion in this chapter is confined to the diagnosis of nutritional deficiency. The most helpful diagnostic indices of nutritional status are the physical examination findings noted in the preceding section. Laboratory investigations should include serum albumin and protein determination, although there are some limitations to their utility, as they may be normal even with significant malnutrition. They can be low in circumstances of excess losses or decreased synthesis. Before parenteral nutrition is given, it is important to check baseline levels of liver function tests, as well as levels of serum urea, electrolytes, and minerals (specifically, calcium, phosphorus, and magnesium). A chest x-ray will be needed to confirm the adequate placement of the total parenteral nutrition (TPN) catheter tip.

Management of Undernutrition and Malnutrition

Methods of Feeding

Oral feeding

Indirect methods of improving the caloric content of the food being given orally include cup and spoon feeding. Oral supplements may also need to be given. Antiemetics may be given for nausea and vomiting, or agents to help improve gastric emptying can be tried. If all these fail to improve the patient's nutritional status, the next step will be to give enteral feeding. Normally available local foodstuffs can be used if their caloric value can be determined. These can be blended and fed to the patient as needed.

Enteral feeding

Tube feedings can be delivered either as bolus or by slow infusion, depending on the patient's nutritional requirements, the composition of the feed being given in terms of solute load, and the capacity of the child's stomach to accommodate the quantities being fed. Various available commercial preparations can be used. In resource-poor settings, a dietitian can be engaged who will be able to use locally available foodstuffs to prepare high-energy blends to which additional nutrients can be added based on any identified deficiencies. It is important when enteral feedings are being given to ensure that the required amount of energy is actually being delivered.[6,9,10]

Parenteral feeding

Parenteral feeding can be given as an adjunct to other nutrition or as total parenteral nutrition if the period of starvation is prolonged or if enteral feeding is going to be impossible. Administration can be by a peripheral line for those requiring immediate support but whose conditions are expected to improve within 1–2 weeks.[11] Lower dextrose concentrations of no more than 12.5% dextrose should be given through a peripheral vein. A peripheral vein can be used only for short-term infusion and must be checked on a frequent basis and discontinued immediately if there are any signs of thrombophlebitis. A catheter can also be placed through a peripheral vein and then advanced until it is in a central position. The pressure from these catheters correlates well with centrally inserted catheters.[12]

Administration can also be through a centrally placed venous line. It is important to ensure that the tip of the central catheter is adequately placed before the solutions are infused. With centrally placed catheters, it is possible to give higher concentrations of dextrose and thus deliver more calories.

In all cases, nutritional support must include lipid, an energy source (usually dextrose), and amino acids. In environments where not all of these preparations are available, anecdotal experiences suggest some benefit in the use of alternative sources, including aliquots of fresh frozen plasma in the short term for small babies or intravenous preparations of amino acids, which can be administered with dextrose preparations in the short term.

Parameters for Monitoring Nutritional Outcomes

Nutritional outcomes are monitored, including a daily assessment of the overall clinical status of the patient, the state of hydration, and weight change. Ideally, it is also necessary on a daily basis to estimate electrolyte, creatinine, and urea levels; serum glucose levels; and magnesium, phosphorus, and calcium. Once the patient has stabilised, these parameters can be assessed much less frequently.

Postoperative Complications

Complications of Enteral Feeding

Complications with enteral feeding are less common than with parenteral nutrition. Such complications are summarised here. If the feeding contains an excess of electrolytes, these can be absorbed into the circulation, resulting in electrolyte imbalance. The concentration of the feeding or the rate of feeding may not be tolerated, with resultant nausea, abdominal cramps, vomiting, diarrhoea, or—less often—constipation. These are usually managed symptomatically, and often just a dilution of the solution given by introducing water into the mixture or slowing the rate of delivery will resolve the problem over a period of time. Rarely will the feeding have to be discontinued. Pulmonary aspiration may occur if amounts fed are not controlled.[9] This is particularly true if the patient has swallowing problems and therefore cannot protect the airway.

If there is any question about satisfactory placement of the tip of the enteral tube, a simple plain radiograph of the abdomen will be able to confirm the placement of the catheter if it is radio-opaque. If the tube is not radio-opaque, a small amount (5 ml) of contrast can be placed in the catheter prior to the x-ray.

Complications of Parenteral Feeding

Complications of parenteral feeding are numerous and include bacteraemia and septicaemia, air embolus, pneumothorax, hypo- or hyperglycaemia, thrombosis, hyperosmolality, metabolic acidosis, and hyperammonaemia. Other complications include cholestasis, migration of the catheter, and catheter blockage. Each complication has to be managed on its own merits. The metabolic complications, such as hypo- or hyperglycaemia and metabolic acidosis, can be managed by adjusting the parenteral nutrition solution. The most serious complication is sepsis, for which antibiotics are given first and then adjusted based on the organisms identified by blood culture. If the patient continues to have fevers or is clinically deteriorating, the parenteral catheter will need to be removed and the sepsis controlled before consideration is given to placing a new catheter, depending on the condition of the patient.

Poor nutrition in the surgical patient affects the clinical course of the disease and the clinical outcome of the patient.

Prevention of Poor Nutrition

Nutrition starts in utero. Attention must be given to appropriate educational programmes to ensure that pregnant women are well nourished and eating suitably balanced diets. This can involve addressing nutritional taboos, such as the belief that if the mother eats eggs in pregnancy, the delivery will be difficult.

Nutrition for children younger than five years of age must ensure adequate intake of calories, minerals, and vitamins that will maximise their growth. Specific known dietary deficiencies peculiar to some areas (e.g., iodine deficiency, which causes specific surgical problems) need to be addressed.

Preoperative assessment of surgical patients must include their nutritional status, and any deficiencies identified must be corrected wherever possible before surgical intervention is undertaken. Where this is not possible, postoperative management must include special attention to nutritional correction.

Ethical Issues

Traditionally and culturally, food and water are considered basic to the needs of each individual person. The modern practice of delivering nutrition and fluids via enteral and parenteral routes now challenges these values, adding on religious and moral dimensions as well as playing out issues of human rights. This is particularly the case when children have complex congenital abnormalities with poor prognosis. Decisions on starting or stopping feeding by oral, enteral, or parenteral means in most countries in Africa requires physicians to adhere to strict institutional policies, which should be developed for this purpose, as the increasing possibility of legal challenges cannot be ruled out.[13] More complex discussions of specific issues is beyond the scope of this book. Additionally, resource constraints in the region would affect the range of options available to the surgeon and the available modes of administration in terms of equipment availability.

Evidence-Based Research

Tables 6.5 and 6.6 present, respectively, a guideline for nasojejunal tube placement and a review of various feeding issues in preterm babies.

Table 6.5: Evidence-based research.

Title	Naso-jejunal tube placement in paediatric intensive care
Authors	McDermott A, Tomkins N, Lazonby G
Institution	The General Infirmary at Leeds, UK
Reference	Paediatr Nurs 2007; 19(2):26–28
Problem	In critically ill children, intragastric feeding is often poorly tolerated.
Intervention	A guideline for bedside nasojejunal tube (NJT) placement has been developed by a multidisciplinary group.
Comparison/control (quality of evidence)	Audit of the practice was carried out after the implementation of the guidelines. Fifty-eight percent of the children would have definitely or probably started on parenteral nutrition.
Outcome/effect	Reduction in requests for NJT placement under x-ray screening and reduction in the use of medication for the placement.
Historical significance/comments	Improved tolerance of enteral feeding for better nutritional outcomes in intensive care units.

Table 6.6: Evidence-based research.

Title	Feeding issues in preterm infants
Authors	Cooke RJ, Embleton ND
Institution	Ward 35, Leazes Wing, Royal Victoria Infirmary, Newcastle upon Tyne, United Kingdom
Reference	Arch Dis Child Fetal Neonatal Ed 2000; 83:F215–F218
Problem	Ensuring that the nutritional intake of sick preterm infants meets requirements for sustained growth.
Intervention	Review of various practices to ascertain whether there are any differences in outcomes among the different practices.
Comparison/ control (quality of evidence)	The relation between measurements of knee-heel and crown-heel length is not consistent, as shown in some studies. These were thought to be the most sensitive indices of the adequacy of nutrient intake. There is no benefit in feeding formula with a protein/energy ration of 2.8 g per 100 kcal until term. Same results are obtained with a similar P/E ration if the infants are fed until between 3 to 9 corrected months.
Outcome/ effect	Feeding practices in preterm infants vary quite widely among special care baby units. Practices must be audited as a basis for their continuance.
Historical significance/ comments	Different studies over a period of time have arrived at different conclusions.

Key Summary Points

1. Preoperatively, most patients in most countries in Africa are frankly malnourished or borderline malnourished, which has implications for postoperative outcomes, including various degrees of poor wound healing.

2. If surgery is elective, it is better to improve on nutritional status preoperatively. This is the best opportunity to maximise postoperative outcomes.

3. If surgery is emergent, supplemental nutrition should be offered as soon as possible.

4. Patients undergoing surgery who will suffer long periods of ileus postoperatively require careful planning for nutritional support.

5. Patients with high metabolic requirements postoperatively also require nutritional support.

6. Enteral feeding is always preferred, offering fewer complications.

7. Necessary baseline tests include serum electrolyte estimation, serum protein levels, and liver function.

8. Attention to nutrition has to start in utero, with education dispelling any nutritional myths for pregnant women.

9. Nutrition in children younger than 5 years of age must ensure adequate intake of calories, which will allow maximum growth of the individual as well as the required intake of minerals and vitamins to maximise their growth. Locally available foodstuffs can be used for this.

10. Institutional policies must be developed to address ethical issues in order to protect physicians.

References

1. World Bank. Repositioning Nutrition as Central to Development: A Strategy for Large Scale Development, 2006. P 43.

2. American Gastroenterological Association Medical Position Statement: guidelines for the use of enteral nutrition. Gastroenterology 1995; 108(4):1280–1281.

3. Campbell SE, Avenell A, Walker AE. Assessment of nutritional status in hospital in-patients. QJM 2002; 95(2):83–87.

4. Johnson LR. Regulation of intestinal growth. In: Green M, Greene HL, eds. The Role of the Intestinal Tract in Nutrient Delivery. Academic Press, 1984, Pp 1–15.

5. Kerner JA, Manual of Pediatric Nutrition, John Wiley & Sons, 1983.

6. Skipper A, Dietitian's Handbook of Enteral and Parenteral Nutrition, 2nd ed. Aspen Publishers, 1998.

7. Marian M. Pediatric nutrition. Nutr Clin Pract 1993; 8:199–209.

8. Jelliffe DB, Jelliffe EFP, eds. Anthropometry: major measurements. In: Community Nutritional Assessment, 1st ed. Oxford University Press, 1989, Pp 68–104.

9. Foster BJ, Leonard MB. Measuring nutritional status in children with chronic kidney disease. Am J Clin Nutr 2004; 80(4):801–814.

10. de Oliveira Iglesias SB, Leite HP, Santana e Meneses JF, de Carvalho WB. Enteral nutrition in critically ill children: are prescription and delivery according to their energy requirements? Nutr Clin Pract 2007; 22(2):233–239.

11. McWhirter JP, Hill K, Richards J, et al. The use, efficacy and monitoring of artificial nutritional support in a teaching hospital. Scott Med J 1995; 40(6):179–183.

12. Alansari M, Hijazi M. Central venous pressure from peripherally inserted central catheters correlates well with that of centrally inserted catheters. American College of Chest Physicians, 2004 (poster presentation).

13. Paris JJ. Withholding or withdrawing nutrition and fluids: what are the real issues? Health Prog 1985; 22–25.

CHAPTER 7
HAEMOGLOBINOPATHIES

G. Olufemi Ogunrinde
Rebecca Inglis

G. Ifeyinwa Onimoe
Richard Onalo

Introduction

Children with haemoglobin disorders are more likely than the general population to need to undergo surgery during their lifetimes to treat the common surgical manifestations of their condition. However, they are also more likely to experience complications as a result of that surgery, with complication rates as high as 32% in patients with sickle haemoglobinopathies. Careful peri- and postoperative management is required to minimise the risk of complications. Furthermore, the prevalence of haemoglobinopathies, with an estimated 269 million carriers worldwide, means that the possibility of an undiagnosed haemoglobin disorder should be considered prior to undertaking a surgical procedure in any child.

Demographics

The haemoglobinopathies are the most common genetic disorders worldwide. One in 20 people are carriers of a defective haemoglobin gene, and 300,000 babies are born each year with a major haemoglobin disorder. Africa is disproportionately affected, shouldering two-thirds of the disease burden, with sickle cell disease particularly prevalent.

The distribution of sickle cell disease across the continent is influenced by the resistance to severe malaria conferred by carrying a single copy of the sickle cell gene. Even though malaria resistance does not extend to those affected by homozygous sickle cell disease itself, the survival advantage for carriers means that the sickle cell trait is selected for in areas where malaria is endemic. As a result, sickle cell disease is more prevalent in sub-Saharan Africa, particularly those countries bordering the equator. Sickle cell disease is an especially significant problem in Nigeria, where 24% of the population are carriers and the condition affects 2 in every 100 live births. This means that in Nigeria alone, 150,000 children are born with sickle cell anaemia each year.

Aetiology/Pathophysiology

Haemoglobinopathies are disorders that affect the globin part of the haemoglobin molecule. Genetic defects can lead to either decreased globin *synthesis*, producing the thalassaemia syndromes, or abnormal globin *structure*, resulting in disorders that include sickle cell disease (SCD).

The haemoglobin molecule comprises four globin chains (two alpha and two beta chains), which are genetically coded: different types combine to make different subtypes of haemoglobin. Of note, two distinct globin chains (each with its individual haem molecule) combine to form a haemoglobin.

Sickle cell disease is caused by an abnormal beta chain due to an amino acid substitution, valine for glutamic acid at β6. Other structural qualitative haemoglobinopathies include haemoglobin C (glutamic acid to lysine at β6) and haemoglobin E (lysine for glutamic acid at β 26). Sickle cell disease comprises a group of clinical disorders, which includes homozygous sickle cell anaemia (HbSS), sickle cell haemoglobin C disease (HbSC), sickle cell thalassaemia disease (HbS/β thal) and other compound heterozygous conditions. The carrier state, sickle cell trait HbAS, is not usually associated with increased morbidity or mortality.

As a result of the abnormal globin protein, both the haemoglobin molecules and the erythrocytes that contain them are unstable and can break down under predisposing conditions (hypoxia, acidosis, hypertonicity), releasing free haemoglobin radicals that lead to oxidative stress on the vascular endothelium. This sets up a chronic inflammatory process in the vasculature of patients with SCD, and this is thought to be the starting point for many of the pathological processes observed. The abnormal globin chain also causes the red cells to become less deformable and to stick more readily to the vascular endothelium. The downstream result is vaso-occlusion, leading to pain, ischaemia, and infarction, which can occur anywhere in the body, including the bones, abdominal viscera, and penile vasculature. Accelerated haemoglobin breakdown also leads to chronic haemolysis and a persistent state of anaemia.

Chronic haemolysis is also a central feature of the thalassaemias, and the major clinical manifestations of these conditions relate to variably severe anaemia. Other complications occur due to iron overload with end organ damage due to iron deposition.

The laboratory tests required to make a diagnosis of a haemoglobinopathy are described in Table 7.1. An important part of the diagnostic process is having a high index of suspicion in at-risk populations. The possibility of an undiagnosed haemoglobinopathy should be actively considered in any child who could potentially require surgery.

Table 7.1: Laboratory Investigations for the haemoglobinopathies.

Investigation	Typical finding
Full blood count	Normocytic anaemia (SCD) Microcytic anaemia* (thalassemia/HbSC)
Blood film	May show sickled erythrocytes, target cells, and nucleated red cells in sickle cell disease. Basophillic stippling is a nonspecific finding in some thalassaemias.
Haemoglobin electrophoresis	Demonstrates a single band of HbS in sickle cell anaemia or HbS with another mutant haemoglobin in compound heterozygotes. A raised level of HbA2 is consistent with β-thalassaemia.
Red cell staining	Reveals aggregates of β globin protein in α-thalassaemia
Sickle solubility and instability tests	A number of rapid screening tests are available for the detection of sickle haemoglobin. Although helpful in some settings, their use is not appropriate for definitive diagnosis because they miss other variants
DNA analysis	Often not required, but may be helpful in ascertaining diagnosis of thalassaemias.

* Iron studies should be sent to exclude iron deficiency.

Surgical Manifestations of Sickle Cell Disease

Acute Abdominal Pain

Acute abdominal pain in children with sickle cell disease presents a significant diagnostic challenge. Painful vaso-occlusive crises can mimic surgical pathologies and are difficult to differentiate on clinical grounds. Diagnosis is further confounded by the range of abdominal disease seen in this population. Important differentials to consider are shown in Table 7.2.

Acute Splenic Sequestration Crisis

Acute splenic sequestration is a life-threatening complication of sickle cell disease. It mainly occurs in children with homozygous sickle cell disease (HbSS) who have not undergone autosplenectomy and older patients with HbSC disease or HbSβ thalassaemia. It affects between 7% and 30% of children with sickle cell anaemia and is less common in other forms of SCD. It is the second most common cause of death in children with sickle cell anaemia under the age of 10. Acute hepatic sequestration is much rarer, but has also been described in this population (Figure 7.1).

In acute splenic sequestration, splenic outflow obstruction leads to massive sequestration of red cells and platelets in the spleen, often causing a significant decrease in circulating blood volume. Patients present with abdominal pain and distention and signs of haemodynamic compromise. The diagnosis is based on evidence of acute splenic enlargement accompanied by a rapid decrease in the haematocrit, usually to half the patient's "baseline value", as well as brisk reticulocytosis with increased nucleated red cells and moderate to severe thrombocytopaenia.

Acute splenic sequestration is a medical emergency, and treatment in the form of blood transfusion should be instigated rapidly to restore circulating volume and replenish red cell mass. Adequate analgesia is also important.

Patients who recover from a first episode of acute splenic sequestration have a 50% chance of having further episodes. Two possible management strategies can prevent this: children can be enrolled in a transfusion programme or undergo a splenectomy. There is no high-quality evidence to support one of these approaches over the other, and both are associated with potential complications.

The particular concern following total splenectomy is infection, so partial splenectomy has been proposed as an alternative to retain some immune function. A recent case series by Vick et al. showed that sickle cell patients who underwent a partial splenectomy were not subject to increased rates of infection. Nevertheless, a theoretical risk of seques-

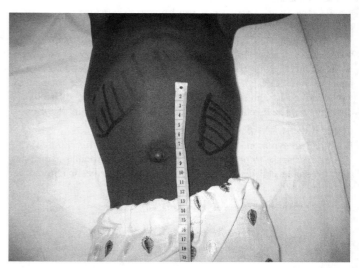

Figure 7.1: Acute liver enlargement should raise suspicions of a hepatic sequestration crisis.

Table 7.2: Differential diagnosis of acute abdominal pain in sickle cell disease.

Cause	Frequency	Characteristic features	Investigations
Vaso-occlusive painful crises	Very common	May mimic acute surgical disease with guarding and distention; often attributed to micro-infarcts of mesentery and abdominal viscera	A specific cause is rarely identified
Gallstone disease			
Biliary colic	Relatively common	Epigastric pain that comes on gradually over several hours and subsides over a similar period	Pigment stones may be visible on a plain abdominal radiograph
Acute cholecystitis	Relatively common	Persistent right upper quadrant pain with or without guarding; possible fever	Ultrasound shows pericholecystic fluid and thickening of the gallbladder
Cholangitis	Uncommon	Right upper quadrant pain with or without guarding; fever and rigors; jaundice	Ultrasound shows dilatation of the common bile duct
Acute splenic sequestration	Common, occurring in up to 30% of patients	Left upper quadrant pain; acute splenic enlargement; hypovolaemic shock	Falling haemoglobin, often with a 2 g/dl drop below baseline; thrombocyopaenia; erythrocytosis
Liver Disease			
Acute sickle hepatic crisis	Common, affecting approximately 10% of patients	Right upper quadrant pain; low-grade fever; nausea; increasing jaundice; tender hepatomegaly	Mild to moderate elevation of liver transaminases, bilirubin level generally less than 15 mg/dl (257 µmol/l)
Hepatic sequestration	Uncommon	Right upper quadrant pain, acute liver enlargement, hypovolaemic shock	Falling haemoglobin; thrombocytopaenia; erythrocytosis
Sickle cell intrahepatic cholestasis	Rare	Right upper quadrant or epigastric pain; acute liver enlargement; fever; nausea and vomiting	Significant hyperbilirubinaemia
Viral hepatitis	Increased risk due to multiple transfusions	Malaise; jaundice; low grade fever; tender hepatomegaly	Elevated liver transaminases; positive viral serology
Pancreatitis	Increased risk due to pigment gallstones	Epigastric pain radiating through to the back; fever; nausea and vomiting	Raised amylase
Appendicitis	Less than in general population	Right iliac fossa pain with or without guarding; nausea and vomiting; fever	
Ischaemic colitis	Rare	Sudden onset of abdominal pain and distention; can pass bloody stool	Raised lactate
Urinary tract infection	Common	Dysuria, frequency, fever	Positive urine dip and culture

tration in the splenic remnant still exists, so this approach needs further evaluation. In the meantime, splenectomy should generally be reserved for selected patients with recurrent splenic sequestration crises or those who develop red cell alloantibodies following transfusion therapy.

Gallstone Disease

Pigment gallstones are a frequent complication of sickle cell disease because continuous haemolysis leads to increased bilirubin excretion and subsequent stone formation. Although many children are asymptomatic, they can experience the full range of gallstone disease from biliary colic to cholangitis.

Management of the acute complications of gallstones is the same as in the general population, and elective cholecystectomy is recommended in patients with symptomatic cholelithiasis. The management of asymptomatic gallstones is less clear, but many would advocate cholecystectomy to avoid subsequent difficulty in distinguishing acute cholecystitis from vaso-occlusive painful episodes.

Orthopaedic Manifestations

Bone-related symptoms are the most common reason for children with sickle cell disease to present to hospital. The osteoarticular manifestations of sickle cell disease can be classified as acute or chronic, as shown in Table 7.3.

Table 7.3: Osteoarticular manifestations of sickle cell disease.

Acute
Vaso-occlusive crises (including dactylitis and diaphyseal infarction)
Osteomyelitis
Septic arthritis
Pathological fractures
Chronic
Avascular osteonecrosis
Chronic arthritis
Osteoporosis
Osteomyelitis

Acute

In a child presenting with acute bone pain, the most important distinction to make is between bone infarction and bone infection. Although the vaso-occlusive crises that lead to bone infarction are up to 50 times more common than osteomyelitis, there is potential for extensive damage to the bone and surrounding structures as well as overwhelming sepsis if an infection remains untreated.

It is difficult to distinguish between the two conditions on clinical criteria alone because the archetypal features of osteomyelitis—namely, pain, swelling, and fever—are also common in vaso-occlusive crises. A history of a painful episode that has lasted longer than 1 to 2 weeks or pain in a distribution that does not conform to previous painful crises should raise suspicions of an alternative underlying cause. Infection is not the only differential; stress fractures should also be considered.

Both vaso-occlusive crises and osteomyelitis are most common in the long bones of the arms and legs, but can involve any part of the skeleton. Dactylitis, with swelling of the hands or feet, occurs in young children between the ages of 6 months and 4 years, and can be one of the earliest signs of sickle cell disease. Careful examination should be made for evidence of a draining sinus or bony deformity, which would suggest chronic or subacute bone infection. Adjacent joints should be assessed for evidence of an effusion, and the range and ease of movement noted.

Preliminary laboratory investigations are often unhelpful in distinguishing infection from infarction because both conditions can cause a leucocytosis with raised inflammatory markers. Blood cultures taken before the commencement of antibiotics can be invaluable, as can culture of a bone or joint aspirate if there is evidence of fluid accumulation.

Imaging investigations are also confounded by the similarity between the radiographic appearances of bony infarction and infection. Plain radiographs can be normal in the early stages of both conditions, and the periositis and osteopaenia seen in acute osteomyelitis can also occur in vaso-occlusion. The imaging modality of choice for suspected osteomyelitis is magnetic resonance imaging (MRI), where it is available, but even this is not 100% specific for differentiating infection from infarction. Ultrasonography, which is showing promise in the diagnosis of osteomyelitis in children in particular, should be used to guide any aspiration procedures.

The management of vaso-occlusive crises is largely supportive, focusing predominantly on pain management. By contrast, the first line management of osteomyelitis requires urgent parenteral antibiotics, ideally directed at whatever organism has been isolated. When antibiotics are being started empirically, it is important to bear in mind that patients with SCD are more predisposed than the general population to contracting *Salmonella* osteomyelitis. Other organisms that cause bone infection in this population include *Staphylococcus aureus*, *Haemophilus influenzae*, and *Escherichia coli*. Third-generation cephalosporins are often used in this setting, and treatment should continue for at least 6 weeks.

Surgical drainage is generally believed to be required only in those cases of osteomyelitis that are not responding to antibiotics or where there is evidence of abscess formation. However, the exact timing and method of surgical intervention remains controversial.

Chronic

Avascular osteonecrosis is the most common chronic complication of sickle cell bone disease and is believed to affect up to 41% of these patients. It occurs when repeated bone infarction leads to destruction and breakdown of an area of bone, and it most often occurs at the femoral head. Other areas affected include the head of the humerus, the knee, and the small joints of the hands and feet.

Sufferers describe pain and limited movement at the affected joint; examination may reveal localised tenderness, with restriction of both active and passive joint movements. Initial investigations should include a plain radiograph, which may be diagnostic in more advanced cases, showing flattening or collapse of the articular surfaces and subchondral radiolucency. Less advanced cases may show evidence of sclerosis. MRI is the second-line investigation of choice.

When considering treatments for avascular necrosis in patients with SCD, it is important to note the differences between this population and nonsickle patients with the same condition. Not only is the pathophysiology of osteonecrosis in SCD thought to differ from that of osteonecrosis from other causes, but the quality of the surrounding bone is often much poorer in this group of patients. Combined with their increased anaesthetic risk, this makes SCD patients less attractive surgical candidates.

A lack of quality data currently precludes any definitive recommendations for the surgical management of avascular necrosis in patients with SCD. The available data confirm a high rate of surgical complications and procedure failures. Much interest has been shown in hip core decompression as a measure to prevent progression of early femoral head disease; however, the only randomised controlled trial that has been carried out failed to provide a clear mandate for this procedure. In fact, the only intervention that has been shown to be effective in preventing progression is bed rest. Clearly, a more feasible long-term solution needs to be found.

Genitourinary Manifestations

The most common genitourinary manifestations of sickle cell disease are haematuria, urinary tract infection, and priapism. The haematuria is often painless and is thought to result from microinfarctions of the renal papillae. Management is predominantly conservative.

Urinary tract infection (UTI) is more common in patients with SCD compared to the general population. The reason for this is remains unclear, but children found to have a UTI should undergo the same careful urological evaluation as nonsickle children.

Priapism is a well-recognised complication of SCD and can be challenging to manage. The condition involves prolonged and painful penile erection, which can lead to irreversible fibrosis and impotence if it persists. About 90% of cases lasting longer than 24 hours have been associated with subsequent erectile dysfunction. Priapism occurs most commonly in children aged 5–13 years (and in adults aged 21–29 years) and affects 28% of the male paediatric sickle population. The majority of children presenting with priapism have sickle cell disease.

The most important history to obtain in a patient presenting with priapism pertains to the duration of the current episode and to previous episodes and their treatment. Alternative causes of priapism, including trauma, drugs, and malignancy, should be excluded.

Examination generally demonstrates rigid corpora cavernosa with a soft glans penis and corpus spongiosum. Involvement of the glans can suggest corporeal infarction.

Investigations should seek to establish or exclude the diagnosis of a haemoglobinopathy in all cases of priapism if this is not already known. Many centres recommend blood gas analysis of blood aspirated from the corpus cavernosum to exclude nonischaemic causes of priapism. Compared to the ischaemic, low-flow priapism most typical in SCD, nonischaemic priapism is a high-flow state with causes that include cavernous artery fistulas. It is normally relatively pain-free and will often resolve without treatment. In ischaemic priapism, aspirated cavernosal blood is expected to appear dark in colour with an oxygen saturation of less than 4 kPa (30 mm Hg) and a pH < 7.25. Where the resources are available, this analysis can be supplemented by colour duplex ultrasonography.

The evidence base for the management of priapism is poor; as a result, considerable variation exists in current management practices. The following discussion is derived largely from the American Urological Association guidelines, which are based on a review of the limited evidence and consensus opinion.

Initial management for all sickle patients presenting with priapism should involve analgesia and hydration. In the past, additional measures, including ice packs, heat packs, and spinal anaesthesia with hypotension, have been advocated, but these measures are now thought to be counterproductive. The role for blood transfusion in this setting, although commonly used, is unproven, and in some cases, transfusion has been associated with serious adverse effects.

Priapism that persists for greater than 4 hours requires urgent focal treatment that should be carried out in conjunction with the systemic treatments described above. The initial intervention can be either a therapeutic aspiration of corporeal blood or an intracavernous injection of a sympathomimetic agent. Both procedures can be carried out under local anaesthetic, following a dorsal nerve block or a penile shaft block.

A therapeutic aspiration is often carried out first, using an 18- or 19-gauge butterfly needle inserted into either corpora cavernosa. Blood can then be aspirated, accompanied by irrigation with saline if so desired. If this procedure fails to achieve detumescence, it should be followed by the intracavernous administration of phenylephrine, an α-1 adrenergic agonist. Depending on the age of the child, a small quantity of the drug diluted in normal saline can be injected with careful monitoring for any side effects including hypertension or arrhythmias. This can be repeated every 3–5 minutes, as required, for approximately 1 hour before an assessment of the treatment's efficacy is made.

Surgery should be considered only if these measures are unsuccessful. The aim of the surgery is to allow the blood from the engorged corpora cavernosa to return to the systemic circulation, most commonly via the corpus spongiosum. A cavernoglanular shunt is the easiest to perform and has the fewest complications. It can be performed with a large biopsy needle (Winter shunt) or a scalpel (Ebbehøj shunt) inserted percutaneously through the glans. It can also be performed by excising a piece of the tunica albuginea at the tip of the corpus cavernosum (Al-Ghorab procedure). If such measures fail to achieve detumescence, a more proximal procedure to create a cavernospongiosal shunt (Quackel's procedure) or to anastomose the saphenous vein to one of the corpora cavernosa (Grayhack procedure) may be warranted.

Recurrent priapism is a common problem, and much effort has been focused on developing a preventive therapy. Gonadotropin-releasing hormone analogues and, more recently, 5α-reductase inhibitors appear to be effective in controlling recurrent priapism, but they have significant side effects and are not currently licensed for use in children. Phosphodiesterase inhibitors are also under evaluation.

Skin

Leg ulcers are less common in children than in adults and affect approximately 3% of patients between the ages of 10 and 19 years with sickle cell anaemia. The ulcers occur spontaneously or as a result of local trauma with subsequent infection and skin necrosis, but no specific organisms have been incriminated. The majority of ulcers are located on the lower leg (Figure 7.2); they can also involve the dorsum of the foot and, more rarely, the sole. Ulcers typically persist for prolonged periods of time and take up to 16 times longer to heal than venous ulcers.

Surgical intervention can be required to debride infected necrotic ulcers or for skin grafting in intractable cases. Various techniques have been deployed, including myocutaneous flaps and split thickness skin grafts but, as with other surgery in this population, such procedures are plagued by a poor success rate.

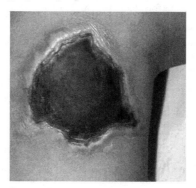

Figure 7.2: Leg ulcer in a patient with sickle cell disease.

Surgical Manifestations of the Thalassaemias

Compared to sickle cell disease, there are relatively few surgical manifestations of the thalassaemias. As in SCD, chronic haemolysis can lead to gallstone formation and symptomatic gallstone disease may require cholecystectomy. Splenectomy is sometimes carried out to treat painful splenomegaly or hypersplenic pancytopaenia; it can also be in used to decrease a patient's transfusion requirement.

Postoperative Complications

Patients with sickle cell disease clearly experience a higher rate of postoperative complications than the general population. Observed complications include the acute chest syndrome, painful vaso-occlusive crises, neurological events, acute kidney injury, and postoperative infections. The high postoperative complication rate has traditionally been attributed to unfavourable intraoperative conditions precipitating erythrocyte sickling and leading to vascular occlusion and subsequent end organ damage. Preventive measures have therefore focused on measures designed to prevent sickling.

Newer models of sickle cell disease have suggested, however, that chronic vascular inflammation and endothelial dysfunction may instead underlie many of the pathological processes. The logic behind measures aimed primarily at preventing sickling has been called into question. An example of such a measure is the common practice of exchange transfusion prior to undertaking surgery. The idea is to dilute the sickle haemoglobin with normal red cells, thereby decreasing the risk of intraoperative sickling. Nevertheless, there is no evidence to suggest the superiority of this approach over a simple "top-up" transfusion; indeed, the case for universal preoperative transfusion remains to be definitively proven (see Table 7.4).

It has been suggested that laparoscopic surgery could diminish the risk of sickle-related complications for patients undergoing abdominal surgery, but this has not been demonstrated to date. Patients undergoing laparoscopic surgery have been shown to have shorter hospital stays, however, so, where feasible, a laparoscopic approach should be considered.

Current advice for the perioperative management of children with sickle cell disease is as follows:

- All teams involved in the patient's surgery should be aware of the diagnosis of sickle cell disease and the need for special attention.

- Preoperative assessment should consider the following indicators of increased operative risk in patients with sickle cell disease:
    - frequent recent hospitalisations;
    - sickle cell lung disease;
    - history of early onset dactylitis (a predictor of severe disease);
    - coexisting chest or urinary tract infection; and
    - previous stroke.

- Simple transfusion to achieve a haemoglobin concentration of approximately 10 g/dl should be performed before all but the lowest risk procedures.

- Careful attention should be paid to avoiding hypoxia, although this should not preclude the use of opiate analgesia for pain management or anxiolytic medication, if required.

- Dehydration and hypothermia should be avoided.

- Early mobilisation, effective postoperative pain control, and chest physiotherapy with incentive spirometry may decrease the risk of chest complications.

Prevention

Many of the conditions discussed in this chapter are unavoidable manifestations of a group of complex multisystem diseases. A number of measures could improve the outcomes for these children, however, including those listed here.

- Early diagnosis of a haemoglobinopathy is essential for appropriate management; the onus lies with the medical team to suspect it in at-risk groups and with certain typical presentations.

- Education of patients and their parents about their condition can help to avoid dangerously late presentations. Parents of infants with sickle cell disease should be taught how to palpate their infants' spleens and when to suspect a splenic crisis; warning signs of other serious complications should also be discussed.

- Penicillin prophylaxis reduces the incidence of infection in children with sickle cell anaemia and heterozygotes with HbS-β^0 thalassaemia. This preventive treatment should be started between 2 and 4 months of age and continued at least until the age of 5.

- All children with sickle cell disease and splenectomised children with thalassaemia should receive immunisation against pneumococcus, *H. influenzae*, meningococcus, influenza, and *Salmonella typhi* (in endemic areas) as well as routine vaccines. Hepatitis B vaccination should be considered in all children with a haemoglobinopathy.

- Careful foot care and well-fitting shoes can help to prevent the development of leg ulcers.

Evidence-Based Research

Table 7.4 presents a study comparing preoperative transfusion regimes for patients with SCD.

Table 7.4. Evidence-based research.

Title	Preoperative blood transfusions for sickle cell disease
Authors	Hirst C, Williamson L
Institution	AstraZeneca, Alderley Park, UK.
Reference	*Cochrane Database of Systematic Reviews* 2001, Issue 3.
Problem	There is a high rate of perioperative complications in patients with sickle cell disease.
Intervention	Preoperative blood transfusion.
Comparison/ control (quality of evidence)	This study is a meta-analysis of two randomised controlled trials comparing an aggressive preoperative transfusion regimen, designed to decrease the sickle haemoglobin level to less than 30%; a conservative regime, designed to increase the haemoglobin level to 10 g/dl; and a group receiving no preoperative transfusion.
Outcome/ effect	The study found that the conservative transfusion regime was as effective as the aggressive regimen in preventing surgical complications, and was associated with fewer transfusion-related adverse events. There was insufficient evidence to demonstrate a clear advantage to preoperative blood transfusion compared with a nontransfused group.
Historical significance/ comments	The potential risks associated with blood transfusions vary significantly according to the setting. In areas of the world where resources are limited, and clean, infection-free blood products cannot be guaranteed, a risk-benefit analysis is likely to favour less frequent usage of preoperative transfusions.

Key Summary Points

1. Haemoglobinopathies (sickle cell disease/thalassaemias) are associated with increased morbidity and mortality.

2. Due to the surgical manifestations of haemoglobinopathies, surgical intervention is a common occurrence and is associated with a higher risk of complications for these patients than for the general population.

3. Basic knowledge of the pathophysiology of sickle cell disease and the principles behind its clinical management is essential for the paediatric surgeon to achieve successful outcomes in sickle cell patients under their care.

4. A multidisciplinary team approach is needed.

5. Careful perioperative management is required to minimise the risk of surgical complications, including the consideration of blood transfusion prior to surgical procedures, paying careful attention to oxygenation and hydration in the intra- and postoperative period, providing adequate pain control, and encouraging early mobilisation.

Suggested Reading

Ahmed S, Shahid RK, Russo LA. Unusual causes of abdominal pain: sickle cell anemia. Best Pract Res Clin Gastroenterol 2005; 19(2):297–310.

Almeida A, Roberts I. Bone involvement in sickle cell disease. Br J Haematol 2005; 129(4):482–490.

Al-Mousawi FR, Malki AA. Managing femoral head osteonecrosis in patients with sickle cell disease. Surgeon 2007; 5(5):282–289.

Badmus TA, Adediran IA, Adesunkanmi AR, Katung IA. Priapism in southwestern Nigeria. East Afr Med J 2003; 80(10):518–524.

Bruno D, Wigfall DR, Zimmerman SA, Rosoff PM, Wiener JS. Genitourinary complications of sickle cell disease. J Urol 2001; 166(3):803–811.

Burnett AL. Therapy insight: priapism associated with hematologic dyscrasias. Nat Clin Pract Urol 2005; 2(9):449–456.

de Gheldere A, Ndjoko R, Docquier PL, Mousny M, Rombouts JJ. Orthopaedic complications associated with sickle-cell disease. Acta Orthop Belg 2006; 72(6):741–747.

Firth PJ. Anaesthesia for peculiar cells—a century of sickle cell disease. Br J Anaesth 2005; 95(3):287–299.

Martí-Carvajal AJ, Solà I, Agreda-Pérez LH. Treatment for avascular necrosis of bone in people with sickle cell disease. Cochrane Database Syst Rev 2009; (3):CD004344.

Montague DK, et al. American Urological Association guideline on the management of priapism. J Urol 2003; 170:1318–1324.

Owusu-Ofori S, Riddington C. Splenectomy versus conservative management for acute sequestration crises in people with sickle cell disease. Cochrane Database Syst Rev 2002; (4):CD003425.

Rachid-Filho D, Cavalcanti AG, Favorito LA, Costa WS, Sampaio FJ. Treatment of recurrent priapism in sickle cell anemia with finasteride: a new approach. Urology 2009; 74(5):1054–1057.

Riddington C, Williamson L. Preoperative blood transfusions for sickle cell disease. Cochrane Database Syst Rev 2001; (3):CD003149.

Schrier SL, Angelucci E. New strategies in the treatment of the thalassemias. Annu Rev Med 2005; 56:157–171.

Trent JT, Kirsner RS. Leg ulcers in sickle cell disease. Adv Skin Wound Care 2004; 17(8):410–416.

Trent RJ. Diagnosis of the haemoglobinopathies. Clin Biochem Rev 2006; 27(1):27–38.

Vick LR, Gosche JR, Islam S. Partial splenectomy prevents splenic sequestration crises in sickle cell disease. J Pediatr Surg 2009; 44(11):2088–2091.

World Health Organization. Report by the Secretariat of the Fifty-ninth World Health Assembly A59/9, 2006.

Zuckerberg AL, Maxwell LG. Preoperative assessment. In: McInerny T, Adam H, Campbell D, Kamat D, Kelleher K, eds. AAP Textbook of Pediatric Care. American Academy of Pediatrics, 2008, chapter 62.

CHAPTER 8
WOUND HEALING

Richard F. Carter
Benedict Nwomeh
David A. Lanning

Introduction

A wound occurs when normal anatomic structure and function are disrupted by injury.[1] The reparative response to injury is a primitive host defense mechanism designed to restore tissue structural integrity, provide a physical barrier against infection, and return damaged tissue to its normal state. Regeneration, which is distinct from repair, is a process in which there is loss of structure and thus function, but the organism has the sophisticated capacity to replace that structure by recreating exactly what was there before the injury occurred.[2]

Epidermis—and to some extent, nerve—can be partially regenerated after injury in humans. In addition, compared to adults, the foetus has the capacity to heal wounds by a process that closely resembles regeneration, with only a minimal scar response.[3] However, adult humans have adopted a wound-healing strategy that trades the accuracy of regeneration for the speed of repair.[4] This process produces scarring and, for practical purposes, as long as the scar tissue is adequate to maintain structure and does not inhibit the function of the organ involved, it is considered a normal repair process. However, when scar tissue is either inadequate or excessive, wound repair is considered abnormal. Abnormal wound healing ranges from deficient tissue formation in diabetic wounds and sacral pressure ulcers, to excessive scarring in keloids, burn contractures, pulmonary fibrosis, and liver cirrhosis.

Understanding the basic mechanisms involved in normal wound healing and tissue response to injury is critical in surgical treatment and management. Further, elucidating the molecular aspects of foetal response to tissue injury, which leads to scarless wound repair, may provide insights to new wound-healing therapies. This chapter briefly outlines common wound-healing problems encountered in caring for paediatric patients, current cellular and molecular aspects of normal and pathologic wound healing, a brief description of foetal wound healing, and essential aspects of care and treatment. Although the emphasis is on cutaneous healing, it is important to note that all tissues respond to injury in a fundamentally similar manner.

Physiology of Wound Healing

Wound healing is the body's response to injury. The injury may be acute or chronic and may involve multiple tissues. Normal healing occurs by an overlapping sequence of events involving cellular migration and proliferation, soluble factors such as growth factors (GFs) and cytokines, and matrix components acting in concert to repair tissue damage[5] (Figure 8.1). The healing response can be described in four broad, overlapping phases: haemostasis, inflammation, proliferation, and remodelling. This dynamic process optimally leads to restoration of tissue integrity and function.

Haemostasis

The initial response to tissue damage and vessel injury is bleeding, which leads to platelet aggregation and platelet plug formation (Figure 8.2). The haemostatic process is initiated and fibrin binds to the platelet plug, forming a matrix for the cellular response leading to healing.[6,7]

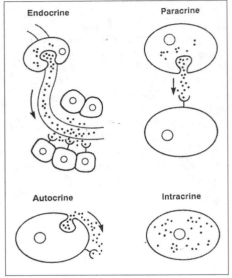

Source: Modified from Cohen IK, Diegelmann RF, Crossland MC. Wound care and wound healing. In: Schwartz SI, et al., eds. Principles of Surgery, 6th ed. McGraw-Hill Inc., 1994.

Figure 8.1: Cell signaling in cytokines.

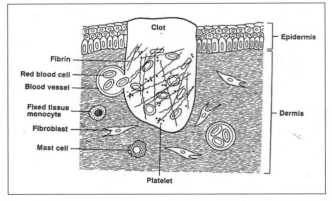

Source: Modified from Cohen IK, Diegelmann RF, Crossland MC. Wound care and wound healing. In: Schwartz SI, et al., eds. Principles of Surgery, 6th ed. McGraw-Hill Inc., 1994.

Figure 8.2: Immediately after injury, platelets release coagulation factors and cytokines to initiate the wound-healing process.

Inflammation

The inflammatory response begins when GFs, chemoattractant mediators, and chemoactivators are released during platelet degranulation and initiate chemotaxis of inflammatory cells to the site of injury and proliferation of inflammatory cells locally. A short period of local

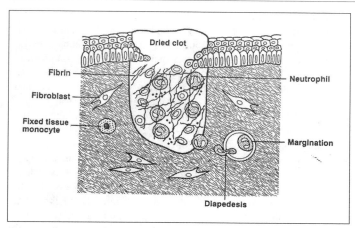

Source: Modified from Cohen IK, Diegelmann RF, Crossland MC. Wound care and wound healing. In: Schwartz SI, et al., eds. Principles of Surgery, 6th ed. McGraw-Hill Inc., 1994.

Figure 8.3: Within 24 hours following tissue injury, neutrophils attach to the endothelium (margination) and then move through the vessel walls (diapedesis) to migrate (chemotaxis) to the wound site.

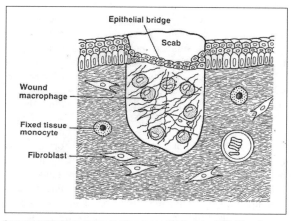

Source: Modified from Cohen IK, Diegelmann RF, Crossland MC. Wound care and wound healing. In: Schwartz SI, et al., eds. Principles of Surgery, 6th ed. McGraw-Hill Inc., 1994.

Figure 8.4: The proliferation phase is characterised by the movement of macrophages into the wound site, which in turn attracts fibroblasts. The fibroblasts then repair the wound by producing new connective tissue.

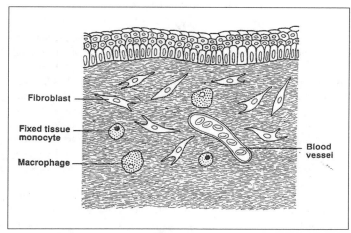

Source: Modified from Cohen IK, Diegelmann RF, Crossland MC. Wound care and wound healing. In: Schwartz SI, et al., eds. Principles of Surgery, 6th ed. McGraw-Hill Inc., 1994.

Figure 8.5: The remodelling phase is characterised by an equilibrium between collagen synthesis and collagen degradation in an effort to re-establish the connective tissue matrix that was destroyed by the tissue injury.

vasoconstriction at the site of injury is followed by vasodilatation, which increases local blood flow to the area. Vascular permeability is increased through activation of the complement pathways and coagulation cascade. There is an influx of cells and substrates necessary for healing, including early neutrophil scavengers, plasma proteins, and activated complement fragments.

A predominance of neutrophils within the first 24 hours act to sterilise the wound (Figure 8.3). After 2–3 days, the cell population shifts to a predominance of macrophages derived from resident macrophages and monocytes that are attracted to and infiltrate the wound. Macrophages continue phagocytosis and secrete GFs and cytokines, which induce fibroblast proliferation, angiogenesis, and production of extracellular matrix. Lymphocytes begin to appear in small numbers, but little is understood about their role in the wound-healing process.

Proliferation

The proliferative phase begins with formation of a fibrin, fibronectin glycosaminoglycan, and hyaluronic acid matrix that is initially populated with platelets and macrophages. The various GFs secreted by the macrophages enhance fibroplasia, and there is migration of fibroblasts into the wound using the fibrin and fibronectin matrix as a scaffold. The fibroblasts proliferate in response to GFs and become the predominant cell type by the third to fifth day following injury (Figure 8.4).

Fibroblasts entering the wound proliferate and synthesize extracellular matrix (ECM) components at the site of injury. There is interaction between the fibroblasts and the ECM through transmembrane receptors called integrins. Ligands for the integrin receptors include GFs, ECM components, and other cells. Ligand binding leads to structural change in the cytoplasmic domain of the receptor and phosphorylation. Signal transduction leads to transcription factor synthesis and gene expression.

Collagen is the predominant ECM protein deposited at the wound. The collagen molecule is a triple helical structure abundant in two unique amino acids, hydroxyproline and hydroxylysine. The hydroxylation process that forms these two amino acids requires ascorbic acid (vitamin C) and is necessary for stabilisation and cross-linking of collagen.[8] During the initial phases of healing, there is an abundance of type III collagen, which is composed of thin fibrils and is relatively pliable. Type I collagen is also formed, and with remodelling it becomes the most abundant form found in normal adult wounds at a 4:1 ratio with type III collagen. Type I collagen is relatively rigid and imparts high tensile strength to the tissue.[5]

Angiogenesis occurs with formation of new capillary networks through endothelial cell division and migration. This new vasculature allows delivery of nutrients and removal of by-products. Granulation tissue may accompany the process in wound healing by secondary intention. This tissue is a dense population of blood vessels, macrophages, and fibroblasts with a loose connective tissue matrix. The presence of granulation tissue is used as a clinical indicator that a wound is ready for skin grafting.[9]

Throughout this phase, wound contracture occurs, which leads to the surrounding skin being pulled circumferentially toward the wound bed. This decreases the wound size and helps it close more rapidly. Epithelialisation also occurs within hours after injury. The epidermis thickens at the wound edges, and basal cells enlarge and migrate over the defect. Cell adhesion glycoproteins, such as fibronectin and tenascin, form the framework to facilitate the epithelial cell migration.

Remodelling

Collagen accumulation in the wound reaches a maximum at 2–3 weeks after injury, and the transition to remodelling begins. There is a balance between synthesis, deposition, and degradation during this time (Figure 8.5). The tensile strength of the wound increases as the initially randomly deposited collagen fibrils are replaced by organised fibrils with more cross-linking. Lysyl oxidase is the major enzyme responsible for ensuring cross-linking of fibrils.

The normal adult 4:1 ratio of type I to type III collagen is restored during remodelling. Equilibrium is established as new collagen is formed and collagen is degraded. The matrix metalloproteinases (MMPs)—collagenases, gelatinases, and stromelysins—degrade the ECM components and are in part responsible for establishing a balance between collagen deposition and degradation.

Wound tensile strength increases for up to 1 year after injury. The tensile strength of wounded skin at best reaches 80% of unwounded skin.[10] The ultimate outcome of adult wound healing is formation of a scar. A scar can be defined morphologically as a lack of organisation compared to the surrounding tissue; it is characterised by disorganised collagen deposition.[11] Collagen of a scar is in densely packed fibers and not the reticular pattern seen in unwounded skin. The final scar is brittle, less elastic, and lacks such appendages as hair follicles or sweat glands.

Foetal Wound Healing: Scarless Repair

Foetal wound healing differs from that of adults in a number of aspects. There is minimal inflammation during foetal healing. The minimal cellular infiltration seen is predominantly mononuclear cells with few neutrophils. Collagen is deposited in a more organised and rapid fashion and has an increased type III to type I ratio. Further, collagen is deposited in a reticular pattern, indistinguishable from surrounding tissue, and has greater tensile strength than that for adult wounds.[3]

Research has demonstrated lower amounts of transforming growth factor-β (TGF-β) types 1 and 2 and decreased ratio of total TGF-β1 and TGF-β2 released from foetal platelets.[12] These factors are thought to be in part responsible for the absence of inflammatory infiltrate and fibrosis in foetal wound repair. In the midgestational foetal rabbit, incisional wounds heal without fibrosis or scar formation, and there is no evidence of wound contracture. The ECM consists mostly of hyaluronan without evidence of collagen deposition, and fibroblasts are present only at the wound margin.[13,14]

The foetal environment may also contribute to the quality of wound healing. However, adult skin transplanted into foetuses in utero does not heal differently than as seen in normal adults.[15] Also, a marsupial foetus heals without scar formation even in the absence of amniotic fluid.[16,17] A sterile environment is important in foetal healing. If a stimulus is provided, such as bacteria-soaked sponges, an inflammatory cascade can be initiated, resulting in extensive inflammation, fibrosis, and scar formation.[18]

The genes and complex cell signalling pathways that regulate the mechanisms resulting in the regenerative type of wound healing seen in the foetus, however, remain unknown. A better understanding of the biology of scarless foetal wound repair may help in the development of therapeutic strategies that can be used to minimise scar formation.

Clinical Wound-Healing Problems

Many pathological processes are characterised by either abnormal collagen deposition or degradation. Insufficient collagen deposition could manifest as abdominal wound dehiscence or leaking intestinal anastomosis, two common examples of deficient healing that cause severe morbidity and frequent mortality. Chronic wounds, such as venous stasis ulcers, diabetic ulcers, and pressure sores, similarly result from inadequate collagen synthesis, although excessive collagen degradation may be the more important factor.[19] In contrast, accumulation of collagen due to excessive deposition or impaired degradation can distort normal tissue architecture, compromise function, and produce a fibrotic state characteristic of such conditions as keloids, hypertrophic burn scars, pulmonary fibrosis, oesophageal strictures, and hepatic cirrhosis. Acute wounds are discussed in the chapters on trauma and burns. The following discussion concentrates on conditions of excessive scarring (keloid and hypertrophic scars) and those of deficient healing (chronic wounds).

Hypertrophic Scars and Keloids

Keloids and hypertrophic scars are challenging complications of wound healing frequently encountered by paediatric surgeons in Africa. Lesions are more common in individuals with darker complexions, with a family history, at a younger age, and in areas exposed to stretch or tension. The overall incidence of keloid formation in wound healing is estimated at 4.5–16%.[11] The incidence of keloids was 6.2% of 4,877 people in a western Nigerian community,[20] and as high as 16% in Zaire.[21] Although the incidence of hypertrophic scars is unknown, it is thought to be higher than keloids. Keloids and hypertrophic scars present functional as well as cosmetic problems. Management remains controversial; however, some recent guidelines have been established.[5]

Normal wounds have stop signals to halt the repair process when the defect is closed and re-epithelialisation is complete. When these signals are absent or altered, the healing process continues and may result in excessive scarring. Prominent scars may be cosmetically and physically challenging for the patient.

Hypertrophic scars are defined as scars confined to the boundaries of the original wound. They are an example of excessive healing, and histologically contain an overabundance of dermal collagen. Hypertrophic scars are usually self-limited and can regress. The scar will tend to fade and flatten. Improvement in scar appearance has been obtained with pressure garments, topical silicone gel, or re-excision.[8]

Keloids are uncommon forms of excessive scarring and predominantly occur in dark-skinned individuals with a genetic predisposition to them. The incidence is as high as 16% in African populations.[5,8,22] In contrast to hypertrophic scars, keloids overgrow the original wound boundaries and rarely regress. Keloids may behave as benign tumours and extend into or invade surrounding tissue. Histologically, keloids are rich in collagen, as collagenases cannot keep up with collagen deposition.

The exact cause of hypertrophic scar and keloid formation is unknown, and treatment is difficult. Recent recommendations from an international advisory panel provide several treatment guidelines.[5] They suggest that first line therapy for immature hypertrophic scars and keloids should be silicone gel sheeting. If scars are resistant, intralesional injection of corticosteroids is indicated. For first-line treatment failures of hypertrophic scars, surgical excision with postoperative silicone gel sheeting should be considered. Larger hypertrophic scars may benefit from Z-plasty, excision, and grafting or flap coverage. Large keloids are more challenging because of their postsurgical recurrence. Some newer treatments, such as local radiation therapy, bleomycin, or 5-flourouracil treatment, may have roles in keloid management.[23]

Chronic and Complex Wounds

Chronic wounds can be defined as those failing to proceed through an orderly and timely process to produce anatomic and functional integrity, or proceeding through the repair process without establishing a sustained result.[1] Practically, a chronic wound is one that has failed to heal within 3 months.[24] The cellular, biochemical, and molecular events that characterise chronic wounds have been well defined, including prolonged inflammatory phase, cellular senescence, deficiency of growth factor receptor sites, deficient fibrin production and growth factor release, and high levels of proteases.[25] Chronic wounds are frequently caused by vascular insufficiency, chronic inflammation, repetitive tissue insults, or underlying pathology.

"Complex wound" is a term used to group acute or chronic wounds that are nonhealing or difficult to treat. They show extensive loss of integument, are frequently complicated by infection, demonstrate circulatory impairment, and are often associated with systemic pathology.[26] Recognising chronic or complex wounds, identifying the underlying causes for poor healing, and early intervention are crucial to decreasing morbidity and mortality. The majority of chronic

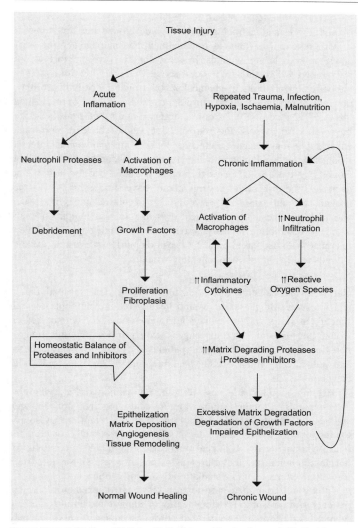

Source: Nwomeh BC, Yager DR, Cohen IK. Physiology of the chronic wound. Clin Plast Surg 1998; 25(3):341–356.

Figure 8.6: Pathophysiology of chronic wounds: the final common pathway.

wounds require surgical procedures such as multiple debridements, skin grafting, or flap coverage to facilitate healing.[27] Chronic wounds in African children are often the outcome of poorly treated and infected traumatic wounds and chronic fungal and mycobacterial infections. A detailed discussion of these chronic infections is beyond the scope of this chapter. Chronic wounds due to diabetes and venous stasis are more common in adult patients. Chronic pressure ulcers are common, and are used in the next section as examples to explain some of the pathophysiological events in chronic wounds.

Pressure Ulcers

The term "pressure ulcer" is preferred to the older term "decubitus ulcer", which was derived from the Latin word *dêcubitus*, meaning "lying down, being bedridden". These ulcers are characterised by deep tissue necrosis and loss of volume that is disproportionately greater than the overlying skin defect.[28]

Pressure ulcers are serious and frequent occurrences among children who are immobile and debilitated, including those who have been hospitalised for a long period. Patients with spinal cord injuries are particularly vulnerable to the formation of pressure ulcers. Several primary aetiological factors are important in the formation of pressure ulcers. Pressure over bony prominences is a key factor, but shear forces, friction, and moisture are also important in the development of pressure ulcers.[29]

External pressure will impede blood flow when it exceeds capillary pressure. In the skin, midcapillary pressure is approximately 20 mm Hg. In contrast, the forces of compression exerted on the overlying bony prominence, such as the ischial tuberosity in a recumbent person, can be as great as 2,600 mm Hg. This amount of external pressure produces venous and lymphatic obstruction, which increases total tissue tension and may progress to arterial occlusion. As a consequence of tissue ischaemia, toxic metabolites accumulate in the tissue spaces and are a major source of noxious stimuli. In normal individuals, such noxious stimuli signal a sense of discomfort and pain. With an intact neurological system, the response to pain is an instant change in posture, which relieves the pressure and reverses the adverse metabolic changes induced by ischaemia. Intermittent relief of pressure as high as 240 mm Hg minimises the tissue damage, and demonstrates the value of intermittent postural change as an effective means of protection from pressure-induced necrosis.[30]

Muscle and subcutaneous tissues are more susceptible to pressure-induced injury than is the skin. Fixation of the skin by an unyielding fascia also predisposes it to damage. The friction between the skin and the bed sheet when a patient is dragged across the bed can remove the protective outer layers of the stratum corneum, thereby accelerating the onset of ulceration. Shearing forces generated in the subcutaneous tissue due to this friction can also cause stretching and angulation of vessels, leading to thrombosis and ischaemia.

Pathobiology of Chronic Wounds

In normally healing wounds, acute inflammation with neutrophil infiltration brings neutrophil-derived matrix protease enzymes to debride the wound and pave the path for new tissue deposition, remodelling, and epithelisation. The regulatory processes that prevent excessive matrix degradation include various protease inhibitors derived from the serum or secreted by cells at the wound site. An optimal mix of various growth factors, matrix-degrading enzymes, and their inhibitors create a physiologic environment for normal healing.

In chronic wounds, the smoothness and orderliness of the healing process is disrupted by some underlying abnormality that prolongs the inflammatory phase and produces a cascade of tissue responses that perpetuates the nonhealing state (Figure 8.6). Repeated trauma, foreign bodies, pressure necrosis, infection, ischaemia, and tissue hypoxia also amplify the chronic inflammatory state characterised by excess neutrophils, macrophages, and lymphocytes. Fragments of dead tissue, bacterial products, and foreign bodies are powerful chemoattractants sustaining a continued influx of inflammatory cells, which in turn produce a variety of growth factors, cytokines, and matrix-degrading enzymes. Among the most potent of these enzymes are elastase (Figure 8.7) and the matrix metalloproteinases, which are present in large amounts in chronic wounds.[31]

Given the low levels of protease inhibitors in these wounds, the proteolytic enzymes gain the upper hand in degrading all protein elements found in the tissue, including collagen, fibronectin, and growth factors. Under these conditions, matrix deposition does not gain a foothold, and epithelialisation proceeds slowly. It is quite clear how such a scenario can create a vicious cycle capable of perpetuating wound chronicity. Therefore, any effective intervention must include a strategy for disrupting this cycle and setting the wound on a permanent path toward healing. Wound debridement can achieve this objective by removing the proteolytic triggers and restoring a wound microenvironment that favors healing.

Principles of Therapy

Identifying and treating all the factors that negatively impact wound healing requires detailed patient evaluation and careful thought. Ensuring good nutrition and adequate systemic and peripheral perfusion are key to promoting wound healing. Treatment of underlying medical problems that may affect healing is also important.

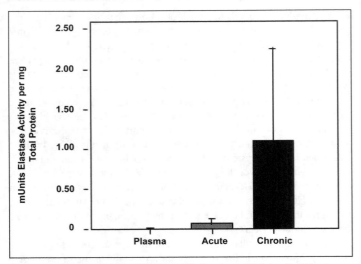

Source: Yager DR, Chen SM, Ward BS, Olutoye OO, Diegelmann RF, Cohen IK. Ability of chronic wound fluid to degrade peptide growth factors is associated with increased levels of elastase activity and diminished levels of proteinase inhibitors. Wound Repair and Regeneration 1997; 5:23.

Figure 8.7: Levels of elastase activity are significantly higher in chronic wound fluid compared with acute wound fluid. Elastase activity was determined by a colorimetric assay using methoxysuccinyl-ala-ala-proval-p-nitoanilide substrate.

Prevention is the best treatment for hospital-acquired ulcers. Assess patients daily for pressure ulcer risk, and evaluate at-risk areas frequently. This includes visualisation of the back and sacrum, areas under blood pressure cuffs, tracheostomy sites, oral and nasal tubes, oxygen delivery devices, arm boards, and cast edges. Apply protective padding to at-risk sites, turn and reposition patients every 2 hours; specialty beds that redistribute weight may be used. If an ulcer does develop, clean the site regularly, debride necrotic tissue, manage bacterial colonisation and infection, and maximise nutritional status.

Maintaining a physiologic local wound environment helps to create conditions conducive to rapid repair and restoration of function. Topical wound management allows manipulation to positively influence the local environment. This includes cleansing, preventing and managing infection, debridement, protecting periwound skin, and use of dressings to mimic skin and create a more physiologic local environment. Take measures to create adequate moisture level, control temperature, establish physiologic pH, ensure good local blood flow, and control bacterial burden.

For local wound care, a variety of dressing choices exist. Common components include hydrogel (glycerin), foam (polymers), hydrocolloid (carboxymethylcellulose), collagen, alginate, cellulose, cotton, rayon, and transparent dressings (polyurethane). Saline-moistened gauze placed in the wound bed and covered by a semiocclusive dry dressing is a simple and effective wound care option. Ultimately, the choice of dressing is based on numerous factors, including clinical indications, patient and caregiver needs, product availability, health care setting, and cost.

Surgery remains an important aspect of wound care. This is particularly true for chronic and complex wounds. Surgical debridement helps to create a wound bed with more physiologic conditions. Skin grafts and tissue flaps can be used to replace missing tissue, fill defects, and cover underlying structures. Surgical decision making for wound care should include a complete patient assessment incorporating comorbid conditions and nutritional status. Further, decision making should involve a wound assessment that includes causative factors, tissue condition, and chronicity. Finally, selection of the wound closure method should be made preoperatively to decrease blood loss, ensure optimal and adequate donor sites, and minimise ischaemic times.

Negative Pressure Wound Therapy
Newer devices and technology have been developed and are thought to provide potential advantages for treatment and management of large, complex, and chronic wounds. In particular, negative pressure wound therapy (NPWT) is thought to be beneficial by removing fluid, increasing perfusion, applying mechanical stretch triggering cellular proliferation, and reducing wound size through equal distribution of mechanical forces.[32,33] Data on NPWT from randomised controlled trials is scarce; however, case reports and retrospective studies have demonstrated enhanced healing in acute traumatic wounds, chronic wounds, infected wounds, wounds secondary to diabetes, sternal wounds, and lower limb wounds.[34] NPWT does appear to prepare a wound bed for surgery and decrease time to healing. Several studies have shown that NPWT can provide safe and cost-effective wound care in children and provide such patient advantages as less frequent dressing changes, outpatient management, resumption of daily activities, and a high degree of patient tolerance with decreased pain.[35-37] It can be particularly useful in large wounds and in chronic or nonhealing wounds.

Nutrition in Wound Healing
Nutrition is fundamental to cellular function and tissue survival, repair, and integrity. All phases of wound healing require nutrients for cell function and survival. Inadequate nutrition is associated with decreased wound tensile strength and longer healing times. Optimisation of nutrition of all paediatric surgical patients is essential for surgical care and will directly impact tissue healing from visceral anastomosis to cutaneous tissue.

Healing requires adequate protein, fat, carbohydrates, vitamins, and minerals: Proteins supply amino acids required for collagen synthesis. Carbohydrates and fats provide an important energy source to support wound repair. Vitamin C is an essential cofactor for hydroxylation during collagen synthesis. Vitamin A is required for normal epithelialisation and proteoglycan synthesis. Zinc is important for cell proliferation and granulation tissue formation.

Initial and continued nutritional assessment of paediatric surgical patients is important to provide the proper support and ensure adequate wound healing for both acute and chronic wounds. Assessment may include body mass index and laboratory data such as serum albumin and prealbumin.

Paediatric versus Adult Wounds
Although wound healing in neonates and children follows the same orderly progression of events as that for adults, tissue defects generally tend to close faster.[38] In children, fibroblasts are present in greater numbers, collagen and elastin are more rapidly produced, and granulation tissue forms faster than it does in adults.[39] Distinct intricacies of the neonatal and paediatric populations, such as epidermal and dermal immaturity, a high body surface-to-weight ratio, sensitivity to pain, and an immature immune system, create additional levels of complexity.[39]

There is a paucity of research in paediatric wound care to guide practice, and few wound care products have been studied in children. Due to the lack of guidelines and evidence-based practice, it is important to be mindful that the normally rapid wound-healing response of children can be delayed by a number of factors, including impaired perfusion, infection, prolonged pressure, oedema, poor nutrition, and the wound macro- and micro-environment.

Conclusion
Treatment starts with thorough patient and wound assessment. Monitor wounds frequently and evaluate treatment daily. Select and adjust wound care regimens based on patient condition, wound status, and resources. When necessary, timely surgical intervention is essential to ensure optimal healing. In many cases, such as wounds from burns, trauma, and hospital-acquired pressure ulceration, policies and guidelines leading to prevention are the best first steps.

As care providers, it is important to approach our patients with compassion and understanding. Treatment of physical and emotional pain is essential. We must provide the best care within our means and recognise when to transfer patients with greater needs. Finally, we must recognise and adequately control pain for our patients. Pain management should be an integral part of wound care and a regimen selected to achieve successful healing while treating the pain associated with the injury and caused by wound care measures.

Table 8.1: Evidence-based research.

Title	Enteral nutritional support in prevention and treatment of pressure ulcers: a systematic review and meta-analysis
Authors	Stratton RJ, Ek AC, Engfer M, et al.
Institution	Institute of Human Nutrition, University of Southhampton, Southhampton General Hospital, Southhampton, UK
Reference	Ageing Res Rev 2005; 4(3):422–450
Problem	Evaluation of nutritional support in patients with, or at risk of developing, pressure ulcers.
Intervention	Enteral nutritional support.
Comparison/ control (quality of evidence)	Fifteen studies (including eight randomised controlled trials (RCTs)) of oral nutritional supplements (ONS) or enteral tube feeding (ETF), were included in the systematic review.
Outcome/ effect	Meta-analysis showed that oral nutritional supplements (250–500 kcal, 2–26 weeks) were associated with a significantly lower incidence of pressure ulcer development in at-risk patients compared to routine care (odds ratio 0.75, 95% CI 0.62–0.89, 4 RCTs, n=1224, elderly, postsurgical, chronically hospitalised patients). Enteral nutritional support, particularly high protein ONS, can significantly reduce the risk of developing pressure ulcers (by 25%).
Historical significance/ comments	This highlights the need for nutritional optimisation of patients to prevent pressure ulcers and to aid in healing.

Evidence-Based Research

Table 8.1 presents an evaluation of enteral support in patients at risk of developing or who already have pressure ulcers. Table 8.2 presents a study of negative pressure wound therapy.

Table 8.2: Evidence-based research.

Title	Negative pressure wound therapy after severe open fractures: a prospective randomized study
Authors	Stannard JP, Volgas DA, Stewart R, et al.
Institution	Division of Orthopaedic Surgery, University of Alabama at Birmingham, Birmingham, Alabama, USA
Reference	J Orthop Trauma 2009; 23(8):552–557
Problem	Treatment of significant wounds related to trauma.
Intervention	Negative pressure wound therapy (NPWT).
Comparison/ control (quality of evidence)	Twenty-three patients with 25 fractures were randomised to a control group and underwent irrigation and debridement followed by standard dressing, with repeat irrigation and debridement every 48–72 hours until wound closure. Thirty-five patients were randomised to the NPWT group and had identical treatment except that NPWT was applied to the wounds between irrigation and debridement procedures until closure.
Outcome/ effect	There was a significant difference between the groups for total infections (P = 0.024). The relative risk ratio was 0.199 (95% confidence interval: 0.045–0.874), suggesting that patients treated with NPWT were only one-fifth as likely to have an infection compared with patients randomised to the control group.
Historical significance/ comments	NPWT represents a promising therapy for severe wounds after high-energy trauma.

Key Summary Points

1. Understanding the basic mechanisms involved in normal wound healing and tissue response to injury is critical in surgical treatment and management.

2. The healing response involves four broad, overlapping phases: haemostasis, inflammation, proliferation, and remodelling. This dynamic process optimally leads to restoration of tissue integrity and function.

3. Identifying and treating all the factors that negatively impact wound healing requires detailed patient evaluation and careful thought.

4. Surgery remains an important aspect of wound care, particularly for chronic and complex wounds.

5. Elucidating the molecular aspects of foetal response to tissue injury, which leads to scarless wound repair, may provide insights to new wound-healing therapies.

References

1. Lazarus GS, et al. Definitions and guidelines for assessment of wounds and evaluation of healing. Wound Repair Regen 1994; 2(3):165–170.

2. Gross RJ. Regeneration versus repair. In: Cohen IK, Diegelmann RF, Lindblad WJ, eds. Wound Healing: Biochemical and Clinical Aspects, WB Saunders, 1992, Pp 20–39.

3. Olutoye OO, Cohen IK. Fetal wound healing: an overview. Wound Repair Regen 1996; 4(1):66–74.

4. Lee, R.C., Doong, H., Control of matrix production during tissue repair. In: Anderson DK, Lee RC, Mustoe TA, Siebert, JW, eds. Advances in Wound Healing and Tissue Repair, World Medical Press, 1993, Pp 1–25.

5. Keswani SG, Crobleholme TM. Wound healing: cellular and molecular mechanisms. In: Oldham KT, Colombani PM, Foglia RP, Skinner MA, eds. Principles and Practice of Pediatric Surgery, Lippincott Williams and Wilkins, 2005, Pp 223–238.

6. Schilling JA. Wound healing. Surg Clin North Am 1976; 56(4):859–874.

7. Weigel PH, Fuller GM, LeBoeuf RD. A model for the role of hyaluronic acid and fibrin in the early events during the inflammatory response and wound healing. J Theor Biol 1986; 119(2):219–234.

8. Fine NA, Mustoe TA. Wound healing. In: Greenfield LJ, Mulholland MW, Lilemoe MD, Oldham KT, eds. Surgery Scientific Principles and Practice. Lippincott Williams and Wilkins, 2001, Pp 69–85.

9. Lorenz HP, Longaker MT. Wounds: biology, pathology, and management. In: Norton JA, Chang AE, Lowry SF, Mulvihill SJ, Pass HI, Thompson RW, eds. Essential Practice of Surgery: Basic Science and Clinical Evidence, Springer, 2003, Pp 77–88.

10. Levenson SM, et al. The healing of rat skin wounds. Ann Surg 1965; 161:293–308.

11. Rockwell WB, Cohen IK, Ehrlich HP. Keloids and hypertrophic scars: a comprehensive review. Plast Reconstr Surg 1989; 84(5):827–837.

12. Olutoye OO, et al. Lower cytokine release by fetal porcine platelets: a possible explanation for reduced inflammation after fetal wounding. J Pediatr Surg 1996; 31(1):91–95.

13. Haynes JH, Krummel TH, Schatzki PF, Flood LC, Cohen IK, Diegelman RF. Histology of the open fetal rabbit wound. Surg Forum 1989; 40:558–560.

14. Krummel TM, et al. Fetal response to injury in the rabbit. J Pediatr Surg 1987; 22(7):640–644.

15. Longaker MT, et al. Adult skin wounds in the fetal environment heal with scar formation. Ann Surg 1994; 219(1):65–72.

16. Armstrong JR, Ferguson MW. Ontogeny of the skin and the transition from scar-free to scarring phenotype during wound healing in the pouch young of a marsupial, *Monodelphis domestica*. Dev Biol 1995; 169(1):242–260.

17. Block M. Wound healing in the new-born opossum (*Didelphis virginianam*). Nature 1960; 187:340–341.

18. Frantz FW, et al. Biology of fetal repair: the presence of bacteria in fetal wounds induces an adult-like healing response. J Pediatr Surg 1993; 28(3):428–433; discussion 433-434.

19. Yager DR, Nwomeh, BC. The proteolytic environment of chronic wounds. Wound Repair Regen 1999; 7(6):433–441.

20. Oluwasanmi JO. Keloids in the African. Clin Plast Surg 1974; 1(1):179–195.

21. Marneros AG, et al. Clinical genetics of familial keloids. Arch Dermatol 2001; **137**(11):1429–1434.

22. Murray JC, Pinnell SR. Keloids and excessive dermal scarring. In: Cohen IK, Diegelmann RF, and Lindblad WJ, eds. Wound Healing, Biochemical and Clinical Aspects, Saunders, 1992, Pp 500–509.

23. Ball CS. Global issues in pediatric nutrition: AIDS. Nutrition 1998; 14(10):767–770.

24. van der Werf TS, et al. Mycobacterium ulcerans disease. Bull World Health Organ 2005; 83(10):785–791.

25. Doughty D, Sparks-Defriese B. Wound-healing physiology. In: Bryant RA, Nix DP, eds. Acute and Chronic Wounds: Current Management Concepts. Mosby, 2007, Pp 56–81.

26. Ferreira MC, et al. Complex wounds. Clinics (Sao Paulo) 2006; 61(6):571–578.

27. Jones KR, Fennie K, Lenihan A. Evidence-based management of chronic wounds. Adv Skin Wound Care 2007; 20(11):591–600.

28. Falanga V. Chronic wounds: pathophysiologic and experimental considerations. J Invest Dermatol 1993; 100(5):721–725.

29. Nwomeh BC, Yager DR, Cohen IK. Physiology of the chronic wound. Clin Plast Surg 1998; 25(3):341–356.

30. Dinsdale SM. Decubitus ulcers: role of pressure and friction in causation. Arch Phys Med Rehabil 1974; 55(4):147–152.

31. Nwomeh BC, et al. MMP-8 is the predominant collagenase in healing wounds and nonhealing ulcers. J Surg Res 1999; 81(2):189–195.

32. Frantz R, Broussard C, Mendez-Eastman S, Cordrey R. Devices and technology in wound care. In: Bryant RA, Nix DP, eds. Acute and Chronic Wounds: Current Management Concepts. Mosby, 2007, Pp 427–460.

33. Jones SM, Banwell PE, Shakespeare PG, Advances in wound healing: topical negative pressure therapy. Postgrad Med J 2005; 81(956):353–357.

34. Mendonca DA, Papini R, Price PE. Negative-pressure wound therapy: a snapshot of the evidence. Int Wound J 2006; 3(4):261–271.

35. Baharestani MM. Use of negative pressure wound therapy in the treatment of neonatal and pediatric wounds: a retrospective examination of clinical outcomes. Ostomy Wound Manage 2007; 53(6):75–85.

36. Caniano DA, Ruth B, Teich S, Wound management with vacuum-assisted closure: experience in 51 pediatric patients. J Pediatr Surg 2005; 40(1):128–132.

37. McCord SS, et al. Negative pressure therapy is effective to manage a variety of wounds in infants and children. Wound Repair Regen 2007; 15(3):296–301.

38. Bale S, Jones V, Caring for children with wounds. J Wound Care 1996; 5(4): 177–180.

39. Baharestani MM. An overview of neonatal and pediatric wound care knowledge and considerations. Ostomy Wound Manage 2007; 53(6):34–36, 38, 40, passim.

CHAPTER 9
VASCULAR ACCESS IN CHILDREN

James O. Adeniran
Hugo A. Heij

Introduction

Every child presenting to the paediatric surgeon will require vascular access at one time or another during the management of the child's surgical condition. Vascular access becomes critical in patients brought to the hospital as emergencies because many of them may have been on treatment in private hospitals for some time, and the obvious veins have been used already. This common task may be even more daunting with factors such as restlessness due to the clinical pathology, shock, unavailability of appropriate catheters, obese patients, and children with multiple limb injuries.[1] It is therefore important for the paediatric surgeon to be familiar with how to gain access to the vascular tree as and when necessary.

The first part of this chapter considers peripheral vascular access, and the second part considers central vascular access. Indications, techniques of catheter insertion, complications and management of these complications, and the cost-benefit aspect in the African setting are discussed.

Peripheral Vascular Access

Indications for Africa

Virtually all patients presenting to a paediatric surgeon need blood tests for diagnosing their ailments, assessing their fitness for anaesthesia, and use in postoperative management. Accurate figures for Africa are not known, but in the United States an estimated more than 200 million peripheral catheters are placed annually.[2] Vascular access is one of the new tools that enables the neonatologist and paediatric surgeon to provide ongoing therapy for very ill babies, at the same time allowing invasive monitoring of the clinical condition.[3] Many patients present to the paediatric emergency room with intestinal obstruction as neonates with anorectal malformations, Hirschsprung's disease, or bowel atresias.[4] Older patients present with peritonitis, usually due to typhoid or appendix perforation.[5] Some patients also present with multiple trauma, and others may present with sickle cell disease in crises. These patients need urgent vascular access for administration of fluids, blood products, drugs, and nutritional formulas.[3]

Venous Access

Venous access is needed for administration of drugs during resuscitation, induction and maintenance of anaesthesia, during cytotoxic therapy, and in haemodialysis. Stem-cell harvest for research and bone marrow transplantation in cases of leukaemias also need venous access. Nutritional support can be given to many patients through peripherally inserted central catheters. Other indications and uses for venous access are shown in Table 9.1.

Aterial Access

Arterial access is used much less in developing countries, not because the indications are lacking, but because the necessary equipment is not available. Arterial sampling for O_2 estimation and cardiovascular monitoring in very ill children, especially those who need ventilation, needs arterial access. Various radiological procedures for diagnosis and treatment are becoming popular in children. Children bleeding from

Table 9.1: Indications for peripheral vascular access.

Indications	Uses
Venous blood sampling	For various diagnostic tests
Resuscitation	Fluids, blood and blood products in:
	Intestinal obstruction
	Peritonitis
	Trauma
	Preoperative work-up
Administration of other products	Drugs during resuscitation
	Drugs during anaesthesia
	Correction of anaemia/coagulation defects
	Parenteral nutrition
	Cytotoxic drugs
Use as central venous access	

the gastrointestinal tract may need digital substraction angiography (DSA) for diagnosis and management. Many advanced liver and renal tumours can now be embolised by using the arterial route with excellent palliation.

Physiology

The French physiologist Jean Marie Poiseuille[6] in 1839 defined resistance through a vessel as:

$$\text{Resistance} = 8 \text{ (viscosity) (catheter length)} / \pi r^4$$

Resistance through the catheter decreases as the length of the catheter decreases and the radius r increases. Maximum flow is therefore best when the catheter is short and wide.

Sites of Peripheral Vascular Access

Venepuncture
Umbilical vein
The umbilical vein may remain patent for up two weeks.[7] It is easily cannulated in neonates and is used extensively in third-world countries for venous blood sampling, infusion of crystalloids and colloids, administration of drugs, and exchange blood transfusion. The technique is described below. Portal vein thrombosis can follow prolonged use; therefore, a peripheral vein should be secured as soon as possible. Platelets should not be infused through the umbilical vein.[7]

Upper limb
The upper limb is the preferred site for cannulation in children. Because the dorsal venous arch starts from the dorsum of the wrist, this site is most commonly attempted first in most children. Two or three veins may be found at the radial and ulna borders. The origin of the cephalic vein may be seen over the snuff box in older children. The cephalic and basilic veins and one or two veins crossing them may be visible at the cubital fossa.

Lower limb

In the lower limb, two veins are usually visible at the lateral border of the dorsum of the foot, and one at the medial border of the tibia. The long saphenous and femoral veins may not be readily visible in most children unless light-complexioned, but they are anatomically just medial to the femoral artery, which is easily palpable at the groin.

Scalp

The superficial temporal vein is usually prominent in the crying child, and easy to cannulate by using the butterfly needle.

Arterial punctures

Although the radial artery at the wrist may be big enough in older children, the femoral artery at the groin is most commonly used in younger children. The superficial temporal artery is small but easily palpable.

Bone punctures

The medial border of the tibia is subcutaneous throughout its length. The proximal part of this subcutaneous border just below the tibia tuberosity opens into a wide marrow from which blood could be aspirated for investigations. Fluids, blood, and drugs could also be rapidly infused for resuscitation.

Technique of Venepuncture

Umbilical vein

The umbilical stump of a neonate has two small thick-walled umbilical arteries, and a large, thin-walled umbilical vein, enmeshed in Wharton's jelly (Figure 9.1).

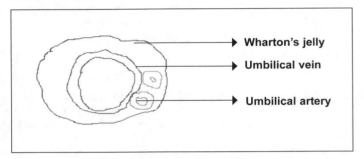

→ Wharton's jelly

→ Umbilical vein

→ Umbilical artery

Source: Courtesy of Dr. Adeyinka A. Adesiyun, University of Ilorin Teaching Hospital, Ilorin, Nigeria.

Figure 9.1: Transverse section of a neonate's umbilicus.

The baby should be kept warm under a radiant warmer and loosely restrained. The umbilical cord, clamp, and surrounding skin is cleaned with a suitable antiseptic. A size 5 or 6 feeding tube is recommended for cannulation. This tube is primed with normal saline with a 5-ml syringe attached. The base of the umbilicus is tied loosely with a sterile piece of umbilical tape or 2'0 silk suture to control bleeding. The umbilical cord is now transected about 3 cm from the base. The vein is picked with forceps and the catheter inserted and advanced until blood flows back freely into the catheter. Saline in the syringe is injected and should flow without resistance. The catheter is secured by two purse-string silk sutures at the base of the umbilicus, and further taped at several points to the skin of the abdomen.

Cannulation at the wrist

The first attempt at cannulation at the wrist should be successful in the "virgin" wrist if appropriate steps and precautions are followed. All necessary equipment should be assembled, including tourniquet, sterile swabs, appropriate catheters, infusion fluids, and plaster to anchor the catheter. Adequate illumination is also necessary. The site chosen for cannulation should be cleaned with an antiseptic solution to prevent introduction of organisms ab initio. It is also important for the clinician to wear protective gloves to prevent contacting diseases such as hepatitis or human immunodeficiency virus (HIV). In venepuncture of the wrist in young children, the wrist could be palmar-flexed and the

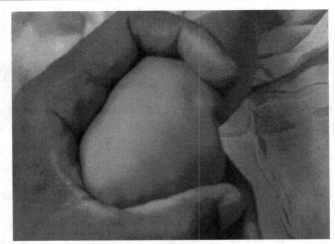

Figure 9.2: Technique of venepuncture at the wrist.

index finger used as a tourniquet while the rest of the hand steadies the child's wrist (Figure 9.2).

If a vein is not immediately visible, the limb can be placed dependent for a couple of minutes before a tourniquet is applied or the wrist can be slapped gently.

An older patient can be asked to grip and relax the fingers for a few minutes. Topical venodilatation may be achieved by topical application of 4% nitroglycerin ointment for 2–4 minutes.[8] Ultrasound, using a handheld Doppler, can be used to locate forearm veins in obese patients.[9] The visible or palpable vein is cleaned with antiseptic fluid. The catheter is then inserted until blood fills the chamber. The hub of the catheter is then withdrawn a little and the rest of the catheter inserted. The infusion fluid is then connected to allow the fluid to open up the rest of the vein. The catheter can then be advanced as far as desirable. Because many children are restless, a small cardboard may be used as a splint. If two or three attempts on one wrist are not successful, the other wrist should be tried by a more experienced person.

Cannulation at other sites

If attempts at both wrists are not successful, the ante-cubital fossa should be tried next. If a tourniquet is applied just above the ankle and the foot is planter-flexed and turned to equinus position, one or two veins may be visible on the dorsum of the foot. The superficial temporal vein over the temple is easily cannulated in children. As the child cries, the superficial temporal artery is easily palpable and provides a guide to the vein, which is just anterior to it. A scalp vein needle can be used for short periods or a cannula for longer periods.

Technique of Arterial Punctures

Intraarterial cannulation allows the clinician to continuously monitor the cardiovascular status of patients and to obtain blood samples for blood gases necessary for ventilatory support and acid-base management. The umbilical artery at the umbilical stump can be easily cannulated in neonates.[3] The radial artery at the wrist and the femoral artery at the groin can also be cannulated percutaneously and for radiological procedures. Dorsalis pedis and posterior tibial arteries can also be used. The brachial artery is usually avoided because of poor collateral circulation; similarly, the superficial temporal arteries are avoided to prevent cerebral infarcts.

For arterial cannulation of limbs, an Allen's test is first performed.[7] In this test, both arteries that supply a limb are compressed for a few minutes. One artery is then released. If the collateral circulation is adequate, the extremity should flush in colour within 5 seconds. The artery can be accessed by either a Seldinger technique[10] or by a cutdown. Blood products, pressors, calcium boluses, and sodium bicarbonate should not be infused through arterial catheters.

Venous Cutdown

A cutdown may be necessary to establish a rapid vascular access, for example, when all visible superficial veins may have been used or the patient comes in shock. The long saphenous vein, either near the ankle or at the groin, the femoral vein at the groin, and the basilic vein at the elbow or the cephalic vein at the delto-pectoral grove are all suitable sites. The area around the chosen vein is cleaned and draped aseptically, then infiltrated with a suitable local anaesthetic. A transverse incision is made only in the skin over the vein. A haemostat is then used to widely open the subcutaneous tissues. The vein is usually then visible. The distal end of the vein is ligated. A small needle is passed transversely across the vein, and the part of the vein superficial to the needle is transected. A suitable catheter is then inserted and anchored with stitches. The transverse skin incision is closed with one or two stitches. The catheter is anchored to skin with both stitches and plaster.

Intraosseous Infusion

The bone marrow space is a rich, noncollapsible venous network.

Intraosseous infusion is a quick method of resuscitating children in shock when immediate intravenous access fails. Crystalloids, colloids, drugs (including anaesthetic drugs), and blood can be given rapidly through this route.[11] The flat, anteromedial, subcutaneous, upper aspect of the tibia 1–3 cm below the tibia tuberosity is usually used (Figure 9.3). Other sites that could be used are:

• the midline of the distal femur 3 cm proximal to the femoral condyles;

• distal tibia proximal to the medial malleolus;

• anterior superior iliac spine;

• lateral malleolus; or

• proximal humerus distal to deltoid insertion.

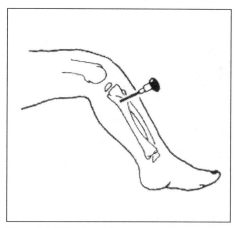

Figure 9.3: Technique of intraosseous infusion.

The chosen site is cleaned and draped, and a little local anaesthetic is given. A Jamshidi needle (which has a trochar), or bone marrow needle, or any size 13–18 butterfly needle can be used. The needle is introduced perpendicular to the skin, then angled away from the growth plate until a "give" is felt. The trochar is then removed. Blood should be aspirated to confirm that the needle is in the marrow. The infusion fluid can then be connected. Sterile gauze and plaster are used to secure the needle. The intraosseous route is for emergency only, and should not be used for more than 2–3 hours. As soon as possible, it should be replaced by a suitable intravenous site.

Complications of Peripheral Vascular Access

Infection/cellulitis

Although our bodies do not normally react to catheters, they are, never-theless, foreign bodies. Catheters should therefore be retained only for as long as necessary. Feeding and drugs should be changed to the oral route as soon as possible. After 2–3 days, signs of inflammation may appear at the site of cannulation. These include pain, redness, and swelling. If the redness appears other than along the site of cannulation, cellulitis is setting in, and the site of cannulation will need to be changed. If the catheter is being used for parenteral nutrition, intravenous antibiotics may be given in an attempt to salvage the line. If the catheter is planned for long-time use, it may be advisable to give regular antibiotics through the vein from the beginning.[12] The presence of infection elsewhere, prolonged hospital stay, immunosuppression, and poor catheter care all contribute to catheter-related sepsis.

Thrombosis/thrombophlebitis

Thrombosis can occur in a catheter, and the thrombus can dislodge to distant parts with grave consequences to the patient. Early signs of thrombosis are inadequate flow in the infusion fluid and extravasation. Use of silicone catheters, parenteral nutrition, and diabetes may predispose the patient to thrombosis. Aortic thrombosis can complicate umbilical artery cannulation, which may lead to leg or bowel gangrene. If persistent blanching of skin of the leg occurs, the catheter may need to be removed. Regular flushing with normal saline, heparin, or urokinase may serve as a preventive. After the catheter has been removed, the vein may become a painful, fibrotic, noncompressible "cord". This is thrombophlebitis. Only painkillers are necessary, as the condition usually settles with time.

Extravasation/skin necrosis

When a new catheter is inserted in a vein, sterile water or saline should be injected first and must be seen to flow freely before the injection of drugs. If this is not done, drugs containing calcium, bicarbonate, or thiopentone, and drugs for chemotherapy can extravasate into subcutaneous tissues, causing necrosis. The dorsum of the hand and foot are common sites. If a toxic drug is given accidentally, application of ice packs to the area, subcutaneous irrigation with water or saline, and injection of hyaluronidase or steroid may reduce the amount of tissue damage.[12] If frank skin necrosis occurs, debridement, sometimes with delayed skin grafting, may be necessary.

Cannula dislodgement/fracture/embolisation

Catheters need to be anchored properly with plaster, and cutdowns should be secured with stitches. Brisk bleeding can occur when an arterial catheter inadvertently dislodges. Pressure for a couple of minutes will usually stop the bleeding. Appropriate splints are necessary in restless children. If frequent intravenous injections are necessary in a restless or shocked patient, or if a patient is receiving rapid intravenous infusions, a second line should be considered. Fracture of a cannula with embolism at distant sites has been reported.

Complications

Complications of peripheral cannulation include:

• haemorrhage/failed cannulation;

• air embolus during catheter insertion, tube change, or tube removal;

• infection/cellulitis;

• thrombosis/thrombophlebitis;

• extravasation/ skin necrosis;

• cannula dislodgement/fracture/embolisation;

• injury to surrounding structures (artery, nerve, solid organs);

• compartment syndrome/osteomyelitis; and

• ugly scars from subcutaneous extravasation, when debridement and skin grafting have been done.

Care should be taken not to injure the corresponding artery, especially during cutdowns. Once the vein is exposed, the artery should be clearly palpated before any vessel is ligated. Complications from intraosseous infusions are rare, but skin necrosis, compartment syndromes, and osteomyelitis can occur.

Central Venous Access

This section discusses the purposes of central venous access (CVA), the techniques and devices tailored to the purposes, and the complications (both short- and long-term). For long-term central venous access, an operating theatre and general anaesthesia with fluoroscopy are ideal, and will give the best results. The cost-benefit aspect of CVA in the African setting is addressed in the final paragraph.

Incidence/Prevalence in the African Setting

Percutaneously placed short-term central venous catheters (CVCs) have been the primary means of central venous access in critically ill children.[13] Central venous access for administration of drugs or blood products can be required urgently in patients with severe trauma or other life-threatening conditions. A chronic need for CVA will arise in patients with oncological or intestinal conditions and for total parental nutrition.[13] About 5 million CVCs are inserted in the United States annually.[2] The role of the paediatric surgeon in CVA is to offer service to paediatric doctor colleagues, and the need for CVA will depend on the type of paediatric (surgical) practice.

The main patient categories are oncology, congenital intestinal malformations, and short bowel syndrome, with lesser demands from haematology (sick cell disease) and orthopedics (intravenous antibiotics for septic arthritis and osteomyelitis). Devices and facilities for CVA are expensive, so the applicability also depends on financial considerations.

Applications and Indications

The indications of central venous access include:

- rapid infusion of intravenous fluids and blood products;

- frequent blood sampling/blood transfusions;

- administration of substances that are likely to damage peripheral veins, such as cytotoxics or hyperosmolar parenteral nutrition (PN);

- long-term administration of drugs (antibiotics) or blood products, obviating the need for repeated venepunctures in children;

- central venous pressure and haemodynamic monitoring of acutely ill patients; and

- haemodialysis.

Clinical Considerations

Need for emergency central venous access

In patients with life-threatening conditions, the need for CVA is obvious at presentation. Although large-bore peripheral cannulas may be used for initial access in the emergency room, CVA will be required as soon as the patient is admitted to the intensive care unit (ICU). Four routes are available for transcutaneous insertion of a central venous catheter:

1. cephalic or basilic veins in the arm;

2. internal jugular vein;

3. subclavia vein; or

4. femoral vein.

The advantages and disadvantages of these routes are summarised in Table 9.2.

Long-term Use of Central Venous Access

Long-term CVA is mainly required for administration of cytotoxics and/or parenteral nutrition. The techniques of insertion and the devices are different from those used in emergency CVA.

Table 9.2: Advantages and disadvantages of different routes for central venous access.

Access	Advantages	Disadvantages
Arm veins	Simple to access, veins visible, and palpable Not close to vital organs Comfortable for patient	Failure to achieve central position High incidence of thrombosis Low maximum infusion rates
Internal jugular	Simple to insert Direct route to central veins High flow-rate Low risk of thrombosis Low risk of pneumothorax	Uncomfortable for patient High rate of long-term complications Tunneling to chest wall more difficult
Subclavian/axillary	Less patient discomfort Lower risk of long-term complications	Curved incision route Difficult to access Higher rate of pneumo/haemothorax
Femoral	High flow rate Good for dialysis Easy insertion	Higher rate of infection/thrombosis More discomfort for patient Difficult in obese patients

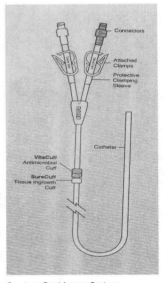

Courtesy: Bard Access Systems.

Figure 9.4: A double-lumen Hickman catheter.

Types of Catheters

A typical catheter for long-term use (such as seen in Figure 9.4) has the following essential features:

- Is manufactured from soft silicon rubber or polyvinyl chloride (PVC).

- Is chemically inert, nonthrombogenic, flexible, and radio-opaque.

- May have single-, dual-, or triple-lumen, which allows simultaneous infusion or infusion of incompatible solutions.

- Has a Dacron cuff (e.g., SureCuff®), which has a matrix that expands after insertion and into which subcutaneous fibrous tissue grows for good anchorage.

- Is a VitaCuff®, which incorporates an antimicrobial collagen sponge designed to prevent infection.

• Has a plastic area where clamps can be applied.

• Has connectors.

• Costs about US$135 (100 euros) each.

Broviac® catheters

Long-term, tunneled catheters have been available since 1968. In 1973, Broviac[14] made the first important improvement to the design by producing a catheter with an internal diameter of 1.0 mm, which facilitates repeated blood sampling.

Hickman® catheters

Robert Hickman,[15] a paediatric nephrologist at the Seattle Children's Hospital, modified the Broviac catheter with subcutaneous tunneling and a Dacron cuff that forms an infection barrier. Broviac and Hickman catheters are open-ended and can be cut to the desired length. The major difference between the Broviac and the Hickman is the internal diameter: the Broviac is 1.0 mm, and the Hickman is 1.6 mm.

Groshong® catheters

The Groshong catheter has a design similar to the Hickman but has a formed blunt end with a slit-like orifice just proximal to the distal end. This acts like a valve, which stops back-bleeding, prevents air entry and embolism from negative intrathoracic pressure, and obviates the need for a heparin lock because saline can be used instead. An external clamp, which may damage the catheter, is therefore unnecessary. Groshong catheters cannot be used to monitor central venous pressure due to the valve function. The valves may, however, produce intermittent boluses of fluid or drugs, which may make these catheters unsuitable for inotropic or vasopressor infusion.

The advantages of Groshong catheters are that they are flexible and the insertion site is removed from the exit site. These assist in the prevention of systemic infection. Once the tissue adheres to the Dacron cuff, another barrier to infection is created. The secured cuff also prevents catheter dislodgment.

The main disadvantages of Groshong catheters are that, being outside the body, they provide vehicles for infection. They also require frequent flushes and dressing changes. There are also limitations for swimming and bathing. The catheters are not suitable for dialysis as they are not designed for high-flow blood withdrawals.

Port-a-Cath®

Port-a-Cath[16] catheters are silicon catheters connected to self-sealing injection ports that are completely inserted under the skin. The intravascular segment is similar to the Hickman catheter. The port is a small metal, plastic, or titanium "drum" or reservoir that has a membrane through which the vein can be accessed by using a special Huber-type needle. Suture holes in the base of the port are anchored to fascia layers with nonabsorbable sutures.

The Port-a-Cath catheter has the following features:

• lightweight, durable titanium portal reservoir, which provides gouge resistance and long-term durability;

• contoured shape, designed for patient comfort and ease of portal palpation;

• needle-stop titanium reservoir floor, which creates positive tactile feedback when the accessing needle makes contact;

• distinct rounded septum ring, designed to assist in septum location;

• high compression SECUR SITE® septum captured in titanium, designed for needle retention and stability;

• bevelled suture holes, designed for ease of suturing;

• ULTRA-LOCK® catheter connector integrated with portal, for ease of system assembly; and

• magnetic resonance imaging (MRI)-compatible portal systems.

The two main advantages of Port-a-Cath catheters are that no part of the catheter is exposed, so the infection rate is low, and that catheter displacement and venous occlusion are uncommon. Other advantages are that the catheter requires flushing only every 5–6 weeks, regular dressing is not required after the incision has healed, and the patient can bathe or swim. The Port-a-Cath can be used for brief general anaesthesia (e.g., lumbar puncture).

The two main disadvantages of these catheters are that insertion is time-consuming and that general anaesthesia is necessary for insertion and removal. Another disadvantage is that the assessing needles have fine bores, so blood transfusion is slow. These catheters are very costly, at about US$675–1350 (500–1000 euros) each.

Peripherally Inserted Central Catheters

Peripherally inserted central catheters (PICC) are fine-bore soft catheters that are passed from cubital veins up the axillary vein into a central vein. They are used as alternatives to Hickman catheters. They generally have higher rates of phlebitis, occlusion, and thrombosis than tunneled catheters.

Surgical Techniques

Insertion of central venous catheter in emergency situations

To be considered a central line, the tip of the catheter must be located in the vena cava, subclavian, brachiocephalic, innominate, or iliac veins.

The safest technique for insertion of a CVC via the transcutaneous route into the internal jugular vein, subclavian, or femoral vein is by the Seldinger[10] method. Complete catheter sets, including aspiration needle, guidewire, dilatator, peel-away sheath, and polyurethane catheter, are available as packs from several companies. In young children, the procedure is best performed under general anaesthesia, but in older or very sick patients, the site can be infiltrated with local anaesthetics. The veins are easier to cannulate by using ultrasound guidance.

Important steps in inserting a central venous line are listed below. These are essentially the steps in the Seldinger technique:

1. Explain the procedure (including possible complications) to the patient.

2. Have the patient or parent sign a consent form.

3. Get all necessary equipment—port, catheter, saline, syringes, heparin solutions, etc.

4. Scrub and down surgical gown and gloves (an assistant may be necessary).

5. Open the port and catheter and flush with heparinised saline. Make sure all connections are working properly.

6. Prep the patient with povidone iodine and drape the required field.

7. Identify the landmarks and infiltrate the required area with local anaesthetic.

8. Place the patient in the Trendelenburg position.

9. Insert an 18-gauge (20G for infants) needle into the chosen vein until blood is freely aspirated (ultrasonic guidance may be helpful).

10. Remove the syringe while retaining the needle.

11. Insert the J-shaped end of the guide wire into the needle (check the position with fluoroscopy, if available).

12. Remove the needle.

13. Advance the dilatator over the guide wire and remove the dilatator.

14. Insert the catheter over the guide wire.

15. Suture the catheter in place.

16. If a port is needed, dissect the subcutaneous tissue with mosquito artery forceps and bluntly with finger to accommodate the port.

17. Flush all ports with heparinised saline.

18. Give the patient intravenous antibiotics.

19. Take a chest x-ray to confirm the final position and rule-out pneumothorax.

Percutaneous insertion into internal jugular vein

The internal jugular vein (IJV) is the most frequently chosen site for insertion of central venous catheters.[17] The right IJV is commonly used because most practitioners are right handed, and the right vein is wider than the left[18] and has a more direct route to the superior vena cava and the right atrium. The right lung is also lower than the left so that injury to the lung is less, and the thoracic duct is on the left side. The risk of pneumothorax is less with IJV cannulation. If there is carotid artery injury, manual compression can easily control the haemorrhage.

For the cannulation, a sandbag is placed behind the patient's shoulders, and the head is turned to the contralateral side. The patient is placed in the Trendelenburg position, and the field cleaned with antiseptic solution. The carotid artery is palpated and gently pushed away at the level of insertion. The vein is approached at 30° to the sagittal plane at the medial border of the sternomastoid midway between the thyroid cartilage and the hyoid bone in the direction of the ipsilateral nipple. If the syringe is aspirated during insertion, the vein should be entered within 2–4-cm depth. The Seldinger technique is then followed. Easier cannulation is now advisable with ultrasonic guidance by using a handheld Doppler probe.[19–21] This not only reduces the number of needle passes to locate the vein, but also decreases the risk of injury to the carotid artery.[21,22]

Percutaneous insertion into subclavian vein

The subclavian vein (SCV) may be preferred for central venous access if, for example, the patient has a cervical spine injury, or if the line is for long-term use (e.g., dialysis, feeding) and this site may be more comfortable for the patient.[17] The risk of long-term complications is lowest with SCV cannulations.

The SCV is the continuation of the axillary vein and originates at the lateral border of the first rib. The SCV passes over the first rib anterior to the subclavian artery, to join with the internal jugular vein at the medial end of the clavicle. The external jugular vein joins the SCV at the midpoint of the clavicle.

The patient is placed supine in the Trendelenburg position. The head is turned to the contralateral side (if C-spine injury has been excluded). The Seldinger technique is adopted.

The needle is introduced 1 cm below the junction of the middle and medial thirds of the clavicle. The needle is directed medially, slightly cephalad, and posteriorly behind the clavicle towards the suprasternal notch. The needle is slowly advanced while gently withdrawing the plunger. When a free flow of blood appears, the Seldinger approach is followed, as detailed previously. The catheter tip should lie in the superior vena cava above the pericardial reflection. A chest x-ray is done to confirm position and exclude pneumothorax. A major disadvantage of this route is that if there is injury to the subclavian artery, direct pressure cannot be easily applied to control bleeding.

Percutaneous insertion into femoral vein

The femoral route is useful in emergency situations or the patient is coagulopathic,[17] but incidences of infection and thrombosis are the highest in this technique.

The long saphenous vein joins the popliteal vein to form the femoral vein, which accompanies the femoral artery in the femoral triangle. To access the vein, the artery is first felt by palpation. Then, keeping a finger on the artery, a needle attached to a 10-ml syringe is introduced at 45 degrees, 1.5 cm medial to the femoral artery pulsation, 2 cm below the inguinal ligament, until blood is aspirated. The Seldinger technique is then continued as described above.

Insertion of catheter for long-term use

The main difference between long-term and short-term catheters is the application of tunnelled catheters in the former situation, which allows long-term (months or even years) use. The central venous access can either be an external silastic catheter (Broviac or Hickman) or an internal device, where the catheter is connected to a subcutaneous reservoir or port (Port-a-Cath).[23]

For long-term central venous access, either the transcutaneous (Seldinger) route described above or the open approach can be used. The open approach allows the use of smaller veins that can be sacrificed, such as the external jugular vein in the neck, the cephalic vein in the deltopectoral fossa, the great saphenous vein, or the epigastric vein in the groin. The open approach requires an "entrance" site where the catheter is inserted into the vein, and an "exit" site where the catheter exits the chest wall, with a tunnel between the two. If the open approach is used for large veins (internal jugular or femoral), a purse-string suture should be put in the anterior wall of the vein and the catheter inserted in the centre.

Complications of Central Venous Access

Catheter clotting and other complications cost the health care system in the United States about one billion dollars annually.[2] Prevention of complications such as those described in the following subsections is the best way to "manage" CVCs.

Haemorrhage/haematoma

Brisk bleeding may occur with CVA, especially if the adjacent artery is injured. Pressure for a few minutes should control the bleeding. Pressure may be difficult to apply if the subclavian artery is injured.

Catheter-related sepsis

In general, CVA has great advantages but requires special facilities, carries significant risks of complications, and is associated with considerable financial costs. The insertion of a foreign body with direct access to the circulation can be considered a cordial invitation to microorganisms to invade the patient. Oncologic patients receiving cytotoxics that depress the bone marrow are particularly at risk of sepsis. Line infection is therefore the most frequent complication leading to early removal of the system. Infection may occur either at the time of insertion or later during changes of connections. Catheter-related infection rates vary from 3% to 60%.[24,25] The infection can be at the exit site, in the tunnel, or catheter-related. Exit-site infections are usually due to *Staphyloccoccus epidermidis*, and can usually be managed by local wound care. Tunnel or pocket infection relates to suppuration in the subcutaneous tunnel relating to the foreign body. The port will need to be removed with antibiotic treatment. Catheter-related sepsis (especially in patients receiving parenteral nutrition) is the most serious of the catheter-related sepsis.

Depending on the clinical condition of the patient, a trial treatment with broad spectrum antibiotics (e.g., amoxicillin, metronidazole, and gentamicin) should be started in all children with fever and a CVC in situ. Fifty percent or more of the CVC can be salvaged with this policy. If the clinical condition does not improve after 24 hours, removal of the CVC should be considered. A layer of glycoprotein (the glycocalix) forms on the silastic wall of the catheter, which harbours bacteria that are protected from antibiotics. The use of ethanol both as prophylactic and therapeutic modalities in patients with repeated CVC infections has been proposed.

If the catheter is removed due to sepsis, either the tip of the catheter can be rolled on to a plate for culture[26,27] or the lumen of the catheter can be flushed with a nutrient broth (the Cleri technique),[28] which is then cultured. The blood through the catheter can also be sampled and cultured before removal.[29] Kite[30] and others have proposed using a small brush to sample endoluminal organisms without removal of the catheter. Due to the risk of bacterial embolisation, this method has not gained routine use, especially in the intensive-care setting.[31] The risk of infection can be reduced by strict adherence to a protocol and reduction of the number of caretakers that manipulate the line.

Thrombosis

The second commonest complication is thrombosis with or without obstruction of the catheter. It is thought that thrombosis starts at the site of the venepuncture and then migrates along the catheter to eventually occlude the tip. Ultrasound examination of CVCs shows that more than 50% have thrombus at the tip of the line.[31] However, clinically manifest thrombosis is rare and occurs mainly in newborns and infants. So far, no studies support the use of prophylactic anticoagulants. If thrombosis is diagnosed, intravenous heparin should be started and anticoagulant treatment with warfarin continued for 3 months. Increasingly more data have now become available on the long-term sequelae of CVC, particularly in oncologic patients. Significant postthrombotic signs and symptoms occur in less than 10%.

Malposition

Malposition is any tip position other than in the superior or inferior vena cava. Placement or migration of the catheter tip into the right atrium may cause cardiac arrhythmias or myocardial erosion. Damage to the wall of the superior vena cava and leakage of fluid into the pericardial space resulting in tamponade have been reported. Also, catheters in the right atrium may be associated with thrombus formation and valvular damage. If the tip is not in a large vessel (and blood cannot be aspirated freely), there is a substantial risk of thrombosis and perforation with extravasation into the pericardial or pleural space.

Obstruction of catheter

Obstruction of the central venous cannula can be caused by administration of incompatible mixtures that form debris. Also, the CVC should be rinsed after withdrawal of blood, and care should be taken to keep the CVC open by continuous flow of infusion. If the CVC is not in use, it should be filled with a heparin solution. If the CVC is blocked, it can sometimes be unblocked by pushing normal saline with a small (2-ml) syringe. Although this manoeuver can be successful, it may result in rupture of the CVC.

Pinch-off

The term "pinch-off" refers to entrapment of subclavian catheters between the clavicle and the first rib. Over time, repeated compression causes catheter fracture, resulting in extravasation of fluids, or catheter breakage and embolisation.

Ethical Issues

The cost-benefit aspect of central venous access in the African setting is addressed in this final paragraph. The use of central venous catheters in the long term is in itself not lifesaving and is potentially dangerous. The advantages are that the caretakers always have CVA, even when the child is asleep. This obviates the need for multiple attempts to set up intravenous lines, allowing normal day-to-day activities and administration of drugs as prescribed on time. It reduces patient (and parent) anxiety, resulting in a better atmosphere. The price of all these benefits is—apart from the financial burden [Broviac, US$200 (150 euros); Port-a-Cath, US$675 (500 euros); use of operating theatre, US$1350 (1000 euros); plus cost of treatment of complications]—also the risk of potentially life-threatening complications. The balance will have to be found for each individual centre and patient.

Evidence-Based Research

Table 9.3 presents a prospective Brazilian study of complications of CVC placement in children.

Table 9.3: Evidence-based research.

Title	Central venous catheter placement in children: a prospective study of complications in a Brazilian public hospital
Authors	Cruzeiro PCF, Carmagos PAM, Miranda ME
Institution	Pediatric Surgical Services, Clinics Hospital, Federal University of Minas Gerais, Belo Horizonte, Minas Gerais, Brazil
Reference	Pediatric Surg Intl 2006; 22:536–540
Problem	This study evaluates the complications of percutaneously placed central catheters in a public hospital.
Study design	Prospective study.
Length of study	Eight months.
Results	155 catheters (130 in neck, 25 in groin) were placed in 127 patients. The cannulation success rate was 81.9% at the first attempt and 100% at the second attempt.
Complications	Perioperative complications: haematomas, 6 (3.9%); arterial puncture, 3 (1.9%). Complications with catheter in situ: mechanical, 51(32.9%); infections, 33 (21.3%).
Outcome/ effect	Age, sex, type of catheter, and primary diagnosis were not associated with complications. There was no pneumothorax, hemothorax, or hydrothorax, and no mortality.
Conclusions	Knowledge of anatomy and familiarity with the Seldinger technique improve the success rate. Percutaneously placed central venous catheters produce satisfactory results in paediatric patients.

Key Summary Points

1. Virtually every child will need vascular access.

2. Maximum flow is achieved with catheters that are wide and short.

3. The umbilical vein can be used for up to 2 weeks in neonates for administration of colloids or crystalloids, and for exchange blood transfusion.

4. The back of the hand is the most commonly used site for venous access in infants.

5. The antecubital fossa, dorsum of the foot, and snuffbox can be accessed in older children.

6. The long saphenous vein at the ankle or at the groin, the femoral vein, antecubital veins, and the cephalic vein are suitable for venous cutdowns.

7. The intraosseous space is a rich, noncollapsible venous network.

8. The upper surface of the tibia, iliac crest, lateral malleolus, and upper femur can be used for bone punctures.

9. The internal jugular vein, subclavian vein, and femoral vein are suitable for central venous access.

10. The Seldinger technique is used for inserting central cannulas.

11. Common complications of vascular access include haemorrhage, line infection, and thrombosis.

References

1. Mbamalu D, Banerjee A. Methods of obtaining peripheral venous access in difficult situations. Postgrad Med J 1999; 75:459–462.

2. Laguna Medical Systems: The Coding Edge Archives. Available at: http://www.lagunamedsys.com/edgearchive/TOC.

3. Jona JZ. Vascular access in the newborn. In: Prem Puri, ed., Newborn Surgery. Arnold, 2003, Pp 120–129.

4. Adeniran JO, Odebode TO. Congenital malformations in paediatric and neurosurgical practices: problems and pattern (a preliminary report). Sahel Med J 2005; 8:4–8.

5. Adeniran JO, Taiwo JO. Typhoid intestinal perforation in children in Ilorin: salmonella versus the surgeon: who is winning the race? Trop J H Sci 2007; 15:61–65.

6. Poiseuille. Available at: http://galileo.phys.virginia.edu/classes/311/notes/.

7. Hansen AR, Greene A, Puder M. Vascular access. In: Hansen AR and Puder M, eds., Manual of Neonatal Surgical Intensive Care. BC Decker Inc, 2003, Pp 117–129.

8. Michael A, Andrew M. The application of emla and glycerine trinitrate ointment prior to venepuncture. Anaesth Intens Care 1996; 24:360–364.

9. Whiteley MS, Chang BP, Marsh HP, Williams AR, Marton HC, Horrocks M. Use of hand-held Doppler to identify "difficult" forearm veins for cannulation. Ann R Coll Surg Engl 1995; 77:224–226.

10. Seldinger SI. Catheter replacement of the needle in percutaneous arteriography. Acta Radiol 1953; 39:368.

11. Intraosseous route. Available at: http://en.wikipedia.org/wiki/main_Page.

12. Barnett AM, Squire R. Vascular access. In: Stringer MD, Oldham KT, Mouriquand PDE, eds. Pediatric Surgery and Urology. Long-term Outcomes. Cambridge University Press, 2006, Pp 947–957.

13. Sol J, van Woensel J, van Ommen C, Bos A. Long-term complications of central venous catheters in children. Paediatrics and Child Health 2007; 3:89–93.

14. Broviac J, Cole J, Scribner B. A silicon rubber right atrial catheter for prolonged parenteral alimentation. Surg Gynecol Obstet 1973; 136:602–606.

15. Hickman R, Buckner C, Clift R, Sanders J, Stewart P, Thomas E. A modified right atrial catheter for access to the venous system in marrow transplant recipients. Surg Gynecol Obstet 1979; 148:871–875.

16. Bard Access Systems. Available at: http://www.bardaccess.com/picc_hick_buv_leon.php.

17. Duffy M, Sair M. Cannulation of central veins. Anaesth Intensive Care Med 2007; 8:17–20.

18. Lobato EB, Sulec CA, Moody RL. Cross sectional area of the right and left internal jugular veins. J Cardiothorac Vasc Anesth 1999; 13:136–138.

19. Denys BG, Uretsky BF, Reddy PS. Ultrasound-assisted cannulation of the internal jugular vein. A prospective comparison to the external landmark-guided technique. Circulation 1993; 87:1557–1562.

20. Caridi JG, Hawkins IF Jr, Wiechmann BN. Sonographic guidance when using the right internal jugular vein for central vein access. Am J Roentgenol 1998; 171:1259–1263.

21. Keenan SP. Use of ultrasound to place central lines. J Crit Care 2002; 17:126–137.

22. Gilbert TB, Seneff MG, Becker RB. Facilitation of internal jugular venous cannulation using an audio-guided Doppler ultrasound vascular access device: results from a prospective, dual-center, randomized, cross-over clinical study. Crit Care Med 1995; 23:60–65.

23. Bernacle A, Arthurs AJ, Rowbuck D, Hiofns MP. Malfunctioning central venous catheters in children: a diagnostic approach. Pediatric Radiology 2008; 38:363–378.

24. Anderson A, Krasnow S, Boyer M. Thrombosis: the major Hickman catheter complication in patients with solid tumour. Chest 1989; 95:71–75.

25. Green F, Moore W, Strickland G, McFarland J. Comparison of a totally implantable access device for chemotherapy (Port-A-Cath) and long-term percutaneous catheterization (Broviac). South Med J 1988; 81:580–603.

26. Hartman G, Shochat S. Management of septic complications associated with silastic catheters in childhood malignancy. Pediatr Infect Dis J 1987; 6:1042–1047.

27. Maki D, Weise C, Sarafin H. A semiquantitative culture method for identifying intravenous catheter related infection. N Engl J Med 1977; 296:1305–1309.

28. Cleri D, Corrado M, Seligman S. Quantitative culture of intravenous catheters and other intravascular inserts. J Infect Dis 1980; 141:781–786.

29. Blot F, Nitenberg G, Chachaty E. Diagnosis of catheter-related bacteraemia: a prospective comparison of the time to positivity of hub-blood versus peripheral-blood cultures. Lancet 1999; 354:1071–1077.

30. Kite P, Dobbins B, Wilcox M. Evaluation of a novel endoluminal brush method for in-situ diagnosis of catheter-related sepsis. J Clin Pathol 1997; 50:278–282.

31. McLure H, Juste R, Thomas M, Soni N, Roberts A, Azadian B. Endoluminal brushing for detection of central venous catheter colonization—a comparison of daily vs single brushing on removal. J Hosp Infect 1997; 36:313–316.

CHAPTER 10
ANAESTHESIA AND PERIOPERATIVE CARE

Mark Newton
Stella A. Eguma
Olamide O. Dairo

Introduction

The practice of providing surgical anaesthesia for children dates back to 1842, when Dr. Crawford Long used ether for an amputation on an 8-year-old boy. Since that event, many paediatric patients have been administered anaesthesia with ether. Today, however, essentially all of the anaesthetic drugs used in the adult population are used in paediatrics. Major steps forward—such as the use of endotracheal intubation (1936), the Jackson-Rees modification of the T-piece (1950), the precordial stethoscope (1953), the use of muscle relaxants (1940s), and the introduction of the newer inhalation anaesthetic agents (1960s)—have allowed the administering of anaesthesia to become safer.

Today, anaesthesia is provided for the paediatric patient on a daily basis in many hospitals throughout the world, despite ongoing challenges. In Africa, for example, the paediatric patient presents for surgery with a pathophysiological picture that can be very different from that of a similar patient in the typical Western hospital setting. The addition of malnutrition, tropical diseases such as tuberculosis and malaria, delayed presentation, poor primary care, and chronic disease states can compound the acute surgical problem that is prompting intervention. In many African settings, the basic hospital infrastructure, theatre supplies, and essential monitoring equipment—all of which make paediatric anaesthesia safer—are commonly unavailable. Anaesthesia supplies appropriately sized for neonates and small children, such as endotracheal tubes, blood pressure cuffs, and even small syringes that allow for safe anaesthesia care, are not available in many hospitals. These issues, as they relate to providing anaesthesia care for neonates and paediatric patients who require surgery in the African setting, challenge even the most skilled of anaesthesia care providers.

This chapter provides an overview of some of the challenges when providing anaesthesia care for children in Africa. The chapter reviews the cardiac, respiratory, and renal differences of children in comparison to adults. Additionally, it addresses preoperative assessment, including guidelines for nothing by mouth (NPO, or *nil per os*), general and regional anaesthesia, intraoperative monitoring, airway management, and postoperative care.

Differences in Anatomy and Physiology

Cardiovascular Function

Neonatal myocardial function demonstrates a cardiac output that is relatively fixed due to the inability of the neonate to increase the stroke volume, which would allow for a higher cardiac output. The neonate cardiac muscle has fewer contractile elements per gram of tissue when compared to an adult heart; this affects the neonate's ability to compensate for hypovolaemic states. Also, the parasympathetic nervous system is more developed than the sympathetic nervous system until the age of 6 months, when the two systems become more balanced. This imbalance in the autonomic nervous system in the neonate predisposes the neonate to bradycardia during times of stress, even with simple airway suctioning, and certainly during airway intubation attempts. This difference between the neonate and the adult is evident during times of

hypovolaemia, such as during intestinal obstruction, many neonatal emergencies, and delayed medical management for many surgical cases because neonates cannot increase their heart rates sufficiently to overcome the decrease in stroke volume.

Congenital heart disease (CHD) is common in the neonatal surgical patient in comparison to the normal population. Many congenital surgical problems have associated cardiac anomalies; therefore, any neonate presenting for surgery needs to have an appropriate cardiac exam. If a murmur is present, then a further work-up may be indicated prior to surgical intervention, and anaesthetic adjustments must be made in an effort to maximise the oxygen delivery and blood pressure. A chest x-ray and oxygen saturation determination will help to determine the need for further more specialised work-up, if available. The need for antibiotic coverage perioperatively should be considered in all patients with a cardiac defect. Currently, an antibiotic given preoperatively either 60 minutes orally or 30 minutes intravenously (IV) will cover the risk of endocarditis.[1]

Respiratory Function

The neonatal airway's narrowest location is the cricoid cartilage and not the vocal cords, as it is in the adult. Also, the glottis is more anterior, with the epiglottis being less rigid, which tends to occlude the airway opening when attempting an intubation. All of these anatomical differences between a neonate and an adult can result in a more difficult intubation when attempting to place the endotracheal tube, but with a skilled anaesthesia care provider, this also can become routine. The induction and intubation of a neonate requires special care because the oxygen saturation will decrease much faster than in an adult patient due to the higher neonatal oxygen consumption and high minute ventilation/functional residual capacity (FRC) ratio in the neonate. A premature infant will have an immature chemoreceptor ventilatory drive and at times slow respiratory effort with an elevation in carbon dioxide levels. For many premature infants, apnea, which is cessation of ventilation for 20 seconds with bradycardia, can be a serious postoperative problem that needs careful monitoring.[1]

Renal Function

The newborn's immature renal function can contribute to many fluid and electrolyte problems in the surgical patient. Glomerular filtration rates (GFRs) reach adult levels by 1 year of age, and the newborn's inability to concentrate urine certainly affects the ability of the newborn to respond to times of hypovolaemia. The infant's inability to balance sodium levels appropriately prompts careful attention to the balance of sodium because the renal system's immaturity results in an overall sodium loss.

Temperature Regulation

Temperature regulation differences result in the newborn having hypothermic periods in the perioperative period. The infant's relatively large surface area, inability to shiver, large head size (related to heat loss), and poor insulation can cause dangerously low temperature levels, which can cause hypoventilation and even cardiac arrhythmias. The room temperature for the newborn needs to be closely monitored; in areas where the outside environment has more impact on the theatre temperature, the use of warming pads and even small heating units may need to be utilised to maintain the patient's body temperature. The use of the type of heating pad that can be purchased in most African capital cities needs to be monitored in the theatre setting, as this pad can cause burns in the neonate if the controls and the patient's temperature are not monitored diligently. Also, the use of warmed fluids at appropriate levels needs to be considered in any theatre where paediatric surgery is more common.

Haematology

The red blood cells in the newborn are very different from those of adult haemoglobin because fetal haemoglobin dominates, and at 6–8 months of age, this subunit of haemoglobin is absent. Foetal haemoglobin has a higher affinity for oxygen; hence, the oxygen-carrying capacity is higher. Many paediatric patients in the African setting may present for surgery with a relative anaemia, and some may need further investigations. Although nutritional causes of anaemia need to be considered first, there are many potential causes, such as malaria, sickle cell disease, intestinal worms, and even drug-induced anaemias. Many paediatric patients can have elective surgery when their haemoglobin is less than 8 gm/dl, but these patients will have a better postoperative course with supplemental oxygen. In the context where sickle cell haemoglobin analysis is not available, blood is given to sickle cell disease patients who present for surgery with a haemoglobin level below 8g/dl.

Preoperative Assessment and Preparation

The emotional stress evident in the eyes of the paediatric patients and parents in the preoperative setting prompts one to make every effort to alleviate this aspect of the anaesthesia and surgical experience. The preparation by the anaesthesia care provider should include a preoperative visit at which the provider determines the need for surgery, the physiological implications for anaesthesia, the necessary laboratory evaluations, and the psychological condition of the patient and family. If this is done in advance, and all questions by the family as well as the surgical team are answered, then the overall care of the paediatric patient will improve. The patient may indeed benefit from a preoperative sedative or other medication so that the transfer from floor care to the theatre care will be smoother.

Psychological factors, which include the patient's age, the cultural norms for surgery, the impact of previous medical care prior to the patient arriving at the institution, and the pathophysiological condition of the patient, all impact the preoperative preparation. Children between the ages of 6 months and 5 years tend to demonstrate the most fear when presenting to the theatre setting. A carefully arranged preoperative environment that can help with these fear issues may allow for easier transfer to the operating theatre. Also, a good physical exam that includes the cardiorespiratory system, nervous system, and gastrointestinal system will allow the anaesthesia care provider the opportunity to develop an anaesthesia plan that is more informed and safe.

Disorders of the central nervous system (CNS) are common in the paediatric patient; trauma—which is very high in this population in every country in the world—can produce closed head injury patients who present in the acute and the chronic phases of trauma. Seizure disorders with anticonvulsant drugs need to be evaluated for their efficacy and such haematologic side effects as low platelets. Cerebral palsy, neuromuscular diseases, and polio are all common aetiologies for a paediatric patient who presents for an orthopaedic procedure or an emergency surgery, and special care needs to be taken in the anaesthesia plan for such populations.

The incidence of congenital cardiac diseases is more common in the paediatric surgical patient than it is in the general population. If a murmur is discovered in the preoperative work-up, it needs to be evaluated. Even a pulse oximetry reading that is normal rules out many

intracardiac shunt lesions, which can be very helpful information for the anaesthesia plan. Respiratory problems, such as adenoid hypertrophy, cleft palate, upper airway infections, and asthma, are commonly seen in the surgical patient and add to the anaesthesia risks. Typically, if a patient presents with an acute productive cough, fever, or wheezing, then elective surgeries need to be cancelled for a minimum of 2 weeks to allow for resolution of the underlying infectious process and the corresponding airway effects. For the preterm infant, the incidence of apnoea and bradycardia increases the need for cardiorespiratory monitoring in the postoperative period for 12–24 hours, depending upon the severity of the problem.

Fasting Guidelines

The preoperative NPO guidelines for surgical procedures for the paediatric population will be different from those for the adult population. An infant younger than 12 months of age can have breast milk or clear liquids up to 4 hours presurgery. After the age of 12 months, clear liquids up to 4 hours and solids (including formula) up to 6 hours presurgery are allowed. All children on diets with fatty foods need to wait 8 hours after a solid meal for elective surgery. Of course, emergency surgery cases need to proceed without consideration of the NPO status, and precautions should be taken to avoid pulmonary aspiration of gastric contents. The glucose status of a neonate who presents for surgery and has had an intravenous line needs close evaluation so that hypoglycaemia does not interfere with the anaesthesia management.

Premedication

The use of preanaesthetic medication to remove anxiety is common in the paediatric population. The use of anticholinergics, benzodiazepines, and narcotics can be adjusted by the anaesthesia care provider to produce the desired effect with weight-appropriate doses. There are risks involved in a setting with few nurses per patient population in the ward, as an elevated dose of the drug may be given inadvertently because the doses are small volumes for the paediatric patient and the side effects may be difficult to detect.

Premedication should be individualised to each patient on the basis of age, weight, level of anxiety, previous anaesthetic experience, allergies, and expected level of cooperation. The oral route remains the commonest way of giving premedication. It has the advantage of being painless, but may have an unpredictable onset or a bitter taste. Midazolam, a short-acting water-soluble benzodiazepine, is widely used for premedication in paediatric practice. It has a fairly reliable onset and duration of action and can be given through a variety of routes, including oral, nasal, sublingual, rectal, intravenous, and intramuscular (IM). It does not appear to prolong recovery room stay or time to hospital discharge. Other commonly used premedication drugs include fentanyl, ketamine, sufentanil, clonidine, and, increasingly, dexmedetomidine. Although some of these agents may not be available, each institution needs to assess its drug availability and budget and then seek an alternative to these agents if they are available.

Premedications should be avoided in the patient with elevated intracranial pressure and carefully titrated in the patient with congenital heart disease as well as the severely depressed child who presents for emergency surgery. The generalities that are presented in this section prompt anaesthesia care providers and surgeons to carefully assess their specific clinical situations and then determine whether the use of premedication is safe and advantageous for their specific population of paediatric patients.

Anaesthetic Management

At the end of the preoperative assessment, an anaesthetic plan is made that takes into consideration the medical condition of the child, the needs of the proposed surgical operation, and a way of allaying any anxiety being felt by the parents and the child. All medications and materials, including blood and intravenous fluids, must be ready before induction begins. All equipment, including the anaesthetic machine, must be checked and confirmed to be working properly.

Adequate preoperative preparation (including building rapport with the patient) and the rational use of premedication will facilitate safe and atraumatic induction of anaesthesia.

Induction of Anaesthesia

Like premedication, induction of anaesthesia should be tailored to the individual patient. The same factors used to determine suitable premedication come into play when choosing an induction method. Inhalational and intravenous routes of induction are more common than rectal and intramuscular routes, although ketamine can be used in the paediatric population when an IV line is not in place or not needed for a very short procedure such as a dressing change.

Because of their fear of needles, inhalational induction is most common for children up to 10 years of age (and perhaps even well into the teenage years) who are undergoing elective surgery. This method is particularly useful because inhaled anaesthetic drugs increase in concentration in the alveoli of children more rapidly than they do in adults. Inhalational induction should be a slow, smooth process with care taken to keep the airway patent at all times. Sevoflurane is replacing halothane as the agent of choice because it appears to have fewer cardiovascular side effects while being faster in onset and recovery. However, many anaesthesia care providers in developing countries may not have access to sevoflurane, and halothane will be the available agent. Halothane in the hands of a trained paediatric anaesthesia care provider will allow for a very smooth induction with the patient ventilating spontaneously, but very careful cardiac monitoring needs to be vigilantly performed.

Intravenous induction is the method of choice when there is a pre-existing IV or when inhalational induction is contraindicated (e.g., in the event of trauma or any full stomach scenario). Thiopentone, ketamine, and propofol remain the main induction agents. Etomidate, when available, can also be useful. Intramuscular induction is often used in the older uncooperative child who cannot be reasoned with, such as a child with autism or mental retardation. In settings where resources are limited, intramuscular ketamine can be useful for very short procedures such as circumcision and wound debridement.

If the patient is cooperative, monitors are applied before induction; otherwise, they are put on as early as possible during induction and kept on until the patient is fully awake. The use of a precordial stethoscope and, if available, a pulse oximeter can provide sufficient monitoring for the induction period, allowing one to assess the airway and cardiac system with limited monitoring equipment.

Maintenance of Anaesthesia

The anaesthetic may be continued by using inhalational agents, intravenous agents (including muscle relaxants and opioids), or a combination of these agents in a balanced technique. During this stage, the airway is kept patent by either a face mask, a laryngeal mask airway (LMA), or an endotracheal tube.

Airway Management

One of the greatest challenges in paediatric anaesthesia is the management of the airway, particularly in neonates. Combinations of anatomical, physiological, and developmental factors conspire to make airway management in children more difficult than that in adults. Normal respiratory rates are 40 per minute in neonates and 20–30 per minute in infants. The smaller size of the paediatric airway means that any small decrease in diameter, such as occurs from secretions, bronchconstriction, oedema, or compression, may more readily lead to significant airway obstruction. Respiration is mainly diaphragmatic in infants; therefore, any slight abdominal distention will greatly embarrass respiration. Oxygen consumption in the neonate is approximately 7 ml/kg per minute, as opposed to 3–4 ml/kg per minute in the adult. For infants

and children, the higher oxygen requirements per kilogram produce hypoxia more rapidly when there is airway obstruction. Perioperative paediatric airway obstruction occurs commonly when the consciousness level is depressed and the airway is not properly positioned to maintain its patency.[2]

Airway Maintenance Equipment

Paediatric airway equipment is usually designed to minimise trauma, dead space, airway resistance, and rebreathing. Equipment for airway maintenance includes face masks (Figure 10.1), oropharyngeal and nasopharyngeal airways (Figure 10.2), breathing circuits and Ambu bags, laryngoscopes, endotracheal tubes, and laryngeal mask airways.

Face Masks

Face masks come in different sizes (00 for neonates, 0 for infants, 1 for small children, 2 for bigger children), shapes, and colours (see Figure 10.1). The neonatal face mask has minimal dead space and is designed to limit rebreathing. It must fit closely over the mouth and nose without obstructing the nares.

Breathing Circuits

The Ayre's T-piece breathing circuit (Figure 10.3) is used for children weighing less than 20 kg because it is a low-resistance circuit. For children weighing more than 20 kg, an adult circuit (Bain or Magill) can be used. The Ayre's T-piece can be used for both spontaneous and assisted ventilation.

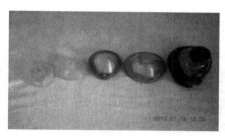

Figure 10.1: Various sizes of paediatric masks.

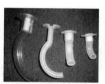

Figure 10.2: Oropharyngeal airway.

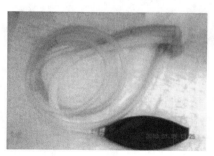

Figure 10.3: An Ayre's T-piece.

Laryngoscopes

The relatively high position and inclination of the larynx in infants make a straight laryngoscope blade (e.g., the Miller 0 (Figure 10.4) or the infant Magill) a good choice, whereas children older than 1 year of age can generally be managed with a curved blade (e.g., size 2 Macintosh (Figure 10.5)).

Laryngeal Mask Airways

LMAs (Figure 10.6) are useful airway management tools. They are less traumatic than endotracheal tubes and do not require laryngoscopy to insert. They do not, however, protect against regurgitation and aspiration. Sizes 1, 1½, 2, 2½, and 3 can be used in children from 2 months to 12 years of age, according to the weight of the child.

Endotracheal Tubes

Endotracheal tubes used for children younger than 6 years of age are usually uncuffed. Table 10.1 provides a guide for choosing an appropriate endotracheal tube.

Mask Ventilation

Due to the neonate's relatively large head, a small roll should be positioned under the shoulders to prevent hyperflexion of the head and align the axis of the mouth, pharynx, and larynx to allow for easy flow of air. For the older child, no pillow or roll is needed. An appropriately sized oropharyngeal airway can improve mask ventilation.

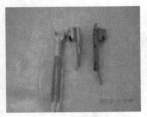

Figure 10.4: Miller's blades and handle.

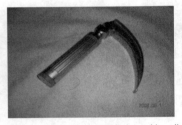

Figure 10.5: Macintosh blade and handle.

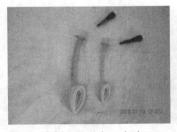 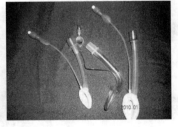

Figure 10.6 Laryngeal mask airways.

Table 10.1: Endotracheal tube sizes for children.

Age	Size of endotracheal tube (mm)
Premature	2–2.5
Full-term newborn	3.0
6–12 months	3.5
1–2 years	4–4.5
>2 years	4.5 + [age (in years) ÷ 4]

Laryngoscopy and Intubation

The airway should be ventilated in all but the shortest of procedures because the paediatric airway is very prone to obstruction during anaesthesia. For neonates and infants, a slight external pressure on the larynx helps to bring the glottis into view. A small leak should be allowed around the tube to prevent oedema formation and postoperative airway obstruction, which may follow prolonged intubation.[3] If the patient is at risk of aspiration, a pharyngeal gauze pack should be placed around the tube.

A gaseous induction using 100% oxygen with halothane is the technique of choice in small children and those with difficult airways. The aim is to attain a plane of anaesthesia that is deep enough to allow laryngoscopy. Once the pupils become constricted and central, laryngoscopy and orotracheal intubation can be performed. Suxamethonium at a dose of 2 mg/kg can be used to facilitate intubation. Atropine (0.02 mg/kg) or glycopyrrolate (0.01 mg/kg) should be given to prevent bradycardia and to dry secretions. Both lungs should be auscultated for bilateral air entry after intubation, and the endotracheal tube should be secured firmly in position.

Signs of respiratory obstruction include an increase in respiratory rate (>50 per minute in an infant and 30 per minute in a child); a "see-saw" pattern of chest and abdominal breathing movements; flaring of the alar nasi; and the use of accessory muscles of respiration (sternomastoids, scalene muscles) resulting in suprasternal, intercostal, and subcostal retraction.

In acute airway obstruction, for which one cannot intubate or ventilate, cricothyrotomy may be the only option. Cricothyrotomy is difficult in a small child and carries many risks. Where difficult tracheal intubation is anticipated, experienced help should be sought beforehand. There are fibre-optic laryngoscopes suitable for use in children, but this requires expertise and experience and is not an option in emergency airway obstruction.

Muscle Relaxants

Muscle relaxants are used to facilitate tracheal intubation and provide muscle relaxation during surgery, thus permitting lighter planes of anaesthesia and reducing the risk of cardiovascular depression. They are used in intraperitoneal, intrathoracic, and intracranial procedures.

Muscle relaxants are classified into depolarising and nondepolarising groups. Succinylcholine is the only depolarising neuromuscular blocker in use today, and it remains the agent with the quickest onset and shortest duration of action. Unfortunately, succinylcholine is associated with some life-threatening side effects (hyperkalaemia, malignant hyperthermia), and its use has reduced somewhat in recent years.

Nondepolarising muscle relaxants are classified based on structure and mode of elimination. The benzoquinolones are atracurium, cis-atracurium, and mivacurium, which may be available in some African urban centres. The first two are eliminated by Hoffmann degradation and ester hydrolysis by nonspecific plasma esterases. Mivacurium is metabolised by plasma cholinesterase.

The aminosteroids (pancuronium, vecuronium, and rocuronium) are metabolised in the liver, and their inactive end products are eliminated by the kidney.

Monitoring

The purpose of monitoring is to measure physiological variables and to indicate trends of change, thus enabling corrective action to be taken. The anaesthetist remains the most important monitor and must remain in close contact with the patient during all aspects of the anaesthetic.

The precordial (or oesophageal) stethoscope is an invaluable monitor for many paediatric anaesthetists. It provides a direct way to continuously monitor heart rate and rhythm as well as breath sounds; it allows early detection of changes in the rate and character of these sounds.

The electrocardiogram (ECG) is useful for diagnosing rate-related arrhythmias, especially bradycardia and supraventricular tachycardia (SVT). The ECG is an index of electrical activity. A normal waveform may exist, however, in the presence of reduced cardiac output, so the ECG should be interpreted in the context of other information obtained from monitors of the patient's circulation.

The patient's circulation may be monitored by observation of the peripheral perfusion, peripheral pulse, blood pressure, urine output, and arterial oxygen saturation. Observation of the patient's extremities yields information about the state of the patient's circulation. When the skin is warm and dry all the way to the fingers and toes, one can infer that tissue perfusion and therefore cardiac output is adequate. Cool extremities thus indicate hypovolaemia and reduced cardiac output. Palpation of peripheral pulses is another way of obtaining the same information. As intravascular volume decreases, the pulse volume decreases, especially in the wrists and feet. Adequate production of urine implies adequate renal perfusion and probably adequate perfusion of other vital organs. Measurement of urine output is particularly indicated in critically ill or shocked patients or when massive fluid shifts are expected. A urine output of 0.75–1 ml/kg per hour is desirable. Blood pressure provides another indirect means of measuring circulating blood volume and cardiac output due to the relationship.

Blood Pressure = Cardiac Output × Peripheral Resistance.

Methods of measuring blood pressure range from palpation and auscultation to direct intraarterial manometry.

A pulse oximeter measures oxygen saturation continuously and thus provides another indirect assessment of the function of the circulatory system. Estimation of blood loss is a useful monitor in maintaining the overall integrity of the cardiovascular system.

Apart from monitoring the patient's colour, respiratory rate, and breathing pattern, auscultation of both lungs should be performed frequently.

Airway pressure monitors and disconnection alarms are desirable in ventilated patients. A capnograph, when available, can be used to confirm correct placement of an endotracheal tube and to continuously assess the adequacy of ventilation.

It is important to remember that monitors only provide information. It is the duty of the anaesthetist to interpret this information and then act appropriately. The postoperative paediatric patient needs close monitoring in the recovery room and wards when narcotics are used for surgical pain management. The vigilance of the nursing staff and anaesthesia care provider will decrease much of the morbidity and mortality associated with many paediatric, and especially neonatal, surgical patients.

Narcotics

Opioids can be titrated for intraoperative and postoperative analgesia, and to provide a smooth awakening from anaesthesia. All the commonly used opioids are used in paediatric practice and, just as in adults, in high doses they all carry the risk of respiratory depression. Fear of this respiratory depression is not a reason to deny children the benefits of opioid pain relief. Careful titration to effect will often eliminate this complication.

Regional Anaesthesia

Regional anaesthesia (RA) is particularly suited to patients undergoing outpatient procedures and peripheral surgery. It has also been suggested that RA may improve pulmonary function in patients who have had thoracic or upper abdominal surgery. Advantages include the reduced need for deeper planes of general anaesthesia in patients who have had a nerve block to supplement their general anaesthesia (GA). RA also allows a pain-free awakening while minimising or avoiding the use of opioids altogether. In addition, there is often early ambulation and excellent postoperative analgesia.

The use of RA, however, has certain limitations in paediatric practice. Except in the older child and adolescent, blocks are rarely performed in the awake child and usually need to be part of a combined technique.

Regional anaesthetic techniques are particularly useful in children at risk for malignant hyperthermia or in those for whom it is necessary

to preserve what little respiratory reserve they have (e.g., children with cystic fibrosis, severe asthma, or neuromuscular disorders).

The two classes of local anaesthetics, esters and amides, exhibit differences in distribution and metabolism in paediatric patients (especially neonates) when compared to adults. Awareness of these pharmacokinetic differences leads to safer use in this vulnerable patient population.

Ester local anaesthetics are metabolised by plasma cholinesterase, which has lower activity levels in neonates and infants up to the age of 6 months. This may theoretically lead to prolonged effects, but in practice, the effects of 2-chloroprocaine given for continuous caudal anaesthesia have been shown not to be prolonged, even when using relatively high infusion rates. In fact, in spite of the low plasma cholinesterase activity, plasma chloroprocaine levels remained low.

Amides are bound by plasma proteins and metabolised by the liver. Neonates have reduced plasma protein concentrations as well as reduced liver blood flow and immature liver enzymes. This all points to increased free drug in the plasma and potential toxicity, although the larger volume of distribution in neonates tends to offset these changes. It is thus important to follow guidelines on maximum recommended doses when doing regional blocks.

Essentially all RA blocks that are useful in the adult population can be used in the paediatric population, with special attention to the toxic drug doses and the anatomical landmarks. Many obstacles in performing RA in the paediatric population may be related to the availability of the appropriate sizes of needles for the patient, especially the neonate. Close post-block monitoring needs to be available. Especially if narcotics are to be used, the nursing staff needs to be carefully educated regarding the signs of toxicity and side effects of these drugs in the paediatric population. Table 10.2 gives the maximum recommended doses for commonly used local anaesthetic agents. Commonly performed regional procedures include caudals, epidurals, spinals, ilio-inguinal blocks, and penile blocks.

Table 10.2: Maximum recommended doses of local anaesthetics.

Local anaesthetic	Maximum dose (mg/kg)
2-Chloroprocaine	20
Lidocaine	7
Mepivacaine	7
Bupivacaine	2.5
Ropivacaine	3.5
Tetracaine	1.5

Postoperative Care

Following the end of the anaesthetic is a period of physiologic stabilisation that typically takes place in a postanaesthetic care unit (PACU), recovery room, or an intensive care unit (ICU). Emergence and recovery describe the transition from the anaesthetic state ultimately to the patient's baseline state. During this period, the patient typically awakens from general anaesthesia and regains protective reflexes.

The immediate postoperative period is a period of maximal hazard that calls for continuous patient monitoring. The commonest complications are airway obstruction, hypoventilation, and hypoxia.

For children who are intubated, the tube should remain in situ until they are fully awake. Laryngospasm is common at extubation, especially in patients who are neither very deeply anaesthetised nor fully awake. The pharynx should be carefully suctioned before extubation. Oxygen should be administered immediately after extubation, and the patient observed for adequate depth of respiration, oxygen saturation, activity, and colour. These children should be cared for by trained staff in the recovery room and should be returned to the ward only after regaining full consciousness and protective reflexes. They should be pain-free, comfortable, have stable vital signs, and there should be no active bleeding from the surgical site.

Perioperative Anaesthesia Complications

Complications may occur during anaesthesia and in the immediate postoperative period. The commonest complication is airway obstruction from failed or difficult intubation, wrong positioning, mucous plug, blood clot, or subglottic oedema following endotracheal extubation.

Table 10.3: Evidence-based research.

Title	Sedation with ketamine for paediatric procedures in the emergency department: a review of 500 cases
Authors	Ng KC, Ang SY
Institution	Department of Emergency Medicine, K K Women and Children Hospital, Singapore
Reference	Singapore Med J. 2002; 43(6):300–304
Problem	The severe shortage of anaesthesia providers in most developing countries leaves the surgeon in the unfortunate position of doubling up as the anaesthetist or using supervising nurses to administer anaesthesia. In this environment, ketamine has proven itself as a good anaesthetic agent with a commendable safety profile. Familiarity with ketamine would seem to be necessary to practice anaesthesia in Africa.
Comparison/ control (quality of evidence)	This is a review article.
Historical significance/ comments	This review article discusses the effectiveness of ketamine for sedation in children during painful procedures. The authors reviewed the use of intravenous and intramuscular ketamine in 500 children for procedures ranging from repair of lacerations, manipulation and reduction of fractures, incision and drainage of abscesses, to removal of foreign bodies. Ninety-six percent of their patients experienced no adverse effect with the use of ketamine and were discharged to home well. Only one patient had adverse effects and had to be admitted overnight. They conclude that ketamine is a relatively safe and effective drug for use in children.

Laryngospasm and bronchospasm may occur, especially if tracheal intubation is attempted under light planes of anaesthesia. Hypothermia and hypoglycaemia are common in preterm neonates and newborns of diabetic mothers. Bradycardia, when it occurs, is a late sign and should be promptly treated with atropine. Nausea and vomiting, postoperative bleeding, pain, and emergence delirium following ketamine anaesthesia are other complications that may be seen in the postoperative period. These can be recognised only by careful monitoring and should be treated promptly.

Most healthy children do well, have an uneventful stay in the PACU, and are quickly reunited with their parents. The need for adequate recovery room nursing care should always be emphasized for the paediatric surgical postoperative patient. The anaesthesia care provider must be readily available in case of a cardiorespiratory event and be in a position to respond quickly with a resuscitation trolley, which should be located in this area of the theatre suite.

Evidenced-Based Research

Tables 10.3 and 10.4, respectively, present a review article on the use of ketamine in children and a discussion of using ketamine in and out of the operating room.

Table 10.4: Evidence-based research.

Title	Ketamine: a new look at an old drug
Authors	Raeder JC, Stenseth LB
Institution	Department of Anesthesia and General Practice Medicine, Ullevaal University Hospital, Oslo, Norway
Reference	Current Opinion in Anaesthesiology 2000; 13(4):463–468
Problem	Although ketamine has proven itself to be a safe general anaesthetic in poorly equipped conditions, recent research suggests more uses both in and out of the operating room.
Historical significance/ comments	This article discusses how the clinical uses of ketamine have expanded beyond dissociative anaesthesia to its effects on immunofunction and more exploration of its analgesic effects. The role of the N-methyl-d-aspartate (NMDA) receptor in analgesia, wind-up phenomena, and possible opioid tolerance hints at more uses for ketamine.

Key Summary Points

1. There are many cardiovascular, respiratory, and renal physiological differences between a neonate and an adult surgical patient.

2. The neonate is more prone than an adult to cardiovascular and respiratory complications in the perioperative setting.

3. Fasting guidelines for the paediatric surgical patients need to be strictly followed to avoid complications.

4. A trained paediatric anaesthesia care provider will need specialized anaesthesia training and skills to decrease the high complication rate seen in paediatric surgical cases.

5. Paediatric patients require supplies and equipment appropriately suited for their size and anatomical differences.

References

1. Ryan JF, Cotes CJ, Todres ID, Goudsouzian N. A Practice of Anaesthesia for Infants and Children, 1st ed. Grune and Stratton Inc., 1986.

2. Cherian VT, Jacob R. Recognition and management of the difficult paediatric airway. In: Jacob R, ed. Understanding Paediatric Anaesthesia, 2nd ed. B.I. Publications, 2008.

3. Rusy L, Usaleva E. Paediatric anaesthesia review. Update in Anaesthesia 1998; 8:2–14.

CHAPTER 11
PAIN MANAGEMENT

Helen Sowerbutts
Kokila Lakhoo

Introduction

Most hospitalized children will experience some pain, either as a result of disease itself or as a result of interventions. A number of studies have demonstrated that the management of pain in children is, unfortunately, often inadequate, especially in the African setting, where resources and skills are limited and overwhelming acute life-saving events override pain management.

Accurately assessing pain and treating it accordingly can be challenging in children due to the different ways in which pain is expressed in the various age groups, compounded by cultural and individual differences in the perception of pain. Effective pain management in children therefore requires much more than just a sound knowledge of analgesic medications; it requires health care professionals to be trained *and* experienced in recognising the degree of pain being experienced by children of different age groups. Health care professionals in Africa must be skilled in using pain assessment tools as well as appreciating the role of social, cultural, and environmental factors in influencing pain perception. Careful consideration must be given to how pain can be prevented and minimised when children are in hospital, and appropriate prescription of analgesics must be combined with a variety of nonpharmacological methods to improve pain perception. Availability of appropriate medications is another limiting factor in African health care systems.[1]

Aetiology/Pathophysiology

Pain can be defined as "an unpleasant sensory and emotional experience associated with actual or potential tissue damage, or described in terms of such damage".[2] This definition highlights an important concept that is especially relevant in children: Pain has both neurological and higher cognitive components. As a result, the degree of pain experienced is not necessarily a reflection of the underlying illness. A relatively minor procedure for one child might cause intense distress for another. Likewise, the health care worker should not underestimate the potential severity of the underlying illness in a child who exteriorises pain to a lesser degree. Factors known to affect a child's pain perception include anxiety, expectation, and previous experience, as well as biological factors such as developmental stage and gender. The role of the family, religion, and culture has also become increasingly recognised in the West[3]; however, this role is less recognised in Africa due to other life-threatening illnesses.

The basic pathways thought to underlie the perception of pain are shown in Figure 11.1. The pathway was originally described by the Melzack-Wall gate control theory in 1965,[4] which states that the detection and transmission of pain from the periphery takes place by A-delta and C nerve fibres that travel to the spinal cord, where a reflex withdrawal arc is triggered. Pain impulses are simultaneously transmitted up the spinal cord to the thalamus and cortex. Various ascending and descending pathways from the cortex and reticular formation allow levels of arousal and higher cognitive functioning to modify the basic pathway.

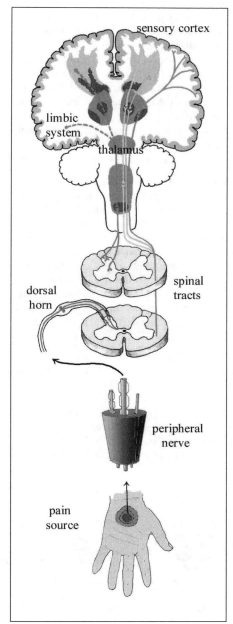

Source: www.perioperativepain.com.

Figure 11.1: Basic pathways involved in the perception of pain.

Inflammatory mediators, such as prostaglandins and bradykinins, have been found to be responsible for stimulating nerve receptors in the periphery. Neurotransmitters, such as endorphins and encephalins, are thought to be at least partly responsible for the central modulation of the pain response. As a result, both the initial inflammatory response and central pathways involved in pain perception are targets for analgesics.

The Importance of Pain Control

Everyone involved in the care of a child is distressed when the child is in pain. It is increasingly being recognised, however, that the deleterious effects of pain are more far-reaching than the immediate psychological dimension. The experience of pain leads to activation of the sympathetic nervous system. This has various potentially harmful effects, including increased myocardial stress and hypertension. In neonates, pain can precipitate apnoeas, and infants may experience syncopal episodes. Pain also leads to activation of the stress axis, which causes increased blood cortisol levels that could impair wound healing. In addition, patients in pain are less likely to mobilise in the postoperative period, putting them at increased risk of atelectasis and chest infections.[5] An increased risk of deep venous thrombosis is also a concern in the adolescent age group. The culmination of these adverse consequences is an increased length of hospital stay and associated increased costs. In addition, longer-term consequences to consider with a child who has suffered a distressing experience include the likelihood that the child will be more distressed and less cooperative in the future.

The Assessment of Pain

The first step towards appropriate pain management is being able to assess how much pain a child is experiencing and why. Naturally, the source of pain should be identified by using investigations appropriate to the differential diagnosis. The accurate assessment of pain in children, however, requires separate consideration of the history of the pain, observation and examination of the child, and the use of validated scoring tools, in addition to knowledge of the underlying cause of discomfort. No single method should be used in isolation. The child and parent should both be consulted; in addition, a range of appropriately trained and experienced health care professionals should be assembled.

History

A good history of pain can aid the clinician in diagnosing the underlying condition as well as in gaining insight into the degree of discomfort. Where possible, the clinician should seek the child's description of the pain. Parental report is also useful. The "SOCRATES" mnemonic is helpful to use whenever taking a pain history—enquiry should be made to the **S**ite, **O**nset, **C**haracter, **R**adiation, **A**ssociated features, **T**emporal features, **E**xacerbating/relieving factors, and the **S**everity of the pain. Questions pertaining to the effect of the pain on the child's level of activity and behaviour are often especially insightful. In particular, the child's ability to partake in usual activities or interest in pleasurable activities should be queried. Enquiry should be made into school absences, sleep disturbance, and reduced interest in feeding, which are often also particularly significant.

In taking the history, the clinician should also attempt to elicit family beliefs and expectations about pain and disease. Previous experiences of the child or other family members may well affect how the child (and parents) responds to pain. Culture also affects how pain is described or even acknowledged.

The signs from the physical examination that can be used to make an assessment of pain largely fall into two categories: physiological and behavioural.

Physiological

First, the cause of pain may be identified, for example, by seeing a visible wound or from palpating abdominal guarding, suggestive of peritoneal irritation. Second, increased heart rate, respiratory rate, and blood pressure are indicative of sympathetic stimulation in response to pain. Such signs are objective and do not require the child's cooperation. They are therefore particularly important in preverbal children, those with physical or mental disability, those with impaired consciousness, and the apparently "stoic" child. However, they are also nonspecific indicators of physiological stress, so these indicators should not be used in isolation. Traditional healer's markings are other good indicators of the site of pain and disease.

Behavioural

Behavioural signs may be generalised responses to pain, such as facial expression, irritability, crying, or lethargy, or may be more specific reactions to certain types of pain, such as ear pulling, assuming certain postures, or refusing to move a certain limb. Although useful, one should not be misled by such signs. There is well-established cultural and even gender-related variation in the degree to which pain is externalised—particularly in the social acceptability of crying. The degree of illness can also influence the extent to which a child is able to express his or her pain. One should always beware of underestimating the degree of pain being experienced in a critically ill child. In some cultures, pain is acknowledged as a sign of weakness, and this taboo needs to be eradicated.

Assessment Tools

Various pain scales have been developed to help measure the degree of pain being experienced by a child. Using such tools has been shown to improve pain management and aid nursing care.[6]

The choice of scale should reflect the nature of pain (for example, acute versus chronic pain), the ethnicity of the child, and—crucially—

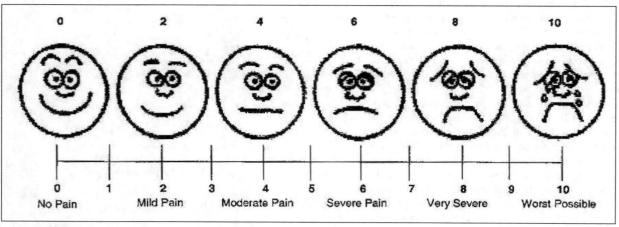

Source: Wong-Baker Faces Pain Scale 1981.

Figure 11.2: Example of pain scale using facial expression of pain severity.

the child's age and developmental level. Children older than 3 years of age are generally considered to have the cognitive ability to use self-report scales. Commonly employed techniques involve the child being asked to point to a photograph or cartoon of a face in various degrees of pain, or the use of linear analogue scales reflecting the continuum of pain intensity. Examples of commonly used tools and the age group for which they are validated include:[7]

• the Oucher Scale, from the age of 3 years;

• the Bieri Scale, from the age of 6 years;

• the Wong-Baker Faces Pain Scale, 8–12 years of age; and

• the Adolescent Paediatric Pain Tool, validated in children from 8 to 17 years of age.

Tools that use cartoon representation of children's faces in various of degrees of pain are likely to be more globally applicable and may be especially useful where resources are limited. An example is shown in Figure 11.2.

For children who are not considered able to verbalise their pain adequately, behavioural scales can be employed. The Faces, Legs, Activity, Crying, and Consolability (FLACC) scale, Toddler-Preschooler Postoperative Pain Scale (TPPPS), and the Children's Hospital of Eastern Ontario Pain Scale (CHEOPS) are generally thought to be suitable from around age 1 to 5 years. Specific scoring systems encompassing behaviour observation and physiological variables should be used in neonates, with separate tools needed for use in premature babies.

Ideally, a variety of different pain scales should be available, with the choice of which scale to use determined on an individual basis. Pain assessment using such tools should be approached with the same attention as that of vital signs: by staff trained in its assessment and who constantly re-evaluate the effectiveness of interventions. Pain flow sheets included in the hospital record may be useful in meeting this goal. Parents should also be educated in the ongoing assessment of their child's pain.

Management

It goes without saying that treatment of the underlying condition is critical to managing a child's pain. This, however, is often not immediately possible and, crucially, many treatments themselves *cause* pain. Adequate symptomatic relief is therefore essential. To control pain effectively, consideration must be given to both pharmacological and nonpharmacological methods of management. The relative use of each should be tailored to the individual child, and each intervention should be modified according to assessments of effectiveness.

Nonpharmacological Techniques

Nondrug methods often do not alleviate pain completely but do help to make it more tolerable by providing the child with coping mechanisms. The hospital environment is often a source of distress in itself, which compounds the experience of pain in children. In recognition of this, attempts should be made to keep to the child's normal routine when in hospital; the number of "new" people tending the child should be minimised and parents should be involved in care as much as possible.

Other nondrug methods can be employed in specific situations—especially in relation to certain procedure-related pain. Distraction is especially useful for short procedures.[8] Methods should be age specific and chosen to reflect the interests of the child. Commonly used examples include videos, games, and books for older children, and bubbles, lights, and music for younger children. Feeding an infant or using a pacifier are simple and inexpensive interventions that have been shown to have analgesic effects.[9] Relaxation techniques, such as gentle rocking and massage, have also been used with some success. Discussion of the procedure, what it involves, and why it is necessary is often useful with older children. Allowing younger children to

familiarise themselves with equipment by first playing with it in a nonpressured environment is also useful to reduce the shock associated with procedures. Employing "play specialists"—specially trained members of staff who are familiar in using a variety of such techniques and able to identify when best to use these—has been shown to reduce hospital length of stay and increase compliance in some hospitals.[10]

Analgesia

The prescription of analgesics should follow the World Health Organization (WHO) pain management ladder (Figure 11.3). A key principle behind this is the cumulative effect of drugs and the step-wise addition of drugs to address pain requirements. Similarly, as pain requirements reduce (for example, in the postoperative period), analgesia should be reduced in a stepwise manner down the ladder. The route of administration, dosage, and timing should be tailored to suit the individual child. In particular, it is important to realise that the gastrointestinal absorption of medications is affected after major surgery, meaning oral administration is often inappropriate in this setting. Age- and weight-appropriate dosages for each analgesic should be calculated for each child on an individual basis.

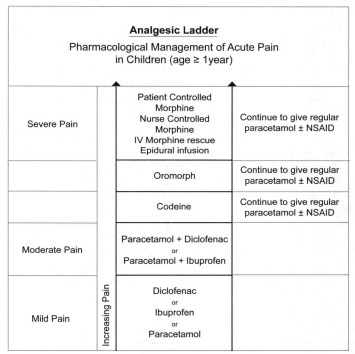

Source: Cross L, Bridge H, ORH & NHS Trusts, Version 1, July 2003.

Figure 11.3: The principles of the WHO analgesic ladder.

Paracetamol is an excellent first-line drug for children with pain. It exists in forms suitable for oral, rectal, and intravenous administration. Rectal absorption is often slow and unpredictable, so this route is less commonly used. Paracetamol is generally well tolerated and low in side effects.

Children who do not get sufficient analgesia from paracetamol alone should also be prescribed a nonsteroidal anti-inflammatory drug (NSAID). Drugs such as ibuprofen and diclofenac work by inhibiting prostaglandin synthesis and reducing inflammation. They are therefore especially valuable in patients with surgical pain. Oral and rectal preparations are available, with rectal diclofenac being particularly well absorbed and of great use in acute pain relief. Caution should be exercised in patients with asthma or with renal or hepatic impairment. These drugs should not be used in patients with known bleeding tendency or those under 3 months of age. Due to the risks of gastric irritation, they should ideally be given with food or milk.

If analgesic requirements are still not met, then codeine, a mild opiate, should be administered. This is generally considered a safe drug with a significantly lower incidence of respiratory depression than other stronger opioids. Nausea and constipation are relatively common side effects that should be anticipated wherever codeine is prescribed. Codeine phosphate is most commonly given by mouth, although rectal preparations are available.

In patients whose pain is still not adequately controlled, or those who are deemed to have severe pain at initial assessment, a strong opioid should be used. The "lower steps" of the analgesic ladder (see Figure 11.3) should always be prescribed as well, with the exception of codeine. Morphine may be administered in oral solution, intramuscularly, or intravenously, depending on clinical need. An intranasal preparation is also now available and is especially useful in the emergency management of acute pain where intravenous access is not always available.[11] Patient-controlled analgesia (PCA) is an alternative mode of administration of intravenous morphine administration by which the patient can choose when doses are given according to need. PCA has been found to produce the same analgesic effect as intramuscular (IM) regimes, but with less sedation.[12]

Morphine has multiple side effects that should be anticipated whenever it is prescribed. Nausea and vomiting are commonplace, so antiemetics should be routinely prescribed on an "as required" basis. Urine retention is a recognised complication, especially in postoperative patients, so many centres routinely catheterise patients until their opiate requirement has ceased. Respiratory depression is the most feared complication associated with the use of morphine. Regular, documented monitoring of sedation level and respiratory parameters should be mandatory, as should the coprescription of "as required" naloxone wherever opioids are prescribed. Concern about respiratory compromise should not, however, influence the decision to use morphine in those who need it. Parents and health care professionals alike should be reassured that dependence is rare in children with surgical pain.

Opioid use in Africa is rare; possible reasons include strict national laws against opioid addiction and misuse of drugs, lack of knowledge, and nonavailability, as reported by WHO.[13] For example, morphine consumption in South Africa for 2004 was 4.6682 mg per capita in comparison to Uganda's 0.4001 mg per capita, Tanzania's 0.3250 mg per capita, and Zambia's 0.0704 mg per capita, and the use of pethidine in Uganda for 2004 was 0.2272 mg per capita, in contrast to South Africa's 3.7694 mg per capita.[14]

Additional Methods of Analgesia
Certain additional techniques are frequently employed in the perioperative period to improve pain management, as described here. Local anaesthetics can be used to create specific nerve blocks to reduce postoperative pain sensation from specific sites. The duration of such blocks depends upon the specific anaesthetic used, but is typically around 6–8 hours. Local anaesthetics now exist in a variety of formats, including gels and creams that can be applied postoperatively as well as solutions that can be infiltrated into operative sites. Local application of anaesthetic creams is particularly useful in procedures involving the skin or mucous membranes, and has been shown to be effective in reducing wound pain in the postoperative period.[15] An advantage of this is that community medical officers can easily acquire and utilise this technique to reduce pain associated with procedures.

When a greater area of analgesic coverage is required, an epidural may be used. This form of regional anaesthesia involves injection of analgesics (usually local anaesthetic with or without opioids) through a catheter placed into the epidural space. Epidurals are especially useful in thoracic procedures and after laparotomy.[16] They are usually inserted in the anaesthetic room and can be linked to a PCA system (where they become patient-controlled epidural analgesia, or PCEA, systems). Their main advantage is that the analgesic action of opioids can be gained without the systemic side effects. However, there are numerous disadvantages to the system. The incidence of postoperative urine retention is reasonably high, so catheterisation is often recommended; epidurals should be avoided in patients at high risk of bleeding or infection; and there is a risk of inappropriate level of blockage, so sensory level should be routinely checked while an epidural is in place.

Ketamine merits special mention with regard to pain control in areas where access to and training in administering other modes of analgesia are limited. This anaesthetic drug has also been shown to have good analgesic properties at subanaesthetic dosages.[17] It can be administered intravenously (IV) or by IM injection, and is generally well tolerated in paediatric patients. Its main adverse effects are transient hypertension, vomiting, agitation on recovery, and hallucinations. Diazepam is coprescribed to buffer the duration and intensity of any side effects.

Prevention
Although it is difficult in practice to completely prevent pain in hospitalised children, several strategies can help to minimise it. Naturally, the accurate diagnosis and prompt treatment of the underlying condition before pain escalates is highly desirable. Regular prescription of analgesia is more effective than medicine given only when pain arises. The clinician should also attempt to recognise the potential for procedures to be painful or distressing and carefully consider which measures are really necessary so that only those that are likely to bring about a change in management are undertaken.

When potentially painful procedures are required, a range of methods can be employed to prevent unnecessary pain. This includes administration of analgesics before an event as well as the use of special additional measures, such as Entonox® in dressing changes of burn patients, or local anaesthetic creams (EMLA®—a eutectic mixture of local anaesthetics—or Amitop®) and cold sprays to minimise discomfort associated with phlebotomy or removal of foreign objects.

In the longer term, minimising pain for paediatric patients will require continued efforts to educate and train staff in its assessment and management. *Crucially, this should involve dispelling such commonly held myths as that infants do not feel pain and the active child is not in pain, and the general feeling that children have to "earn" analgesics before they are given.*

Ethical Issues
The African child is particularly vulnerable to disease and injury, and subsequently to pain and suffering. Factors such as inadequate training, language barriers, cultural diversity, limited resources, and the burden of disease prevent sick and injured children from receiving basic pain care. This situation can be rectified only by providing pre- and postgraduate training on the safe use of analgesic preparations, making drugs available, and gaining government support.

These ethical issues are best summarised in a review titled: "Challenges associated with paediatric pain management in Sub Saharan Africa" in the International Journal of Surgery.[1]

Evidence-Based Research
Table 11.1 deals with a study of postoperative pain relief following inguinal herniotomy.

Table 11.1: Evidence-based research.

Title	A comparison between EMLA cream application versus lidocaine infiltration for post-operative analgesia after inguinal herniotomy in children
Authors	Usmani H, Pal Singh S, Quadir A, Chana RS
Institution	Department of Anesthesia, Jawaharlal Nehru Medical College, Aligargh Muslim University, Aligarh, India
Reference	Reg Anesth Pain Med 2009; 34(2):106–109
Problem	Postoperative pain relief following inguinal herniotomy.
Intervention	Topical application of 5% EMLA cream before surgery or wound infiltration with 1% lidocaine.
Comparison/ control (quality of evidence)	Study group comprised 90 children aged 4–12 years undergoing elective herniotomy under general anaesthetic. Patients were randomly assigned to placebo cream alone, 5% EMLA cream, or placebo cream + 1% lidocaine infiltration after induction of anaesthesia. Operative protocol was standardised among groups. The requirement for postoperative analgesia among groups was compared.
Outcome/ effect	The number of patients requiring fentanyl as rescue analgesia was significantly less in the study groups than in the placebo group. Topical application of EMLA provided postoperative pain relief comparable to infiltration with 1% lidocaine.
Historical significance/ comments	Suggests that the application of local anaesthetic cream is a viable alternative to wound infiltration in the control of postoperative pain. This would be a valuable strategy in settings where clinical training and resources are limited.

Key Summary Points

1. Pain of some degree is almost universal in hospitalised children, either as a result of underlying disease or interventions.

2. The recognition and subsequent management of pain is often inadequate in children.

3. Health care professionals have a moral obligation to provide the best possible management of children's pain and should be trained in pain recognition.

4. The perception and expression of pain is highly dependent on the age and cognitive function of the child.

5. Accurate determination of the level pain is the first step to adequate management and should take into consideration the parent's and child's reports, the change in behaviour of the child, the measurement of physiological parameters and knowledge of the underlying medical condition.

6. Cultural- and age-validated scoring tools should be routinely used in the assessment of pain in children.

7. A combination of pharmacological and nondrug methods should be used for managing pain.

8. Clinicians should anticipate pain in children and minimise the number of potentially painful procedures to which a child is subjected.

References

1. Albertyn R, Rode H, Millar AJ, Thomas J. Challenges associated with paediatric pain management in Sub Saharan Africa. Int J Surg 2009; 7(2):91–93.

2. Merskey H, Bogduk N. Classification of Chronic Pain. International Association for the Study of Pain Press, 1994, P 210.

3. Twycross A, Moriarty A, Betts T. Paediatric Pain Management: A Multi-disciplinary Approach. Radcliffe Medical Press, 1999, Pp 56–76.

4. Melzack R, Wall PD. Pain mechanisms: a new theory. Science 1965; 150:971–979.

5. Eland JM. Pain in children. Nurs Clin North Am 1990; 25(4):871–884.

6. Schofield P. Using assessment tools to help patients in pain. Profession Nurse 1995; 10(11):703–706.

7. Cohen LL, et al. Evidence based assessment of pain. J Pediatr Psychol 2008; 33(9):939–955; discussion 956–957. Epub 2007 Nov 17. Review.

8. Carter. Child and infant pain; Principles of Nursing Care and Management. Chapman and Hall, 1994.

9. Sexton S, Natale R. Risks and benefits of pacifiers. Am Fam Physician 2009; 79(8):681–685.

10. Dix A. Clinical management. Where medicine meets management. Let us play. Health Serv J 2004; 114(5902):26–27.

11. Borland M, Jacobs I, King B, O'Brien D. A randomised crossover trial of patient controlled intranasal fentanyl and oral morphine for procedural wound care in adult patients with burns. Burns 2004; 30(3):262–268.

12. Berde DB, et al. Patient controlled analgesia in children and adolescents: a randomised prospective comparison with intramuscular morphine for post-operative analgesia. Pediatrics 1993; 118:460–466.

13. Adams V, Bertolino M, et al. Access to pain relief—a basic human right. Report for the hospice and palliative care day, 2007. Available from http://www.worldday.org/documents/access_to_relief.pdf.

14. Availability of morphine and pethidine in the world and Africa. Advocacy for palliative care in Africa: a focus on essential pain medication accessibility, 2006. Available from http://www.medsch.wisc.edu/painpolicy.

15. Usmani H, Pal Singh S, Quadir A, Chana RS. A comparison between EMLA cream application versus lidocaine infiltration for post-operative analgesia after inguinal herniotomy in children. Reg Anesth Pain Med 2009; 34(2):106–109.

16. Block BM, Liu SS, Rowlingson AJ, Cowan AR, Cowan JA, Wu CL. Efficacy of postoperative epidural analgesia: a meta-analysis. JAMA 2003; 290(18):2455–2463.

17. Mistry RB, Nahata MC. Ketamine for conscious sedation in pediatric emergency care. Pharmacotherapy 2005; 25(8):1104–1111.

CHAPTER 12
INTENSIVE CARE

Andrew Gustaf Nyman
Alison Shefler

Introduction

Injury or illness is defined as critical when one or more organ systems are either in danger of failing or have begun to fail. In this situation, the possibility of incomplete recovery or death exists. Critical care comprises the monitoring, support, treatment, and interventions for the organ systems in failure. Paediatric critical care not only encompasses bedside management of children with severe, potentially life-threatening medical or surgical illness, but also extends to providing support to the child's family or caregivers. The challenge lies in the complex balance of providing support of single or multiple organ systems in failure while at the same time minimising adverse consequences of treatment. This level of care is usually, but not always, provided in a dedicated paediatric intensive care environment with the capacity to offer sophisticated monitoring, diagnostic and therapeutic interventions, as well as advanced technological support for the critically ill child. When the outcome is poor or death ensues, the critical care focus shifts to palliative and, if necessary, bereavement support. The spectrum of disease in children differs from that of the adult population, as does the paediatric response to illness, surgery, or injury. Congenital abnormalities, genetic syndromes, inborn errors of metabolism, and toxins, as well as trauma, including birth-related and nonaccidental injury, all influence the differential diagnosis of an acutely unwell child. Regardless of the aetiology, basic principles of initial management and stabilisation should be applied in all situations.[1,2]

Approach to the Acutely Unwell Child

Respiratory failure is a common manifestation of critical illness and generally requires early recognition and intervention to prevent progression to full cardiopulmonary arrest, which carries a grave prognosis.[3–9] This section of the chapter therefore begins by outlining the systematic approach that underpins all paediatric life support and intensive care management of the acutely unwell child, namely, addressing the child's airway, breathing, and circulation.[10]

Airway

The goals of airway management are to overcome obstruction, promote adequate gas exchange, and prevent aspiration.

The first priority in the assessment of a critically ill or injured child is to ensure a patent airway. Any compromise to airway patency, either structural or functional, is a potential medical emergency, and it is important to recognise it because failure to establish or maintain the airway can result in or worsen respiratory compromise. Respiratory failure may, in turn, progress to cardiopulmonary arrest; thus, every effort should be made to secure airway stabilisation in a timely manner.

The paediatric airway is more susceptible to airway compromise than that of adults for a number of reasons.[11–15]

- A child's proportionally larger head and prominent occiput result in neck flexion, with the potential for exacerbating upper airway obstruction when lying supine.

- The tongue is relatively large and its muscle tone is reduced.

- The epiglottis is shorter, narrower, and more horizontally positioned than in an adult.

- The larynx is in a more anterior and cephalad position than in an adult.

- The trachea is smaller and narrower.

- The airway is funnel shaped, with the narrowest portion at the level of the cricoid cartilage.

Functional airway compromise results in children with decreased muscle tone in the head and neck. It may be secondary to a decreased level of consciousness and/or the effects of anaesthesia or analgesic or sedative drugs. An inability to maintain a patent airway, even in the absence of a structural abnormality, may present as great a risk as the presence of anatomical obstruction.

Airway compromise may be due to or exacerbated by congenital anomalies, the presence of foreign bodies, or extrinsic compression by structures outside the airway. The most significant difference in the paediatric airway compared to that of adults, and therefore a major contribution to the vulnerability of the airway, is its size and diameter.[15] According to the Hagen-Poiseuille law, which relates to the flow of gas, a change in the radius of the airway has the greatest effect on air flow. As a result, any oedema of the paediatric airway will significantly reduce the calibre of the airway, resulting in a dramatic increase in resistance to air flow and, consequently, the work of breathing. This is particularly important in infants, who are obligatory nasal breathers. Nasal breathing, without any additional obstruction, doubles resistance to flow. The nares in infants and children are significantly smaller than in adults and can account for up to 50% of total airway resistance. With this is mind, it is important to note that simply removing secretions from the nares may result in a dramatic decrease in the work of breathing.[15]

When intervention is required to establish airway patency, a stepwise approach is essential. If basic manoeuvres, such as positioning the head, chin, or jaw, are insufficient, one may have to use airway adjuncts such as a Guedel oropharyngeal airway or a nasopharyngeal airway. For all children who have a potential cervical spine injury, the spine should be adequately immobilised, and unnecessary manipulation should be avoided. Should previous efforts to establish an airway be unsuccessful, endotracheal intubation, laryngeal mask airway, or—rarely—surgical intervention in the form of a tracheostomy may be required, both to establish airway patency and to maintain adequate gas exchange.

Breathing

Acute respiratory failure is a major cause of paediatric morbidity and mortality. It accounts for approximately 30–50% of admissions to paediatric intensive care facilities.[7,16–21] Numerous clinical situations have the potential for progression to respiratory failure, reflecting the complex involvement of the respiratory system with other organ systems. Diagnosis and management of respiratory failure require an understanding of normal respiratory physiology as well the pathophysiological processes occurring in acute medical or surgical disease.

Respiratory failure is inadequate exchange of oxygen and carbon dioxide resulting in failure to meet metabolic demands.

Anatomically, the respiratory system structure comprises the lungs and respiratory pump. The lungs include the airways, alveoli, and pulmonary circulation. Failure in any of these elements may result in abnormal gas exchange, which is manifested by hypoxia; this condition is termed hypoxic respiratory failure. The respiratory pump refers to the thorax, respiratory muscles, and nervous innervations. The inability to effectively pump air into and out of the lungs results in hypoventilation and thus hypercarbia; this condition is termed hypercarbic respiratory failure. Although the two systems can be described separately, the two interact significantly with each other. Failure in one of these systems often results in failure of the other.

To achieve adequate gas exchange, several conditions must be met:

• Adequate gas must reach the alveoli.

• Inspired gas in the alveoli must match the blood distribution within the pulmonary capillaries.

• The alveolar-capillary membrane must permit gas exchange.

A child with a decreased level of consciousness due to any cause—including the postoperative patient under the influence of anaesthetic, analgesic, or sedating drugs—may have inadequate respiratory drive, resulting in an inadequate respiratory rate (see Table 12.1). Acute respiratory distress may result from disease in the large or small airways, the lung parenchyma, the pleural space, or a combination of all of these. Disease in other organ systems, such as cardiac failure or metabolic acidosis associated with diabetic ketoacidosis or toxin ingestion, may give rise to increased respiratory effort. Should any of these disease processes result in inadequate gas exchange, respiratory failure ensues.

Table 12.1: Normal respiratory rate in children.

Age	Breaths per minute
Birth–1 year	20–30
2–5 years	20–25
>5 years	16–20

In addition to the above factors, gas exchange may be affected by systemic processes such as the systemic inflammatory response syndrome (SIRS) seen in sepsis and following cardiac bypass, as well as nonpulmonary factors, including acute blood loss, poor cardiac output (CO), increased oxygen demand, and chronic anaemia. Nutritional deficiencies may contribute to an inability to meet the demands of acute medical or surgical illness.

The most serious manifestation of respiratory insufficiency is hypoxia. Initial compensatory hyperventilation may cause an early drop in $PaCO_2$; however, as these compensatory mechanisms fail, hypercapnia ensues.

Oxygen should be administered to all critically ill or injured children in the highest possible concentration until the assessment of cardiorespiratory status is complete.

The early goal of administering the highest possible oxygen concentration to the acutely unwell patient remains the highest priority, as oxygen delivery to the tissues may be suboptimal in the child with decreased circulating volume or abnormalities in microcirculation, such as may be seen in sepsis, hypovolaemia, or haemorrhage.

Respiratory insufficiency is generally recognised by an early increase in respiratory rate, which may be followed by a decrease in respiratory rate as the child's clinical condition worsens.[22] Apnoea in the small infant is worrying and requires immediate intervention. Cyanosis and tachycardia are early findings, and as hypoxia worsens, progression to bradycardia and cardiac arrest may occur.[23]

Supplemental oxygen can be delivered via many different delivery devices. The choice of device will be dictated by clinical situation and local availability as well as by which device is best tolerated by the child.

Nonrebreathing face mask
A nonrebreathing face mask is the most effective way of delivering oxygen by face mask. It consists of a face mask connected by a unidirectional valve to an oxygen reservoir bag. The unidirectional valve delivers all inhaled gas from the oxygen reservoir and prevents exhaled air from entering the reservoir. The mask must fit snugly over the nose, and the fresh gas flow rate must be maintained to ensure the reservoir remains distended by at least half its volume at all times. In ideal conditions, these masks can provide 100% oxygen; however, it is often slightly less than this in practice.

Venturi masks
The Venturi mask works on Bernoulli's principle, which states that as the velocity of gas increases the pressure surrounding that gas decreases. Oxygen is introduced through a tapered inlet into the device. As the oxygen flows through the narrowed inlet the velocity increases and a resultant decrease in pressure surrounding the stream of gas causes room air to be entrained into the device through side ports in the device. The concentration of oxygen delivered with these devices remains relatively constant. These masks can deliver 24–40% oxygen.

Nasal cannulae
Nasal cannulae consist of two protruding prongs that are placed into the child's nares. The delivered concentration of oxygen depends on the flow rate as well as the child's minute ventilation and the volume of the nasopharynx as these determine the amount of entrained room air. Generally, children accept flow rates of up to 2 litres per minute; flow rates in excess of this are uncomfortable and poorly tolerated. Correctly fitted and at appropriate flow rates, nasal cannulae are often better tolerated than face masks in most children, but they are less suitable when oxygen needs are high.

Oxygen hood, tent, and head box
Oxygen hoods, tents, or head boxes are clear plastic systems that enclose either the head, upper body, or entire body. The child breathes fresh gas supplied into the enclosure. The concentration within the enclosure can be monitored by using a gas analyser. High oxygen delivery is difficult to maintain with this system because gas is lost through leakage; this system may thus be most suitable for small infants. If this system is used, a minimum fresh gas flow of 2–3 l/kg per minute should be used to prevent carbon dioxide retention.

Bag-mask ventilation
Some children require positive pressure ventilation, either to overcome a degree of upper airway obstruction or to provide breathing support. Effective bag-mask ventilation requires a good seal between the mask and face to provide adequate inflation pressures as well as the ability to compress the gas-containing bag in a coordinated manner, which is sometimes better achieved by two health care providers. It is often necessary to gently move the child's head and neck to determine the optimum position to provide effective ventilation. Excessive flexion or extension of the head and neck should be avoided, however, as this often results in airway obstruction. As mentioned previously, for all children who have a potential cervical spine injury, the spine should be adequately immobilised and unnecessary manipulation should be avoided.

The two bags commonly used in bag-mask valve ventilation include the self-inflating bag and the standard anaesthetic circuit. The self-inflating bag consists of a bag, oxygen inlet, connector for the face mask or tracheal tube, pressure relief valve, and a reservoir. The self-inflating bag is relatively easy to use and more available, and when used with the reservoir, it can provide near 100% oxygen. It can provide emergency ventilation without a fresh gas source because the gas movement generated by bag inflation will inflate the chest with room air, even without an external gas source. Because the valve mechanism opens only in response to manual bag inflation, the self-inflating bag is not appropriate to deliver oxygen or continuous positive pressure in the spontaneously breathing child. The bag in a standard anaesthetic circuit, however, requires a constant supply of fresh gas in order for it to fill. The bag must therefore be connected to a fresh gas supply to inflate the lungs via either a face mask or tracheal tube. The advantage of the standard bag over the self-inflating bag is the ability to deliver fresh gas and continuous positive pressure to the spontaneously breathing child and to control the pressures administered with each breath. The system can be difficult to use, however, in all but experienced anaesthetic hands.

Mechanical ventilation

Mechanical ventilation provides a way of supporting the respiratory system while waiting for the natural history of the pathological process to improve or for specific treatment to be effective. The goals of mechanical ventilation are to ensure adequate oxygen delivery, decrease the work of breathing, and ensure adequate elimination of carbon dioxide.[24] Mechanical ventilation is generally provided by using positive pressure-ventilated breaths superimposed on a background of positive end expiratory pressure (PEEP) to maintain alveolar patency during expiration. PEEP can stabilise alveoli, decrease ventilation-to-perfusion (V:Q) mismatch, and reduce the alveolar shear injury incurred through repetitive inflation with positive pressure—the so-called "ventilator-induced lung injury".[25] Excessive PEEP, however, may result in overdistention of recruited alveoli and have a negative impact on cardiac output.

The goals of mechanical ventilation are to optimise alveolar ventilation, maximise V:Q matching, decrease the work of breathing, and minimise the risk of ventilator-associated injury.

The usual starting point when calculating the initial inflation pressure requirement is a simple visual assessment of the amount of pressure required to move the chest. Adjustments can then be made according to the clinical situation and oxygen requirement, and, if available, as dictated by blood gas analysis. If the bedside ventilator system enables tidal volume calculation, the ventilator pressure should be adjusted with the aim of delivering a tidal volume of 5–10 ml/kg. This will vary with chest compliance, but it often requires peak inspiratory pressures in the range of 20–25 cm H_2O, with a PEEP of 3–5 cm H_2O.[26] Higher PEEP may be required to achieve adequate oxygenation when extensive airspace disease or pulmonary oedema is present. Wherever possible, avoid excessive inflation pressures to avoid ventilator-associated lung disease, which has been associated with high inspiratory pressures.[27] Tidal volumes of 6 ml/kg and limiting the peak inspiratory pressure to less than 32 cm H_2O has demonstrated a significant reduction in mortality.[27] In setting the rate, both the inspiratory and expiratory times—that is, the proportion of the respiratory cycle occupied by inspiration and expiration, respectively—can be adjusted. The inspiratory time is usually decided based on the age, size, and disease process of the patient. As a guide, inspiratory times increase from approximately 0.5 seconds in a neonate to 1 second in children older than 5 years of age. A useful starting point is to simply start with a ventilator rate of 20 breaths per minute and adjust as necessary. Small infants and neonates may require a higher starting rate, in the range of 40–60 breaths per minute.

When making adjustments to the mode and frequency of mechanical ventilation, effective oxygenation is determined by manipulations of inspired oxygen (FiO_2) and mean airway pressure (MAP). The factors that most reliably influence MAP are the amount of set PEEP and the inspiratory time. To optimise ventilation and thus carbon dioxide clearance, minute volume should be increased by increasing the peak inspiratory pressure as well as the ventilator rate. Note, however, that changes in mechanical ventilation to achieve improvements in oxygenation and ventilation have an impact on each other as well as on other organ systems, most notably the cardiovascular system. Increasing mean airway pressures, for example, may potentially impede venous return and thus negatively affect cardiac output. With any adjustment, the clinician should establish whether a positive change has been effected with the fewest possible negative clinical consequences.

The inability to achieve effective oxygenation and ventilation by using conventional positive pressure ventilation may suggest the need for nonconventional modalities of ventilator support, such as high-frequency oscillatory ventilation, high-frequency jet ventilation, or extracorporeal membrane oxygenation (ECMO). Generally, these therapies are available mainly as rescue therapy in intensive care centres.

Circulation

Many children with severe disease require cardiovascular monitoring and support. Circulatory compromise frequently accompanies critical illness and may be either a primary cause or be secondary to the presence of untreated respiratory failure and hypoxia. Early recognition and intervention is therefore essential to prevent further progression to circulatory collapse and death. When the cardiovascular system is unable to provide adequate perfusion of end organs to supply adequate oxygen and nutrients to cells, the situation is referred to as shock. Table 12.2 shows a common scheme for the classification of shock.

Table 12.2: Classification of shock.

Shock classification	Aetiology
Hypovolaemic	Haemorrhage Diarrhoea and vomiting Burns Peritonitis
Distributive	Sepsis Anaphylaxis Vasodilating drugs Spinal cord injuries
Cardiogenic	Arrhythmias Cardiomyopathy Myocardial infarction or contusion Congenital structural heart disease Cardiac tamponade
Obstructive	Tension haemo/pneumothorax Flail chest Pulmonary embolism
Dissociative	Anaemia Carbon monoxide poisoning Methaemoglobinaemia

In evaluating a child with signs of shock, the earliest and most sensitive—but not exclusively reliable—sign is tachycardia. This may also be caused by pain, anxiety, fever, or medications, but these causes are often easily excluded. The presence of additional significant signs consistent with inadequate blood supply to end organs, such as altered mental state, poor peripheral skin perfusion due to vasoconstriction, thready rapid pulses that may be difficult to palpate, and decreased urine output as a result of poor organ perfusion, help to establish a diagnosis of shock. Vasodilatation as a sign of shock is less common in children as compared to adults.[28] Metabolic acidosis commonly accompanies suboptimal perfusion due to tissue anaerobic metabolism, and the tachypnoea that results may be a useful clinical marker.[29]

It is important to remember that children have robust compensatory mechanisms, and blood pressure may be preserved even in moderate circulatory insufficiency. A fall in blood pressure is a late ominous sign and defines decompensated shock. Normal cardiovascular parameters in children are given in Table 12.3.

Table 12.3: Normal paediatric cardiovascular parameters.

Age (years)	Heart rate (beats per minute)	Mean blood pressure (mm Hg)
Neonate	100–180	40–60
1	100–200	50–100
2	80–160	50–100
5	80–150	60–90
10	60–120	60–90
15	50–120	65–95

Cardiac output depends on the following factors:

• *Preload:* Affected by circulating blood volume and effective delivery to the heart

• *Afterload:* Systolic blood pressure and vascular tone

• *Inotropic state:* Cardiac contractility

• *Chronotropy:* Heart rate as well as rhythm

> In supporting circulation, the goal is to optimise cardiac output. The most common clinical situation resulting in shock is hypovolaemia secondary to dehydration or blood loss.

In surgical pre- and postoperative patients, hypovolaemia may be exacerbated by distributive shock due to losses into third spaces as a result of increased capillary permeability. It is therefore of the utmost importance to restore adequate intravascular volume promptly by using isotonic crystalloid or colloid. If there has been significant haemorrhage, packed red blood cells should be considered. It is essential to rule out a cardiogenic cause of shock to avoid excessive fluid administration and overloading a compromised heart. This is usually distinguishable by clinical examination to rule out signs of heart failure, such as cardiomegaly or hepatomegaly, as well as with electrocardiogram (ECG) monitoring and chest x-ray, which may demonstrate congestive heart failure or pulmonary oedema and an increased heart shadow. In children, distention of neck veins is a less reliable sign.

Fluid resuscitation in an attempt to restore intravascular volume is best initiated by using boluses of 20 ml/kg crystalloid or colloid solutions, titrated to clinical markers of cardiac output (heart rate, urine output, capillary refill, and level of consciousness). Numerous clinical trials have attempted to determine the optimal fluid in paediatric resuscitation. The choice of fluid is controversial, but because no clear benefit has been demonstrated for crystalloid over colloid, the choice must be dictated by availability as well as local policy in the acute situation.[30–34] The femoral vein is frequently used to provide central venous access, enabling administration of vasoactive drugs, parenteral nutrition and drugs in higher concentration than would be tolerated in a peripheral venous cannula.

Large fluid deficits typically exist in sepsis, and initial volume resuscitation usually requires 40–60 ml/kg, but may be as much as 200 ml/kg. It is important to note that at the same time as providing ongoing fluid resuscitation, respiratory support in the form of intubation and ventilation may be required. Airway and respiratory support, if needed,

should be initiated simultaneously, and neither should delay the other. In patients with suspected or known cardiomyopathy, clinicians must be cautious with aggressive fluid resuscitation because overdistention of a poorly functioning myocardium is likely to cause the patient to deteriorate. In these patients, it is often advisable to give smaller fluid boluses and assess their effects on an ongoing basis.

Patients with poor physiological reserve as well as those who do not respond to fluid resuscitation may benefit from invasive haemodynamic monitoring to more accurately titrate their fluid and inotropic therapies.[28,29,35–44]

In evaluating the cardiovascular system, it is important to confirm sinus rhythm on an ECG by establishing that every QRS complex is preceded by a P wave and that every P wave is followed by a QRS complex. More definitive assessment with cardiac ultrasound is helpful but not often available in the acute situation. Arrhythmias are uncommon in critically ill children without structural heart disease, and sinus tachycardia is commonly present. In the presence of tachycardia that persists when measures such as fever, hypovolaemia, anxiety, and pain are controlled. Tachyarrhythmias such as supraventricular tachycardia (SVT), atrial fibrillation, and ventricular tachycardia must be considered.[45]

When measures such as fluid therapy and maintaining sinus rhythm do not produce an adequate cardiac output, the circulation may be supported further by using vasoactive drugs to increase cardiac inotropy and chronotropy and/or vasoconstrict the peripheral vascular system. Invasive pressure monitoring of central venous or arterial pressure, where available, may provide cardiovascular information to further guide volume and pharmacological support. First-line vasoactive drugs commonly used in the intensive care environment include dopamine and adrenaline, both of which increase heart rate and contractility as well as increasing systemic vascular resistance to varying degrees that generally favour increased cardiac output. Noradrenaline is primarily a vasoconstrictor, and its use is limited to the less common situations in which vasodilatation is present, such as in the older child with sepsis or following cardiac surgery when an increase in systemic vascular resistance is desirable. Milrinone, a phosphodiesterase inhibitor, is increasingly used for inotropic support, especially following cardiac surgery when diastolic function in addition to systolic function may be impaired. Most patients will respond to a simple approach using a single inotropic agent. Detailed and repeated clinical examination, haemodynamic monitoring and—if available—cardiac imaging enables vasoactive support with one or more agents tailored according to the patient's individual requirements.[46–49]

Specific Organ System Dysfunction

Neurology

Acute neurological abnormality may result from a primary disorder of the nervous system or from the consequences of severe illness in other organ systems. Children with respiratory or cardiovascular compromise are often hypoxic with varying degrees of impairment of their levels of consciousness. This may range from irritability and lethargy to seizures or coma. Seriously ill children are often hypotonic but may exhibit more worrying signs of abnormal posturing and eventually respiratory arrest. Primary neurological disease, such as acute meningitis or encephalitis, trauma, a mass lesion, or intoxication may present with a similar spectrum of nonspecific abnormalities. In the early stages of assessment, it is important to stabilise airway, breathing, and circulation, as previously noted, to ensure optimal oxygenation of the brain, regardless of aetiology.

Causes of decreased level of consciousness include hypoxia; hypotension or shock; infection; metabolic disturbances (e.g., hypoglycaemia); toxins or drugs; trauma, especially head injury, including nonaccidental injury; and intracerebral haemorrhage.

Once oxygenation and appropriate circulation are restored, the diagnosis may be clarified with a more detailed history and physical examination to elicit specific signs. Radiological imaging, such as computed tomography

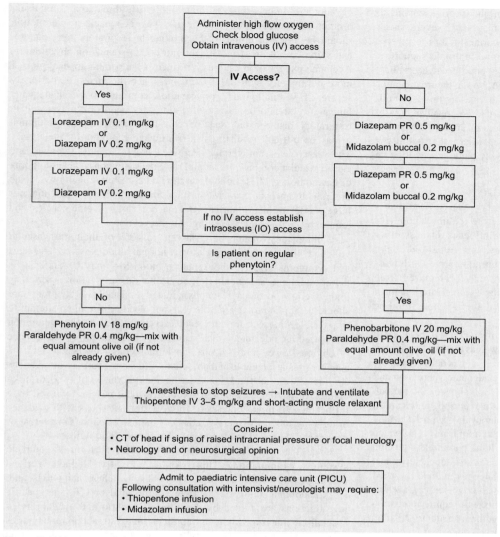

Figure 12.1: Management of status epilepticus in a child.

(CT) of the head, may be required. The diagnosis of central nervous system (CNS) infection generally requires lumbar puncture to assess cell count, protein, and glucose content.

Lumbar puncture should be performed in a controlled manner, provided there are no contraindications,[50] such as focal neurological signs, raised intracranial pressure (ICP), cardiovascular instability, coagulopathy, local skin infection over the proposed puncture site, suspected spinal cord mass or intracranial mass lesion, or spinal column deformities.

Always defer lumbar puncture in unstable patients, but never delay antibiotic or antiviral treatment, if indicated.

The use of hypotonic fluid is contraindicated when signs of raised intracranial pressure are evident. Hypotonic fluid should generally be avoided in all children with acute neurological disease. This is due to the risk of sudden fluid shifts resulting from changes in plasma osmolality and the potential for rapid increases in intracranial pressure.[51] Not enough data exist to support routine fluid restriction.[52-53] In the setting of acute neurological deterioration with signs of rising intracranial pressure and possible brain stem herniation, the use of hypertonic saline or intravenous mannitol may be warranted.[54]

Seizures are a common feature of both primary and secondary CNS abnormality. It is important to address the underlying cause, which mirrors the differential diagnosis of decreased level of consciousness, and establish oxygenation and circulation as detailed above. If appropriate, specific therapy should be instituted as soon as possible (e.g., the treatment of hypoglycaemia with a dextrose infusion of 5–10 ml/kg of 10% dextrose solution). The treatment for a prolonged seizure or recurrent seizures is indicated in Figure 12.1.[55-57]

Although the paediatric CNS may be relatively immature, children do still have appropriate response to pain. It is therefore important to remember that critically ill children who require invasive diagnostic or therapeutic procedures, or intubation and mechanical ventilation, require appropriate analgesia and sedation. In addition to the obvious benefits of analgesia and sedation, there is evidence to support decreased morbidity and mortality following cardiac surgery in infants treated with effective analgesia.[58-60] In the intensive-care setting, opioids, such as morphine and fentanyl, are commonly used for analgesia, whereas sedation is commonly achieved with benzodiazepines, such as midazolam or diazepam.

Infection

Bacterial, viral, fungal, and protozoal infections are responsible for more than 60% of deaths worldwide. Acute respiratory infections are among the leading cause of childhood mortality and account for almost two million childhood deaths annually. Approximately 70% of these deaths occur in Africa. The most important causes of death in the developing world continue to be malaria, pneumonia, malnutrition, and HIV-related illnesses.[61-63]

In evaluating a child with severe infection, the priority remains to ensure adequate airway, breathing, and circulation. If severe shock is present in the setting of infection, it is important to aim to reverse the shock with aggressive fluid resuscitation and inotropic support, if required, with the ultimate goal of achieving age-appropriate heart rates, normal blood pressure, and capillary refill time.[64] As in the treatment of hypovolaemia, boluses of crystalloid or colloid totalling up to 200 ml/kg may be required, and inotropic support should be considered early in patients unresponsive to two or three boluses of 20 ml/kg. Specific infections may dictate variations in management after initial stability is established. The site of infection as well as likely pathogens will guide the choice of antimicrobial therapy.

Postoperative Care

Following major elective or emergency surgery, the child probably will be haemodynamically unstable and therefore require support for one or more organ systems. Other factors that influence this instability include the age, underlying nutritional status, and premorbid health of the patient; the length of the operation; intraoperative cardiovascular status; and fluid losses. Intensive care may be required from the immediate postoperative period, but delayed deterioration must always be anticipated in high-risk cases and these patients should be monitored accordingly.

In caring for high-risk patients, the degree of support will be dictated by the specific set of clinical circumstances as well as the local resources. Attention must be paid to ensure that adequate oxygen is delivered to the recovering patient. This involves also ensuring adequate ventilation and circulation and appropriate monitoring of the vital signs of the patient. Fluid balance is important in the perioperative period, and careful attention to and monitoring of intake and output are required. Many abdominal surgical procedures result in patients requiring a prolonged period of nutritional support; if available, total parenteral nutrition should be considered in patients who are unable to adequately meet their nutritional demands enterally. Other challenges include the need for total immobility following complex reconstructive surgery, such as repair of an oesophageal atresia. These patients will require intubation and ventilation over several days in order to maintain adequate sedation, analgesia, and muscle relaxation. Finally, it is important that each child be regularly and adequately assessed for pain and distress so that appropriate analgesia and/or sedation may be administered.

Trauma

Traumatic injuries are a cause of significant childhood morbidity and mortality worldwide. Children are particularly vulnerable to traumatic brain as well as major organ injury due to their relatively immature and elastic skeleton and their inability to withstand large blunt forces.[65–67] It is paramount that the initial resuscitation and stabilisation of a critically injured child be both methodical and thorough in order to recognise and institute appropriate therapy in a timely manner. In children who die immediately or soon after an injury, the predominant causes of death are airway compromise resulting in hypoxia, hypovolaemic shock, and injury to the brain and cervical spine. Children are extremely vulnerable to cerebral hypoxia; it is therefore understandable that airway management and attention to respiratory function are the most critically important aspects of resuscitation and ongoing management of the seriously injured child.[10] Attention to these areas of care enable optimal oxygenation and ventilation and minimise secondary injury to the brain and other vital organs. The cervical spine should be immobilised by using either manual in-line stabilisation or on a firm surface with the neck placed in a hard collar of the appropriate size, with lateral support using firm blocks and straps. These cervical spine precautions should remain until such injuries have been excluded clinically, radiologically, or both. With attention to the cervical spine, the airway may be secured by simple airway manoeuvres, or require more specialised equipment or intervention in the form of oral endotracheal intubation.[68]

Thoracic injury may be potentially life-threatening, requiring prompt recognition and treatment.[69] The adequacy of ventilation should be assessed clinically by looking at respiratory rate, pattern, and symmetry of chest movement and breath sounds on auscultation. Adequate oxygenation can be confirmed if the patient appears pink or more definitively with pulse oximetry. Once the airway is definitely secure, if ventilation and oxygenation continue to be inadequate, lung injury should be suspected. Pulmonary contusion may result in respiratory distress and may be confirmed radiologically, although it may be difficult to distinguish from acute aspiration or atelectasis. The presence of unilaterally decreased breath sounds, hypoxia, and cardiovascular compromise should raise the suspicion of pneumothorax or haemothorax. These conditions should be treated urgently by needle or drain thoracocentesis. Mediastinal injuries with the potential for large vessel or major airway trauma are surgical emergencies and require prompt imaging and surgical intervention.[70]

Children are capable of losing up to 40% of their intravascular volume while maintaining a relatively normal blood pressure. The signs and symptoms of early shock due to blood loss may be subtle; it is therefore important to begin fluid resuscitation early, before a seriously injured child becomes haemodynamically unstable. Direct pressure should be applied to any visible external bleeding site in an attempt to stop the bleeding. Secure intravenous access should be sought; common veins used include antecubital, saphenous, and femoral. In the absence of obvious lower limb fracture, an intraosseous (IO) needle into the anterior tibia is a reliable and potentially life-saving form of intravenous (IV) access. Initial fluid resuscitation should consist of two 10-ml/kg boluses of isotonic crystalloid solution, which may be followed by a further two 10-ml/kg boluses of fluid. If signs of shock with evidence of ongoing blood loss persist, consider the use of either O-negative or type-specific packed red blood cells for further fluid boluses.

Once the child is physiologically stable, perform a complete systemic examination. This would normally include various radiological investigations of the cervical spine, chest, and pelvis, and, if intrabdominal injury is suspected, ultrasound or CT. The specific investigations are guided by the clinical scenario and availability of specialised imaging. Many intrathoracic and intraabdominal injuries may be managed conservatively; however, some surgical intervention may be required. Bowel injury may present in a delayed fashion, requiring surgery some time after the initial injury. Detailed surgical management of specific injuries is beyond the scope of this chapter, and is addressed in relevant chapters of this book.

Challenges of Paediatric Critical Care

The biggest challenges for health care providers in the developing world include improving primary care and public health efforts, such as immunisation and sanitation, as well as ensuring universal access to health care.[71]

The provision of critical care and the limited means available to run a dedicated critical care environment suitable for children from infancy to adolescence present an ethical dilemma when multiple health care demands coexist. In an attempt to address such dilemmas, certain units have developed intensive care admission criteria that would not exist in the developed world. Examples of these criteria include refusing admission to an augmented or critical care environment in patients known to be infected with human immunodeficiency virus (HIV) as well as refusing admission to a critical care environment in patients who present acutely to a health care centre and would require transfer to the regional paediatric intensive care unit (PICU). This is particularly evident in sub-Saharan Africa, where there is a huge burden on health as a result of the HIV epidemic.[61–62]

Approximately two million children worldwide have HIV; of these, 90% live in sub-Saharan Africa. Although the rate of annual HIV-related deaths in children is gradually decreasing, approximately

300,000 children continue to die of AIDS-related illnesses worldwide every year.[63]

Paediatric critical care in developing countries is necessarily highly centralised. Most developing countries have large centres that provide varying degrees of tertiary medical care, including paediatric critical care. However, the resources available to these tertiary centres are extremely inconsistent and unpredictable; as a result, the medical capabilities differ widely across centres and countries.[72]

In an attempt to provide critical care for children, hospitals must use existing resources to the best of their ability, including, for example, using existing theatre facilities as an environment to care for critically ill children in the short term or combining adult, paediatric, and neonatal critical care.

In view of the limited availability of paediatric critical care in developing countries, it is important to define priorities and recognise those children who might benefit from being transferred and admitted to a dedicated unit. The additional costs incurred by safe and effective transport of the most vulnerable paediatric patients are a major consideration in the decision-making process and undoubtedly will influence the allocation of limited resources. Determining those admission criteria will depend on local as well as wider factors within a defined geographical area.

Unfortunately, data available on the provision of paediatric critical care in the developing world are lacking. Only the most sophisticated and developed units with dedicated resources for expensive diagnostic and therapeutic drugs and equipment tend to publish data, thereby creating a publication bias.[1] As a result, published data may not reflect the true spectrum of the clinical workload.

Conclusion

Many complex factors affect the ability to provide dedicated paediatric critical care units. Much of the modern infrastructure may be out of reach to units due to cost. Caring for paediatric patients during acute critical illness or injury as well as following major surgery can be both challenging and rewarding. Attention and priority should be at maintaining a secure airway, followed by providing adequate respiratory and cardiovascular support. Detailed clinical history, examination, and, where possible, further investigations will provide clearer diagnostic information in the aim of providing definitive care. Paediatric critical care not only provides the management of children with severe medical or surgical illness, but frequently goes beyond cure to encompass holistic care of the patient and family.

Evidence-Based Research

Tables 12.4 and 12.5 present evidence-based reviews of ventilation strategies and sepsis management, respectively.

Table 12.4: Evidence-based research.

Title	Review of paediatric intensive care ventilation practice
Authors	Turner DA, Arnold JH
Institution	Harvard Medical School and Department of Anesthesia, Division of Critical Care Medicine, Children's Hospital, Boston, Massachusetts, USA
Reference	Curr Opin Crit Care 2007; 13(1):57–63
Problem	Review current paediatric ventilation strategies and evidence.
Outcome/ effect	Mechanical ventilation with pressure limitation by using low tidal volumes has become the main form of ventilation in paediatric intensive care units.
Historical significance/ comments	Various ventilator strategies such as high-frequency oscillatory ventilation, airway pressure release ventilation, and adjuncts such as surfactant, need further evaluation.

Table 12.5: Evidence-based research.

Title	Clinical practice parameters for hemodynamic support of pediatric and neonatal septic shock: 2007 update from the American College of Critical Care Medicine
Authors	Brierley J, Carcillo JA, Choong K, Cornell T, DeCaen A, Deymann A, et al.
Institution	American College of Critical Care Medicine, Mount Prospect, Illinois, USA
Reference	Crit Care Med 2009; 37(2):666–688
Problem	Clinical guidelines required to promote best practices and improve patient outcomes in paediatric and neonatal septic shock.
Intervention	Extensive literature search with experts in field grading evidence.
Comparison/ control (quality of evidence)	Compares centres that implemented previous guidelines.
Outcome/ effect	Early use of paediatric and neonatal sepsis guidelines was associated with improved outcome.
Historical significance/ comments	Continue to support the early use of age-specific therapies to attain time-sensitive goals. Compared to adults, children require proportionally larger quantities of fluid in resuscitation for sepsis. Early use of inotropic support is recommended.

Key Summary Points

1. Respiratory failure is a major cause of paediatric morbidity and mortality worldwide, and early intervention is essential to prevent progression to cardiopulmonary arrest.

2. Oxygen should be administered to all critically ill or injured children in the highest possible concentration until the assessment of cardiorespiratory status is complete.

3. International consensus guidelines on the management of paediatric and neonatal septic shock provide a clear treatment framework, demonstrating that aggressive fluid management of hypovolemic and septic shock has a positive impact on outcome.

4. Whenever possible, efforts should be made to minimise inflation pressures in positive pressure ventilation to protect the patient from lung injury.

5. The degree of intensive care support is dictated by the specific set of clinical circumstances as well as the local resources.

References

1. Wheeler DS, Wong HR, Shanley TP. Pediatric Critical Care Medicine. Basic Science and Clinical Evidence. Springer-Verlag London Limited, 2007.

2. Macnab A, Macrae D, Henning R. Care of the Critically Ill Child, 1st ed. Churchill Livingstone, 15 September 1999.

3. Hickey RW, Cohen DM, Strausbaugh S, Dietrich AM. Pediatric patients requiring CPR in the prehospital setting. Ann Emerg Med 1995; 25:495–501.

4. Innes PA, Summers CA, Boyd IM, Molyneaux EM. Audit of pediatric cardiopulmonary resuscitation. Arch Dis Child 1993; 68:487–491.

5. Thompson JE, Bonner B, Lower GM. Pediatric cardiopulmonary arrests in rural populations. Pediatrics 1990; 86:302–306.

6. Teach SJ, Moore PE, Fleischer GR. Death and resuscitation in the pediatric emergency department. Ann Emerg Med 1995; 25:799–803.

7. Peters MJ, Tasker RC, Kiff KM, Yates R, Hatch DJ. Acute hypoxic respiratory failure in children: case mix and utility of respiratory indices. Intensive Care Med 1998; 24:699–705.

8. Sirbaugh PE, Pepe PE, Shook JE, et al. A prospective, population-base study of the demographics, epidemiology, management, and outcome of out-of-hospital pediatric cardiopulmonary arrest. Ann Emerg Med 1999; 33:174–184.

9. Young KD, Seidel JS. Pediatric cardiopulmonary resuscitation: a collective review. Ann Emerg Med 1999; 33:195–205.

10. Advanced Life Support Group (ALSG). Advanced Paediatric Life Support. The Practical Approach, 4th ed. BMJ Books, 4 February 2005.

11. Brown OE. Structure and function of the upper airway. In: Westmore RF, Muntz HR, McGill TJI, eds. Pediatric Otolaryngology. Principles and Practice Pathways. Thieme Publishers; 2000: 679–688.

12. Eckenhoff J. Some anatomic considerations of the infant larynx influencing endotracheal anesthesia. Anesthesiology 1951; 12:401–410.

13. Cote CJ, Ryan JF, Todres ID, Groudsouzian NG, eds. A Practice of Anesthesia for Infants and Children, 2nd ed. WB Saunders, 1993.

14. McNiece WL, Dierdorf SF. The pediatric airway. Semin Pediatr Surg 2004; 13:152–165.

15. Dickinson AE. The normal and abnormal pediatric upper airway. Recognition and management of obstruction. Clin Chest Med 1987; 8:583–596.

16. Rotta AT, Wiryawan B. Respiratory emergencies in children. Respir Care 2003; 48(3):248–258; discussion 258–260.

17. Flori HR, Glidden DV, Rutherford GW, Matthay MA. Pediatric acute lung injury: prospective evaluation of risk factors associated with mortality. Am J Respir Crit Care Med 2005; 171(9):995–1001. Epub 23 December 2004.

18. DeBruin W, Notterman D, Magid M, Godwin T, Johnston S. Acute hypoxic respiratory failure in infants and children: clinical and pathological characteristics. Crit Care Med 1992; 24:699–705.

19. Timmons OD, Havens PL, Fackler JC. Predicting death in pediatric patients with acute respiratory failure. Pediatric Critical Care Study Group, Extracorporeal Life Support Organization. Chest 1995; 108(3):789–797.

20. PICANet National Report 2006–2008. Available at: http://www.picanet.org.uk/Documents/General/Annual 20report_2009/PICANet 20National 20Report 202006 20-202008_new.pdf.

21. Hoyert DL, Kung H-C, Smith BL. Deaths: preliminary data for 2003. Natl Vital Statistics Rep 2005; 53(15):1–48.

22. Taussig LM, Landau LI. Pediatric Respiratory Medicine. Mosby, 1999.

23. Zaritsky A. Cardiopulmonary resuscitation in children. Clin Chest Med 1987; 8:561–571.

24. Wheeler DS, Wong HR, Shanley TP. Pediatric Critical Care Medicine. Basic Science and Clinical Evidence. Springer-Verlag London Limited, 2007, Pp 299 –307.

25. Gattinoni L, Carlesso E, Cadringher P, Valenza F, Vagginelli F, Chiumello D. Physical and biological triggers of ventilator-induced lung injury and its prevention. Eur Respir J Suppl 2003; 47:15s–25s.

26. Tobin MJ. Principles and Practice of Mechanical Ventilation. McGraw-Hill, 1994.

27. Network TA. Ventilation with lower tidal volumes as compared with traditional tidal volumes for acute lung injury and the acute respiratory distress syndrome. N Engl J Med 2000; 342:1301–1308.

28. Ceneviva G, Paschall JA, Maffei F, Carcillo JA. Hemodynamic support in fluid-refractory pediatric septic shock. Pediatrics 1998; 102(2):e19.

29. Carcillo JA, Pollack MM, Ruttimann UE, Fields AI. Sequential physiologic interactions in pediatric cardiogenic and septic shock. Crit Care Med 1989; 17(1):12–16.

30. Cochrane Injuries Group Albumin Reviewers. Human albumin administration in critically ill patients: systematic review of randomised controlled trials. BMJ 1998; 317(7153):235–240.

31. Finfer S, Bellomo R, Boyce N, French J, Myburgh J, Norton R. A comparison of albumin and saline for fluid resuscitation in the intensive care unit. N Engl J Med 2004; 350(22):2247–2256.

32. Upadhyay M, Singhi S, Murlidharan J, Kaur N, Majumdar S. Randomized evaluation of fluid resuscitation with crystalloid (saline) and colloid (polymer from degraded gelatin in saline) in pediatric septic shock. Indian Pediatr 2005; 42(3):223–231.

33. Schroth M, Plank C, Meissner U, Eberle KP, Weyand M, Cesnjevar R, et al. Hypertonic-hyperoncotic solutions improve cardiac function in children after open-heart surgery. Pediatrics 2006; 118(1):e76–e84.

34. Ngo NT, Cao XT, Kneen R, Wills B, Nguyen VM, Nguyen TQ, et al. Acute management of dengue shock syndrome: a randomized double-blind comparison of 4 intravenous fluid regimens in the first hour. Clin Infect Dis 2001; 32(2):204–213.

35. Nhan NT, Phuong CXT, Kneen R, et al. Acute management of dengue shock syndrome: A randomized double-blind comparison of 4 intravenous fluid regimens in the first hour. Clin Infect Dis 2001; 32:204–212.

36. Carcillo JA, Davis AI, Zaritsky A. Role of early fluid resuscitation in pediatric septic shock. JAMA 1991; 266:1242–1245.

37. Lee PK, Deringer JR, Kreiswirth BN, et al. Fluid replacement protection of rabbits challenged subcutaneous with toxic shock syndrome toxins. Infect Immun 1991; 59:879–884.

38. Ottoson J, Dawidson I, Brandberg A, et al. Cardiac output and organ blood flow in experimental septic shock and treatment with antibiotics, corticosteroids, and fluid infusion. Circ Shock 1991; 35:14–24.

39. Wilson MA, Choe MC, Spain DA. Fluid resuscitation attenuates early cytokine mRNA expression after peritonitis. J Trauma 1996; 41:622–627.

40. Boldt J, Muller M, Heesen M. Influence of different volume therapies and entoxifylline infusion on circulating adhesion molecules in critically ill patients. Crit Care Med 1998; 24:385–391.

41. Zadrobilek E, Hackl W, Sporn P, et al. Effect of large volume replacement with balanced electrolyte solutions on extravascular lung water in surgical patients with sepsis syndrome. Intensive Care Med 1989; 15:505–510.

42. Carcillo JA, Tasker RC. Fluid resuscitation of hypovolemic shock: acute medicine's great triumph for children. Intensive Care Med 2006; 32(7):958–961.

43. Pladys P, Wodey E, Betremieux P. Effects of volume expansion on cardiac output in the preterm infant. Acta Paediatr 1997; 86:1241–1245.

44. Ranjit S, Kissoon N, Jayakumar I. Aggressive management of dengue shock syndrome may decrease mortality rate: a suggested protocol. Pediatr Crit Care Med 2005; 6(4):412–419.

45. Reinelt P, Karth GD, Geppert A, Heinz G. Incidence and type of cardiac arrhythmias in critically ill patients: a single center experience in a medical-cardiological ICU. Intensive Care Med 2001; 27(9):1466–1473.

46. Coffin LH Jr, Ankeney JL, Beheler EM. Experimental study and clinical use of epinephrine for treatment of low cardiac output syndrome. Circulation 1966; 33(4 Suppl):I78–I85.

47. Richard C, Ricome JL, Rimailho A, Bottineau G, Auzepy P. Combined hemodynamic effects of dopamine and dobutamine in cardiogenic shock. Circulation 1983; 67(3):620–626.

48. Stopfkuchen H, Racké K, Schwörer H, Queisser-Luft A, Vogel K. Effects of dopamine infusion on plasma catecholamines in preterm and term newborn infants. Eur J Pediatr 1991; 150(7):503–506.

49. Duggal B, Pratap U, Slavik Z, Kaplanova J, Macrae D. Milrinone and low cardiac output following cardiac surgery in infants: is there a direct myocardial effect? Pediatr Cardiol 2005; 26(5):642–645.

50. Ward E, Gushurst CA. Uses and technique of pediatric lumbar puncture. Am J Dis Child 1992; 146(10):1160–1165.

51. Pollock AS, Arieff AI. Abnormalities of cell volume regulation and their functional consequences. Am J Physiol 1980; 239(3):F195–F205.

52. Duke T. Fluid management of bacterial meningitis in developing countries. Arch Dis Child 1998; 79:181–185.

53. Singhi SC, Singhi PD, Srinivas B, et al. Fluid restriction does not improve outcome of acute meningitis. Pediatr Infect Dis J 1995; 14:495–503.

54. Guidelines for the acute medical management of severe traumatic brain injury in infants, children, and adolescents. Chapter 11, Use of hyperosmolar therapy in the management of severe pediatric traumatic brain injury. Pediatr Crit Care Med 2003; 4(3 Suppl):S40–S44.

55. Morrison G, Gibbons E, Whitehouse WP. High-dose midazolam therapy for refractory status epilepticus in children. Intensive Care Med 2006; 32(12):2070–2076.

56. Qureshi A, Wassmer E, Davies P, Berry K, Whitehouse WP. Comparative audit of intravenous lorazepam and diazepam in the emergency treatment of convulsive status epilepticus in children. Seizure 2002; 11(3):141–144.

57. Appleton R, Choonara I, Martland T, Phillips B, Scott R, Whitehouse W. The treatment of convulsive status epilepticus in children. Members of the Status Epilepticus Working Party. Arch Dis Child 2000; 83(5):415–419.

58. Anand KJ, Hansen DD, Hickey PR. Hormonal-metabolic stress responses in neonates undergoing cardiac surgery. Anesthesiology 1990; 73(4):661–670.

59. Anand KJ, Hickey PR. Halothane-morphine compared with high-dose sufentanil for anesthesia and postoperative analgesia in neonatal cardiac surgery. N Engl J Med 1992; 326(1):1–9.

60. Anand KJ, Hickey PR. Pain and its effects in the human neonate and fetus. N Engl J Med 1987; 317(21):1321–1329.

61. Jeena PM, McNally LM, Stobie M, et al. Challenges in the provision of ICU services to HIV infected children in resource poor settings: a South African case study. J Med Ethics 2005; 31:226–230.

62. Frey B, Argent A. Safe paediatric intensive care. Intensive Care Med 2004; 30:1041–1046.

63. 2008 Report on the global AIDS epidemic. Available at: http://www.unaids.org/en/KnowledgeCentre/HIVData/ GlobalReport/2008/2008_Global_report.asp.

64. Brierley J, Carcillo JA, Choong K, et al. Clinical practice parameters for the hemodynamic support of pediatric and neonatal septic shock: 2007 update from the American College of Critical Care Medicine. Crit Care Med 2009; 37(2):666–688.

65. Walker ML, Storrs BB, Mayer T. Factors affecting outcome in the pediatric patient with multiple trauma. Further experience with the modified injury severity scale. Childs Brain 1984; 11(6):387–397.

66. Mayer T, Walker ML, Johnson DG, Matlak ME. Causes of morbidity and mortality in severe pediatric trauma. JAMA 1981; 245(7):719–721.

67. Luerssen TG, Klauber MR, Marshall LF. Outcome from head injury related to patient's age. A longitudinal prospective study of adult and pediatric head injury. J Neurosurg 1988; 68(3):409–416.

68. Chiaretti A, De Benedictis R, Della Corte F, Piastra M, Viola L, Polidori G, Di Rocco C. The impact of initial management on the outcome of children with severe head injury. Childs Nerv Syst 2002; 18(1–2):54–60. Epub 18 December 2001.

69. Sartorelli KH, Vane DW. The diagnosis and management of children with blunt injury of the chest. Semin Pediatr Surg 2003; 13:98–105.

70. American College of Surgeons. Advanced Trauma Life Support, 7th ed. American College of Surgeons, 2002.

71. Sachdeva RC. Intensive care—a cost effective option for developing countries? Indian J Pediatr 2001; 68:339–342.

72. Mathivhal LR. ICU's worldwide: an overview of critical care medicine in South Africa. Crit Care Med 2001; 2:108–112.

CHAPTER 13
ETHICS OF PAEDIATRIC SURGERY IN AFRICA

Daniel Sidler   Benedict C. Nwomeh
Sharon King   Peter F. Omonzejele

Introduction

A paediatric surgeon not only has the responsibility to care for the young and developing patient but equally has the duty to counsel and care for the concerned parents—and sometimes their broader family members, who all live within a very specific cultural milieu with its value systems and demands. Besides surgical skills, therefore, a paediatric surgeon needs to be aware of the psychological, cultural, and ethical issues involved with the care of patients and their families. At times, this can be quite challenging.

Paediatric surgery has a long and interesting history of profound concern with providing quality of care and the many potential ethical dilemmas encountered. Old traditions as well as new technological developments can present with a quagmire of ethical dilemmas, and modern paediatric surgeons should be aware of these issues and have the cognitive and emotional maturity as well as the skills to carry out their duties in the most professional manner.

This chapter can only be a very short introduction to some important ethical issues, concentrating on the often neglected African aspects.

History

Historically, the Hippocratic Oath defined the ethical principles guiding medicine, instructing physicians to use their knowledge and skills for the benefit and protection of their patients. Over the years, a collaborative process has evolved, incorporating ethical principles of patient autonomy, respect for persons, nonmaleficence, beneficence, and justice.[1] In this model, the physician contributes medical knowledge, skill, and judgment; the patient or patient advocate personally evaluates the potential benefits and risks inherent in the proposed treatment.

Western medical ethics may be traced to guidelines on the duty of physicians in antiquity, such as the Hippocratic Oath and early rabbinic and Christian teachings. From the medieval and early modern period, the field is indebted to such Muslim physicians as Ishaq bin Ali Rahawi, who wrote the *Conduct of a Physician*, the first book dedicated to medical ethics, and al-Razi; Jewish thinkers such as Maimonides; Roman Catholic scholastic thinkers such as Thomas Aquinas; and the case-oriented analysis (casuistry) of Catholic moral theology. These intellectual traditions still continue today in Catholic, Islamic, and Jewish medical ethics.

In modern times, five main reasons have been constitutive for the birth of a discipline of biomedical ethics expressed succinctly by Isaiah Berlin[2]:

> I wish my life and decisions to depend on myself, not on external forces of whatever kind. I wish to be the instrument of my own, not other men's act of will. I wish to be a subject, not an object; to be moved by reasons, by conscious purposes which are my own, not by causes which affect me, as it were, from outside. I wish to be

somebody, not nobody—a doer, deciding, not being decided for, self-directed and not acted upon by external nature or by other men.

This is in stark contrast to the African philosophy of Ubuntu, which basically says that one's humanity is dependent on the appreciation, preservation, and affirmation of the other person's humanity, as was well expressed by Dzobo in 1992[3]: *"We are, therefore I am, and since I am, therefore we are."*

Before we go into the discussions of what constitutes African ethics, we need to clarify the use of that term in this context. The entire African continent cannot be said to have identical cultural ethics. However, ethical themes and values are similar "in their essentials, as African cultures, metaphysics, attitudes are at least very similar".[4] For the purpose of this chapter, the generalisation to African ethics based on similar African cultures is therefore acceptable. This applies with the exception of North Africa, where cultures and ethics are more in line with Islamic injunctions.

African ethics (also known as African traditional ethics) is communal in outlook; it defines moral precepts and values that Africans abide by consciously or unconsciously in their day-to-day living. Those moral precepts are defined and founded on communal values. Hence, Africans have the saying that "one can only dance well when one dances in line with the drum beat of the community". This means that what is considered good or bad is what the community considers as such. For instance, amongst the Esan people of southern South Nigeria, *ebeme* and *agbonsi* (the good and worthy life) are understood in terms of the communal good. This means that the realisation and actualisation of the self is expected to be through and within the community and not outside of the community.

However, this does not mean that the self is suppressed in favour of the community. Rather, it means that in the actualisation of the self, the community should and indeed must be taken into consideration. As a result, community recognition and appreciation are highly important in African communities, and a member cannot be recognised by the community if his or her moral values are personal and subjective and at variance with those of the community. This is important, as "morality in African traditional thought is essentially interpersonal and social, with a basis in human well-being".[5]

African ethics is based on a communal and utilitarian foundation. In traditional African societies, the good aims for greater benefits to the generality of the community, and is therefore not based on religious or divine injunctions as such. "The gods may only be relevant when it comes to the use of divination and application of sanctions, that is, if a member of the society errs against the norms of the society and he is unrepentant".[6] This belief implies that the consequences of one's actions rather than the alignment of such action with his or her religious faith determine praiseworthiness from a community perspective.

Western-Style Medical Ethics

Let us first look at the Western style of medical ethics and at the five important constitutive points and discuss how we could apply these principles to an African context:

1. growth of the middle class with its new value system of individualism, utilitarianism, and a culture of consumerism;

2. disenchantment of the world, leading to a decline of a reliance on myths, religions, and ideologies, leading to an increased rational and practical approach to life;

3. increased influence of feminism, giving rights to women;

4. fragmentation of society into different spheres, such as human rights, morality, religion, politics, jurisdiction, family, school, etc. as well as the super-specialisation within medicine; and

5. new belief or ideology of a technoscientific progress into utopia.

Such faith in a utopia achievable by technoscientific progress boosted the scientific enterprise enormously. Such scientific discoveries were not only embraced with enthusiasm, but created an equal amount of controversy. Medical progress (e.g., haemodialysis becoming possible with the development of the arteriovenous shunt, or techniques of cardiopulmonary resuscitation), together with the perennial problem of limited resources, raised a set of very difficult considerations, such as who should live, who should die, and who should decide?

Such positive development was not without serious abuse of physician power, as is highlighted by the Tuskegee study. One of US president Bill Clinton's more convincing apologies in recent times was that made on 16 May 1997, for the infamous Tuskegee Syphilis Study. From 1932 to 1972, hundreds of poor black farm workers with syphilis were deliberately left untreated, with the supposed goal of studying the natural history of the disease. Participants received free food and transportation to encourage them to join a study they were told was aimed at curing their "bad blood". In fact, government officials went to inordinate lengths over the decades to ensure that these men received no treatment at all, even after the discovery of penicillin. It is inexplicable that such a study went on for more than 40 years (1930–1970), even after a treatment for syphilis was found. It is unlikely, even after the Nuremberg Code and the Universal Declaration of Human Rights (1948), that people would be safe from unethical research practices.

Recent research on male circumcision as a prevention of human immunodeficiency virus (HIV) (3 randomised controlled trials (RCTs) in South Africa, Kenya, and Uganda) requires assessment of the research outcome for the female partners of those men who were HIV positive at the time of circumcision, to realise that a Tuskegee could be repeated. It has been suggested that the female partners of the HIV-infected men who were circumcised had not been informed that they were part of a study. The outcome of the study as reported by Dr. Wawer,[7] showed that the HIV incidence of those female partners increased by 60% over a period of two years.

Informed Consent

In the Western world, a specific style of conversation between the patient and doctor has developed whereby the patient is encouraged to take a more active, informed position within the decision-making process.[8] Some physicians, however, still point out that they can solve all difficult questions without discussing them with the patient or the patient's proxy by relying solely on their own professional expertise. It is important, however, to be aware that professional expertise is not without value judgements. Therefore, the physician-patient relationship has been described as an often-conflicting power dichotomy. An extreme on the side of patient autonomy denies any room for physician decision making.[9] Such an extreme approach had been called the informative, or engineering, model of the patient-physician relationship, whereby the "physician's role is to disclose factual information about

diagnosis, prognosis, treatment options, etc. A patient's role, on the other hand, is to inform his or her physician about values and preferences concerning treatment".[10] The assumption here seems to be that all value-judgements should be the patient's responsibility. Such an assumption, however, is illusionary because value-free information is impossible to attain.[10]

More important are five consequences of this informative model. (1) It impoverishes the patient-physician relationship by discouraging doctors from empathising with their patients because such empathy is considered undesirable and might negatively influence the doctor's professional attitude. (2) It stops any discussion between the patient and doctor from the beginning, preventing doctors from questioning perceived strange and irrational patient treatment demands and preferences. (3) It prohibits physicians from sharing their acquired personal experiences and moral beliefs. (4) It completely misinterprets patients' preferences as ready-made and given; it does not acknowledge or allow patient preferences to develop or to be adjusted during the course of illness and therapy. (5) It deals with the patient-doctor relationship and their respective preferences and attitudes as if there were no overall, encompassing societal good to be considered; it completely ignores that both patient and doctor have their preferences imprinted by society and need them to be adjusted from time to time by the overall good of society.

Paternalism, as the opposite of the informative model, often involves some form of interference with or refusal to conform to patients' preferences. "Paternalism, then, is the intentional overriding of one person's known preferences or actions by another person, where the person who overrides justifies the action by the goal of benefitting or avoiding harm to the person whose will is overridden."[1]

Within the African context, paternalism has hardly been contested. It is still common and easy for physicians to ignore and neglect patient autonomy. Apart from the cultural divide and lack of exposure to each other's value systems, there is an underlying assumption that medical knowledge and technology could be too complex to understand for patients in general, and African patients in particular. Patients easily develop unrealistic expectations of modern medicine and adopt a cowed role, trusting their doctors' expertise unconditionally.

We suggest that the dichotomy between autonomy and paternalism be abandoned altogether to favour a model of deliberation wherein patient and physician interact, share and finally make the decision together. Both parties ought to accept moral responsibility to arrive at a decision. Such a solution is more than just the consensus of two positions and suits the African context and philosophy of Ubuntu. The deliberation model points to the urgent need for democratisation of Western medicine and its institutions.

Giving informed consent for a procedure on a child has its own set of problems. It is morally advisable, if a child has the cognitive and emotional maturity to understand the situation, that his or her assent should be sought as well as the consent of the parents or legal proxy. Parents, however, do not have the right to refuse or give consent to surgical procedures if doing so would be detrimental or of no immediate benefit to the child. Paediatric surgeons should be familiar with each country's individual legislation.

The ethical justification of informed consent is respect for the patient's and family's autonomy and for the right of the patient or proxy to make informed decisions. Informed consent is, therefore, one of our main duties as paediatric surgeons, and this usually means obtaining parental consent.

Informed consent includes a three-tier cascade, each step presupposing the previous one.

1. *Determination of the patient's competence to give consent:* Competence is a prerequisite to be able to give informed consent. A competent patient needs to be able to grasp the essentials of what is explained, to think rationally and logically, and to come to an

apparent rational decision. Competence can be limited according to the circumstances of the patient, both intrinsic (mental) and extrinsic (specific law or rule, such as incarceration or institutionalisation).

2. *Provision of adequate information:* Information forms the foundation upon which the competent patient can make a decision. Such information must include a full explanation of the proposed techniques as well as information about the chances of success, incidence of complications, risks involved, available alternatives and their relative risks and complications, costs involved, and the role of each member of the surgical team. Risks include those inherent to the procedure and disease, compounded by host risks relating to underlying disease and comorbidity, as well as those inherent to the particular environment where surgery is to be performed (e.g., inexperienced surgeon, new procedure, and so on).[11]

3. *Decision making:* Based on the information supplied and the patient's competence, the patient or proxy can make a voluntary decision without coercion to undergo (or defer) a treatment. The patient or proxy should be informed of the consequences of that decision and his or her right to withdraw such consent at any stage and to seek a second opinion.

Within clinical practice, the process of informed consent presents several inherent problems:

1. *The timing of obtaining consent:* Under ideal circumstances, the taking of informed consent should occur a few days prior to surgery to facilitate unhurried, uncoerced decision making; to obtain more information; to discuss the matter with family members; and to review the decisions made. In the case of an emergency, this might be impossible, but this does not absolve the surgeon of the responsibility to obtain informed consent to whatever extent possible. We address the subject of informed consent during emergency surgery later in this chapter.

2. *The complexity of the disease and its modern surgical treatment:* Paediatric surgery has become a mature discipline in its own right,[12] and the technological options have been growing. Not all options are currently available in some African countries due to resource constraints. Some patients might therefore decide to have their elective surgery performed in another country.

3. *The extent of information necessary:* Any information that the patient might need, or reasonably use, to make a decision is appropriate. As a general guideline, the more serious a condition and the higher the probability of risk and complications, the greater is the need to inform the patient. However, forcing unwanted information onto a patient could cause unnecessary anguish and could be interpreted as psychological battery.

4. *Risk disclosure:* A reasonable question is whether it serves the patient's interest to disclose all complications and how much patients actually understand the statistics. The ideal would be to provide institutional outcome figures. As an alternative to quoting actual figures of complication risks, a verbal scale from very high, to moderate, to very low, to negligible could be used.

5. *The use of aids and pamphlets:* The South African Health Professions Council (HPCSA) guidelines advocate the use of "up-to-date written material, visual and other aids to explain complex aspects of . . . treatment where appropriate and/or practicable".

6. *Who should take the consent?* Without a doubt, the surgeon doing the procedure is the best person to obtain consent. The surgeon should inform the patient about the risks and complications that could arise from the procedure.

7. *Costs:* It is the duty of the surgeon to inform the patient or parents/caregivers about the costs to be incurred and how they are expected to pay.

8. *Research:* These points do not apply fully to research on patients.

In summary, the patient's cooperation is important before performing any procedure. The aim is not to impress or dominate, but to inform. The surgeon should use understandable and down-to-earth language, tapered to the level of the patient's and parents' understanding, to discuss:

- all invasive procedures and those realistically expected;
- all common and serious complications; and
- all options and alternatives.

The basic idea of the process of informed consent–taking is that the surgeon should have made as sincere an attempt as possible to come as close to the ideal, given the limitations of time, language, and cultural difficulties.

HIV, Ethics, and the Paediatric Surgeon

Why is human immunodeficiency virus/acquired immune deficiency syndrome (HIV/AIDS) such a major issue for society and for medicine? One of the reasons is the sheer magnitude of the pandemic, especially in sub-Saharan Africa. The vast majority of affected people are poor and thus easily subjected to discrimination. Another is the fact that it is a sexually transmitted disease, and as such is viewed as morally reprehensible. People affected by HIV/AIDS are often seen as blameworthy, and AIDS is viewed as punishment for moral transgression. Grayling writes that AIDS is seen as "evidence of God's wrath, justly provoked by our sins".[13]

HIV is different from other epidemics because it affects mainly young adults and has a long incubation period with a very high mortality. Additionally, the HIV outbreak has occurred at a time when medicine is very technology driven, and advances in medical and surgical treatment may expose health care workers (HCWs) to great risk from blood and other body fluids.[14]

The surgeon is a unique medical professional in that "any operation performed harms before healing....Consequently, by striving to minimise this necessary temporary injury to the patient while maximising the therapy's curative potential, surgeons have forever engaged in ethical deliberations".[15] The Cambridge Textbook of Bioethics describes the surgeon as being the patient's advocate "in the purest sense"[15] because the surgeon protects the patient's values as well as his or her physical health.

In the context of HIV, it is important to consider whether surgery poses an additional risk to the HIV-infected person, and to weigh the relative risks and benefits.[16] There is also the issue of personal risk to the surgeon, and whether the HCW can refuse to treat an HIV-infected patient. This hotly debated subject in the ethics literature in the late 1980s and early 1990s has become a nonissue with the advent of antiretroviral treatment (ART) and postexposure prophylaxis.[14]

By virtue of its high prevalence in Africa, the surgeon inevitably will encounter many moral dilemmas associated with HIV/AIDS. In this chapter, we address the following ethical dilemmas in the context of HIV/AIDS and medical care: HIV testing and informed consent; confidentiality, privacy, and the duty to warn; and justice, discrimination, and access to ART. We also touch on the debate around the ethics of neonatal circumcision as prevention for HIV.

HIV Testing and Informed Consent

Usually, in-depth discussion and consent for blood tests is not required. However, HIV historically was considered to be different because treatment was not available early in the AIDS epidemic, and HIV was associated with psychosocial risks and discrimination with regard to employment and access to health insurance.[17] International and national guidelines state that HIV testing should be done only with the informed consent of the patient (if old enough to consent) or the parent, and after pretest counselling. This approach to HIV testing, together with respect for confidentiality, constitutes a strict advocacy view of the rights of the individual. The issues of consent in children, particularly in the African setting, have already been addressed in the first part of this chapter, and they also apply here. The age at which a child can consent to HIV testing depends on the child's maturity and understanding. New legislation in South Africa places this age at 12 years. There is an increasingly strong movement, both internationally and locally, to advocate for "opt-out" testing, where HIV testing becomes part of routine medical care unless patients refuse it. The problem for Africa is that antiretroviral therapy is not universally available, making it difficult to legislate "opt-out" testing. The current approach is to recommend voluntary testing except in very limited emergency situations.

Confidentiality, Privacy, and the Duty to Warn
The stigma and discrimination associated with HIV/AIDS necessitate confidentiality and privacy of information. If privacy of medical information is assured, it is more likely that patients will be prepared to be tested, and it promotes patient autonomy and trust in the clinical relationship.

An important consideration for the paediatric surgeon is that a diagnosis of HIV in a young child implies, in the majority of cases, that the mother is HIV infected. This impacts on confidentiality regarding the mother's status and relationships and gives rise to a set of ethical and moral dilemmas.

Conflict may arise in the clinical situation where HCWs demand to know the status of patients as they believe themselves to be at risk of being infected. This is of particular importance in the case of surgeons, who are at even greater risk of becoming infected due to the nature of their work. With the adoption of universal infection control precautions, however, the risk of HIV transmission should be minimised, provided the necessary resources are available.[18]

But what about HIV-infected HCWs? Do they also have a duty to disclose their HIV status to patients or to health authorities? Should this form part of the informed consent process? Disclosure may jeopardise HCWs' ability to practice and their careers, and so the general guideline is that HCWs may continue to practise without disclosure, but with restrictions so as to avoid situations in which the patient may be at high risk of becoming infected.[16]

Justice, Discrimination, and Access to Treatment
The reality of medical practice in Africa is that it mostly occurs in resource-constrained environments. It is inevitable that distributive justice will play an important role in ensuring the fair distribution of these resources. Public policy dictates that those patients who would benefit the most should have access to ART, and that eligibility criteria are just.[19] At the same time, people admitted to the ART programme are expected to be compliant; resistant viral strains have been identified in patients who have not been on ART.[14] The rights of the individual to access therapy have to be weighed against the rights of the community put at risk by noncompliant patients. How does one manage a young child who is dependent on the caregiver for access to ARTs, but whose caregiver is not an adherent to therapy? Should the child be removed from the caregiver?

HIV-infected individuals have been subjected to discrimination in society as well as by the health care system.[18] This discrimination results in patients being deprived of services and care, which may cause them to lose faith in the system. Children may be denied access to certain health services (e.g., intensive care or surgery) because of their HIV status. It is difficult for the individual surgeon unilaterally to make difficult decisions, and policymakers increasingly have adopted the approach of "accountability for reasonableness" to prioritise services.[16]

Neonatal Circumcision for the Prevention of HIV
A full discussion of circumcision to prevent HIV is beyond the scope of this chapter. Three studies from Africa have demonstrated a protective effect of circumcision against heterosexual HIV acquisition in adult males, and this finding has been extrapolated to a recommendation to perform mandatory neonatal circumcision in sub-Saharan Africa.[20] The argument that "newborns are extremely resilient and are programmed for stress" to support the neonatal timing of circumcision[21] does not take into account the ethical issues surrounding the removal "of healthy tissue from patients who are unable to consent to the procedure".[22] Extrapolating the

weak protective effect in a selective adult population to infant circumcision without any supportive data[23] may not be appropriate.

Informed Consent during Emergency Operations
Among the several legitimate exceptions to the right of informed consent are public health emergency, medical emergency, the incompetent patient, patient waiver of consent, and therapeutic privilege.[24] When immediate action must be taken to prevent death or other serious harm to the patient, the emergency exception mandates that appropriate care not be delayed.[24,25] Informed consent under this condition is based on the legitimate presumption that the child or legal proxy would allow treatment if the opportunity existed, so consent is implied. The exercise of the emergency exception imposes responsibility on the paediatric surgeon to be reasonably certain that immediate intervention is essential to preserve life or to prevent serious harm to the child. In addition, the paediatric surgeon must reach the judgment that treatment cannot be safely delayed to obtain informed consent.[26]

Consideration of informed consent during emergency surgery might be met with some cynicism because the imperative to save life is seen as overriding patients' autonomy. Surgical emergency creates a special challenge insofar as decisions must be made in a relatively short period of time. Submitting a child to emergency surgery is one of the most profound and emotionally exhausting tasks most parents will encounter. Added to the stress of sudden illness and the distress caused by pain or other acute symptoms in their child, parents may have little time to grasp the important information required to give an informed consent. However, only the occasional situation (e.g., haemorrhagic shock) justifies the emergency exception. In the majority of children undergoing urgent or emergency surgery (e.g., appendectomy), there is quite often ample time for preoperative education of the family and informed consent.

In Western countries, a surgical emergency rarely absolves the surgeon of the requirement to obtain consent. We propose that African paediatric surgeons observe this practice as a moral and ethical necessity, even though they may not yet have a legal obligation to do so. If the parent(s) or the family members are not present, the surgeon can decide according to the best interest's paradigm. Some hospitals will have their own regulations, such as that the superintendent can give consent to an emergency procedure as long as there is evidence that the staff has tried to contact the family members. Telephonic consent is acceptable.

Informed consent during paediatric surgery emergencies has been the subject of a detailed review, including practical guidance on the methods of preoperative education that can be adopted in the emergency surgery setting and areas in which further research might help to improve this important aspect of surgical care.[27]

Informed Child Assent
Strictly speaking, only those patients who have appropriate decisional capacity and legal empowerment can give their informed consent. Under common law in most countries, the decision-making responsibility falls generally to parents or other surrogates. Because no one—not even the most well-meaning parent acting in a surrogate capacity—can always assure that the child's best interests are being represented, the doctrine of informed consent has limited direct application to children.[28] Although informed permission given by parents does not satisfy the strict moral standards of the doctrine of informed consent, it is sufficient for ethical—and is often required for legal—purposes. In addition, older children and adolescents should be involved, to the greatest extent possible, in their own decision making. Depending on the circumstances, the *assent* of the paediatric patient should be sought, appropriate to their development, age, and understanding, and often in conjunction with informed permission from the parent or legal guardian. In many Western countries, the requirement for informed child assent has been codified, but in all cases, doctors should carefully listen

to the opinion and wishes of children who are not able to give full consent and should strive to obtain their assent. The consent/assent process must promote and protect the dignity, privacy, and confidentiality of the child and his or her family.

Conclusion

This chapter has addressed some of the ethical issues that the paediatric surgeon may encounter. The relationship is three-pronged: the child-patient, the decision maker (parent/caregiver), and the surgical team. It is important that the surgeon be aware of the ethical issues and moral dilemmas influencing this relationship, and that the child's best interests remain paramount. In many African countries, resource constraints also play an important role; here the surgeon must weigh the risks and benefits of surgery to the patient and advocate for the patient where appropriate. There is also an obligation for the experienced surgeon to convey knowledge, skills, and values to other staff and to the public.

Evidence-Based Research

Table 13.1 presents an expert opinion on European guidelines regarding informed child assent.

Table 13.1: Evidence-based research.

Title	Informed consent/assent in children. Statement of the Ethics Working Group of the Confederation of European Specialists in Paediatrics (CESP)
Authors	De Lourdes Levy M, Larcher V, Kurz R
Institution	Ethics Working Group of the CESP, Department of Paediatrics, University Hospital Graz, Graz, Austria; University Clinic of Pediatrics, Hospital de Santa Maria, Lisbon, Portugal; Queen Mary's School of Medicine and Dentistry, London, UK
Reference	Eur J Pediatr 2003; 162(9):629–633
Problem	A report by a working group of experts assembled from several European countries providing paediatric health care practitioners with guidelines on informed consent and assent.
Intervention	Expert opinion.
Outcome/ effect	Consent or assent is required for all aspects of medical care, for preventive, diagnostic, or therapeutic measures and research. The consent/assent process must promote and protect the dignity, privacy, and confidentiality of the child and his or her family.
Historical significance/ comments	This report extends and clarifies similar guidelines issued by the American Academy of Paediatrics, Committee on Bioethics.[28]

Key Summary Points

1. Surgeons should be aware of the specific cultural, psychological, and ethical milieu to which the child and family belongs.

2. Practice should be guided by the ethical principles of patient autonomy, respect for persons, nonmalfaisance, beneficence, and justice.

3. African ethics is based on communal, rather than individual, values.

4. Informed parental consent should always be obtained before surgical procedures to whatever extent possible even in emergencies.

5. Informed child assent should be sought, as appropriate to the child's development, age, and understanding.

References

1. Beauchamp TL, Childress JF. Principles of Biomedical Ethics, 5th ed. Oxford University Press, 2001.

2. Berlin I, Hardy H. Liberty: Incorporating Four Essays on Liberty. Oxford University Press, 2002.

3. Dzobo NK. The image of man in Africa. In: Wiredu K, Gyekye K, eds. Person and Community (Ghaniaian Philosophical Studies). Council for Research in Values and Philosophy, 1992; Pp 132–145.

4. Tangwa G. The traditional African perception of a person: some implications for bioethics. Hastings Center Report 2000; 30:5.

5. Omoregbe, J. Ethics: A Systematic and Historical Study. Joja Educational Publishers, 1998.

6. Omonzejele, P. African ethics and voluntary euthanasia. Medicine and Law Journal 2004; 23.

7. Wawer MJ., et al. Circumcision in HIV-infected men and its effect on HIV transmission to female partners in Rakai, Uganda: a randomised controlled trial. The Lancet 2009; 374(9685):229–237.

8. Katz J, Capron AM. The Silent World of Doctor and Patient. Johns Hopkins University Press, 2002, Pp 1–264.

9. Lelie A, Verweij M. Futility without a dichotomy: towards an ideal physician-patient relationship. Bioethics 2003; 17:21–31.

10. Veatch RM, Stempsey WE. Incommensurability: its implications for the patient/ physician relation. J Med Phil 1995; 20:253–269.

11. McIlwain J. Level of risk (letter), MPS Africa Casebook 2003; 3:26.

12. Moore SW, Sidler D, Rode H. Paediatric surgery: birth of a new specialty or a coming of age? Editorial. SAMJ 2008; 98(4):1.

13. Grayling AC. The Form of Things. Phoenix Publishing, 2006.

14. Bryan CS. HIV/AIDS and bioethics: historical perspective, personal retrospective. Health Care Analysis 2002; 10:5–18.

15. Andrews J, Zaroff L. Surgical ethics. In: Singer PA, Viens AM, eds. The Cambridge Textbook of Bioethics, Cambridge University Press, 2008.

16. Mielke J, Kalangu KKN. The surgeon and human immunodeficiency virus. World J Surg 2003; 27:967–971.

17. Wolf LE, Lo B. Ethical dimensions of HIV/AIDS. HIV InSite Knowledge Base Chapter 2001. Available at: http://hivinsite.ucsf.edu/InSite (accessed 26 February 2006).

18. Gostin LO, Webber DW. HIV infection and AIDS in the public health and health care systems: the role of law and litigation. In: Beauchamp TL, Walters L, eds. Contemporary Issues in Bioethics, 6th ed. Wadsworth/Thomson, 2003.

19. Moodley K. HIV/AIDS in South Africa—an exploration of the ethical options. In: Moodley K, Pienaar W, eds. Medical Ethics Student Manual, Stellenbosch University, Cape Town, 2008.

20. Clark P, Eisenman J, Szapor S. Mandatory neonatal circumcision in sub-Saharan Africa: medical and ethical analysis. Med Sci Monit 2007; 13(12):RA205–RA213.

21. Schoen EJ. Should newborns be circumcised? Yes. Can Fam Physician 2007; 53:2096–2098.

22. Andres D. Should newborns be circumcised? No. Can Fam Physician 2007; 53:2097–2099.

23. Van Howe RS, Svoboda JS. Neonatal circumcision is neither medically necessary nor ethically permissible: a response to Clark et al. Med Sci Monit 2008; 14(8):LE7–LE13.

24. Faden RR, Beauchamp TL: A History and Theory of Informed Consent. Oxford University Press, 1986.

25. American College of Emergency Physicians. Code of ethics for emergency physicians. Ann Emerg Med 1997; 30:365–372.

26. Moskop JC: Informed consent in the emergency department. Emerg Med Clin North Am 1999; 17:327–340.

27. Nwomeh BC, Waller AL, Caniano DA, Kelleher KJ. Informed consent for emergency surgery in infants and children. J Pediatr Surg 2005; 40(8):1320–1325.

28. Committee on Bioethics, American Academy of Pediatrics. Informed consent, parental permission, and assent in pediatric practice. Pediatrics 1995; 95:314–317.

CHAPTER 14
PSYCHOLOGICAL ISSUES IN PAEDIATRIC SURGERY

Akanidomo J. Ibanga

Hannah B. Ibanga

Introduction

The last few decades have been marked by tremendous improvement in the successful performance of most paediatric surgical procedures. This improvement is in terms of both increased knowledge and skills of attending physicians and updated surgical equipment now available for a variety of procedures. This has resulted in a higher survival rate as well as a reduction in the associated risk. Despite these improvements, however, many children and parents still experience high levels of distress when children are awaiting an invasive surgical procedure.[1-4] This chapter looks at issues in paediatric surgical practice that make it stressful not only for the child awaiting surgery but also for the child's parents. We first look briefly at the classifications of surgical procedures and the sources of stress for the child and parents. We then look at the commonly reported stress-related emotional experience, first for the child and then for the parents, and how this relates to prognosis. This discussion is followed by elaborating more on the conditions in sub-Saharan African countries that contribute to possible heightened levels of stress, and we draw this chapter to its conclusion by looking at some evidence-based efforts to reduce surgery-related stress and how effective or feasible the application of these may be in the sub-Saharan health care environment.

Overview of Surgical Procedures

Many parents who may be present during ward rounds or may have overheard discussions or may have had consultations with their child's physician come across terms that refer more to the type of surgery for the child. They may thus hear the surgery being referred to as either major, minor, emergency, elective, or required. It is outside the scope of this chapter to discuss these in detail, but it suffices to briefly describe these terms here.

Major Surgery

Surgery is regarded as major when it involves the head, neck, chest, or abdomen. Examples of these would be surgical operations involving organ transplants or repair of congenital malformations, heart disease, or correction of foetal developmental problems. In comparison to other forms of surgery, this class usually involves a higher risk and longer hospital stay, both pre- and postoperatively.

Emergency (Urgent) Surgery

Emergency surgery is carried out with a focus on correcting a life-threatening condition. Examples of these would be a result of an accident (motor vehicle or many forms of domestic accidents) or where there is an intestinal obstruction or any other life-threatening condition.

Elective Surgery

Unlike the previous surgeries, elective surgery does not correct a life-threatening condition and is not an absolute necessity for the health of the child. It is, however, a surgery that is carried out with the hope of improving the child's quality of life. Surgery to remove a hernia or tonsils, as well as circumcision, would fall under this class.

Required Surgery

Any procedure that is required in order to improve the quality of life for the child is termed required surgery. Required surgery does not need to be done immediately, as is the case for emergency surgery. In this situation, more time is available to plan and prepare the child and parents involved for the surgery

Minor Surgery

Minor surgery is a term reserved for invasive procedures that have a short recovery time. These operations can actually be carried out in an outpatient basis, or the child can go home the same day in most cases. The recovery time for the child to return to normal functioning is usually very short. Although listed as a minor procedure, it is not considered so by parents whose children are awaiting these procedures.

Stress and Anxiety

Irrespective of the class of invasive procedure a child is to undergo, many children and their parents find it stressful. LeRoy and his colleagues[5] looked at different sources of stress for children who were awaiting an operation as well as their parents, and came up with a slightly different list for each of them. The sources of stress for children include: (1) physical harm or injury, resulting in discomfort, pain, mutilation, or death; (2) separation from parents and dealing with strangers in the absence of a familiar, trusted adult; (3) fear of the unknown; (4) uncertainty about limits and acceptable behaviour; and (5) loss of control, autonomy, and competence. In contrast, the sources of stress for parents and guardians include: (1) concern about the possibility of physical harm or injury resulting in discomfort, pain, mutilation, or death to the child; (2) alterations in the parenting role; (3) lack of information; (4) the intensive care unit (ICU) environment; and (5) postoperative changes in the child's behaviour, appearance, or emotional responses.

Anxiety is the most commonly reported stress-related emotion experienced by children awaiting surgery and their parents. Brophy and Erickson,[6] in their survey of those awaiting elective surgery, found that 60% of the children reported being anxious. Note that this was for elective surgical procedures, which are simple and preplanned; for these children to still experience anxieties or fears of compromised physical integrity as well as death, it would be logical to assume that the reported percentage would greatly increase were we to survey those awaiting more complex surgical procedures. In the following subsections, we briefly look at the child's and parents' anxieties and how these affect surgical outcomes. We highlight our need to have a greater understanding and to develop a response to help alleviate these anxieties.

Children's Anxiety

Numerous researchers[7-9] have found an association between preoperative anxiety and negative postsurgical outcomes. When a child is about to undergo surgery, for instance, and is to be anaesthetised, the child who is anxious at this stage is very uncooperative, often making the process more pronounced and prolonged. The greatest risk of noncooperative behaviour is with children between the ages of 2 and 6 years. Preoperative anxiety has also been linked to disturbances at recovery from the effects of anaesthesia.[10–12] Disturbances in the child's postsurgical behaviour have also been recorded;[13,14] for a small group of these children, this problem can be long lasting.

Other multiple adverse outcomes associated with the child's anxiety include increased postoperative pain and delirium[15,16] as well as postsurgical maladaptive behavioural changes.[17,18] Psychosocial adjustment problems are a major concern.[19–21] Notably, these changes are not limited to those awaiting or having undergone an invasive procedure; as pointed out by Vernon,[22] these changes are also evident in children who have been hospitalised without necessarily undergoing any surgical procedure.

An understanding of the effects that a child's level of anxiety has on postsurgical outcomes drives the need to direct efforts that would attempt to reduce preoperative anxiety for these children. Reducing the level of anxiety a child may have in regard to the process may help in facilitating postsurgical recovery for that child.[23–25]

Success in reducing the level of stress experienced, however, depends on a number of factors. This would include the physician's knowledge as well as skills in working with children or liaising with their parents in reducing surgery–related anxiety. Some parents may need guidance in what to say to the child, how much detail to include, the possible presences of a parent at anaesthetic induction, and so forth. Incorporating working with parents and their children to reduce surgery-related anxiety into the routine clinical practice would help circumvent some postsurgical complications that may arise, reduce readmission rates, and shorten hospital contact days.

Parental Anxiety

As mentioned earlier, parents of children undergoing surgery often experience considerable stress themselves. Maligalig[26] found that parents were anxious about anaesthesia and associated risks, how the child would respond to the surgical experience, and their own inadequacy in taking care of the child when discharged from the hospital. The level of anxiety experienced by parents, however, is affected by several factors. Mothers, for instance, experience a greater degree of anxiety than do fathers.[27,28] This may be due to maternal instinct or, as discussed later, the meaning and essence of the child in that family, and the apportioning of blame when the child becomes ill.

The anxiety experienced by parents and their ability to manage it is also related to the coping style adopted. Coping loosely refers to a parent's ability to see the problems as manageable, even in the face of its being unpleasant. When faced with a problem, over time, there are generally two response or coping behaviors—a problem-focused or an emotion-focused strategy. Thus, responses may be predominantly problem-focused or predominantly emotion-focused. People who use problem-focused strategies in coping are likely to be characterised as exhibiting approach behaviours. These individuals would seek health- and procedure-related information about the surgery and they generally would be more anxious prior to the procedure.[29] In contrast, people who adopt emotion-focused strategies are characterised by avoidance of health-related information and denial of the stress. These individuals are more likely to exhibit greater anxiety after the event than before it.

What this implies is that to help people cope with their anxieties, it would be best to know how they predominantly respond to problems. Once we can identify this, we can tailor interventions that are congruent with their response (coping) styles. Providing those who respond with a problem-focused strategy with information and elaborating on the medical equipment and procedure to be undertaken would help alleviate some of these anxieties. This approach, however, would have the opposite effect for those who respond with an emotion-focused strategy. For those parents, it would be best to build in activities that would enable deliberate avoidance or refocusing (distraction) from the procedure. A simple way to identify parents' predominant coping

styles in a clinical setting is to note those parents who exhibit high information-seeking behaviour or a high need to monitor the child's progress. These parents are most likely adopting a problem-focused approach and would benefit greatly from information about the procedure and what the likely outcomes and potential side effects of the procedure may be.

MacLaren and Kain,[30] in their comparative study of mothers of children undergoing minor outpatient surgery and other women awaiting surgery, found that the mothers of these children were more anxious than the women who themselves were undergoing minor operations, but equally as anxious as women awaiting major surgery. These findings lend credence to earlier studies,[14,15] which found that mothers of children sought more preoperative information concerning their child's surgery than adult patients who were themselves awaiting surgery.

The focus on the parents' anxiety in regard to the child's surgical procedure is important for several reasons. As pointed out by Piira et al.,[31] parents play a critical role in managing the child's pain in the aftermath of surgery; they are responsible for collaborating with health care professionals in making decisions and choices regarding the child's health and would need to be competent and prepared to do so. If the parents' anxiety and distress are high, their understanding may be hindered and their level of cooperation may be inadequate for the proper management of the child. Thus, parents should be adequately informed and in a frame of mind to give consent.

A high level of parental anxiety during communication with physicians may affect both their ability to communicate their concerns and ask questions and their understanding of the physicians' explanations and prescriptions. This then runs the risk of poor postsurgical management of the child. As pointed out by Montgomery et al.,[32] there may be a need to engage parents identified as anxious in a different kind of information-sharing process.

Additionally, high parental preoperative anxiety is associated with high preoperative anxiety in children undergoing surgery;[10,33–35] it would be correct to assume that a reduction in parental anxiety would lead to better outcomes for the children. Children have a tendency to evaluate and validate their experience based on the responses of the adults around them; often, these are the child's parents. This is seen in babies just learning to walk: whether a fall is worthy of tears or they should just pick themselves up and carry on with what they were engaged in has much to do with the response of the parent or the attending adult. Where the adult response is shock and concern, it triggers a cry for help; where the adult response says pick yourself up, it often leads to less of a tragic response.

For children who may be experiencing a particular event for the first time, which in this case is surgical, the cue to how to respond is to gather from the adults in that environment their anxiety or fears about the event, which is usually evident to the child, and to respond with a similar degree of anxiety. Because of this dependence on parents for guidance in coping with new or stressful situations, the focus and the need to address parental anxiety in this situation is all the more pertinent.

Peculiar Stressors in Sub-Saharan Africa

Conditions that are peculiar to sub-Saharan Africa contribute particular stressors to people living in that region. These include the cost of surgical operations, availability of surgical services, essence of children in the Nigerian cultures, and stigmatisation. These are discussed more elaborately in the following subsections.

Cost of Procedure

Cost is particularly stressful in the sub-Saharan region. This region is characterised by difficult economic and health conditions: a low per capita gross domestic product, a negative economic growth rate, low life expectancy at birth, and catastrophic maternal and infant mortality.[36] These factors give insight to the stress that paediatric surgery poses for parents and children. First, the cost of a surgical procedure and its management can be prohibitive. The cost is borne solely by the parents or guardians of the child. Many of these parents are living below the poverty line; thus, having the added stress of how to fund the surgery and purchase the needed postsurgical management for the child may be an overbearing burden. Ameh et al.[37] have pointed out that the inability of parents to carry the financial burden has led to their removing the child from the hospital prior to completion of postsurgical management. Coupled with this is the difficulty that often arises when trying to access blood products or antibiotics that are needed for the child. These are all implicated in the development of postsurgical complications. Having health insurance would help to reduce this cost, but not many of these countries offer insurance, and for others, such as Nigeria, it is still in its infancy and not accessible for most children presenting for surgical diagnoses.

Accessibility of Surgical Services

There are only a few qualified paediatric surgeons in sub-Saharan Africa, and for most part these surgeons work in tertiary health care institutions located in urban town centres. Many of these facilities are not adequately funded and many are outdated. The additional and almost nonexistent primary and secondary health care system is weak.[38] The 2003 data for Nigeria, for instance, shows the ratio of paediatric surgeons to a child as 1 surgeon for every 2.2–2.7 million children. This ratio varies greatly across the regions of the country with more of the surgeons being located in the southern, more affluent area.

This picture is reflective of most other sub-Saharan countries. By implication, many hospitals in these countries do not have a resident paediatric surgeon; in these instances, paediatric surgical cases are handled by general practitioners, who are more competent in dealing with adult patients and often with equipment that is meant for adult surgical procedures. Gaps currently exist in postoperative pain management for adults, so by implication this is even more so for pain management in children.[39]

Parents are often aware of the shortage of personnel and associated issues and their implications for their child's successful surgical operation. Additionally, in this climate, where services are scarce, getting the desired treatment often implies relocating with the child, at least temporarily, to the towns where the hospitals are situated. This, as earlier pointed out, has cost implications that are borne by the parents. The absence of funds or inability to access these facilities leads to added stress for the parents and child.

Meaning and Essence of Children in the Sub-Saharan Cultures

In many of the sub-Saharan countries, great value is place on having children; in the more traditional settings, the norm was to have many children. For instance, the ideal family size in a Yoruba monogamous marriage is five to eight living children. Economic factors affecting family income and ability to cater for large families, as well as conflicts leading to relocation of families, has affected the desired number of children per household. In some countries in the sub-Saharan region, smaller family size is the norm. Even though there is reduction in the number of children per household in some of these countries, Woldemicael[40] has pointed out that children are still greatly valued. The value assigned to children also has a bearing on the economic benefits that they bring to the family. They are seen as additional sources of income, and increase the likelihood that one would be successful, thus bringing honour to the family. The pressure to have a child in these countries is thus enormous, and the health and status of the child takes on different meanings and makes any illness or need for surgery of particular concern for the parents or guardians.

This bias becomes even more pertinent, depending on the gender of the child. Across the sub-Saharan region, there is a preference for a male child; a male child is considered a major asset to the parents for both social and economic reasons.[41-43] Hake[44] has pointed out that this gender preference is based on the roles of sons in farming, trading, giving support in old age, and providing proper burial rites. In some instances, this desire for a male child has led to marital breakdown and divorce or marriage to a second wife, so in an attempt to have a male child, a woman ends up having ten or more children, which increases the chance of having malformed babies.[45]

In this climate, the male child's health takes on additional psychological meaning for the parents, and his welfare plays a very prominent role in the family's functioning. The high expectations that arise from this lead to increased preoperative anxiety for the parents and, depending on the age of the child, may bring additional emotional guilt in considering what the parents may be going through as a result of his condition. This may be both in terms of financial sacrifices that the parents are making for this procedure and the possible ridicule and discrimination that the family on the whole may be experiencing.

Discrimination and Stigmatisation

In situations where the expectations are high, so also is the pressure to have children and the possible discrimination that can arise as a result of this. A woman with children is accorded respect; a woman who does not have children is at a higher risk of being disrespected or excluded at certain social forums. She is often ridiculed and jeered by her mates for not having children and sometimes specifically for not having a male child.

There is an added complication for children born with some medical condition that may require surgery, either corrective or due to events occurring in early childhood, that may lead to the child being disfigured. In the traditional setting, any person that does not meet the norm and cannot play along with other children for medical or other reasons is teased, challenged, made fun of, ridiculed, and generally isolated or stigmatised.[46–48] These children, by reason of their condition, are likely to be competitively denied basic needs of appropriate clothing, good feeding, sound education, and emotional support. This discrimination and stigmatisation may be generalised to the whole family, so the child's siblings are teased and spoken of in derogatory terms. This leads to fear and anxiety for both parents and children, even more so when a surgical procedure alters in some way the child's functioning or physique. There is the fear of how the child will recover and adjust to the fact of not being able to move around. Thus, having to undergo an invasive procedure in any of these conditions is met with great anxiety and anticipation.

The discrimination experience and the treatment of children with disabilities are due to ignorance, superstition, and taboos.[49] This may be the result of cultural beliefs that attribute the cause of the disability either to a warning curse from God, family sins, offences against the gods, witches or wizards, adultery, misfortune, ancestors, a misdeed in a previous life, an evil spirit, or the killing of certain forbidden animals.[50]

In certain situations, it is not so much the illness as it is the particular invasive approach or associated issues that lead to the heightened level of stigma that is experienced. Archibong and Idika,[46] in their prospective study between 1992 and 2001 of treatment for anorectal malformations in a tertiary referral centre in South-Eastern Nigeria, found cultural beliefs implicated in the loss of 11 (20%) of their surgical cases. A common procedure for treatment of anorectal malformation is for the child to undergo an initial colostomy. This process allows for adequate weight gain, reduces possible postoperative complications, and increases the success of perineal abdominal pull-through. The authors, however, found that the practice of wearing a colostomy bag was detested by some families and that it was considered by society to be a bad omen and therefore stigmatised. They believed that the deaths of the 11 children in the course of treatment were due largely to neglect of the child by family members, fuelled by the superstitious beliefs and negative attitudes.

Also, due to the condition and how it is viewed by the parents or society, children may be brought to the hospital late or be removed from the hospital without permission. Thus, even though the children are valued, this value seems to depend on the child being well and conforming to what is expected of a "normal" child. At a certain level, children undergoing these various procedures may come to understand the way their condition is viewed by members of the family and society at large. Where this is not viewed positively, or is associated with stigma and discrimination, children may grow up feeling guilty for bringing this upon the family. They may thus feel responsible for the ridicule and embarrassment and may even misinterpret possible misunderstandings that occur as a natural part of growth for a nuclear unit. These feelings of guilt may have long-term implications for a child's development.

Psychological Preparation for Paediatric Surgery

Over the last four decades, a number of efforts have focused on alleviating the potential trauma experienced by parents and their children as they await or undergo an invasive surgical procedure. These efforts also aim to maximise the effect of medical treatment.[51] Thus, children (and their parents) are prepared for surgery in an attempt to prevent or decrease the severity of associated distress. These preparatory interventions range from pharmacological (administration of premedication) to psychosocial approaches, the latter of which has been the focus of this chapter.

In looking at the psychological preparation of children for surgery, various authors have presented slightly different paths. For instance, Vernon et al.[22] reviewed existing preparatory programmes and highlighted three main themes that were evident in these programmes: (1) giving information to the child, (2) encouraging emotional expression, and (3) establishing a relationship of trust and confidence with the hospital staff. These three themes were later expanded by Elkins and Roberts[52] to include (4) preparing parents and (5) providing or teaching coping strategies to parents and children.

In a more recent review, Maclaren, and Kain[30] adopted a historical approach, suggesting that preparation programmes moved through three different phases: information orientation and design in the 1960s, aimed at facilitating emotional expression and trust between the parties; modelling and stress-point nursing procedures in the 1970s; and then in the 1980s came the teaching of children skills and the involvement of parents. They concluded that evidence supports the development of coping skills as being the most effective preoperative preparation. This is followed by modelling, play therapy, an operation room tour, with the least effective being print media.

In discussing preoperative psychological preparation, we now look briefly at the various programmes with a focus on what is involved and how they attempted to accomplish this.

Giving Information to the Child

One of the major sources of distress is the child's lack of information or unfamiliarity with the hospital and surgical process.[22] It would then be natural to expect that simply providing the child with accurate information in a format that the child could understand would go a long way in addressing this. Providing information is not that simple, however, and does not relate in a direct way to the reduction in the levels of experienced distress. One possible explanation for this may be the fact that coping strategy affects the way we respond to the timing of information provided. As discussed earlier in the context of adult coping responses, people tend to predominantly respond in two ways; problem-focused or emotion-focused. This is also applicable to children. For instance, if a child's predominant response is emotion-focused, which tends towards avoidance, the presentation of information prior to the procedure may cause more distress than otherwise. In this instance, it may be better to help the child with refocusing (distraction) techniques. If the child copes by using predominantly information-seeking approaches, however, then the provision of medical information in regard to the procedure will help alleviate the anxiety experienced by the child.

The second issue to take into consideration is the timing of providing information. Intuitively, it would appear that the earlier the children and parents are given information and taken through the preparatory process, the better the outcome. This is not necessarily so. A review of the evidence shows that for invasive procedures, the timing for giving information to the child depends on the child's age. For children younger than 6 years of age, it is optimal to start 1–5 days prior to the procedure, but for children who are older than 6 years of age, the best results are obtained when they are informed a week before the surgery. Information given prior to this time leads to heightened anxiety levels for school-age children.[53,54] It would appear that in situations in which there is a limited time for preparing the child of school age, a more beneficial approach may be to use distraction and refocusing techniques.

Using developmentally appropriate language not only allows the child to gain a sense of mastery but also facilitates the child's greater understanding of the procedure, correcting any misinformation that may have existed. In many instances, this would involve working with parents on how to best communicate with their child regarding the upcoming procedure.

Given that the parents' high levels of distress can be transmitted to the child, which increases the likelihood of multiple negative surgical outcomes,[55] it is important that addressing parents' distress be made a primary focus in its own right.[10,56] There is therefore a need to target parents for specific anxiety reduction interventions. Parents should be offered support with more access to the physician to communicate their fears and clarify their own understanding of the situation. Many parents may have an external perception of control of their child's health—which is peculiar to sub-Saharan Africa. These parents should be assigned a small task, such as monitoring the child's temperature, from the beginning of the child's hospitalisation.[57] This serves to link the parents' perception of internal control and the child's health condition.

In giving information to parents, the paediatrician must also recognise the predominant coping strategy adopted by the parents, which affects their response to the given information. In a clinical context, for instance, it is easy to identify parents who use a predominantly information-focused approach because they will manifest a high degree of information-seeking behaviour. These parents can then be provided with detailed procedural information. Providing them with accurate information would help reduce the level of anxiety experienced and make them more prepared to offer the needed support to the child. In contrast, parents who predominantly use an emotion-focused approach could be given basic information and helped in refocusing while they support their child.

Using a Variety of Channels in the Provision of Information

There are different channels through which information is provided to children and their parents. Information could be written with enhanced visual images for a target audience of either the child or parents. This is a facility used by many hospitals, which provide leaflets or send information out to parents and children prior to their surgical procedure. Written information alone, however, has not proven to be very effective in preparing the child or parent for surgery.

Other channels for passing information to parents and children include using multimedia facilities such as videos of hospital procedures and hospitals in general, giving tours of the hospital, discussion with the paediatrician or health care professional, and engaging the children in play sessions or puppet through which the child displays emotions and feelings that may expose fears and thus allow them to be addressed. McEwen et al.[58] exposed parents to an 8-minute informative video in addition to normal preoperative preparations. They found that those parents who were exposed to the video film showed both a reduction in the desire for information as well as a greater reduction in postoperative anxiety.

Offering Play Therapy

Some hospitals provide a designated area with toys for children to play with and personnel to oversee this process. Usually, the aim of this is threefold: First, it provides an avenue for a child's emotional expression, thus revealing fears and conceptions that the child may have that could then be corrected. Second, it provides information in a format that would be easy for the child to understand. Last, it creates an avenue to help build the confidence of the child and establish a trusting relationship between the child and hospital personnel. In preparing the child for surgery, surgery- or hospital-related props are used. Hence play may involve the use of miniature versions of hospital equipment, such as syringes, masks, surgical implements, toy stethoscopes, dolls, intravenous lines, and the like. Play therapy often involves the use of a specialist, and it offers the chance to evaluate the current level of the child's knowledge, misconceptions, and coping level.[5]

Providing Psychological Interventions

Psychological intervention involves teaching the child and parents actual techniques that help them to anticipate, recognise, and manage stress-related surgical experiences. The child is taught actual life-coping skills in these sessions. Some of the interventions that have been used include a progressive muscle relaxation technique, positive self-instruction, guided imagery, conscious breathing exercises, and refocusing. For the most part, these skills are taught by mental health professionals in sessions that last an average of 15–45 minutes, depending on the capabilities of the individual or the attention span if it is a child. Often there is a need for the child or parent to actively rehearse this procedure after the sessions for maximal mastery and to get the desired effect.

Providing Models and Counselling for Children and Their Parents

The modelling and counselling approach is theoretically grounded in the social learning approach, which points to the ability to learn from observing others engaging in a particular behaviour. In this light, children awaiting a surgical procedure are exposed to models that have undergone similar procedures and responded positively to it. To be effective in getting the children to identify and desire to behave in a similar manner, the models are usually people the children can easily identify with by reason of age, gender, race, and other similar characteristics. The children may be exposed to the models through write-ups, videos, photographs, or film. This is more effective for children who have no previous medical experience.[9,59]

Closely related to this is having the children or parents interact either formally or informally with people who are in the same or similar circumstances or who have previously undergone the experience that they are awaiting. This could be in the form of group therapy or sessions, where people come together and are exposed to others facing similar situations to help them not feel alone. A wider application of this is in more developed societies is getting people involved in online or Internet forums to discuss and ask other people who may have had certain experiences what their advice would be. Although interactions of this nature have not been tested in all settings and for all conditions, evidence[60,61] shows that people do welcome online interactions of this nature and find them extremely useful.

Conclusion

It is important to point out that hospitals differ in regard to recommended practices in preparing a child for an invasive procedure. Some have formal policies on some of these procedures, whereas others rely more on the clinical judgement of the attending health care professional and what is feasible within that setup. For instance, the United States and United Kingdom vary vastly on the issue of parental presence (or absence) during anaesthetic induction. Kain et al.[50] found that 85% of anaesthetists in the UK allowed parents to be present during anaesthetic induction in 75% of the cases, but a much lower percentage

was obtained for the USA, where only 58% of the respondents allowed parents to be present in less than 5% of the cases. This could be a result of inconclusive evidence concerning the advantages (alleviating child's anxiety and gaining cooperation)[62] or disadvantages (making the anaesthetist nervous or causing child to be stressed from the parents' own response).[63] It could also be that the difference reflects the fear of litigation or other possible legal proceedings that may exist.[53]

In their review of preoperative preparation programmes for children, Watson and Visram[64] concluded that these programmes are not universally helpful in reducing anxiety or postoperative behaviour problems. What we do know is that some programmes have better outcomes than others and that they need to be tailored to the individual child, taking into account the child's age, previous hospital experiences, and temperament.

A gap still exists, however, in transferring the results obtained in clinical research trials to routine clinical settings. Many of these preparation programmes have been evaluated in the controlled environments of clinical research trials, where factors are manipulated to allow for clearer understanding; in routine clinical settings, these factors may not necessarily be the same, thus leading to potentially different results.[15] Bridging this gap is a necessity.

Generally speaking, however, in the developed countries such as the United States and in Europe, there is a continuous search for ways of incorporating these evidence-based findings into routine clinical settings to improve the lot of both children and parents awaiting invasive surgical procedures. For paediatric surgeons in the sub-Saharan region, in contrast, the greater challenge and focus are on providing basic health and counselling services for this group.

In the sub-Saharan region, the compounding factor is the acute shortage of paediatric surgeons and other supporting health care professionals. In the more developed settings, where the ratio of children to paediatric surgeons is much lower, the inability to adequately prepare a child and parents for invasive procedures is due largely to a lack of time. The high volume of ambulatory patients seen in surgical units and the policy at some institutions to forgo a separate preoperative visit, as is typical for inpatient surgical procedures, is common. Clinicians who work with families in the ambulatory setting have an increased burden of identifying family needs and providing interventions to parents and children in a very brief time period. As expected, the situation in sub-Saharan Africa can be considered a lot worse because the child-to-surgeon ratio is so much larger.

In addition to these challenges are specific considerations when implementing preparatory programmes in sub-Saharan Africa. Notably, evidence on the effectiveness of these programmes is from the industrialised world and may not necessarily be applicable in sub-Saharan practice. Several questions arise that would be worth considering: Do children in sub-Saharan Africa respond to information in the same way as do children in the more developed societies, or are they more dependent on their parents and guardians in determining how they respond to new situations? Are the hospitals equipped to offer the preoperative preparatory sessions that are required, and do they have mental health workers or other professionals that can facilitate these sessions, or will preoperative preparation be a part of the paediatricians already overcrowded role? Are there plans in place to confront fundamental societal beliefs and values that may, as in the earlier described case, affect the acceptance of certain procedures that have been found effective for managing or treating certain conditions? A great need exists for research with a focus on finding brief cost-effective preoperative programmes that are relevant for surgical practice in the sub-Saharan region. Raising the bar to a point where every child has access to a well-thought-out preoperative programme will continue to be a challenge, but nevertheless one that African nations should strive to overcome.

Evidence-Based Research

Table 14.1 presents evidence-based research on the effect on anxiety of using preoperative preparation for parents of elective surgery patients.

Table 14.1: Evidence-based research.

Title	The effect of videotaped preoperative information on parental anxiety during anesthesia induction for elective paediatric procedures
Authors	McEwen A, Moorthy C, Quantock C, Rose H, Kavanagh R
Institution	The Royal Alexandra Hospital for Sick Children, Dyke Road, Brighton, UK
Reference	Pediatr Anesth 2007; 17:534–539
Problem	Cost effectiveness of routine antenatal screening.
Intervention	Preoperative preparation for parents.
Comparison/ control (quality of edvidence)	Parents were randomly assigned to either the experimental group, which was exposed to an 8-minute preoperative preparation video in addition to normal preoperative procedures; or the control group, which received only the normal preoperative preparation.
Outcome/ effect	Statistically significant differences were found between parents who were exposed to normal preparation and those who, in addition to this, watched an 8-minute video. Parents who watched the video in comparison to controls showed significantly greater reductions in their desire for information as well as their levels of anxiety (as measured by the Preoperative Anxiety and Information Scale).
Historical significance/ comments	This study shows an innovative cost-effective approach to addressing parental anxiety in regard to children who are awaiting surgery. A well-presented 8-minute video had the additional effect of providing answers to questions that parents may have had, and a reduction in the desire for information was also evident in this group.

Key Summary Points

1. Many children and their parents experience high levels of distress when awaiting an invasive paediatric surgical procedure.

2. Anxiety is the most commonly reported stress-related emotion that is experienced.

3. Preoperative anxiety is associated with a number of negative postsurgical outcomes.

4. Many of Africa's less resourced countries have peculiar challenges that heighten the level of the anxiety experience.

5. Reducing the level of distress is paramount in facilitating postsurgical recovery for the child.

6. Various preparatory programmes exist, but they are not universally helpful. Programmes need to take into consideration the child's age, sex, previous hospital experience, and temperament, as well as factors that are related to parental status, well-being, and anxiety level.

7. Many programmes that have proven effective in a clinical research setting must be effectively transferred to routine clinical settings.

8. With the peculiarities of the African continent, it is crucial for further research to be done in the area of presurgical stress and anxiety.

9. We must raise the bar to every African child having access to a well-thought-out preoperative programme.

References

1. Landolt M, Boehler U, Schwager C, Schallberger U, Nuessli R. Post traumatic stress disorder in paediatric patients and their parents: findings from an exploratory study. J Paed Child Health 1998; 34:539–543.

2. Landolt MA, Vollrath M, Ribi K. Incidence and associations of parental and child posttraumatic stress symptoms in paediatric patients. J Child Psychol Psychia 2003; 44:1199–1207.

3. Hug M, Tonz M, Kaiser G. Parental stress in paediatric day-case surgery. Ped Surg Intl 2005; 2:94–99.

4. Li HCW, Lam HYA. Paediatric day surgery: impact on Hong Kong Chinese children and their parents. J Clin Nurs 2003; 12:882–887.

5. LeRoy S, Elixson, EM, O'Brien P, Tong E, Turpin S, Uzark K. Recommendations for preparing children and adolescents for invasive cardiac procedures: a statement from the American Heart Association Pediatric Nursing Subcommittee of the Council on Cardiovascular Nursing in collaboration with the Council on Cardiovascular Diseases of the Young. Circulation 2003; 108:2550–2564.

6. Brophy C, Erickson M. Children's self-statements and adjustment to elective outpatient surgery. J Dev Beh Pedia 11; 1990:13–16.

7. Bush JP, Melamed BG, Sheras PL, Greenbaum PE. Mother-child patterns of coping with anticipatory medical stress. Health Psych 1986; 5:137–157.

8. Jay SM, Ozolins M, Elliott CH, Caldwell S. Assessment of children's distress during painful medical procedures. Health Psych 1983; 2:133–147.

9. Melamed BG, Dearborn M, Hermecz DA. Necessary considerations for surgery preparation: age and previous experience. Psychosomatic Med 1983; 45:517–525.

10. Kain ZN, Wang SM, Mayes LC, Caramico LA, Hofstadter MB. Distress during the induction of anesthesia and postoperative behavioral outcomes. Anesth Analg 1999; 88:1042–1047.

11. Holm-Knudsen RJ, Carlin JB, McKenzie IM. Distress at induction of anaesthesia in children. A survey of incidence, associated factors and recovery characteristics. Paed Anaes 1998; 8:383–392.

12. Kotiniemi LH, Ryhanen PT, Moilanen IK. Behavioural changes in children following day-case surgery: a 4-week follow-up of 551 children. Anaesthesia 1997; 52:970–976.

13. Eckenhoff JE. Relationship of anesthesia to postoperative personality changes in children. Amer J Dis Childhood, 1958; 86:587–591.

14. Meyers E, Muravchick S. Anesthesia induction techniques in pediatric patients: a controlled study of behavioral consequences. Anesth Analg 1977; 56:538–542.

15. Kain ZN, Caldwell-Andrews AA, Maranets I, McClain B, Gaal D, Mayes LC, Feng R, Zhang H. Preoperative anxiety and emergence delirium and postoperative maladaptive behaviors. Anesth Analg 2004; 99:1648–1654.

16. Kain ZN, Mayes LC, Caldwell-Andrews AA, Karas DE, McClain BC. Preoperative anxiety, postoperative pain, and behavioral recovery in young children undergoing surgery. Pediatrics 2006; 118:651–658.

17. Campbell IR, Scaife JM, Johnstone JM. Psychological effects of day case surgery compared with inpatient surgery. Arch Dis Childhood 1998; 63:415–417.

18. Kotiniemi LH, Ryhanen PT, Moilanen IK. Behavioural changes in children following day-case surgery: a 4-week follow-up of 551 children. Anaesthesia 1997; 52:970–976.

19. Utens EM, Verhulst FC, Meijboom FJ, et al. Behavioural and emotional problems in children and adolescents with congenital heart disease. Psychol Med 1993; 23:415–424.

20. Casey FA, Sykes DH, Craig BG, et al. Behavioral adjustment of children with surgically palliated complex congenital heart disease. J Pediatric Psych 1996; 21:335–352.

21. Lavigne JV, Faier-Routman J. Psychological adjustment to pediatric physical disorders: a meta-analytic review. J Pediatric Psych 1992; 17:133–157.

22. Vernon, DTA, Schulman JL, Fooley JM. Changes in children's behavior after hospitalization. Amer J Dis Children 1966; 111:481–497.

23. Bondy L, Sims N, Schroeder DR, Offord KP, Narr BJ. The effect of anaesthetic patient education on preoperative patient anxiety. Reg Anesth Pain Mgmt 1999; I24:158–164.

24. Devine EC. Effects of psychoeducational care for adult surgical patients: a meta-analysis of 191 studies. Patient Educ Couns 1992; 19:129–142.

25. Kain Z, Caramico L, Mayes L, Genevro J, Bornstein M, Hofstadter M. Preoperative preparation programs in children: a comparative study. Anesth Analg 1998; 87:1249–1255.

26. Maligalig RM, Parents' perceptions of the stressors of pediatric ambulatory surgery. J Post Anesth Nurs 1994; 9:278–282.

27. Ben-Amitay Kosov I, Reiss A, Toren P, Yoran-Hegesh R, Kotler M, Mozes T. Is elective surgery traumatic for children and their parents? J Paed Child Health 2006; 42:618–624.

28. Norberg AL, Lindblad F, Boman, KK. Parental traumatic stress during and after paediatric cancer treatment. Acta Oncologica 2005; 44:382–388.

29. Miller SM, Roussi P, Altman D, Helm W, Steinberg A. Effects of coping style on psychological reactions of low-income, minority women to colposcopy. J Reprod Med 1994; 39:711–718.

30. MacLaren J, Kain ZN. A comparison of preoperative anxiety in female patients with mothers of children undergoing surgery. Anesth Analg 2008; 106(3):810–813.

31. Piira T, Sugiura T, Champion GD, Donnelly N, Cole ASJ. The role of parental presence in the context of children's medical procedures: a systematic review. Child: Care, Health Dev 2003; 31:233–243.

32. Montgomery C, Lydon A, Lloyd K. Psychological distress among cancer patients and informed consent. J Psychosom Res 1999; 46:241–245.

33. Bevan JC, Johnston C, Tousignant G. (1990). Preoperative parental anxiety predicts behavioural and emotional responses to induction of anaesthesia in children. Can J Anaesth 1990; 37:177–182.

34. Kain ZN, Mayes LC, O'Connor TZ, et al. Preoperative anxiety in children, predictors and outcomes. Arch Pediatr Adolesc Med 1996; 150:1238–1245.

35. Kain Z. Perioperative information and parental anxiety: the next generation. Anesth Analg 1999; 88:237–239.

36. World Health Organization. World Health Statistics 2008. Available at http://www.who.int/whois/whostat/2008/en/index.html (accessed 3 September 2009).

37. Ameh EA, Adejuyigbe O, Nmadu PT. Pediatric surgery in Nigeria. J Pediatr Surg 2006; 41:542–546.

38. Ouro-Bang'Na Maman AF, Koumenou E, Gnassingbe K, Chobli M, et al. Anesthesia for children in sub-Saharan Africa—a description of settings, common presenting conditions, techniques and outcomes. Pediatric Anesth 2009; 19:5–11.

39. Ouro Bang'Na Maman AF, Agbe´tra N, Moumouni I, et al. Prise en charge de la douleur post-ope´ratoire au Togo: connaissance et attitude des prescripteurs. Can J Anesth 2006; 53:529–531.

40. Woldemicael G. Recent fertility decline in Eritrea: is it a conflict-led transition? Demog Res 2008; 18:27–57.

41. Campbell EK, Campbell PG. Family size and sex preferences and eventual fertility in Botswana. J Biosoc Sci 1997; 29:191–204.

42. Mwageni EA, Ankomah A, Powell RA. Sex preference and contraceptive behaviour among men in Mbeya region, Tanzania. J Fam Plan Reprod Health Care 2001; 27:85–89.

43. Olusoye S. The girl child: a blessing or an abomination. Nigeria's Pop 1993; (Oct–Dec):41–42.

44. Hake JM. Child-Rearing Practices in Northern Nigeria. Ibadan University Press, 1972.

45. Gupta B. Incidence of congenital malformations in Nigerian children. W Afr Med J 1969; 8:22–27.

46. Archibong AE, Idika IM. Results of treatment in children with anorectal malformations in Calabar, Nigeria. S Afr J Surg 2004; 42(3):88–90.

47. Bender RE. The Conquest of Deafness. The Press of Case Western Reserve University, 1970.

48. Goffman E. Stigma, Notes on Management of Spoilt Identity. Prentice-Hall, 1963.

49. Ojofeitimi, Oyefeso. Beliefs, attitudes and expectations of mothers concerning their handicapped children in Ile-Ife, Nigeria. J Royal Soc Promotion Health 1980; 100:101–103.

50. Onwuegbu OL. The Nigerian Culture: Its Perception and Treatment of the Handicapped. Unpublished essays, Federal Advanced Teachers' College for Special Education, Oyo, Oyo State, Nigeria, 1977.

51. Kenny TJ. The hospitalized child. Pediatr Clin N A 1975; 22:583–593.

52. Elkins PO, Roberts MC. Psychological preparation for pediatric hospitalization. Clin Psychol Rev 1983; 3:275–295.

53. Kain ZN, Mayes LC, O'Connor TZ, Cicchetti DV. Preoperative anxiety in children. Predictors and outcomes. Arch Pediatr Adoles Med 1996; 150:1238–1245.

54. Faust J, Melamed BG. Influence of arousal, previous experience, and age on surgery preparation of same day of surgery and in-hospital pediatric patients. J Consult Clin Psych 1984; 52:359–365.

55. Skipper JK, Leonard RC. Children, stress, and hospitalization: a field experiment. J Health Soc Behav 1968; 9:275–287.

56. Cassady JF Jr, Wysocki TT, Miller KM, Cancel DD, Izenberg N. Use of a preanesthetic video for facilitation of parental education and anxiolysis before pediatric ambulatory surgery. Anesth Analg 1999; 88:246–250.

57. Scrimin S, Haynes M, Altoè G, Bornstein, MH, Axia G. Anxiety and stress in mothers and fathers in the 24h after their child's surgery. Child: Care, Health Dev 2009; 35:227–233.

58. McEwen A, Moorthy C, Quantock C, Rose H. Kavanagh R. The effect of videotaped preoperative information on parental anxiety during anesthesia induction for elective pediatric procedures. Pediatric Anesth 2007; 17:534–539.

59. Klorman R, Hilpert PL, Michael R, et al. Effects of coping and mastery modeling on experienced and inexperienced pedodontic patients' disruptiveness. Behav Ther 1980; 11:156–168.

60. Briery BG, Rabian B. Psychosocial changes associated with participation in a pediatric summer camp. J Pediatr Psych 1999; 24:183–190.

61. Ibanga AJ, Copello A, Templeton L, Orford J, Velleman R. Web-based support for affected others. A paper presented at the 66th Alcohol Problems Research Symposium, Kendall, 18–19 March 2009.

62. Hannallah RS. Who benefits when parents are present during anaesthesia induction in their children? Can J Anaesth 1994; 42:361–364.

63. Johnston CC, Bevan JC, Haig MJ, Kirnon V, Tousignant G. Parental presence during anesthesia induction. AORN J 1988; 47:187–194.

64. Watson A, Visram A. Children's preoperative anxiety and postoperative behaviour. Paediatr Anaesth 2003; 13:188–204.

SURGICAL INFECTIONS AND INFESTATIONS

CHAPTER 15
COMMON BACTERIAL INFECTIONS IN CHILDREN

Iftikhar Ahmad Jan

Kokila Lakhoo

Introduction

Bacterial infections are the cause of significant mortality and morbidity in children. Infections of surgical importance may affect virtually any organ or tissue in the body. These may be community or hospital acquired. The major groups of community-acquired infections are skin and soft tissue infections, bone infections, and infections of specific organs. Hospital-acquired infections may further be classified as infections of surgical wounds, infections in wards, and infections in immunocompromised and critically ill patients. Bacterial infections are more common at extreme ages, and thus babies less than 2 months of age are highly susceptible to bacterial infection. Other conditions such as malnutrition, immune-deficiency states, and prolonged illnesses, make children more susceptible to acquire infections.

Skin and Soft Tissue Infections

Skin and soft tissue infections are better described according to the depth of tissue involved. Common bacterial infections in children are impetigo, scalded skin syndrome, follicultis, furuncle or boil, carbuncle, erysipelas, necrotising fasciitis, clostridial myonecrosis (gas gangrene), nonclostridial myonecrosis, synergistic gangrenes, lymphadenitis, and abscesses. In addition, ear and throat infections and infections of specific systems (e.g., urinary tract infections, respiratory tract infections) may be important in the management of paediatric surgical patients.

Impetigo

Impetigo is an infection of the superficial layers of the skin. It is caused by a minor breach in skin continuity and is common in babies with poor hygiene, in crowded living conditions, and living in warm and humid areas. Impetigo is a disease of babies and children, and may constitute 4–6% of all bacterial infections in the paediatric population. Underlying conditions, such as eczema, insect bites, small cuts, or abrasions, may initiate the process.

Impetigo may be described as bullous and nonbullous, according to the presentation. Nonbullous impetigo constitutes more than 70% of impetigo infections. It presents as a thick, honey-colored crust on the face or limbs. It may be mildly painful, but other constitutional symptoms are not present. Healing is spontaneous and usually does not lead to scarring, it is mostly caused by *Staphylococcus aureus* or *Streptococcus pyogenes*. Bullous impetigo is less common and is often seen in babies and young children due to their soft skin. It is mostly caused by *Staphylococcus aureus* and presents as blister-like lesions filled with fluid pus. Both varieties of impetigo are diagnosed by the classic appearance, and investigations are not necessary. A swab from the lesion may cause growth of the causative organism. Nasal swabs from patients and mothers may help, however, in identifying the source in patients with repeated appearances of new lesions.

Topical antibiotics, such as fuscidic acid, mupirocin, or polymyxin-B, may help in early healing of the lesions and also make the lesions soft and less irritating. Cases resistant to fuscidic acid due to the widespread topical usage of fuscidic acid have now been reported, however. Some patients with multiple lesions and those not responding to topical antibiotics may need systemic antibiotics and cephalosporins. Amoxil-clavunate will

help in early healing of the lesions. Most impetigos heal without any sequel, but such complications as toxic shock syndrome may be seen in immune-compromised cases. Poststreptococcal glomerulonephritis and rheumatic fever are threats that warrant early and adequate treatment of skin lesions in children.

Folliculitis

Folliculitis is an infection of the hair follicle. It usually presents as a small tender nodule of the hair follicle. It is commonly caused by *Staphylococcus aureus*. Two types of lesions are seen. In superficial folliculitis, multiple hair follicles are involved and cause small pustules at the opening of the adjacent hair follicles. The deeper form of folliculitis affects a single hair follicle and causes local swelling and tenderness. These are usually seen on the scalp in children. There is local tenderness but no fever or other constitutional symptoms. It is usually caused by local trauma, sweating, friction, and local lesions such as eczema. Hot tub folliculitis is caused by *Pseudomonas aeruginosa* and occurs in hot tubs and pools with improper cleaning and disinfection. Folliculitis is a self-limiting condition in most cases but may progress to form furuncle, which is a severe infection of the hair follicle and appendages. The treatment of folliculitis is by cleaning and topical antibiotics. In immunocompromised patients and diabetics, systemic antibiotics should be started to avoid any complications.

Furuncle or Boil

Furuncles are severe infections of the hair follicles, sweat glands, and surrounding tissues. They may occur anywhere in the hair-bearing areas of body, but they are most common on the face, neck, armpits, buttocks, and thighs. *Staphylococcus aureus* is the causative organism in most cases, but other organisms may be involved. Furuncles usually start as painful nodules and develop into large inflamed and tender areas with constitutional symptoms of fever, malaise, and anorexia. They are uncommon lesions in the paediatric population, but may be seen in patients with immune deficiency and diabetes mellitus. Multiple lesions may occur, especially after inadequate treatment. If untreated, the lesion may lead to spreading cellulitis and can be dangerous in areas such as the nose and face, where it may lead to thrombosis of the cavernous sinus with serious consequences.

Diagnosis is obvious by the classic appearance of the lesion, which initially presents as a tender lesion with a wide red indurated area and an obvious central punctum. Pus expressed through the head of the lesion gives relief of symptoms. Furuncles are especially dangerous in immune-compromised patents. Multiple crops of the lesions may occur and combine to form a carbuncle. Furuncles need treatment by oral antibiotics, cloxacillin, amoxicillin clavulanate, macrolides, or cephalosporins. Once the abscess has drained, the patient improves rapidly; however, antibiotics treatment should be continued until complete healing of the lesion to prevent new lesions.

Carbuncle

A carbuncle is a spreading infection in the subcutaneous tissue planes caused by multiple infected hair follicles. Carbuncles are rare in children but may be seen in hairy and immunocompromised patients; these usually occur in the neck. It is characterised by extensive necrosis, with multiple abscesses that drain on the surface by multiple sinuses and ultimately unite to form a large area of tissue necrosis. *Staphylococcus aureus* is the causative organism in most cases. Treatment consists of drainage of abscesses and excision of the dead and necrotic tissue. Intravenous broad-spectrum antibiotics help in the control of infection. Extensive tissue destruction may require skin grafting in few cases.

Cellulitis

Cellulitis is a spreading infection in the subcutaneous tissue planes. It may occur after a small skin breach, especially in immunocompromised children. Insect bites, local trauma, vascular insufficiency, and diabetes are some of the predisposing factors in the causation of celluitis. Cellulitis may also occur secondary to other soft tissue infections such as furuncles or carbuncles. Classic signs of inflammation include redness, pain, swelling, warmth, and loss of function. The skin overlying the affected area is shiny and red. The patient may develop fever with chills, malaise, and body aches. It is important to identify the underlying primary pathology, such as diabetes. Staphylococci, streptococci, and even gram-negative organisms may be responsible for the lesion. The goals of treatment are control of infection and prevention of complications. Treatment includes correction of contributing factors, broad-spectrum antibiotics, and analgesics. Hospitalisation may be required in extensive involvement. Facial cellulitis, also called erysipelas, is a serious condition and needs hospitalisation and intravenous antibiotics. Spreading cellulitis in the floor of the mouth may cause Ludwig's angina, which may threaten the life of the patients due to laryngeal oedema and airway obstruction. Steroids may be required along with antibiotics, and in some cases a tracheotomy may be required to relieve airway obstruction.

Pyomyositis Tropical

Pyomyositis tropical is a fulminant infection of the muscles. It is caused by *Staphylococcus aureus*, but other organisms such as streptococcus and gram-negative organisms may be responsible. Multiple abscesses may be formed in different parts of the body. The child presents with high-grade fever and chills with abscess formation. Abscesses are formed in various muscles of the body. The infective process may affect other tissues of the body; meningitis, pericardial effusions, and endocarditis may be present. Empyema thorax is another serious complication of pyomyositis tropical. The disease is commonly seen in immuncompromised patients, especially those with human immunodeficiency virus (HIV) and those on chemotherapy. Blood cultures will grow the organism and also help in deciding appropriate antibiotics. Antibiotics of choice for pyomyositis tropical are cloxacillin, fuscidic acid, and cephalosporin. Fuscidic acid preparations are expensive and not easily available, but are very effective due to good tissue and bone penetration. A combination of cloxacillin and gentamicin may help to restrain the infection. Draining of abscesses should be performed early and may help prevent extension of the disease to other organs and tissues. See Chapter 19 for additional information.

Clostridia Myonecrosis (Gas Gangrene)

Gas gangrene is a fulminant synergistic infection caused by mixed infections by saccharolytic and proteolytic organisms. The organisms involved are *Clostridium perfirngens*, *Clostridium oedemateins*, and *Clostridium septicum*. Clostridia are facultative anaerobes and grow rapidly in low oxygen. Gas gangrene is commonly seen in war situations; however, in civilian practice it may also be seen after roadside accidents and in dirty and contaminated wounds. Its true incidence is not known, but it may occur in 0.1 per 100,000 per annum.

Indications

The clostridia strains produce various exotoxins and cause extensive necrosis of tissue proteins, fats, and red blood cells. The tissue com-partments become tense and oedematous. Presence of gas in the tissue is responsible for the crepitus seen in these patients. In lacerated, devascularised, and contaminated wounds, the chances of gas gangrene increase manifold. The incubation period varies from 1 day to several weeks, but is usually less than 3 days.

Initially, the wound may not look very bad and there is no smell, but once the process of myonecrosis has initiated, it rapidly progresses to involve the adjacent tissue and foul smell is evident. The affected area becomes tense, oedematous and severely tender. If not treated adequately, the patient may soon develop generalised sepsis and renal shutdown. Death is possible due to multiple organ failure.

Diagnosis and Treatment

Diagnosis is usually obvious by the nature of the trauma and deterioration of the patient's condition a few days after the injury. X-ray will show gas in the tissue with foreign bodies. The aim of management in extensive injury shall be to prevent gas gangrene and aggressive therapy for those who have developed the disease. Prevention and management may be achieved by adequate resuscitation of the patient after injury, thorough debridement of dead and dying tissue, removal of all foreign bodies from the wound, thorough washing of the wound, keeping the haemoglobin to an optimal level for good tissue oxygenation, use of broad-spectrum antibiotics, and prophylactic use of hyperbaric oxygen where facilities are available. The broad-spectrum antibiotics include cover for gram-positive, gram-negative, and anaerobic organisms. Intravenous benzyl penicillin is the drug of choice and should be given to all suspected cases of gas gangrene every 4 to 6 hours. Anti-gas gangrene globulin may also be useful if used early in the course of the illness.

The main focus of management should be to surgically remove all dead and dying tissue. The procedure shall be performed under general anaesthesia and may be repeated after 24 hours to ensure drainage of all infected areas, excision of dead tissue, and amputations if necessary. All wounds must be left open with loose dressing to ensure good circulation and to avoid ischaemia due to compartment syndrome. Where hyperbaric oxygen therapy is possible, it should be given for 1–2 hours at 2.5 atmospheric pressure.

Necrotising Fasciitis

Necrotising fasciitis (NF) is a fulminant soft tissue infection causing extensive fascial, fat, and muscle necrosis. Due to extensive tissue destruction, it has been described as the "flesh-eating disease". The condition is not common and is mostly seen in malnourished, immunocompromised, and debilitated patients. Two types are described: Type-I NF is a polymicrobial synergistic infection caused by anaerobes (bacteroides and peptostreptococci), facultative anaerobes (non–beta-haemolytic streptococci) and *Enterobacter* species (*Escherichia coli*, *Enterobacter*, *Klebsiella*, and *Proteus*). Type-II NF is caused by group A beta-haemolytic streptococcal (GABHS) infection, and is often described as streptococcal myonecrosis. The true incidence of NF is not known; however, the disease is commonly seen in children in the developing countries.

Type-I Necrotising Fasciitis

Various forms of type-I NF include Meleney's progressive bacterial gangrene, Fournier's gangrene, cancrum oris, and noma vulva. In children, severe systemic diseases, such as gastroenteritis, sepsis, gut perforations, and omphalitis, may predispose the patient to infective gangrene. Type-I NF involves the abdominal wall, perineum, groin, and postoperative wounds. Rarely, it may affect the oral cavity. In newborn babies, umbilical infection secondary to poor hygiene can cause rapidly spreading gangrene of the umbilicus. Initially, erythema and hyperaemia develop in the affected area and rapidly spread to local tissue necrosis and may spread to the abdominal and chest walls. Most babies have polymicrobial infections. Multiple organisms are usually recovered from the patients, and the number of isolates varies from two to six, averaging 3.5 isolates per specimen. Patients need aggressive supportive therapy along with a combination of antibiotics from gram-positive, gram-negative, and anaerobic coverage. Usually, a combination of third-generation cephalosporin with metronidazole is used. Extensive tissue debridement is necessary in most children. Mortality remains high, and more than 50% of patients with Type-I NF may die secondary to overwhelming sepsis.

Meleney's progressive bacterial gangrene is a form of necrotising fasciitis caused by microaerophilic streptococci, aerobic staphylococci, bacteroides, and gram-negative organisms. It is usually seen as a complication after abdominal surgery, especially after bowel surgery, abdominal abscess drainage, mass abdominal closure under tension, and surgical drains. The symptoms appear one to two weeks after the initial procedure. The skin around the wound becomes red and tender, with a foul-smelling discharge. Wide areas of skin and tissue necrosis then occur, and the patient may become very sick and toxic. Aggressive resuscitation and use of a combination of broad-spectrum antibiotics are necessary. Wound debridement should be done as soon as the patient is stable, and the wounds left open for adequate drainage of infected material. With the removal of dead and necrotic tissue, the patient's condition may improve. Mortality, however, remains high, especially in diabetics, immunocompromised patients, and malnourished children. See Chapter 21 for additional information.

Fournier's gangrene is a polymicrobial synergistic gangrene. This usually affects the perineal area (Figure 15. 1). It starts as a small itching area, which forms a small ulcer, and then widespread tissue necrosis occurs. The condition is initially painful but pain subsides with the loss of skin and subcutaneous tissue.

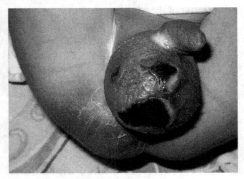

Figure 15.1: Fournier's gangrene.

Cancrum oris and noma vulva are mucocutaneous gangrenes affecting the mouth and vulva. These occur in severely malnourished children with infectious diseases such as gastroenteritis, measles, and chicken pox. A polymicrobial fulminant infection occurs, causing extensive skin and soft tissue necrosis. The progression of the inflammatory process is rapid, and extensive tissue destruction may be noted in a few days. This may cause serious disfigurement of the face, and extensive surgical procedures may be required later to cover the facial defects. The patient should be managed by correction of malnutrition, control of infection with broad-spectrum antibiotics, and tissue reconstruction. Corrective surgery should be performed only when the patient has fully recovered, to avoid any recurrence.

Type-II Necrotising Fasciitis
Children with varicella zoster infection are at a high risk of developing GABHS-associated necrotising fasciitis. Children younger than 10 years of age who have chicken pox have a 58-fold risk of developing invasive GABHS infections. The infections usually appear 4–6 days after the onset of a rash in children with chicken pox and may cause widespread tissue necrosis. Mortality is high, and aggressive management is needed to control infection and save the life of the patient. Mortality in children after NF may be from 10% to 20%. The clinical presentation in GABHS-associated necrotising fasciitis may start as the flu-like symptoms of fever with chills, malaise, and pain, but the patient soon develops signs of toxicity, tachypnoea, local tenderness, and erythema. Severe pain in the affected area with constitutional symptoms is an important indicator of a rapidly developing fulminant infection. Local signs, such as redness, induration, skin color changes, and pouring of pus, are indicative of serious tissue infection.

Nosocomial Infections
Nosocomial infections are those caused by a hospital stay but not related to the patient's original condition. Infections are considered nosocomial if they appear after 48 hours in hospital or within 30 days after discharge from hospital. Nosocomial is a Greek word and comes from *nosos*, which means "disease", and *komeo*, which means "care". Nosocomial infections are now considered one of the major causes of morbidity and mortality in patients with prolonged hospitalisation. In developed countries, the incidence of nosocomial infections ranges from 7% to 14%; it is higher in developing countries with limited resources. The most common sites of nosocomial infections are the urinary tract, surgical wounds, cannula sites, and respiratory tract. There are at least five modes of transmission of infections in admitted patients, including direct and indirect contact, droplet infections, as well as airborne, vehicle-borne, and vector-borne infections.

Direct contact between patients (hand shaking, sitting together, or sharing beds) may transfer bacteria from one patient to another. In these cases, the patient harboring the bacteria acts as a source and the one infected is the target. Indirect infection occurs by the use of various intermediate substances, such as infected instruments, gloves, syringes, dressings, and so forth. Droplet infections occur by cross infection when coughing, sneezing, and talking. Vectors (e.g., flies, mosquitoes, and rodents) may also cause transmission of infection in the admitted patients. Vehicle-borne infections are secondary to food products, water, and ward equipment. Hospital staff who are harbouring the infection are another important source of infection. The incidence of nosocomial infections rises with the duration of the stay in hospital.

Various factors, such as premature birth, advanced age, immunodeficiencies, indwelling catheters, prolonged antibiotic therapy, and repeated blood product transfusions, predispose patients to nosocomial infections. The most important factor, however, is the lack of cleanliness in the wards. Prevention is the mainstay in warding off nosocomial infections. Prevention may be achieved by avoiding direct contact among patients and isolating patients with any active infection. Open wounds and contaminated utensils are the main cause of cross infections in the hospitals. All patients with open wounds should be treated with utmost care; any cross contamination may be avoided by using disposable lines, gloves, and gowns. In case of an outbreak of ward infections, the wards should be closed immediately and properly fumigated, and all trolleys, beds, and utensils should be fumigated. Any source of infection in the ward staff should be identified by nasal swabs and armpit cultures, and staff with positive cultures should be treated before returning to work. Staphylococci are the commonest organisms that may stay for a long time in the naris of carriers. In affected patients, local fuscidin crème should be used until the cultures are negative.

It has now been proven without a doubt that the incidence of nosocomial infections can be minimised significantly by hand washing before coming in contact with the patients. Therefore, hand washing must be ensured in all wards, and hand-washing areas should be present in accessible locations in the wards. Cholorhexidine lotion may help in the prevention of infection if the water supply is scarce. In developing countries, the use of disposable gloves may not be possible for all patients, but must be used for patients with open and infected wounds, for the safety of the other patients as well as the treating personnel.

Abscesses
An abscess is a collection of pus in a cavity surrounded by a pyogenic membrane. Pus is composed of necrotic leucocytes, tissue cells, and bacteria. Abscess formation occurs secondary to bacterial invasion of tissue. The bacteria multiply rapidly in the tissue and initiate an inflammatory

response, which includes increased blood flow in the tissue and attraction of inflammatory cells, especially leukocytes. The capillary becomes porous, and plasma proteins, especially fibrinogen, is released into the tissue spaces. Fibrinogen forms a fibrin plug to restrain the invading organism. The neutrophils start phagocytosis of bacteria, release proteolytic enzymes, and ultimately undergo necrosis. The abscess cavity is isolated from the surrounding tissue by the formation of pyogenic membrane. The proteolytic enzymes digest the dead tissue and give liquid consistency to pus. With the progression of the inflammatory process, granulation tissue is formed around the abscess cavity. The granulation tissue helps to prevent the spread of bacteria and inflammatory processes into the surrounding tissue, but it also prevents adequate concentration of antibiotic penetration into the tissue, making antibiotics less effective. Bacteria have a limit to proliferation, and after the maximum number of bacteria per unit volume has been achieved, further proliferation is stopped. Bacteria become less active and thus less vulnerable to antibiotics. The production of various enzymes, such as beta-lactamase, also cause a breakdown of the antibiotics. As the inflammatory process progresses, macrophages appear in the inflammatory zone and start the process of demolition. These macrophages then replace the neutrophils within the pyogenic membrane and ultimately start healing by secondary intention to leave a residual scar.

Locations

Abscesses may form anywhere in the body (Figures 15.2 and 15.3). The main sources of abscess formation are open or penetrating wounds, local extension from an adjacent focus of infection, haematogenous spread, or infections via lymph vessels and lymph nodes. The infecting organism varies according to the site and source of infection. Most abscesses on the skin and subcutaneous tissue are caused by *Staphylococcus aureus*. Causative organisms in deep abdominal abscesses depend upon the source of infection. In colon and appendix perforations, the abscess is usually polymicrobial and may cause fulminant infection or serious necrotising fasciitis. This form of infection is not common in the paediatric population; however, malnourished, immunocompromised children and those on chemotherapy are at a high risk of such infections.

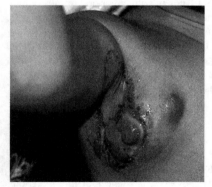

Figure 15.3: Axillary abscess.

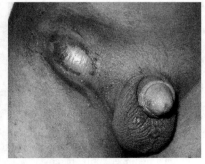

Figure 15.2: Groin abscess.

Diagnosis

The diagnosis of a surface abscess is obvious by its classic appearance, local pain, redness, tenderness, and central yellow punctum, from which it may drain if not treated adequately. An internal abscess may be difficult to diagnose due to overlapping symptoms with the preceding illness. The key diagnostic features are persistent fluctuant pyrexia, chills, and lack of appetite.

Treatment

Treatment of abscesses anywhere in the body is drainage. This holds true for most abscesses except for small lesions. If not drained in time an abscess tends to find its own path in the area of least resistance. It may therefore drain itself externally onto the surface, or internally as seen in subcutaneous tissue abscesses, or internally into other hollow organs such as the gut or urinary bladder. Spontaneous drainage of an abscess may have serious consequences, and every effort shall be made to control infection and drain the abscess surgically. This may be achieved for surface abscesses by making an incision, or for internal abscesses, by percutaneous drainage by ultrasound or computed tomography (CT) guidance. In some cases, an internal abscess will need exploration if it is not in an accessible area for percutaneous drainage. The surface abscess cavity should not be closed after drainage, as pus continues to form for days and weeks, and even after adequate drainage this may cause a recurrence in closed wounds. Repeated drainage of an internal abscess may be required. All abscesses must be sent for culture and sensitivity to ensure proper antibiotic coverage after drainage.

The role of antibiotics in an abscess is to control spread of infection. Once the abscess has been drained, the patient usually recovers rapidly, but antibiotics should be continued to prevent the spread of infection, especially in debilitated and immunocompromised patients.

Intraabdominal Abscess

Intraabdominal abscesses are commonly seen as a sequel of abdominal surgery; however, gut conditions, such as Crohn's disease, ulcerative colitis, and abdominal malignancies, may also cause a primary intraabdominal abscess. Abdominal abscesses are also seen after gut perforations secondary to trauma, penetrating injuries, and infective processes such as necrotising enterocolitis, enteric fever, and appendicitis. Immunocompromised patients are at a high risk of developing abdominal abscesses. In these patients, due to their altered immunological response, gut flora may grow rapidly and bacterial translocation may cause intraloop abscesses. The clinical features of intraabdominal abscesses depend upon the causative factors. In postoperative cases and bowel resection, the patient may initially show good recovery, but between 5 and 10 day postoperative, the patient develops intermittent fever, local tenderness, abdominal distention, and a palpable lump in the abdomen. In pelvic abscesses, rectal examination will reveal a tender bulge anteriorly. Subphrenic abscesses may also cause respiratory symptoms and breathing difficulty. Abscesses have the history of incidence secondary to penetrating injury or abdominal surgery, with or without gut perforation. Patients with inflammatory bowel disease (e.g., ulcerative colitis and Crohn's disease) will experience a deterioration in their general condition. Plain abdominal x-ray will show dilated gut loops due to the ileus and elevation of the hemidiaphragm in subphrenic collections. Ultrasonography will show the size and dimension of collection, but an abdominal CT scan may be required to evaluate the exact anatomy of the abscess cavity and its extension. Most localised intraabdominal abscesses may now be treated with ultrasound- or CT-guided aspiration along with broad-spectrum antibiotics. Open external drainage may also be required in patients who fail to improve after percutaneous aspiration or those forming repeated abscesses.

Cold Abscess

Cold abscess is the name given to a specialised form of abscess caused by *Mycobacterium tuberculosis*. Unlike acute pyogenic abscess, cold abscess has an insidious onset. It usually affects the neck area but may form abscess in areas such as the spine and psoas muscle. The patient usually has clinical features of tuberculosis, with anorexia, weight loss, low-grade fever and night sweats, but these may be absent in some cases. In the neck, the cold abscess usually affects the jugulo digastrics lymph nodes, which are initially enlarged. Over a period of months the lymph nodes become fluctuant and show signs of a localised abscess, but acute signs are classically absent. The abscess may burst if left untreated, and a persistent sinus then develops. Usually, infected patients have multiple sinuses that not only cause significant disfigurement but also are a source of infection for other people. Paraspinal cold abscesses are usually due to caries of the spine. The lumbar area is mostly affected. A classic example is psoas abscess, with visible fluctuant swelling in the inguinal region. The diagnosis is often easy due to the classic presentation; however, confirmation is by high erythrocytes sedimentation rate, positive tuberculin test and isolation of gram-positive rod from the pus staining. Fine-needle aspiration cytology will help in confirming the diagnosis by the identification of caseating granuloma and rarely acid-fast bacilli. Lymph node biopsy is confirmatory and is usually taken during drainage of a large cold abscess.

Treatment of tuberculosis abscess depends upon the causative organism. Most cases are due to *Mycobacterium tuberculosis*, and a four-drug therapy is usually curative. Many patients, after good initial response, unfortunately stop the treatment, and these patients are at high risk of developing resistant strains of *Mycobacterium tuberculosis*. Treatment is then by culture and sensitivity of the pus, and treatment may have to be given for a long time. Infections caused by atypical mycobacterium are now on the rise due to the bovine strain of mycobacterium. Treatment is by extensive local excision and use of erythromycin.

Post-BCG Tuberculosis Lymphadenitis

BCG is a tuberculosis vaccine. Post-BCG abscess is the name given to a specialised form of cold abscess seen in babies who have been vaccinated for tuberculosis. There is usually a history of delayed healing of the BCG vaccination site for several weeks or months. This is followed by an enlargement of the regional lymph nodes and then suppuration and abscess formation. Axillary lymph nodes on the affected side are usually involved, but other nodes (e.g., preauricular nodes) have also been affected in some patients. The baby is usually symptom free except for the fluctuant swelling in the axilla. Final-needle aspiration cytology will show green-yellow pus with acid-fast bacilli on microscopy, and caseating granulaomas may be visible on histology in intact nodes. Treatment is by aspiration of the nodes followed by single- or two-drug antituberculous therapy. The response is quick, and 3-6 months of treatment is sufficient for a permanent cure. In large abscesses, drainage or local excision of the affected nodes may be necessary.

Liver Abscess

Liver abscess in children is not uncommon in developing countries. Two main forms are seen: pyogenic liver abscess and amoebic liver abscess. In adults, liver abscesses are usually seen as an extension of infections from other viscera, such as appendicitis, ulcerative colitis, hepatobiliary calculi, enteric fever and penetrating injuries. In children, liver abscesses usually occur from hematogenous spread. Many of these children also have underlying immune deficiencies; chronic granulomatous disease in childhood has shown a strong association with pyogenic liver abscesses. Liver abscesses are also seen in children who are on chemotherapy or on immunosuppression for transplant surgery. Rarely, liver abscesses may occur after hepatobiliary surgery, such as biliary atresia and choledochal cyst.

The classic presentation of pyogenic liver abscess is high-grade fever with chills, abdominal pain, tender hepatomegaly, and jaundice. A high leukocyte count is suggestive, but in some patients the leukocyte count may not be very high. Nearly half of the patients will have positive blood cultures. Liver function tests are often marginally deranged. Diagnosis is confirmed by ultrasonography, and a CT scan will help in differentiating this from other cystic lesions. Serological tests for amoebae may be performed to exclude amoebic liver abscess. The treatment of liver abscess is drainage of the abscess, which may be performed either percutaneously under ultrasound or CT guidance. Where facilities for such treatment are not available, open drainage may be required. Complications of percutaneous drainage may be seen in nearly 4% of patients.

Staphylococcus aureus is the commonest organism isolated from liver abscesses. Other organisms, such as pseudomonas, *E. coli*, streptococci, and even bacteroides and *Candida*, may be isolated from pus cultures. Multiple organisms are seen in a significant number of patients. Patients with pyogenic liver abscess should be treated with broad-spectrum antibiotics with coverage for gram-positive, gram-negative, and anaerobic organisms. These may later be adjusted according to the sensitivity report, but they usually need long-term treatment. The abscess cavity gradually regresses, and thus ultasonography may show activity for a long time, but that does not mean the patient has active infections.

Amoebic Liver Abscess

Amoebic liver abscess is caused by *Entamoeba histolytica*, which causes colitis with diarrhoea and colicky abdominal pain.The stools are stained with mucus and blood, but some patients may be asymptomatic and act as chronic carriers. Transmission is through the faeco-oral route. The protozoa find their way through the gut mucosa into the portal circulation and into the liver, where they multiply rapidly and cause abscess formation. Due to the necrosis of the liver substance, the pus has an anchovy-chocolate-like appearance. The right lobe is commonly affected, but the disease may involve any lobe of the liver. If the abscess is not treated in time, it may have a tendency to burst into the pleural and peritoneal cavities. The consequences may be disastrous, and the patient may present with severe respiratory symptoms or may go into shock. Children with amoebic liver abscesses look unwell. Due to the prolonged infective process, the patients are anorexic and lose weight, and they have abdominal pain, tender hepatomegaly, and fever Leukocytosis is present, and stool examination may show cysts of *Entamoeba histolytica*.

Ultrasonography and CT scan will suggest the diagnosis of liver abscess. Diagnosis of amoebic liver abscess can be confirmed by serological tests such as an indirect haemagglutination test or growth of organisms from pus. Once a diagnosis is made, treatment with either oral or intravenous metroneidazole may be started. Many amoebic liver abscesses will resolve with medical treatment only; however, it takes a long time and may need external drainage. The treatment of choice for amoebic liver abscess is ultrasound- or CT-guided aspiration of the abscess along with metronidazole therapy. Some patients may need open drainage of the liver abscess if these measures fail.

Central Venous Line Infection

In the paediatric population, central venous access may be required in a variety of situations. With the use of small-calibre lines, such as percutaneously inserted central (PIC) venous lines, the incidence of line sepsis has decreased significantly; however, incidences of line infections in short- and long-term lines may still occur. The signs of line sepsis may not be easy to identify in patients with other sources of infection. Redness over the skin, fluctuating or persistent pyrexia, and generalised sepsis may be indicative of line sepsis. Definitive diagnosis is made by the culture of similar organisms from the peripheral blood, entry site of the line, and blood from the line. Any temporary line should immediately be removed, along with treatment with broad-spectrum antibiotics. In patients who have had long-term lines inserted (e.g., Hickman, Broviac, or portcath lines), salvage of the line may be attempted by giving high-dose broad-spectrum antibiotics through the line. If, however, the symptoms persist, then removal of the line should not be delayed. Serious consequences secondary to line sepsis include bacteria endocarditis, multiple abscesses, and meningitis. If a line is broken or damaged with significant sepsis, it may be replaced over a guide wire under antibiotic cover.

Evidence-Based Research

Table 15.1 compares the healing effects of honey versus EUSOL, and Table 15.2 presents evidence-based research on perianal abscess and fistula-in-ano in children in Zaria, Nigeria.

Table 15.1: Evidence-based research.

Title	Comparison of healing of incised abscess wounds with honey and EUSOL dressing
Authors	Okeniyi JA, Olubanjo OO, Ogunlesi TA, Oyelami OA
Institution	Department of Paediatrics and Child Health, Obafemi Awolowo University, Ile-Ife, Ilesa, Nigeria.
Reference	J Altern Complement Med 2005; 11(3):511–513.
Problem	Healing of wounds post abscess drainage
Intervention	To clinically compare the healing of abscess wounds dressed with either crude undiluted honey or Edinburgh University solution of lime (EUSOL).
Comparison/ control (quality of evidence)	A prospective clinical randomized study. LOCATION: The Isolation Children's Ward of the Wesley Guild Hospital, Ilesa, an affiliate of the Obafemi Awolowo University, Ile-Ife, Nigeria. SUBJECTS: 32 Nigerian children with 43 pyomyositis abcesses. INTERVENTIONS: All subjects had fresh surgical incisions and drainage of the abcesses and a 21-day course of ampicillin plus cloxacillin (Ampiclox) and gentamicin; the wounds were left to close spontaneously with twice-daily wound dressing with packing of the abscess cavity with either honey- or EUSOL-soaked gauze in two randomized treatment groups. OUTCOME MEASURES: The clinical conditions of the wound sites were documented on days 1, 3, 7, and 21 as either clean or dirty, dry or wet, granulation tissue present or absent, and epithelialisation present or absent. The length of hospital stay was also measured. RESULTS: Honey-treated wounds demonstrated quicker healing, and the length of hospital stay was significantly shorter in patients with honey-treated wounds than those treated with EUSOL (t = 2.45, p = 0.019).
Outcome/ effect	Honey is a superior wound dressing agent compared to EUSOL. Honey is recommended for the dressing of infected wounds, even more so in tropical countries, where it is most readily available.

Table 15.2: Evidence-based research.

Title	Perianal abscess and fistula in children in Zaria
Authors	Ameh EA
Institution	Paediatric Surgery Unit, Department of Surgery, Ahmadu Bello University Teaching Hospital, Zaria, Nigeria.
Reference	Niger Postgrad Med J 2003; 10(2):107–109.
Problem	Perianal abscess and fistula in ano in African children
Comparison/ control (quality of evidence)	Perianal abscess (PAA) and fistula-in-ano (FIA) are not uncommon in children, but reports from tropical Africa are uncommon. In a period of 17 years, 17 children aged 12 years and younger were treated for these conditions in Zaria, Nigeria. There were 14 boys and 3 girls, aged 4 months to 12 years (median age, 3 years), Eight had PAA (median age, 3 years), 5 ischiorectal abscess (median age, 5 years) and 4 FIA (median age, 10 months). FIA followed pull through for anorectal malformation in two patients, and in one it was preceded by PAA. PAA was associated with chronic fissure-in-ano in one patient and uncontrolled diabetes mellitus in one. One 16-month-old girl with an ischiorectal abscess developed severe perineal necrotising fascitis and separation and retraction of the anorectum. *Escherichia coli* was cultured in two patients with abscesses, and *Staphylococcus aureus* in another two. Culture was sterile in seven patients with abscesses. Treatment was by adequate incision and drainage for abscesses. Fistulectomy was the treatment for FIA, but in one patient a diversion colostomy was performed in addition, as the fistula was a high one. The child who developed necrotising fascitis had debridement and a diversion colostomy. FIA recurred in one patient, necessitating repeat fistulectomy. Although the number of patients is small, perianal sepsis appears to be less common in the Tropical African environment compared to developed countries. Some differences are highlighted.

Key Summary Points

1. Bacterial infections are the cause of significant mortality and morbidity in children.

2. Infections of surgical importance may affect virtually any organ or tissue in the body.

3. Infections may be community or hospital acquired.

4. Bacterial infections are more common at extreme of ages, and thus babies younger than 2 months of age are highly susceptible to acquire bacterial infection.

5. Other conditions such as malnutrition, immune-deficiency states, and prolonged illnesses make the children more susceptible to acquire infections.

Suggested Reading

Chauhan S, Jain S, Varma S, Chauhan SS. Tropical pyomyositis (myositis tropicans): current perspective. Postgrad Med J 2004; 80(943):267–270.

Cole C, Gazewood J. Diagnosis and treatment of impetigo. Am Fam Physician 2007; 75(6):859–864.

Jain SK, Persaud D, Perl TM, et al. Nosocomial malaria and saline flush. Emerg Infect Dis 2005; 11(7): 1097–1099..

Legbo JN, Legbo JF. Bacterial isolates from necrotizing fasciitis: a clinico-pathological perspective. Niger J Med 2007; 16(2):143–147.

Moazam F, Nazir Z. Amebic liver abscess: spare the knife but save the child. J Pediatr Surg 1998; 33(1):119–122.

Pereira FE, Musso C, Castelo JS. Pathology of pyogenic liver abscess in children. Pediatr Dev Pathol 1999; 2(6):537–543.

Steer AC, Danchin MH, Carapetis JR. Group A streptococcal infections in children. J. Paediatr Child Health 2007; 43(4): 203–213.

Swiss NOSO. Swiss Hand Hygiene Campaign, fact sheet. Available at www.swisshandhygiene.ch and www.swiss-noso.ch. Accessed 5 October 2009.

CHAPTER 16
SURGICAL SITE INFECTION

Abdulrasheed A. Nasir
Sharon Cox
Emmanuel A. Ameh

Introduction

Infection is the clinical manifestation of the inflammatory reaction incited by invasion and proliferation of microorganisms.[1] Despite modern surgical techniques and the use of antibiotic prophylaxis, surgical site infection (SSI) is one of the most common complications encountered in surgery. SSI places a significant burden on both the patient and health system,[2] especially in Africa where resources are limited. SSI occurs in up to 40% of surgical procedures, delaying recovery by one week on average and often resulting in the need for further surgical procedures.[3] It is still a major limiting factor in advancing the horizons of surgery in spite of the progress made in its control. SSI is thus a major cause of morbidity, prolonged hospital stay, and increased health costs.[4]

Demographics

Although a large number of reports on SSI are available in adult literature,[5–8] reports for children are few, and most are from developed countries with an overall incidence of 2.5–20%.[4,9–13] In most of Africa, incidence data are not available, but one hospital-based prospective report suggests an incidence of 23.6%.[14]

Classification

SSIs are defined as infections occurring within 30 days of the procedure and involving the operative area. Where implants have been placed, this time period is extended to 1 year if the infection appears to relate to the procedure.[3]

A system of classification for operative wounds that is based on the degree of microbial contamination was developed by the US National Research Council (NRC) group in 1964.[15] Four wound classes with an increasing risk of SSIs were described: clean, clean-contaminated, contaminated, and dirty (Table 16.1). The simplicity of this system of classification has resulted in its widespread use to predict the rate of infection after surgery.

The term used by the Centers for Disease Control and Prevention (CDC) for infections associated with surgical procedures was changed from surgical wound infection to surgical site infection by the Surgical Wound Infection Task Force in 1992.[16] Infections are classified by the depth of the tissue involved: superficial incisional (skin and subcutaneous tissue), deep incisional (deep soft tissue–muscle and fascia), and organ space[16] (any part of the anatomy opened or manipulated during the procedure other than the incision).

Superficial Incisional SSI

A superficial incisional infection occurs within 30 days after the operation. It involves only the skin or subcutaneous tissue of the incision. At least *one* of the following is present:

- purulent drainage, with or without laboratory confirmation, from the superficial incision;

- organisms isolated from an aseptically obtained culture of fluid or tissue from the superficial incision;

- at least one of the following signs or symptoms of infection: pain or tenderness, localised swelling, redness, or heat *and* superficial incisions deliberately opened by the surgeon, *unless* the incision is culture-negative; or

- diagnosis of superficial incisional SSI by the surgeon or attending physician.

Deep Incisional SSI

A deep incisional SSI occurs within 30 days after the operation if no implant is left in place, or within 1 year if an implant is present. It involves the deep soft tissues (e.g., fascial and muscle layers) of the incision. At least *one* of the following is present:

- purulent drainage from the deep incision but not from the organ space component of the surgical site;

- a deep incision spontaneously dehisces or is deliberately opened by a surgeon when the patient has at least one of the following signs or symptoms: fever (>38°C), localised pain, or tenderness, unless the site is culture-negative;

- an abscess or other evidence of infection involving the deep incision is found on direct examination, during reoperation, or by histopathologic or radiologic examination; or

- diagnosis of a deep incisional SSI by the surgeon or attending physician.

Organ Space SSI

An organ space SSI occurs within 30 days after the operation if no implant is left in place, or within 1 year if an implant is present. It involves any part of the anatomy (e.g., organs or spaces), other than

Table 16.1: Classification of operative wounds based on degree of microbial contamination.

Classification	Criteria
Clean	Elective, nonemergency, nontraumatic case, primarily closed; no acute inflammation; no break in aseptic technique; respiratory, gastrointestinal, biliary, and genitourinary tracts not entered.
Clean-contaminated	Urgent or emergency case that is otherwise clean; elective opening of respiratory, gastrointestinal, biliary, or genitourinary tract with minimal spillage (e.g., appendectomy) not encountering infected urine or bile; minor aseptic technique break.
Contaminated	Nonpurulent inflammation; gross spillage from gastrointestinal tract; entry into biliary or genitourinary tract in the presence of infected bile or urine; major break in aseptic technique; penetrating trauma <4 hours old; chronic open wounds to be grafted or covered.
Dirty	Purulent inflammation (e.g., abscess); preoperative perforation of respiratory, gastrointestinal, biliary, or genitourinary tract; penetrating trauma >4 hours old.

Source: B'ernard F, Grandon J, Postoperative wound infections: the influence of ultraviolet irradiation of the operating room and of various other factors. Ann Surg 1964; 160(Supp 1).

the incision, that was opened or manipulated during an operation. At least *one* of the following is present:

- purulent drainage from a drain that is placed through a stab wound into the organ or space;

- organisms are isolated from an aseptically obtained culture of fluid or tissue in the organ or space;

- an abscess or other evidence of infection involving the organ space that is found on direct examination, during reoperation, or by histopathologic or radiologic examination; or

- diagnosis of an organ space SSI by a surgeon or attending physician.

Risk Assessment

Attempts have been made to derive a clinically useful index that will encompass the major factors influencing wound infection rate and thus predict a patient's risk of developing wound infection in the postoperative period. A multivariate index combining patient susceptibility and wound contamination was developed and tested during the CDC Study on the Efficacy of Nosocomial Infection Control (SENIC).[17] This index involves the following four risk factors:

1. an operation that involves the abdomen;

2. an operation lasting longer than 2 hours;

3. an operation classified as either contaminated, dirty, or infected; and

4. a patient having three or more discharge diagnoses.

Each of these equally weighted factors contributes a point when present, so the risk index values range from 0 to 4. By using these factors, the SENIC index predicted SSI risk twice as well as the traditional wound classification scheme alone. Because this index included discharge diagnoses, some modification and a prospective evaluation of the index became necessary before it could be recommended for clinical use. A further modification of this index was therefore developed. This is the National Nosocomial Infection Surveillance (NNIS) index.[18] The NNIS risk index is operation-specific and applied to prospectively collected surveillance data. The index values range from 0 to 3 points and are defined by three independent and equally weighted variables. One point is scored for each of the following when present:

1. a patient having an American Society of Anesthesiologists (ASA) preoperative score of 3, 4, or 5;

2. an operation classified as either contaminated or dirty; and

3. an operation lasting more than T hours, where T depends on the operation being performed (T approximates the 50th percentile of the duration of a procedure and varies from 1 hour for an appendectomy to 7 hours in organ transplant surgery).

The ASA class replaced discharge diagnoses of the SENIC risk index as a surrogate for the patient's underlying severity of illness (host susceptibility). It has the advantage of being readily available in the chart during the patient's hospital stay. Unlike SENIC's constant 2-hour cut point for the duration of the operation, the operation-specific cut points used in the NNIS risk index increase its discriminatory power. Although their long-term usefulness in predicting postoperative wound infection is still being evaluated, preliminary reports have been validating the usefulness of these indices in adult patients. There is a need to validate these indices in paediatric patients before general acceptance.

In a report on 322 sub-Saharan African children undergoing operation, the SSI rate was 14.3% in clean incisions, 19.3% in clean-contaminated incisions, 27.3% in contaminated incisions, and 60% in dirty incisions. The degree of incisional contamination and a duration of surgery ≥2 hours were important risk factors that were significantly associated with SSI.[14]

In addition to the above general factors, there are important individual patient risk factors that may also affect the incidence of wound infection, such as body mass index (BMI), age, human immunodeficiency virus (HIV), and immune deficiency states.

Pathophysiology

SSI arises secondary to exogenous or endogenous bacterial contamination at the time of the operative procedure. Bacterial proliferation results in tissue reaction and outpouring of inflammatory cells, leading to tissue destruction and pus formation. The presence of local factors such as necrosis, haematoma, and dead space provide bacteria with a milieu for growth, and the presence of other foreign bodies inhibits local tissue resistance.[7] Microorganisms may contain or produce toxins and other substances that increase their ability to invade a host, produce damage within the host, or survive on or in host tissue. Many gram-negative bacteria produce an endotoxin that stimulates cytokine production. The cytokines can trigger a systemic inflammatory response syndrome that sometimes leads to multiple system organ failure.[19]

Patient factors that may possibly increase the risk of an SSI include coincident remote site infections or colonisation, diabetes, systemic steroid use, obesity (>20% ideal body weight), and poor nutritional status.

Clinical Presentation

Nonspecific clinical signs mimicking infection frequently occur in the postoperative period, making the diagnosis difficult. These signs include wound erythema and induration secondary to lymphatic and venous obstruction, fever, and leucocytosis. Most SSIs present from 3 to 14 days postoperatively.

Gram-positive SSIs tend to arise early (3 to 6 days) and are characterised by prominent local signs and symptoms. The wound is indurated, erythematous, and tender. Drainage is purulent and generous. Systemic signs are usually mild and include low-grade fever and irritability.[1] Group A streptococcus SSI typically presents dramatically 24 to 48 hours postoperatively with spreading cellulitis with distinct margins and lymphangitis. Drainage is scant and serous in nature. Systemic signs are prominent with high-grade fever and toxaemia.[1]

Gram-negative SSI tends to arise later, 7 to 14 days postoperatively, and thus could present after discharge from hospital. Local signs are less pronounced. Systemic signs are, however, often more prominent, with high-grade fever and tachycardia. Wound drainage, if present, is sero-purulent and may be foul smelling.

Local Features of SSI
Common local features of SSI include:

- pain and tenderness beyond what is expected for the nature of the surgery, and despite adequate analgesia;

- swelling, induration, and warmth;

- shiny, erythematous skin; and

- purulent discharge.

Systemic Features of SSI
Common systemic features of SSI include:

- pyrexia (≥37.8°C);

- leucocytosis;

- tachycardia;

- tachypnoea;

- vomiting; and

- refusal to feed/anorexia (particularly in neonates and infants).

Complications

If uncontrolled, SSI may progress to life-threatening complications. The severity of each complication depends in large part on the infecting pathogen, the site of infection, the nature of surgery, and the underlying host factors. Due to the frequently delayed presentation of several conditions, and the high prevalence of SSI, complications occur often in sub-Saharan Africa.

Commonly encountered early complications are necrotising fasciitis, wound dehiscence, metastatic abscesses, and septicaemia and organ failure. Delayed or long-term complications include incisional hernia and ugly and/or deforming scars.

Investigations

Although the diagnosis of most surgical site infection is clinical, further investigation may be necessary for planning of treatment and follow-up. Any of the following investigations may be relevant:

1. Any discharge from the wound should be cultured to establish the microbiological profile and organism antibiotic sensitivity of the infection. Tissue biopsy and culture may be helpful in situations where culture of discharge proves contaminated or unable to provide a reliable yield. The culture should involve both aerobic and anaerobic culture.

2. Ultrasonography may be required if subcutaneous or organ space collection is suspected; however, if used too early, this modality may give false positives, as fluid may just be postoperative serous collections rather than pus. It is also useful in monitoring treatment.

3. A computed tomography (CT) scan is rarely necessary but may be helpful in organ space infection, specifically where multiple relook laparotomies and bowel gas distort any ultrasound view or when ultrasonography does not provide conclusive information.

4. A complete blood count will determine whether leucocytosis and neutrophilia are evident, especially when the infection becomes systemic.

5. In persistent/uncontrollable situations, efforts should be made to identify any underlying predisposing factors such as HIV infection, diabetes mellitus, foreign bodies, or anastomotic breakdown and fistula formation.

Management

Specific Treatment

The definitive treatment of SSI is adequate pus drainage. The entire wound must be opened by suture removal for effective drainage. In incisional SSI, the wound is packed with moist gauze or commercial cavity dressing until granulation has appeared. Dressing with native honey has been proven efficient in Africa.[14,20] Depending on circumstances, secondary suture of granulating clean wounds may be possible. Vacuum-assisted dressings have been clinically proven to encourage granulation tissue and wound closure, and in the African setting, the use of wall suction on low pressure suction is perfectly acceptable to achieve adequate vacuum-assisted closure (VAC) dressing.

Even though percutaneous ultrasound-guided drainage may be possible in organ space collections, surgical drainage is often required to remove all collected pus and any dead tissue or slough, and to irrigate the cavity.

General Measures

In most instances, local wound care, as detailed above, may be enough to control the infection. However, if there are systemic features or the infection is not controlled by local measures, then empiric systemic antibiotics, altered when sensitivities become available, should be given. Failure of response within 48–72 hours may suggest underlying deeper abscess requiring drainage or wound exploration for gangrenous complications.[1]

Prevention

Risks

The risk of developing a surgical wound infection is largely determined by three factors:

1. the amount and type of microbial contamination of the wound;

2. the condition of the wound at the end of the operation (largely determined by surgical technique and disease processes encountered during the operation); and

3. host susceptibility, that is, the patient's intrinsic ability to deal with microbial contamination.

These factors interact in a complex manner to result in SSI.[21] Measures intended to prevent surgical wound infections are directed at these. The preoperative hospital stay should be kept as short as possible. Any host factors likely to predispose to SSI, including nutritional issues, medications such as steroids, diabetic control, and remote infections should be properly controlled before embarking on surgery.

Prophylactic Antibiotics

Prophylactic antibiotics are those administered to patients before contamination has occurred. Their role is to minimise postoperative infection in clean or clean-contaminated wounds. The choice and use of prophylactic antibiotics should be guided by the knowledge of site-specific flora (both patient and hospital environment), as well as the nature of the intended surgery, the antibiotic spectrum of cover, toxicity, and pharmacokinetics, with the aim being the highest tissue levels at the time of maximum contamination. If no hollow viscus or mucosal barrier is violated, antibiotics generally need to cover only gram-positive organisms, whereas breach of the gastrointestinal, genitourinary, biliary, and aerodigestive tracts should cover both skin flora and site-specific aerobic and anaerobic organisms, if needed.

Antibiotics should be given parenterally. The first dose should be given not more than 2 hours before the skin incision and is frequently given at the time of anaesthetic induction. Infection risk is higher in procedures lasting more than 2 hours, so antibiotic repetition may be required. It must be emphasized that prophylactic antibiotics should not be a substitute for adherence to strict asepsis in the operating room and meticulous surgical technique.

Operating Environment

The operating team should adhere to a tested scrub protocol using reliable antiseptics. The surgical site should be prepared by using potent and reliable antiseptics appropriate to the site. Every effort should be made to avoid breaking aseptic techniques during the entire procedure.

Most infections are acquired in the operating room, so good surgical practices are crucial to their prevention. Excellent surgical technique is widely believed to reduce the risk of SSI. This includes maintaining effective haemostasis while preserving adequate blood supply, preventing hypothermia, gently handling tissues, avoiding inadvertent entries into a hollow viscus, removing devitalised tissues, using suture material appropriately, eradicating dead space, and appropriately managing the postoperative incision.[21]

Surveillance

The development of an SSI surveillance programme within each unit or hospital is essential for recognition and reduction of surgical wound infections.[22–24] Further research is needed to determine the most practical and sensitive method for general use. Inpatient surveillance must include bedside examination and total chart review, which has a 90% sensitivity,[23] and microbiology report review (sensitivity 33–65%).[24] One infection control nurse for a total of 250 beds, together with an organised surveillance system, can reduce hospital infection rates by up to 32%.[22]

As surgical services improve and move toward ambulatory and day case surgery, 20–72% of surgical wound infections will present clinically only after discharge,[3] so a system of follow-up for case finding and reporting is mandatory in the outpatient population as well. This may include developing communication lines to local clinics or specific outpatient reviews within 2 weeks of discharge.

It is only by monitoring, reporting, and analyzing SSI incidence that procedure- or surgeon-specific trends can be determined and prevention methods put in place.

Evidence-Based Research

At present, there are no randomised control trials on surgical site infection in children. Tables 16.2 and 16.3, which present analyses of paediatric wound infections, are based on reports of large prospective studies on incidence and risk factors of SSIs.

Table 16.2: Evidence-based research.

Title	Pediatric wound infections: a prospective multicenter study
Authors	Horwitz JR, Chwals WJ, Doski JJ, Suescun EA, Cheu HW, Lally KP
Institution	University of Texas-Houston Medical School and Herman Children's Hospital, Houston, Texas, USA; Wilford Hall USAF Medical Center, San Antonio, Texas, USA; Bownman Gray School of Medicine, Winston-Salem, North Carolina, USA
Reference	Annals of Surgery 1998; 227:553–558
Problem	To identify risk factors associated with the development of wound infection in children.
Comparison	Comparing children who developed wound infection and those who did not.
Outcome/effect	The overall incidence of wound infection was 4.4%. The amount of wound contamination (p = 0.006) and duration of operation (p = 0.03) were found to be significantly associated with a postoperative wound infection. There were no significant differences in age, gender, ASA preoperative assessment score, length of preoperative stay, and use of perioperative antibiotics.
Historical significance/comments	This report of a large series of surgical site infection in children with a multicentre approach provides a useful practice guide, although there is the possibility of differences in patient selection and case mix with this approach. The authors recommend prospective surveillance of wound infection in children with feedback to clinicians to reduce the cost of health care associated with wound infection.

Table 16.3: Evidence-based research.

Title	Surgical site infection in children: prospective analysis of the burden and risk factors in a sub-Saharan African setting
Authors	Ameh EA, Mshelbwala PM, Nasir AA, Lukong CS, Jabo BA, Anumah MA, Nmadu PT
Institution	Division of Pediatric Surgery, Department of Surgery, Ahmadu Bello University Teaching Hospital, Zaria, Nigeria
Reference	Surgical Infections (Larchmt) 2009; 10(2):105-9
Problem	There is a lack of data regarding the prevalence and risk factors of surgical site infection in children in Africa. The problem is to determine the burden and risk factors for SSI in children in a major teaching hospital in sub-Saharan Africa.
Comparison	Comparing children who developed wound infection and those who did not.
Outcome/effect	The overall rate of SSI was 23.6%. The SSI rate was 14.3% in clean incisions, 19.3% in clean-contaminated incisions, 27.3% in contaminated incisions, and 60% in dirty incisions (p < 0.05). The infection rate was 25.8% in emergency procedures and 20.8% in elective procedures (p < 0.05). The infection rate was 31% in operations lasting 2 hours or more and 17.3% in operations lasting less than 2 hours (p < 0.05).
Historical significance/comments	This is the first prospective report of SSI in children in sub-Saharan Africa. The burden of SSI is high in the setting. The authors attributed this to the lack of definite infection surveillance/control programmes and the tropical climate. The degree of incisional contamination and a long duration of surgery (≥2 hours) are important risk factors. The report draws attention to the lack of hospital infection control and antibiotic guidelines, and has prompted a proactive approach to these issues.

Key Summary Points

1. Surgical site infections are a major cause of morbidity and increased costs in health care.
2. A multitude of risk factors influence the development of SSIs, and awareness of these will help to promote effective preventive strategies.
3. The degree of wound contamination and duration of surgery are proven risk factors.
4. Surveillance systems that monitor rates of wound infection and provide feedback to clinicians have been shown to contribute to quality improvement and help to prevent and control infection.
5. Antibiotic prophylaxis is not an alternative to maintenance of asepsis.
6. SSIs in children are related more to perioperative factors than to the patients' overall physiologic status.
7. Rigorous adherence to the principles of asepsis by all scrubbed personnel is the foundation of surgical site infection prevention.

References

1. Mollit D. Surgical Infections. In: Ziegler MA, et al. Operative Pediatric Surgery. McGraw-Hill, 2003, Pp 161–178.
2. Wilson AP, Gibbons C, Reeves BC, et al. Surgical wound infection as a performance indicator: agreement of common definitions of wound infection in 4773 patients. BMJ 2004; 329(7468):720.
3. Rode H, Brown RA, Millar AJW. Surgical skin and soft tissue infections. Current Opinion Infect Dis, 1993; 6:683–690.
4. Horwitz JR, et al. Pediatric wound infections: a prospective multicenter study. Ann Surg 1998; 227(4):553–558.
5. Efem, SEE, Akuma AJA, Inyang U. Surgical wound infection rate in Calabar University Teaching Hospital. West Afr J Med 1986; 5:61–68.
6. Ferreira AJ. Surgical wound infection in a general hospital- a preliminary report. West Afr J Surg 1979; 3:57–64.

7.   Lawal OO, Adejuyigbe O, Oluwole SF. The predictive value of bacterial contamination at operation in post-operative wound sepsis. Afr J Med Sci 1990; 19(3):173–179.

8.   Ojiegbe GC, Njoku-Obi AN, Ojukwu JO. Incidence and parametric determinants of post-operative wound infections in a university teaching hospital. Cent Afr J Med 1990; 36(3):63–67.

9.   Bhattacharyya N., Kosloske AM. Postoperative wound infection in pediatric surgical patients: a study of 676 infants and children. J Pediatr Surg 1990; 25(1):125–129.

10. Davenport M, Doig CM. Wound infection in pediatric surgery: a study in 1,094 neonates. J Pediatr Surg 1993; 28(1):26–30.

11. Doig CM, Wilkinson AW. Wound infection in a children's hospital. Br J Surg 1976; 63(8):647–650.

12. Duque-Estrada EO, Duarte MR, Rodrigues DM, Raphael MD. Wound infections in pediatric surgery: a study of 575 patients in a university hospital. Pediatr Surg Int 2003; 19(6):436–438.

13. Uludag O, Rieu P, Niessen M, Voss A. Incidence of surgical site infections in pediatric patients: a 3-month prospective study in an academic pediatric surgical unit. Pediatr Surg Int 2000; 16(5-6):417–420.

14. Ameh EA, Mshelbwala PM, Nasir AA, et al. Surgical site infection in children: prospective analysis of the burden and risk factors in a sub-Saharan African setting. Surg Infect (Larchmt) 2009; 10(2):105-9

15. B'ernard, F, Grandon J. Postoperative wound infections: the influence of ultraviolet irradiation of the operating room and of various other factors. Ann Surg 1964; 160(Supp 1).

16. Horan TC, Gaynes RP, Martone WJ, Jarvis WR, Emori TG. CDC definitions of nosocomial surgical site infections, 1992: a modification of CDC definitions of surgical wound infections. Infect Control Hosp Epidemiol 1992; 13(10):606–608.

17. Haley RW, Culver DH, Morgan WM, White JW, Emori TG, Hooton TM. Identifying patients at high risk of surgical wound infection. A simple multivariate index of patient susceptibility and wound contamination. Am J Epidemiol 1985; 121(2):206–215.

18. Culver DH, Horan TC, Gaynes RP, et al. Surgical wound infection rates by wound class, operative procedure, and patient risk index. National Nosocomial Infections Surveillance System. Am J Med 1991; 91(3B):152S–157S.

19. Demling R, LaLonde C, Saldinger P, Knox J. Multiple-organ dysfunction in the surgical patient: pathophysiology, prevention, and treatment. Curr Probl Surg 1993; 30(4):345–414.

20. Oluwatosin OM. Surgical wound infection: a general overview. Ann Ibadan Postgrad Med 2005; 3:26–31.

21. Mangram AJ, Horan TC, Pearson ML, Silver LC, Jarvis WR. Guideline for prevention of surgical site infection, 1999. Hospital Infection Control Practices Advisory Committee. Infect Control Hosp Epidemiol 1999; 20(4):250–278; quiz 279–280.

22. Holtz TH, Wenzel RP. Postdischarge surveillance for nosocomial wound infection: a brief review and commentary. Am J Infect Control 1992; 20(4):206–213.

23. Lee JT. Wound infection surveillance. Infect Dis Clin North Am 1992; 6(3):643–656.

24. Consensus Paper on the Surveillance of Surgical Wound Infections. The Society for Hospital Epidemiology of America, The Association for Practitioners in Infection Control, The Centers for Disease Control, The Surgical Infection Society. Infect Control Hosp Epidemiol 1992; 13:599–605.

CHAPTER 17
SURGICAL COMPLICATIONS OF TYPHOID FEVER

Emmanuel A. Ameh
Francis A. Abantanga

Introduction

Typhoid fever is a common infection that has continued to be a public health problem in many developing countries,[1, 2] particularly in areas with poor sanitation and limited availability of clean, potable water. The surgical complications of typhoid fever are a cause of significant morbidity and mortality in children in many parts of Africa, particularly in sub-Saharan Africa. The management of intestinal perforation,[3–6] which is the most common surgical complication, has posed a difficult challenge due to its high morbidity and mortality. A controversy remains regarding what should be the best and most effective surgical option for treating these intestinal perforations.

Demographics

The World Health Organization (WHO) conservatively puts the annual global incidence of typhoid fever at 21 million cases, with 1–4% mortality.[2] The disease predominantly affects school-age children (5–15 years of age), although it does occur in younger children.[2]

Children account for more than 50% of all cases of typhoid intestinal perforation (TIP), which is the commonest severe complication of typhoid,[5] with a peak age incidence of 5–9 years. Unlike typhoid fever in adults, which predominantly affects males,[4,7] boys and girls are equally affected.[5,6]

The overall perforation rate of typhoid in children is about 10%, but the perforation rate appears to increase with age, reaching a high of 30% by age 12 years (Table 17.1).[5]

Typhoid fever, with or without intestinal perforation, appears to occur year round,[5,7] but with a slightly higher incidence in the rainy season (Figure 17.1). This is perhaps an indication of the gross defects in sanitation and lack of safe potable water.

Aetiology/Pathophysiology

Typhoid infection is faeco-oral in nature and is due to faecal contamination of food and water. The infection is caused by the bacteria, *Salmonella typhi* (also known as *Salmonella enterica serotype typhi),* a gram-negative rod found only in humans, and rarely by *Salmonella paratyphi.* The mechanism of transmission and causation of the common surgical complications is as shown in the flow chart in Figure 17.2.

Surgical Complications

Typhoid fever is a systemic infection involving virtually all organs to varying degrees. The more common surgical complications include intestinal perforation; intestinal bleeding; cholecystitis (perforation, empyema); osteomyelitis; and abscesses. Rare surgical complications include pancreatitis, hepatic and splenic abscesses, pleural effusion, and orchitis.

Therefore, the following procedures are called for (note the mnemonic BSU):

- Week 1: Take **B**lood for culture.

- Week 2: Take **S**tool for culture.

- Week 3: Take **U**rine for culture.

Table 17.1: Age and sex of typhoid perforation and perforation rate in children.

	Number of typhoid perforations (1987-1996)			Typhoid perforation rate (over 5 years)		
Age (years)	Sex		Total cases (%)	Number of typhoid cases	Total number of perforations	Perforation rate (%)
	Boys	Girls				
<1	1	—	1 (1.6)	25	1	4.0
1–4	1	2	3 (4.7)	120	2	1.7
5–9	25	18	43 (67.2)	194	24	12.4
10–12	7	10	17 (26.6)	41	12	29.3
Total	34	30	64 (100)	380	39	10.3

Source: Adapted with kind permission from Annals of Tropical Paediatrics and International Child Health, Liverpool School of Tropical Medicine.

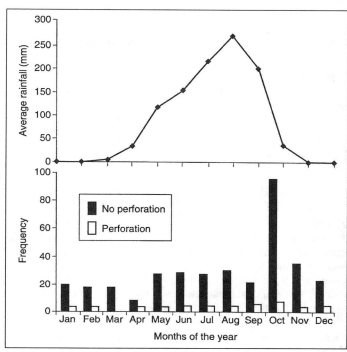

Source: Reproduced with kind permission from Annals of Tropical Paediatrics and International Child Health, Liverpool School of Tropical Medicine.

Figure 17.1: Seasonal distribution of rainfall (top) and typhoid fever in children, with and without perforation (bottom).

Table 17.2: Mechanism of surgical complications of typhoid fever.

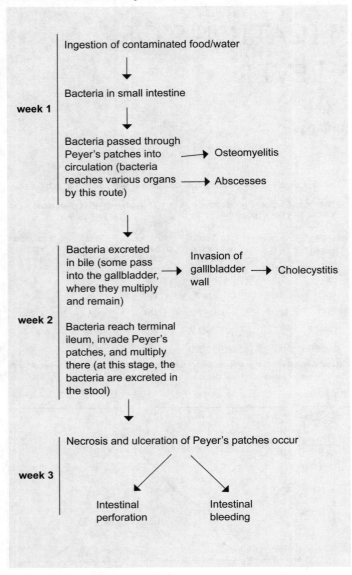

Clinical Presentation

History

Presentation is commonly late;[5] most patients present several weeks after onset of symptoms, frequently after several attempts at treatment with antibiotics or traditional medications. Symptoms may be atypical in infants and toddlers[3,8] younger than 5 years of age. A little less than 10% develop intestinal perforation under medical treatment,[5] and symptoms may be masked in these patients.

The symptoms include:

- Fever and general body weakness: These are usually the earliest symptoms and always precede abdominal pain (in contrast to appendicitis, for which pain precedes fever). Headache frequently accompanies the fever.

- *Abdominal pain* usually begins 2–30 days (median = 9 days)[5] after the onset of fever. The pain is initially vague but gradually becomes generalised. Although typhoid fever without perforation may be associated with some abdominal pain, this is usually not severe, and the onset of increasing abdominal pain frequently signifies that an intraabdominal complication is setting in.

- *Abdominal distention* can be observed.

- *Diarrhoea or constipation:* Diarrhoea may occur in the early stages, but constipation sets in later in the course of the illness.

- *Passage of blood* in the stool may occur, either as frank or altered blood.

- *Jaundice* may be a complaint.

- *Pain* at the site of the abscess or osteomyelitis.

Physical Examination

These patients are usually very ill; common findings include dehydration, pyrexia, pallor from anaemia (about 50% of children with typhoid perforation have a packed cell volume below 30%[3,5]), and wasting, particularly if the illness has gone on for several weeks.

Jaundice may be present. Shock may also be present, as evidenced by tachycardia and hypotension (blood pressure <80/60 mm Hg); shock is present in about 75–80% of children with typhoid perforation.

Abdominal/rectal examination

There is usually distention, but in a few patients distention may not be remarkable. Patients presenting late may have demonstrable anterior abdominal wall oedema. Bowel sounds are diminished or absent in those presenting late.

Generalised tenderness with guarding is present; this finding, however, may not be remarkable, especially in patients who perforate under medical treatment. Abdominal rigidity is present in only one-third of children with typhoid perforation.[5] A dilated and tender gallbladder may be palpable in the right hypochondrium in patients with cholecystitis.

There may be fullness in the recto-vesical or recto-uterine pouch, suggesting a pelvic collection of pus. Blood may be seen on the examining finger in patients with bleeding.

In osteomyelitis or abscess, the affected site should be thoroughly examined.

Respiratory examination

In very ill patients, respiratory function is compromised by chest infection, which is worsened by the marked abdominal distention. Crepitations may be heard, sometimes bilaterally, indicating that pneumonia has set in and is worsening the child's condition.

Evaluation/Investigations

Because a majority of the patients present with an acute abdomen, intestinal perforation and gallbladder involvement need to be excluded. The latter is most important, as cholecystitis may not require urgent surgical intervention. The diagnosis of TIP is often clinical, based on features of peritonitis,[3,7] and investigations are done to support the diagnosis and identify deficits, as well as to ascertain the fitness of the patient for surgery.

1. *Serum electrolytes, urea, and creatinine:* The levels of sodium, potassium, chloride, and bicarbonate are estimated. They are often deranged, especially in those presenting late. Hypokalaemia is a troublesome problem, and metabolic acidosis may be identified. An elevated urea level is an indication of the severity of dehydration as well as renal compromise; the latter is more likely if hyperkalaemia is also present.

2. *Plain radiography:*

- Chest and upper abdomen (erect film): Some patients with intestinal perforation present evidence of air under the diaphragm. This is present in about 55% of children with TIP,[3] but may be as high as 96% in those with typhoid colonic perforation.[9] The extent of pneumoperitoneum is important as it may be necessary to vent the air to improve respiration and reduce hypoxia. Absence of air under the diaphragm, however, does not exclude perforation. Pulmonary consolidation may be present in those with chest infection.

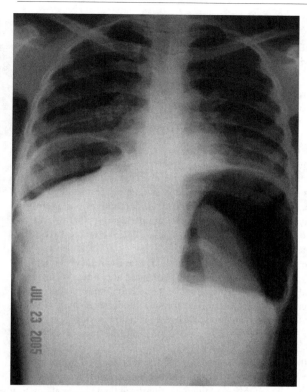

Figure 17.3: Large pneumoperitoneum from typhoid perforation.

- Full abdomen (erect and supine): The intestines may show dilatation and oedematous walls. Frequently, all that can be seen is a diffuse opacity in most of the abdomen, particularly in those presenting late with intraperitoneal collection. Patients who are too sick for erect film should have a lateral decubitus film to identify pneumoperitoneum (Figure 17.3). The shadow of a distended gallbladder may be obvious, suggesting cholecystitis.

3. *Abdominal ultrasonography:* This is to be done only in patients who do not need urgent surgery and in whom the diagnosis is doubtful; it should identify the following , if present: intraperitoneal abscesses and cholecystitis. The usual evidence of cholecystitis in these patients is mainly dilatation, presence of pericholecystic fluid, and oedematous wall. Other intraabdominal conditions can be excluded.

4. *Microbiological cultures:* Blood and urine, as well as an operative specimen of intraperitoneal fluid/pus, are cultured to identify the *Salmonella* organism and any superimposed infections. In one report of children younger than 5 years of age with TIP,[3] *Salmonella typhi* was cultured from the peritoneal fluid in 46%, urine in 36%, and stool in 32%. In patients in whom intraoperative diagnosis of cholecystitis (and its complication) is made, a sample of gallbladder contents is also cultured.

5. *Complete blood count:* A haemogram is done to identify anaemia. The platelet count is ascertained, particularly in patients with evidence of coagulopathy. Although leucopaenia is a more common finding in patients with uncomplicated typhoid fever, leucocytosis and neutrophilia are more common in those with intestinal perforation or cholecystitis.

6. *Blood grouping and cross matching:* These procedures are necessary in most patients for correction of anaemia or intraoperative use.

7. *Widal's test:* Although found to be positive in one report,[3] this test is rather nonspecific and frequently misinterpreted. It has limited use in the management of these patients.

8. *Further investigations:* These will depend on other complications that are suspected. Note that resuscitation takes precedence over these investigations, which should not delay intervention after resuscitation is complete.

Management

1. *Correction of fluid and electrolyte deficits:* Care needs to be taken to achieve adequate correction. A common cause of death is inadequate replacement of fluid and electrolyte deficits. Four to six hours may be needed to achieve adequate correction.

- Dextrose: Intravenous dextrose in 0.18-0.45% N saline is used in children younger than 5 years of age (the amount of saline used will depend on the serum level of Na$^+$). In older children, dextrose in 0.9% N saline is used. Large volumes of fluid may be required: 20 ml/kg by bolus infusion is given initially in severely dehydrated patients and those presenting in shock. Ten ml/kg may be repeated after 1 hour if urine output is not satisfactory (never give bolus infusion of any potassium-containing fluid). Thereafter, adjust infusion to maintain a urine output of 1.5–2 ml/kg/hr.

- Potassium (K$^+$): Once the child is making adequate urine, give at least a daily requirement of K$^+$ (1–2 mmol/kg/day) until a serum biochemistry result is available. Thereafter, any calculated deficit is added to the daily requirement. The amount of potassium required is added to the intravenous fluid and administered over 18 to 24 hours (do not give more than 10 mmol of K$^+$ in an hour unless the child is in the intensive care unit (ICU) and is being monitored using an electrocardiogram (ECG)).

2. *Nasogastric decompression:* An appropriate size nasogastric tube is inserted and the stomach decompressed by low pressure suction or intermittent aspiration. This will also help in reducing the pressure on the diaphragm and improve respiration.

3. *Urethral catheter*: An indwelling urethral catheter is left in place to ensure adequate monitoring of urine output.

4. *Reversal of hypoxia:* Hypoxia is a common problem that may affect the integrity of intestinal anastomosis as well as survival. Respiration may be impaired by abdominal distention, peritonitis, and presence of a large pneumoperitoneum. If the pneumoperitoneum is large (see Figure 17.3), insert a size 16G–18G intravenous cannula in the right or left upper quadrant (depending on the site of maximal air collection) to vent the collected gas (avoid the lower border of the liver, if enlarged). The cannula is removed after adequate venting. This manoeuvre often helps to improve respiration and reduce hypoxia. Administer 100% oxygen by nasal catheter until surgery. Oxygen administration may need to be continued for up to 6 hours postoperatively in very ill children.

5. *Blood transfusion:* This is necessary to correct anaemia if the haemogram is <8 gm/dl (packed cell volume of <24%). Anaemia is always corrected before surgery to minimise hypoxia. A rough estimate for blood transfusion is 20 ml/kg body weight to attempt to correct the anaemia before surgery.

6. *Correction of coagulopathy:* A vitamin K injection, 10 mg daily, is given and maintained for at least 5 days.

7. *Antibiotic therapy:* Intravenous, broad-spectrum antibiotics are commenced immediately when the diagnosis of typhoid is suspected. The antibiotics may need to be changed later if there is no improvement and culture results become available. A commonly used effective antibiotic combination is *one* of the following:

- Chloramphenicol (50–75 mg/kg/24 hours in 6-hour dosing) + gentamicin (3–5 mg/kg/24 hours in 8-hour dosing) + metronidazole (7.5 mg/kg/dose given in 8-hour dosing).

- Amoxicillin [50–75 mg/kg/24 hours in 8-hour dosing (or ampicillin, 50–75 mg/kg/24 hours in 6-hour dosing)] + gentamicin (3–5 mg/kg/24 hours in 8-hour dosing) + metronidazole (7.5 mg/kg/dose given in 8-hour dosing).

- Third-generation cephalosporin + metronidazole.

- A quinolone such as ciprofloxacin[10,11] + metronidazole (IV peri-

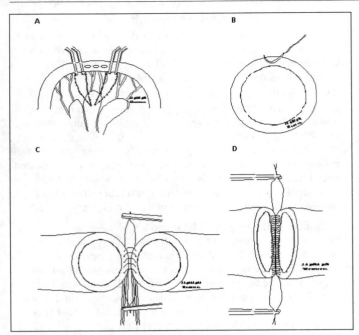

Figure 17.4: Segmental resection of ileum with perforations and end-to-end anastomosis: (A) preparation of bowel with multiple perforations for resection; (B) demonstration of picking only the seromuscular layer; (C) insertion of the posterior seromuscular layer of sutures; (D) posterior seromuscular layer of sutures tied.

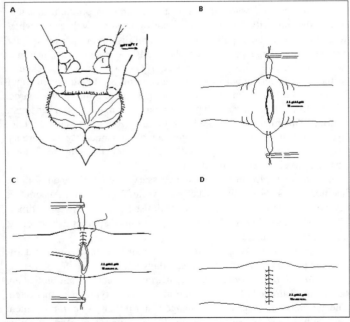

Figure 17.5: Closure of a single ileal perforation in one layer: (A) the perforation on the antimesenteric border of the ileum; (B) after the necrotic edges of the perforation have been excised and stay sutures placed in readiness for a single-layer interrupted seromuscular closure of the perforation; (C) the perforation being closed; (D) the final result of single-layer closure of a typhoid perforation.

operatively). Ciprofloxacin (8–16 mg/kg/24 hours in 2 divided doses IV) and metronidazole as above. Oral ciprofloxacin is given as 10–30 mg/kg in 2 divided doses (this drug combination may be given with or without gentamicin).

The chosen antibiotic regime is continued postoperatively until the temperature returns to normal. Thereafter, the drugs are continued orally (if an oral form is available) for 7–14 days.

Definitive Treatment

Intestinal Perforation

The definitive treatment for intestinal perforation is operative—to evacuate faecal contamination and prevent further contamination. Surgery is done only when the child is adequately resuscitated. Blood transfusions may need to be continued intraoperatively or even post-operatively. If the child is too sick, nonparalysing anaesthesia and hypotension-producing anaesthetic agents (e.g., ketamine hydrochloride) are considered.

For the abdominal incision in small children, a transverse upper or lower abdominal incision is used. If perforated appendicitis is a strong differential diagnosis, a lower transverse incision is more appropriate; if complicated cholecystitis or perforated duodenal ulcer is a strong differential diagnosis, an upper transverse incision is more appropriate. In bigger children (>8 years of age), a long midline incision centred on the umbilicus may provide better exposure.

Once the peritoneal cavity is opened, a specimen of any peritoneal fluid or pus is taken. All peritoneal collections are evacuated. The intestines are thoroughly examined, beginning at the ileocaecal junction until the duodenojejunal junction is reached. The perforation(s) are usually located on the antimesenteric border, and near perforation(s) may also be identified. Leakage from any identified perforation is controlled by a Babcock's forceps clamped lightly over a piece of gauze. Alternatively, the bowel with the piece of gauze over the perforation is handed over to the assistant to put light pressure over it to prevent leakage of intestinal contents while the surgeon continues inspecting the rest of the intestine.

After identifying the perforation(s), the stomach, duodenum, large intestine, liver, and spleen are inspected. Most perforations are located in the last 80 cm of the terminal ileum,[3,5,7] but, rarely, the jejunum and colon (caecum to sigmoid colon)[9] may also be involved. The definitive surgical procedure is decided only after completing the examination of the entire small and large intestines because the sites and number of perforations may dictate the procedure of choice, and there may be areas of impending perforation, which would appear paper-thin on the serosal surface.

Currently, the surgical options are:

1. *Segmental resection of affected intestine* (Figure 17.4): The resected segment should include all perforations and near perforations. The resection margin should be healthy and free of evidence of inflammation such as oedema. Segmental resection is a good choice even for a single perforation. A limited right hemicolectomy may be necessary if the most distal perforation is too close to the ileocaecal junction for safe anastomosis (i.e., <3 cm). The resected length of intestine is always measured and documented. Then intestinal continuity is restored by end-to-end anastomosis. The resected segment is sent to the lab for histopathology.

2. *Simple closure of perforations* (Figures 17.5 and 17.6): This procedure may be used for a single perforation, if perforations are far apart, or if the number of perforations are so numerous that resection may result in a short gut. The edge of the perforation is excised circumferentially (the excised edge is sent to the lab for histopathology). Then simple closure is achieved by a single layer of interrupted, seromuscular stitches.

3. *Enterostomy* (Figure 17.7): An enterostomy is performed if the child is too sick or intestinal oedema is too extensive for safe

anastomosis or simple closure. The perforation (if single) or the proximal and distal ends (following segmental resection) of the intestine are exteriorised as stoma, to be closed at a later date when oedema has subsided and the patient is fit. In very ill patients, a T-tube placed in the lumen after closing all distal perforations has been found to be effective.[12]

Note: Be sure to clean the peritoneal cavity with copious amounts of normal saline.

The fascia and skin are closed; however, if the anterior abdominal wall is oedematous, the skin is left open (delayed primary closure is done after 3 days if there is no wound infection). If the skin is closed in the presence of abdominal wall oedema, surgical site infection frequently occurs.

Where there is severe contamination of the peritoneal cavity with faeculent peritoneal fluid and/or pus, the alternative is to pack the peritoneal cavity with abdominal packs soaked in normal saline and return to close the wound in 48 to 72 hours. This delayed primary wound closure allows a second look to inspect the peritoneal cavity for fluid/pus collection, inspect the suture line or anastomosis for leakage, and repair perforations missed during the first surgery or even reperforations.

Cholecystitis

Cholecystitis and perforation of the gallbladder are important complications[13–15] that occur with increasing frequency. If the diagnosis is certain and no evidence of perforation or gangrene exists, the antibiotics described earlier under "Management" (#7, Antibiotic therapy) are administered and the patient is monitored. If the fever subsides and the child improves, the antibiotics are continued for 7 to 10 days. A cholecystectomy is performed after 6 to 12 weeks.

If the above treatment fails or there is evidence of general peritonitis (perforation or gangrene), treatment is operative. A laparotomy is performed and the specimen of gallbladder contents is sent for culture. A tube cholecystostomy, using a Foley or Malecot catheter, is performed. When all evidence of inflammation has subsided, the tube is removed (note that a tube cholangiogram may be necessary before removal of the tube).

Intestinal Bleeding

After resuscitation, the antibiotics described earlier under "Management" (#7, Antibiotic therapy) are started. The antibiotics are continued for 10 to 14 days after cessation of bleeding. Blood loss may need to be replaced by blood transfusion. The patient is kept in hospital for 5 to 7 days after the bleeding has completely stopped—this is necessary because the bleeding may recur.

Osteomyelitis

Some of the affected patients may have sickle cell disease, which is treated accordingly. Administer chloramphenicol (50–75 mg/kg/24 hr in 6-hour dosing); ampiclox (100 mg/kg/24 hr in 6-hour dosing); or third-generation cephalosporin, initially by intravenous route until temperature returns to normal, then orally for 4–6 weeks. Caution is advised if chloramphenicol is going to be used for a long time.

Any associated abscesses are drained. The affected limb may need to be splinted and elevated until the pain and oedema subside.

Abscesses

Abscesses can occur in any part of the body; they can be superficial or deeply located. The abscess is drained and the patient is given appropriate antibiotics.

Malnutrition

Some of the patients are malnourished or nutritionally depleted. Parenteral nutrition, if available, is given during the acute phase of the illness. When the patient is able to tolerate oral intake, a diet rich in proteins and carbohydrates is given—small, frequent feedings are better tolerated than a large amount at one time.

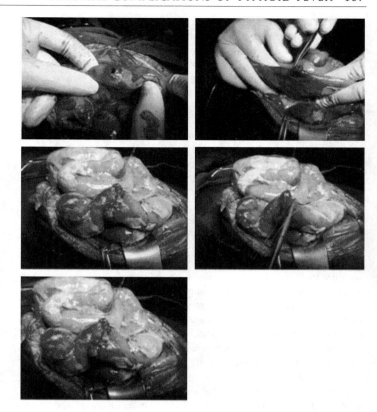

Figure 17.6: Closure of a single ileal perforation after excising the necrotic edges together with the inflamed surrounding area (see Figure 17.5).

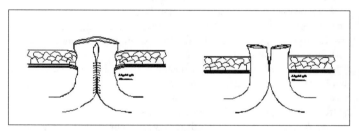

Figure 17.7: Diagrammatic illustration of an enterostomy.

Postoperative Complications

Complications are frequently encountered, particularly in patients who have had intestinal perforation. The more common complications include:

1. *Prolonged ileus* may last for several days and manifest as increasing or persistent nasogastric drainage. Adequate fluid and electrolyte balance, nasogastric drainage, and parenteral nutrition are maintained, and the condition usually resolves on this treatment.

2. *Surgical site infection* is one of the most common complications occurring in 49–59% of patients with TIP.[3–5] Infection is usually superficial in the wound but may be deep. If the infection is deep, anastomotic leakage is suspected. A swab from the wound is cultured to ascertain the microorganisms and their antibiotic sensitivity. Treatment is by local wound care (native honey is quite effective). If the skin was previously sutured, some of the stitches may need to be removed to allow drainage. After the infection is under control, secondary suturing of the wound is performed; if the wound contracts, and the residual wound is small, it is allowed to heal by secondary intention.

3. *Abdominal wound dehiscence* may be partial or complete. This has been reported in 3–14% of children with TIP,[3–5] and is frequently the result of surgical site infection, anastomotic leakage, or intraperitoneal

abscess. These causes are considered and excluded. A reoperation is required: the anastomosis is inspected and handled accordingly if there is leakage; any abscess collection is evacuated and the peritoneal cavity cleaned; the fascia is closed with continuous suturing using appropriate size nonabsorbable suture. Tension-relaxing sutures may need to be applied for 7 to 10 days to take the tension off the fascial closure.

4. *Anastomotic leakage or complete breakdown of the anastomosis* has been reported in about 7% of children with TIP and usually requires relaparotomy. The initial anastomosis is resected and another anastomosis effected. Alternatively, the ends of the intestine are exteriorised as stoma, to be closed at a later date when safe to do so.

5. *Enterocutaneous fistula* will usually close spontaneously with nonoperative management. If there is evidence that it is an end fistula, or if copious intestinal fluid (high output fistula) is discharging through the wound, or if there is peritonitis, relaparotomy is required and the situation is then handled as in the case of anastomotic leakage.

6. *Intraperitoneal abscess* (7–9%)[3,5] usually manifests as a return of fever in a patient who had started to improve. The abscess may be due to a leaking anastomosis or inadequate toileting of the peritoneal cavity with copious amounts of normal saline. Abdominal ultrasonography should confirm the diagnosis. Relaparotomy is required. The anastomosis is inspected to identify any leakage. The abscess is drained and the peritoneal cavity is thoroughly cleaned.

7. *Adhesion intestinal obstruction* may occur several days to years later. It is treated nonoperatively initially (IV fluid resuscitation, analgesics, regular reassessment—preferably by the same surgeon and antibiotics). If evidence of intestinal strangulation or nonoperative treatment fails (intensification of abdominal pain, increased abdominal distention with tenderness and rebound tenderness, and guarding or failure of the general condition of the patient to improve), a relaparotomy is done to release adhesions.

8. *Reperforation* may occur at a new site in 7–9% of children with TIP.[5] It may be the result of an unidentified impending perforation or progression of ongoing infection. A relaparotomy is required and the perforation is handled on its merit.

9. *Hypoproteinaemia* occurs postoperatively in most cases. This manifests in pitting oedema of the feet and ankles. A blood sample is taken for serum proteins, and the condition is treated with fresh blood or fresh frozen plasma (FFP) where available.

10. *Pleural effusion*, although rare, can occur in the postoperative period and is usually unilateral. If the effusion is massive, either it is drained by tapping, or a chest tube is passed immediately for drainage.

Prognosis and Outcomes

Of the children treated for TIP, 53–79%[3,5,6] develop one or more complications. One report suggests that the complication rate may be significantly higher in children younger than 5 years of age.[3] The spectrum of these complications is discussed above.

Mortality from TIP appears to vary widely, ranging from 12% to 41%,[3–5] but a mortality of 0% was reported in children with typhoid colonic perforation.[9] Most mortality is from overwhelming infection, occurring usually after an average of 4–5 days postoperatively. The single most important significant predictor of death in patients with TIP is the duration of abdominal pain after 7 days.[3,5,7] The number of perforations does not appear to significantly affect mortality.

Prevention

Typhoid fever and its complications can be largely prevented by simple public health measures. Current preventive measures include improvements in sanitation and water supply and vaccination.

Improvements in Sanitation and Water Supply

As a faeco-oral infection, typhoid fever is controlled by improvements in sewage and waste disposal, as well as provision of safe potable water. Where piped water is not feasible, provision of bore holes is useful. Community health education regarding waste disposal and discouraging defaecation in the open is relevant.

Vaccination

Although vaccination is not routine at this time, WHO has recommended it as a short-term measure in high-risk areas.[1,2] Two vaccines are considered safe and effective and are presently licenced internationally for those aged >2 years:[2] the injectable Vi polysaccharide and the live attenuated oral Ty21a vaccine (available as a capsule and in suspension). The vaccines are recommended for control of typhoid in high-risk groups and populations as well as for outbreak control. Vaccines may also be offered to travellers to endemic areas. These vaccines are not licensed for use in children aged <2 years. Other improved vaccines are presently being tested, including the Vi-protein conjugate vaccine, which could be useful for children below 2 years of age[1] if eventually licenced.

Evidence-Based Research

The references cited in Tables 17.2 and 17.3 present the effects of operations and surgical management of typhoid perforations in children.

Table 17.2: Evidence-based research.

Title	Comparison of three operations for typhoid perforation
Authors	Ameh EA, Dogo PM, Attah MM, Nmadu PT
Institution	Department of Surgery, Ahmadu Bello University Teaching Hospital, Zaria, Nigeria
Reference	Br J Surg 1997; 84(4):558–559
Problem	Extent of surgery in children with typhoid ileal perforation.
Intervention	Three different operations for typhoid perforation in children.
Comparison/ control (quality of evidence)	Compares three procedures in the operative management of a difficult problem of typhoid ileal perforation in children—simple closure, wedge resection and anastomosis and segmental resection, and anastomosis—by using the same management protocol for all patients.
Outcome/ effect	In all the three operative methods used, the mortality rates were still high, especially so in the wedge resection group. Despite this high mortality, segmental resection with end-to-end anastomosis, where appropriate, gave better results in this study.
Historical significance/ comments	Morbidity and mortality rates in typhoid perforation of the ileum are high irrespective of the surgical procedure used. The need exists to prevent the disease as a whole, but failing that, the management protocol for children with typhoid ileal perforations should include early aggressive resuscitation, antibiotics and analgesics, early limited/minimal surgery, thorough peritoneal toileting (cleaning), blood transfusion and oxygen support (where necessary), and early enteral feeding with supportive care.

Table 17.3: Evidence-based research.

Title	Typhoid colonic perforation in childhood: a ten-year experience
Authors	Chang Y-T, Lin J-Y, Huang Y-S
Institution	Division of Pediatric Surgery, Department of Surgery, Kaohsiung Medical University Hospital, Kaohsiung, Taiwan
Reference	World J Surg 2006; 30:242–247
Problem	The ideal treatment of typhoid colonic perforation in children.
Intervention	Three different ways of surgical management of typhoid colonic perforations in children.
Comparison/ control (quality of evidence)	Compares three methods of surgically treating typhoid colonic perforations in children: primary closure of the perforation with ileostomy, wedge resection and simple closure, and partial colectomy with colostomy.
Outcome/ effect	One hundred percent survival rates, mainly attributed to the institution of total parenteral nutrition (TPN) after sufficient hydration. Another outcome measure was length of hospital stay (LOS), which was shorter for the wedge resection and simple closure group than for the others. Complications were similar to those seen in cases of typhoid ileal perforations.
Historical significance/ comments	Typhoid colonic perforation is rare in the authors' subregion, but it does occur. Paediatric surgeons should be suspicious when the ileum is inspected for perforations and none are found, and should inspect the colon. The small size of the sample in the study notwithstanding, useful lessons are to be learned from it, especially the use of TPN to keep the patients nourished until normal bowel movement is fully recovered, which can definitely play a major role in the survival of patients.

Key Summary Points

1. Diagnosis of typhoid intestinal perforation (TIP) is mostly clinical. Plain erect/supine abdominal x-rays and/or chest x-ray may show pneumoperitoneum in about 75% of patients.

2. Most patients are very ill, anaemic, hypoproteinaemic, malnourished, and may have toxic myocarditis. Prepare them well before surgery.

3. Most patients have fluid and electrolyte imbalance. Initial electrolytes may be normal, but repeat check after resuscitation, as they often become deranged by then. Check electrolytes (esp. K^+, Na^+, and Cl^-) in all patients and correct imbalances before surgery.

4. Give appropriate antibiotics that are effective against *Salmonella typhi* and anaerobes (usually, a minimum of two antibiotics) and analgesics.

5. Eliminate continuous peritoneal contamination by surgery. Simple closure or segmental resection and anastomosis are effective. If the child is too ill, exteriorise the segment of bowel with the perforation as an ileostomy. Thorough peritoneal lavage/ toileting with copious amounts of normal saline is mandatory.

6. Strictly monitor input/output for all children with TIP and at least repeat the haemogram and electrolytes 48 hours after surgery and correct any derangements.

7. Use total parenteral nutrition (TPN) where available, but convert to enteral feeding as soon as practicable.

8. Reassess the child daily to identify any postoperative complications and deal with them as soon as feasible.

References

1. Ochiai RL, Acosta CJ, Danovaro-Holliday MC, et al. A study of typhoid fever in five Asian countries: disease burden and implication for controls. Bull World Hlth Org 2008; 86:260–268.

2. World Health Organization. Typhoid vaccines: WHO position paper. Weekly Epidemiol Rec No. 6, 2008; 83:49–60.

3. Ekenze SO, Ikefuna AN. Typhoid perforation under 5 years of age. Ann Trop Paediatr 2008; 28:53–58.

4. Abantanga FA, Wiafe-Addai B. Postoperative complications after surgery for typhoid perforation in children in Ghana. Pediatr Surg Int 1998; 14:55–58.

5. Ameh EA. Typhoid ileal perforation in children: a scourge in developing countries. Ann Trop Paediatr 1999; 19:267–272.

6. Clegg-Lamptey JNA, Hodasi WM, Dakubo JCB. Typhoid intestinal perforation in Ghana: a five-year retrospective study. Trop Doct 2007; 37:231–233.

7. Meier DE, Tarpley JL. Typhoid intestinal perforation in Nigerian children. World J Surg 1998; 22:319–323.

8. Mahle WT, Levine MM. Salmonella typhi infection in children younger than 5 years of age. Pediatr Infect Dis 1993; 12:627–637.

9. Chang Y-T, Lin J-Y, Huang Y-S. Typhoid colonic perforation in childhood: a ten-year experience. World J Surg 2006; 30:242–247.

10. Drossou-Agakidou V, Roilides E, Papakyriakidou-Koliouska P, et al. Use of ciprofloxacin in neonatal sepsis: lack of adverse effects up to one year. Pediatr Infect Dis J 2004; 23:346–349.

11. Dutta P, Rasaily R, Saha MR, et al. Ciprofloxacin for treatment of severe typhoid fever in children. Antimicrob Agents Chemother 1993; 37:1197–1199.

12. Pandey A, Kumar V, Gangopadhyay AN, Upadhyaya VD, Srivastava A, Singh RB. A pilot study on the role of T-tube in typhoid intestinal perforation in children. World J Surg 2008;32:2607-11.

13. Khanna AK, Tiwary SK, Khanna R. Surgical complications of enteric fever in children. J Pediatr Infectious Diseases 2007; 2:59–66.

14. Saxena V, Basu S, Sharma CLN. Perforation of the gall bladder following typhoid fever-induced ileal perforation. Hong Kong Med J 2007; 13:475–477.

15. Shuka VK, Khamdelwal C, Kumar M, Vaidya MP. Enteric perforation of the gallbladder. Postgrad Med J 1983; 59:125–126.

CHAPTER 18
TUBERCULOSIS

Shilpa Sharma
Devendra K. Gupta

Introduction

Tuberculosis (TB) is a dreadful disease that is still rampant in the developing world.[1-4] It can involve almost any organ or tissue in the body from the brain to the bones. The problem is more significant in children in developing countries, as they are the neglected lot who are often entrapped with infection, be it pneumonia or gastroenteritis. This delays the diagnosis of the disease and increases the tendency of the disease to spread into miliary infection in the sick undernourished child.

Tuberculosis was declared a global public health emergency in 1993 by the World Health Organization (WHO).[5] According to the WHO, developing countries, including India, China, Pakistan, Philippines, Thailand, Indonesia, Bangladesh, and the Democratic Republic of Congo, account for nearly 75% of all cases of TB. There are about 0.5 million deaths worldwide every year from this disease.[6]

Tuberculosis is still a major cause of morbidity in developing countries. Today, 19–43.5% of the world's population is infected with *Mycobacterium tuberculosis*, with more than 8 million new cases of TB occurring each year.[7] The incidence and severity of pulmonary infections such as TB are expected to increase with the increasing incidence of human immunodeficiency virus (HIV) infection.[8] The highest TB incidences and HIV infection prevalence are recorded in sub-Saharan Africa (with about 35% of mothers known to be infected with HIV), and as a consequence, children in this region bear the greatest burden of TB/HIV infection.[9] The incidence is rising in Western countries due to immigration from Third World countries and the rising trend of HIV infection. There has been a decrease in mortality in cases of pulmonary tuberculosis without HIV due to recent improved health care and prompt initiation of therapy.

Diagnosis of tuberculosis in children is difficult because children are less likely to have obvious symptoms of TB. Tubercular infection has been identified in all organs in children. Genitourinary tuberculosis, although rare in children, has vague symptoms and presentation with the delayed diagnosis due to the late presentation leading to cicatrisation sequelae.[10] Children and young adults comprised 70% of the study population in a large series of craniovertebral junction tuberculosis.[11] This chapter focusses only on chest and abdominal tuberculosis.

The children most at high risk for tuberculosis include:

• children living in a household with an adult who has active tuberculosis;

• children of poor socioeconomic status;

• children residing in rural areas;

• undernourished children;

• children living in small enclosed areas and in areas with poor ventilation;

• children living in a high endemic region;

• children infected with HIV or in an immunocompromised state following chemotherapy or prolonged steroid use;

• children with infections such as measles, varicella, and pertussis, which may activate quiescent TB; and

• children with certain human leukocyte antigen (HLA) types that have a predisposition to TB.

Tubercular Bacilli

Mycobacterium tuberculosis is the most common cause of TB. Other rare causes are *M. bovis* and *M. avium*. *M. bovis* infection has been traced to the use of cheese made from unpasteurised milk. *M. tuberculosis* is an aerobic, non–spore-forming, nonmotile, slow-growing bacillus with a curved and beaded rod-shaped morphology. It can survive under adverse environmental conditions. The acid-fast characteristic of the mycobacteria is its unique feature. Humans are the only known reservoirs for *M. tuberculosis*.

Epidemiology

The overall incidence of tuberculosis is as high as 0.7–2 per 1,000 children in the developing countries, with chest, meninges, and lymph nodes being commonly involved.[12] The disease is predominant in females. Infants are more susceptible to tuberculous bacilli and may develop severe extrapulmonary and miliary forms of the disease.[13] Tubercular infection of the abdominal cavity accounts for 15% of all intestinal obstructions.[1,2] It is more common in children, affecting those >5 years of age and particularly those residing in rural areas.[3]

Tuberculosis in infants and children <4 years of age is much more likely to spread throughout the body through the bloodstream. Thus, children are at much greater risk of developing miliary tuberculosis. Hence, prompt diagnosis and treatment of tuberculosis is essential.

Routes of Infection

The route of infection for pulmonary tuberculosis is inhalation of airborne bacteria. After inhalation, the bacilli are usually deposited in the mid-lung zone, into the subpleural distal respiratory bronchiole or alveoli. The alveolar macrophages then phagocytose the inhaled bacilli but are unable to kill them, thus the bacilli continue to multiply unimpeded. The infected macrophages are then transported to the regional lymph nodes. The initial pulmonary site of infection and its adjacent lymph nodes are known as the primary complex or Ghon focus.

Progression of the primary complex may lead to enlargement of hilar and mediastinal nodes with resultant bronchial collapse. Progressive primary TB may develop when the primary focus cavitates and the organisms spread through the contiguous bronchi.

Lympho-hematogenous dissemination of the mycobacteria may occur to other lymph nodes, and regions in the body (e.g., kidney, epiphyses of long bones, vertebral bodies, meninges, and, occasionally, the apical posterior areas of the lungs) or may spread widely as miliary TB. This may occur when caseous material reaches the bloodstream from a primary focus or a caseating metastatic focus in the wall of a pulmonary vein (Weigert focus). Bacilli may remain dormant in the apical posterior areas of the lung for several months, or even years, with later progression of disease.

The gastrointestinal tract is involved in more than 60% of cases of abdominal tuberculosis. The postulated routes of infection into the gastrointestinal tract include:

- hematogenous spread from reactivation of old primary lung focus;

- ingestion of infected sputum from active pulmonary focus;

- contiguous spread from adjacent organs; and

- through lymph channels from infected nodes.

The most common site is the terminal ileum and ileocaecal region due to increased physiological stasis, increased fluid and electrolyte absorption, minimal digestive activity, and an abundance of lymphoid tissue at this site. The other sites, in order of frequency, include the colon and jejunum. Rarely, tuberculosis may involve other areas such as the perianal region, appendix, duodenum, stomach, and oesophagus. The nodal involvement due to tuberculosis is commonly mesenteric or retroperitoneal. The abdominal solid organs (liver, spleen, and pancreas) may also be affected with tuberculosis, but rarely.

Pathophysiology

Nearly all cases of abdominal TB are due to the human strain of *M. tuberculosis*, although atypical mycobacteria account for a few cases. Infection due to the *bovis* species is rare, largely due to the practice of boiling milk. In India, the organism isolated from all intestinal lesions has been *M. tuberculosis* and not *M. bovis*.[14] The peritoneum is commonly involved, although any part of the abdominal cavity, such as hollow viscera, lymph nodes, and solid viscera, may be involved. An accurate diagnosis requires a high index of suspicion, as most of the investigations are nonspecific and less sensitive.

Tuberculous granulomas of variable size are initially formed in the submucosa or the Peyer's patches. Tubercular ulcers are relatively superficial, transversely oriented, and do not penetrate beyond the muscularis. Cicatrical healing of these circumferential ulcers results in strictures. Mesenteric lymph nodes may be enlarged or matted, and may caseate.

A cell-mediated immune response terminates the unimpeded growth of *M. tuberculosis* within 2 to 3 weeks after the initial infection. Cluster of differentiation 4 (CD4) helper T cells activate the macrophages to kill the intracellular bacteria with resultant epithelioid granuloma formation. CD8 suppressor T cells lyse the macrophages infected with the mycobacteria, resulting in the formation of caseating granulomas. Mycobacteria cannot continue to grow in the acidic extracellular environment, and thus most infections are controlled. The only evidence of infection is a positive tuberculin skin (Montoux) test result.

Clinical Presentation

Tuberculosis patients are usually malnourished, as they belong to lower socioeconomic strata. Primary pulmonary tuberculosis may present with generalised symptoms, such as fever of unknown origin, failure to thrive, night sweats, anorexia, significant weight loss, nonproductive cough, or unexplained lymphadenopathy. Pulmonary TB may manifest as endobronchial TB with focal lymphadenopathy, progressive pulmonary disease, pleural involvement, and reactivated pulmonary disease. Progression of the pulmonary parenchymal infection leads to enlargement of the caseous area and may lead to pneumonia, atelectasis, and air trapping in young children. Children usually appear ill with symptoms of fever, cough, malaise, and weight loss. Tubercular pleural effusion may present with acute onset of fever, chest pain that increases in intensity on deep inspiration, and shortness of breath. Fever usually persists for 14–21 days. Reactivation TB usually has a subacute presentation with weight loss, fever, cough, and, rarely, haemoptysis. Reactivation TB typically occurs in older children and adolescents.

Isolated mediastinal tuberculous lymphadenitis is a relatively common entity in children, second in frequency after cervical localisation. In the absence of an accompanying parenchymal lesion, mediastinal tuberculous lymphadenitis may pose a diagnostic dilemma on admission and must be distinguished from other causes of mediastinal masses. Bronchoscopy is suggested as a diagnostic tool when tuberculosis cannot be excluded by radiology or specific tuberculin skin tests (TSTs). Thoracotomy and excision are reported as necessary to treat the obstructive symptoms. Thoracoscopic mediastinal node biopsy has also been reported as feasible in an infant.[15] Infants <6 months of age may present with respiratory failure, requiring ventilatory support.[16]

Extrapulmonary TB includes peripheral lymphadenopathy, tubercular meningitis, miliary TB, skeletal TB, and other organ involvement. Any child with pneumonia, pleural effusion, or a cavitary or mass lesion in the lung that does not improve with standard antibacterial therapy should be evaluated for tuberculosis.

The clinical presentation of abdominal tuberculosis can be acute, chronic, or acute on chronic. Most patients have constitutional symptoms of low- or high-grade fever (40–70%), weight loss (40–90%), night sweats, anorexia, and malaise. The delay in presentation can vary between 1 and 14 months. Abdominal symptoms include diarrhoea, constipation, alternating constipation and diarrhoea, and pain, which can be either colicky due to luminal compromise or dull and continuous when the mesenteric lymph nodes are involved. A physical examination may show features of ascites, lump abdomen, or visible peristalsis with dilated bowel loops. Miliary tuberculosis presenting with multiple intestinal perforations as an initial manifestation of the disease has also been reported in an infant.[13]

Tuberculosis of the Abdomen

Any part of the abdomen may get involved in tubercular pathology. The chronic intestinal lesions produced by tuberculosis are of three types: ulcerative, hypertrophic, and stricturous. The ulcerative form is seen more often in malnourished patients, whereas the hypertrophic form is seen in relatively well-nourished patients. Colonic and ileocaecal lesions are ulcerohypertrophic. In tuberculous peritonitis, the gross pathology is characterised by omental thickening and peritoneal tubercles.[14,17,18]

Peritoneal Tuberculosis

Peritoneal tuberculosis occurs in four forms:

1. *Wet type peritonitis with generalised ascitis*: The distended abdomen is in sharp contrast to that of a malnourished child, with little muscle mass and subcutaneous fat.

2. *Encysted (loculated) ascitis type:* The child may present with an asymptomatic localised abdominal lump, which may be due to loculated ascites, enlarged lymph node, or matted omentum and intestines.

3. *Dry type with adhesions:* The child presents with subacute abdominal obstruction or a history of feeling a moving ball of wind abdominally.

4. *Classic "plastic" form:* This is a fibrotic type with abdominal masses composed of mesenteric and omental thickening, with matted bowel loops felt as lump(s) in the abdomen. The adolescent has gastrointestinal (GI) symptoms along with a doughy feel of the abdomen. The latter is due to diffuse peritonitis with thickening and adhesions of omentum, mesentery, and peritoneum. The classic presentation is, however, with attacks of subacute intestinal obstruction, most of which resolve on conservative management. A lump is found in 25–33% of cases, most often in the right iliac fossa, in ileocaecal and small bowel TB.

A combination of these types is also common. Tubercular peritonitis and nodal forms are more commonly seen in children and adolescents as compared to the gastrointestinal form.

Mesenteric and other lymphadenitis

Nodal forms can present as a lump or intestinal obstruction due to kinks and adhesions. Bowel loops may get involved in the inflammatory process and form a local lump in the right iliac fossa, producing subacute obstruction. Obstructions of the bile duct, pancreatic duct, duodenum, inferior vena cava, or ureter by lymph nodes may also occur, but are rare.

Acute abdomen

Uncommonly, the presentation may be like an acute abdomen, which may be due to rupture of a caseous lymph node, GI perforation, tubercular peritonitis, ruptured mesenteric abscess, or acute obstruction, especially in the presence of stricture. Involvement of the appendix is usually a part of ileocaecal involvement, and rarely may present as an isolated case of acute appendicitis.

Gastrointestinal involvement

The patient may present with nonspecific symptoms of vague abdominal pain, mild discomfort, anorexia, malaise, and fever. After a relay of investigations, if no cause is identified, an exploratory laparotomy is done in view of the persisting symptoms (Figure 18.1). The positive findings may be only congestion and neovascularisation. Symptoms will subside on starting antitubercular treatment.

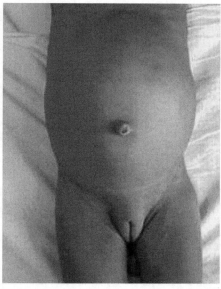

Figure 18.1: A 2-year-old child presenting with subacute intestinal obstruction due to ileocaecal tuberculosis confirmed on laparotomy.

Oesophageo-Gastroduodenal Tuberculosis

Involvement of oesophagus is extremely rare and presents as dysphagia, odynophagia, and a midoesophageal ulcer. Gastroduodenal tuberculosis may present with dyspepsia and gastric outlet obstruction. Surgical bypass has been required in the majority of cases to relieve obstruction, but successful endoscopic balloon dilatation of duodenal strictures has also been done.

Jejunoileal Tuberculosis

Tubercular involvement of the jejunum and ileum may present with malabsorption and subacute intestinal obstruction. On exploration, there may be jejunoileitis with nonspecific inflammatory changes on biopsy.

Terminal Ileal and Ileocaecal Tuberculosis

In India, around 3–20% of all cases of bowel obstruction are due to tuberculosis.[19] Tubercular intestinal stricture presents with recurrent subacute intestinal obstruction in the form of obstipation, vomiting, abdominal distention, and colicky abdominal pain associated with gurgling, feeling like a ball of wind is moving in the abdomen, and visible intestinal loops. Having a chronic inflammatory pathology, tubercular perforations are rare and usually single and proximal to a stricture.

Segmental Colonic Tuberculosis

This type of tuberculosis commonly involves the sigmoid, ascending and transverse colon. Manifestations include chronic constipation, fever, anorexia, weight loss, and change in bowel habits. It may simulate late presentation of Hirschsprung's disease in young children, Crohn's disease, amoeboma, or malignancy in adolescents.

Rectal and Anal Tuberculosis

Rectal tuberculosis is rare and may present with haematochezia, constitutional symptoms and constipation with anal discharge, multiple fistula with ragged margins, or perianal swelling. Digital examination may reveal an annular stricture, which is usually tight and of variable length with focal areas of deep ulceration.

Miscellaneous Presentations

An uncommon presentation of abdominal tuberculosis is as pyrexia of unknown origin. Suggestive hepatomegaly may lead to the diagnosis of hepatic tuberculosis on liver biopsy. The miliary and local forms of hepatic tuberculosis have quite similar clinical presentations and pathological features. Hepatosplenic tuberculosis is common as a part of disseminated and miliary tuberculosis.

Female patients with abdominal tuberculosis may present with menstrual disorders or later with infertility as a result of involvement of the uterus or fallopian tubes.

Investigations

Diagnosis is usually made through a combination of radiologic, endoscopic, microbiologic, histologic, and molecular techniques.

Haematological Tests

Anaemia and hypoalbuminaemia may be associated with tuberculosis due to poor nutrition. Total leucocyte count is raised in half the cases. There may also be associated leucocytosis due to superadded infection along with lymphocytosis suggestive of chronic infection.

A raised erythrocyte sedimentation rate (ESR), although nonspecific, is a very supportive finding and is a good marker to assess the response to treatment. Serologic tests have a limited role due to their inability to distinguish between past and present infections.

Mantoux Test

An induration of less than 6 mm in diameter indicates either (1) an uninfected patient, (2) recent infection, (3) anergy due to malnutrition or disease states such as measles, or (4) overwhelming tuberculosis infection (50% of autopsies proved cases of severe tuberculosis had been Mantoux negative). Induration in the range of 6–9 mm indicates either past infection or a Calmette-Guérin bacillus (BCG) tuberculosis vaccination. It may also be found in some cases of active infection, particularly where atypical mycobacteria are involved. Induration of 10–14 mm in children <5 years of age strongly indicates active infection. Patients with an induration >14 mm are four times more likely to have an active disease than those with a Mantoux test in the range of 10–14 mm. If the patient has been vaccinated with BCG before, then an induration of more than 15 mm at 1 year, or 12 mm at 2 years after vaccination is considered positive.

Specimens for bacteriologic examination include sputum, gastric lavage, bronchoalveolar lavage, lung tissue, and lymph node. Gastric aspirates may be used in place of sputum in children <6 years of age with pulmonary tuberculosis, as they may not be able to cough out sputum. An early-morning sample should be obtained for undiluted bronchial secretions accumulated during the night. As gastric acidity is poorly tolerated by the tubercle bacilli, neutralisation of the specimen should be done immediately with 10% sodium carbonate or 40% anhydrous sodium phosphate. Even with utmost care, the tubercle bacilli can be detected in only 70% of infants and in only 30–40% of children with disease. Sputum specimens and bronchoalveolar lavage may be used in older children. Nasopharyngeal secretions and saliva are not acceptable.

Acid-Fast Bacilli Staining

Acid-fast bacilli (AFB) Ziehl-Neelsen staining provides preliminary confirmation of the diagnosis, although it cannot differentiate *M. tuberculosis* from other acid-fast organisms, such as other mycobacterial organisms or *Nocardia* species. It can give a quantitative assessment of the number of bacilli being excreted (e.g., 1+, 2+, 3+). For a reliable positive result, smears require approximately 10,000 organisms per milliliter. Therefore, the results may be negative in early stages of the disease or with sparse bacilli. A single organism on a slide is highly suggestive and warrants further investigation.

Mycobacterium Culture

Culture of *M. tuberculosis* is the definitive method to detect bacilli and is more sensitive than examination of the smear. Approximately 10 AFB per millimeter of a digested concentrated specimen are sufficient to detect the organisms by culture. A culture also allows identification of specific species and testing for drug sensitivity. Due to the emergence of multidrug-resistant (MDR) organisms, determination of the drug sensitivity panel of an isolate is important so that appropriate treatment can be ensured.

M. tuberculosis is a slow-growing organism, however, so a period of 6–8 weeks is required for colonies to appear on conventional culture media. Conventional solid media include the Löwenstein-Jensen medium, which is egg based, and the Middlebrook 7H10 and 7H11 media, which are agar based. Liquid media (e.g., Dubos oleic-albumin media) also are available, and they require incubation in 5–10% carbon dioxide for 3–8 weeks.

Nucleic Acid Techniques

Nucleic acid techniques include nucleic acid probes and polymerase chain reaction (PCR). Although their sensitivity and specificity in smear-positive cases exceed 95%, the sensitivity of smear-negative cases varies from 40% to 70%.

- *Nucleic acid probes* help advance identification of the *M. tuberculosis* complex. Sensitivity and specificity approach 100% when at least 100,000 organisms are present.

- *PCR nucleic acid amplification tests* allow the direct identification of *M. tuberculosis* in clinical specimens, unlike nucleic acid probes, which require substantial time for bacterial accumulation in broth culture.

Enzyme-Linked Immunoassay Test

A new test, Quantiferon (QFT-g), was approved in 2005 by the US Food and Drug Administration (FDA). The test basically detects the presence of interferon gamma release protein (IFN-g) from the blood of sensitised patients when incubated with the early secretory antigenic target-6 (ESAT6) and culture filtrate protein 10 (CFP10) peptides. The test is as sensitive as, and more specific than, the tuberculin skin test and has been recommended as a screening tool for diagnosing disease as well as infection. No available serodiagnostic test for TB has adequate sensitivity and specificity for routine use in diagnosing TB in children.

Chest Radiograph

Evidence of tuberculosis in a chest radiograph supports the diagnosis, but a normal chest radiograph does not rule it out. It may show signs of active tuberculosis in 15% of patients.[20] The findings can be (1) miliary tuberculosis in a sick child without eosinophilia; (2) atelectasis, emphysema, bronchiectasis, or parenchymal opacity—any of these when present with pleural effusion or hilar lymphadenopathy indicates active disease; or (3) patchy consolidation or infiltration, which can be nonspecific but when associated with a positive Mantoux test and cavitation in the apex indicates activity. Signs of "old" tuberculosis (e.g., obliterated costophrenic angle, calcified hilar lymph nodes, or a fibro-calcific lesion) are present in 20% of patients.[20]

Plain Radiograph Abdomen

An erect radiograph is also invaluable at the time of abdominal pain in demonstrating dilated jejunal and ileal loops with multiple air fluid levels, with an absence of gas in the colon and fixed bowel loop in cases of obstruction, pneumoperitoneum in cases of perforation, and any intussusception. Enteroliths, mottled calcification in the mesenteric lymph nodes, and any evidence of ascitis may be suggested on the plain film.

Contrast Studies

Barium meal and enema are together positive in 80–85% of the cases of GI tuberculosis.

- *Small bowel barium meal:* The radiologic findings that may be seen on a small bowel study include:
  - mucosal irregularity and rapid emptying (ulcerative);
  - flocculation and fragmentation of barium (malabsorption);
  - stiffened and thickened folds;
  - luminal stenosis with smooth but stiff contours ("hour glass-stenosis");
  - dilated loops and strictures;
  - displaced loops (enlarged lymph nodes); and
  - adherent fixed and matted loops (adhesive peritoneal disease).

- *Barium enema:* The following characteristics may be seen:
  - spasm and oedema of the ileocaecal valve (early involvement); characteristic thickening of the ileocaecal valve lips or wide gaping of the valve with narrowed terminal ileum ("Fleischner" or "inverted umbrella sign");
  - "conical caecum", a deformed and pulled-up caecum due to contraction and fibrosis;
  - increased (obtuse) ileocaecal angle and dilated terminal ileum, appearing suspended from a retracted, fibrosed caecum ("goose neck deformity") ;
  - deformed and incompetent ileocaecal valve;
  - "purse string stenosis"—localised stenosis opposite the ileocaecal valve with a rounded-off smooth caecum and a dilated terminal ileum ;
  - "Stierlin's sign"—appears as a narrowing of the terminal ileum with rapid empying into a shortened, rigid, or obliterated caecum; and
  - "string sign"—a narrow stream of barium, indicating stenosis

Both Stierlin and String signs can also be seen in Crohn's disease. Enteroclysis followed by a barium enema may be the best protocol for evaluation of intestinal tuberculosis.

Ultrasonography

Ultrasound is more helpful in peritoneal and nodal tuberculosis, but it may also identify thickened and dilated bowel loops. The following features may be seen:

- Free or loculated ascitis.

- "Club sandwich" or "sliced bread" sign, due to localised fluid between radially oriented bowel loops.

- Lymphadenopathy may be discrete or conglomerated (matted). The echotexture is mixed heterogenous, in contrast to the homogenously hypoechoic nodes of lymphoma. Both caseation and calcification are highly suggestive of a tubercular aetiology.

- Bowel wall thickening—best appreciated in the ileocaecal region.

- Thickening of the small bowel mesentery of 15 mm or more.

- Pseudo-kidney sign—involvement of the ileocaecal region that is pulled up to a subhepatic position.

Ultrasound-guided fine-needle aspiration (FNA) biopsy has been used successfully in the diagnosis of abdominal tuberculosis. Ultrasonography may also be useful for guiding procedures such as ascitic tap and FNA cytology or biopsy from the lymph nodes or hypertrophic lesions.

Computed Tomographic Scan

Ileocaecal tuberculosis is usually hyperplastic and well evaluated on a computed tomography (CT) scan. Circumferential thickening of caecum and terminal ileum, adherent loops, large regional nodes, and mesenteric thickening can together form a mass centred around the ileocaecal junction. A CT scan can also pick up ulceration or nodularity within the terminal ileum, along with narrowing and proximal dilatation. Involvement around the hepatic flexure of the colon is common. Complications of perforation, abscess, and obstruction can also be seen. Tubercular ascitic fluid is of high attenuation value (25–45 HU) due to its high protein content. Thickened peritoneum and enhancing peritoneal nodules may be seen. A smooth peritoneum with minimal thickening and marked enhancement after contrast suggests tuberculous peritonitis, whereas nodular and irregular peritoneal thickening suggests the presence of peritoneal carcinomatosis.[21] Omental thickening is well seen often as an omental cake appearance.[22]

Lymph nodes may be interspersed. The four patterns of contrast enhancement of tuberculous lymph nodes on the contrast-enhanced CT (CECT) have been described as (in order of frequency): (1) peripheral rim enhancement, (2) nonhomogenous enhancement, (3) homogenous enhancement, and (4) homogenous nonenhancement.[23] Different patterns of contrast enhancement may be seen within the same nodal group, possibly related to the different stages of the pathological process. Caseating lymph nodes are seen as having hypodense centres and peripheral rim enhancement. The presence of nodal calcification in the absence of a known primary tumour in patients from endemic areas suggests a tubercular aetiology. CT findings can help differentiate it from other inflammatory and neoplastic diseases, particularly lymphoma and Crohn's disease.[24] In tuberculosis, the mesenteric, mesenteric root, celiac, porta hepatic, and peripancreatic nodes are characteristically involved, reflecting the lymphatic drainage of the small bowel. The tuberculous involvement of the pancreas may show as well-defined hypoechoic areas on ultrasonography and as hypodense necrotic regions within the enlarged pancreas. CT is more accurate than ultrasound in detecting abnormalities such as periportal and peripancreatic lymph nodes and bowel wall thickening. However, bowel wall dilatation can be better appreciated on ultrasound than on a CT scan. Magnetic resonance imaging (MRI), when compared to a CT scan, provides no additional information.[25]

Cytology and Biochemistry of Ascitic Fluid

The ascitic fluid in abdominal tuberculosis is clear or straw-coloured. Its glucose concentration is less than 30 mg/dl, and its high protein content is >3 g/dl, with a total cell count of 150–4000/cu mm, usually more than 1,000/cu mm (consisting predominantly of lymphocytes (>70%)). The ascites-to-blood glucose ratio is less than 0.96.[26] The serum ascitis albumin gradient is less than 1.1 g/dl, and adenosine deaminase levels are above 36 U/l. Adenosine deaminase (ADA) is increased in tuberculous ascitic fluid due to the stimulation of T-cells by mycobacterial antigens. In coinfection with HIV, the ADA values can be normal or low. High interferon levels in tubercular ascitis have been found to be useful diagnostically. Combining both ADA and interferon estimations may further increase the sensitivity and the specificity. The AFB smear and culture are positive in only 10–15% cases, but the yield rises dramatically by culturing a litre of fluid concentrated by centrifugation.[27] Fluorescent staining with auramine-O is superior to Ziehl-Neelsen staining with regard to the positivity and the ease of detection. In children, AFB may be recovered from stomach wash, keeping in mind that scant saprophytic mycobacteria may also be present as normal flora.

PCR conducted with ascites fluid has produced DNA sequences compatible with tuberculosis.[28] PCR can be a rapid and reliable method for identification of peritoneal tuberculosis; acceleration of the diagnostic decision-making process prevents exposure to unnecessary surgery and allows early initiation of antituberculosis treatment.

Imaging Bacterial Infection with Infecton

A new radioimaging agent, Tc-99m ciprofloxacin (Infecton) has been used to detect deep-seated bacterial infections, such as intraabdominal abscesses. Patients with suspected bacterial infection have been subjected to Infecton imaging and microbiological evaluation, reporting an overall sensitivity of 85.4% and a specificity of 81.7% for detecting infective foci.[29] Sensitivity was higher (87.6%) in microbiologically confirmed infections. Infecton may aid in the earlier detection and treatment of deep-seated infections, and serial imaging with Infecton might be useful in monitoring clinical response and optimising the duration of antimicrobial treatment.

Colonoscopy

Although the appearance is nonspecific, colonoscopy has been used for the diagnosis of colonic or ileocaecal tuberculosis. Most commonly, ulcers, strictures, or oedematous and polypoid mucosal folds are seen. Mucosal pinkish nonfriable nodules of variable sizes with ulcerations in between the nodules in a discrete segment of colon, most often in the caecum, are pathognomic. Areas of strictures, pseudopolypoid oedematous folds, and a deformed and oedematous ileocaecal valve may be seen.

Multiple biopsies should be taken from the edge of the ulcers. The tissue should also be examined for AFB smear and culture, as the histology may not be characteristic.

Endoscopic biopsy specimens may be subjected to PCR for detection of AFB.[30] The limitations of colonoscopic biopsy are that previous antitubercular therapy can alter the histology, and that granulomas are often found in the submucosa. Of 82 patients with GI tuberculosis, colonoscopy was diagnostic in only 47.[31]

Laparoscopy

Laparoscopy is a very useful investigation in doubtful cases. Visual appearances have been found to be more helpful than histology, culture, or guinea pig inoculation.[32]

The laparoscopic findings in peritoneal tuberculosis can be grouped into three categories: (1) thickened peritoneum with tubercles, (2) thickened peritoneum without tubercles, and (3) fibroadhesive peritonitis with markedly thickened peritoneum and multiple thick adhesions fixing the viscera.

Markers for Treatment Response

ESR tends to fall with response to antitubercular treatment. A significant decrease in the concentrations of C-reactive protein (CRP), ceruloplasmin, haptoglobin, and alpha-1-acid glycoprotein has been seen with antitubercular treatment.

Differential Diagnosis

Hypertrophic intestinal tuberculosis may mimic malignant neoplasms such as lymphoma or carcinoma. The ulcero-hypertrophic form may mimic inflammatory bowel disease. The nodal form may closely mimic lymphomas. The ascitic form can be difficult to distinguish from malignant peritoneal disease and sometimes ascites due to chronic liver disease. In cases of hepatosplenomegaly, all other causes need to be excluded before considering a tubercular aetiology. Sometimes, when all investigations are negative and TB is strongly suspected, a laparotomy may be indicated.

Treatment

Laparotomy

In circumstances where the clinical suspicion of intraabdominal disease is strong, but results of investigations are equivocal, a diagnostic laparotomy may be a safer option for abdominal tuberculosis. Where clinical suspicion is strong and imaging features are suggestive, a therapeutic trial of antitubercular treatment (ATT) may be justified. However, laparotomy is definitely indicated where the diagnosis is in doubt and if the malignancy cannot be ruled out with certainty. In many patients, it may not be possible to rule out malignancy, even at laparotomy. A frozen section examination may help in such cases. A mesenteric lymph node should preferably be removed in such cases, as caseation and granulomas are much more likely to be present in lymph nodes than in the intestinal lesions. An omental nodule may also be taken for biopsy. The correction of a stenotic bowel lesion may be done if found.

It is important to remember that:

- Laparotomy is better performed under empirical cover of antitubercular drugs for about 2 weeks, wherever feasible.

- The aim of surgery in tubercular abdominal patients is to do minimal intervention and avoid any major operative procedure. Perhaps only a bypass surgery is enough just to relieve the symptoms. Tubercular pathology cannot be eradicated by surgery alone.

- External diversion (ileostomy or double-barrel stoma), internal diversion with side-to-side bowel anastomosis, closure of the perforation, and stricturoplasty are the commonly performed procedures. Surgical resection is less commonly performed.

- Laparoscopy is not indicated due to the high possibility of adhesions inside the peritoneal cavity. The risk of perforation of the bowel is also high while being handled with instrumentation. Tract contamination may result in chronic tubercular fistula.

Medical Treatment

Antimicrobial treatment is the same for pulmonary and abdominal tuberculosis. Medical treatment with a standard full course of ATT is indicated in all patients. In peritoneal tuberculosis, only medical treatment is required. Intestinal tuberculosis is a systemic disease. In GI tuberculosis, surgery may be required and preferably is done 6–8 weeks after starting the antitubercular therapy. Although the use of short course regimens for 6–9 months have been found to be equally effective by few studies, many physicians still extend the treatment duration to 12 to 18 months, according to the conventional regimens in cases of abdominal tuberculosis.[33] This is justified in view of the unpredictable absorption due to the diseased gut and associated symptoms such as vomiting and malabsorption.

The main antitubercular drugs are isoniazid (INH), rifampicin, ethambutol, pyrazinamide (PZA), and streptomycin (SM). Thiacetazone and p-aminosalicylic acid (PAS) are not recommended for use for abdominal tuberculosis. In a study of 350 patients with extrapulmonary tuberculosis (including 47 children),[34] a 9-month regimen using only INH and rifampicin was successful in 95% of the cases, with only 0.7% of the cases relapsing during a follow-up of 9 years.

Patients with peritoneal, nodal, or ulcerative intestinal disease are usually treated with drugs (e.g., ATT). Corticosteroids have also been used to reduce subsequent complications of adhesions in patients with peritoneal disease. No controlled studies have been performed to show the additional benefit of using steroids. Patients with intestinal obstruction due to strictures and hypertrophic lesions require surgical treatment. Successful treatment of obstructing intestinal lesions with ATT alone has also been seen. Patients usually report improvement in systemic symptoms in a few weeks, but relief of intestinal symptoms may require a much longer duration.

Monitoring with liver function tests (LFTs) is necessary, especially if the patient has suspected icterus or malaise, anorexia, or abdominal pain. INH, rifampicin, and pyrazinamide should be discontinued temporarily in the presence of icterus or a threefold rise in transaminases. As the antitubercular therapy causes healing with fibrosis, this may result in further narrowing and intestinal stricture. Therapy can also alter the histopathological picture and may even increase the perforation rate.

Directly Observed Therapy

Since noncompliance to these regimens is a common cause of treatment failure, directly observed therapy (DOT) is recommended. This involves administration of medication under supervision by a health care provider or a nurse. DOT should be used with all children suffering from tuberculosis. The lack of availability of the paediatric dosage forms of most antituberculosis medications necessitates using crushed pills and suspensions. Even when drugs are given under DOT, tolerance of the medications must be monitored closely. Intermittent regimens should be monitored by DOT for the duration of therapy because poor compliance may result in inadequate drug delivery.

Surgery for Pulmonary Tuberculosis

It must be emphasized that medical therapy remains the mainstay of treatment in pulmonary tuberculosis, and surgical treatment is primarily used to handle complications and hasten recovery.

In children, the primary complex is usually directly or indirectly the main etiologic factor responsible for the need for surgical intervention. Indications for surgical intervention are limited in children, and the challenge lies in determining the timing and nature of intervention.

Indications for surgery in paediatric pulmonary tuberculosis include:
- airway obstruction, extrinsic lymph node compression or intraluminal obstruction;
- progressive primary infection-cavity formation;
- posttuberculous bronchiectasis;
- bronchial stenosis/stricture;
- drainage of lung abscess;
- bronchopleural fistula, broncho-oesophageal fistula;
- massive hemoptysis;
- chest wall sinus;
- posttubular constrictive pericarditis;
- fibrothorax/trapped lung;
- suspicion of malignancy;
- pulmonary resection for MDR-TB;
- tubercular rib osteomyelitis; and
- tubercular empyema.

Indications for pulmonary resection in cases of tuberculosis include:
- persistently positive sputum cultures with cavitation after 6 months of continuous optimal chemotherapy with two or more drugs;
- symptomatic bronchiectasis not controlled with conservative measures;
- advanced disease with extensive caseation necrosis;
- massive life-threatening haemoptysis or recurrent severe haemoptysis;
- trapped lung;
- localised disease with resistant organisms (localised disease defined as that encompassing one or two segments of the lung); and
- a mass lesion of the lung in an area of tubercular involvement.

Surgery for Abdominal Tuberculosis

In GI tuberculosis, if symptoms recur after starting drugs, then elective surgery is planned. Emergency surgery may be required in 25–30% of abdominal tuberculosis cases, particularly those who present with perforation, acute intestinal obstruction not responding to conservative measures, acute peritonitis, and, rarely, significant hematochezia (Figure 18.2). Historically, bypassing the stenosed segment was practiced when effective antitubercular drugs were not available, as any surgery involved with side-to-side anastomosis or the resection of the bowel segment was considered hazardous in the presence of active disease. This practice, however, produced blind loop syndrome, fistulas, and recurrent obstruction in the remaining segments. With the advent

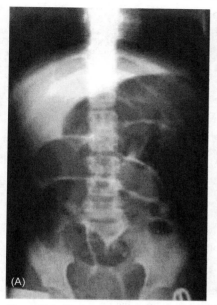 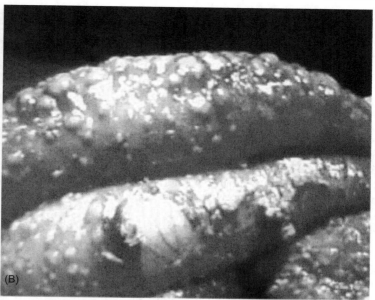

Figure 18.2: (A) X-ray of the abdomen of an 8-year-old boy showing multiple dilated loops of the bowel. The patient presented with distended abdomen, fever, vomiting, and constipation, with similar episodes reported in the past 6 months. (B) Operative findings of 8-year-old patient showing dilated loops of the bowel with multiple caseous granulomas involving the whole intestine. The seromuscular coat was quite inflamed and friable. There was a mass at the ileocaecal junction entrapping the bowel loops, resulting in an acute intestinal obstruction. Adhesionolysis, resection of the mass, and a double-barrel proximal ileostomy were done. Primary anastomosis was avoided because the bowel looked fiery and friable with active tubercular infection (child had not received antitubercular drugs).

of antitubercular drugs, more radical procedures became popular in an attempt to eradicate the disease locally. These procedures were not tolerated well earlier by the malnourished patient. Moreover, the lesions are often widely spaced and not suitable for resection. The abdomen is closed without drainage even in the presence of ascites or peritonitis.

The recommended surgical procedures today are conservative. A period of preoperative drug therapy is controversial; however, 2 weeks of multidrug therapy is considered minimal to reduce the chances of spread of active infection during surgery. Strictures that reduce the lumen by half or more and cause proximal hypertrophy or dilation are treated by strictureplasty. This involves an incision along the antimesenteric side, which is closed transversely in two layers. A segment of bowel bearing multiple strictures or a single long tubular stricture may merit resection, with a 5-cm safe margin. Tubercular perforations are usually ileal and are associated with distal strictures. Resection and anastomosis are preferred because simple closure of the perforation is associated with a high incidence of leakage and fistula formation and thus higher mortality.[35] For ileocaecal tuberculosis, limited resection of the ileocaecal area, rather than formal right hemicolectomy, involves lesser dissection and thus less chance of injury to the duodenum or ureter. For colonic lesions, resection is advocated.

Some obstructing intestinal lesions may also be relieved with antitubercular drugs alone without surgery. The mean time required for the relief of obstructive symptoms is usually 6 months.

Emergency surgery for intestinal obstruction is best avoided, as it carries 18–24% mortality. Thus, every patient who presents with intestinal obstruction should initially be managed conservatively. Tubercular perforations carry high mortality despite surgery. In contrast, elective surgery for GI tuberculosis carries only 0.5–2% mortality. Despite the advent of newer antitubercular drugs, abdominal tuberculosis carries a mortality of 4–12%. This is largely due to associated problems of malnutrition, anaemia, hypoalbuminaemia, and poor wound healing.

Extrapulmonary Tuberculosis

Most cases of extrapulmonary TB, including cervical lymphadenopathy, can be treated with the same regimens used to treat pulmonary TB. Exceptions include bone and joint disease, miliary disease, and men-

ingitis. For these, the recommendation is a 2-month therapy of INH, rifampin, pyrazinamide, and streptomycin once a day, followed by 7–10 months of INH and rifampin once a day.

The other recommended regimen is 2 months of the same four drugs—INH, rifampin, pyrazinamide, and streptomycin—followed by 7–10 months of INH and rifampin twice a week. Capreomycin or kanamycin may be given instead of streptomycin in areas where resistance to streptomycin is common.

Tuberculosis and HIV

The use of a regimen that uses rifabutin instead of rifampin has been advised when treating HIV disease and TB simultaneously.

The treatment regimen for TB initially should include at least three drugs and should be continued for at least 9 months. INH, rifampin, and pyrazinamide with or without ethambutol or streptomycin should be administered for the first 2 months. Treatment of disseminated disease or drug-resistant TB may require the addition of a fourth drug.

The tuberculin skin test, or Mantoux test, which is the standard marker of *Mycobacterium tuberculosis* infection in immunocompetent children, has poor sensitivity when used in HIV-infected children.[9] Novel T cell assays may offer higher sensitivity and specificity, but these tests still fail to make the crucial distinction between latent *M. tuberculosis* infection and active disease, and they are limited by cost considerations.[9]

Symptom-based diagnostic approaches are less helpful in HIV-infected children, as TB-related symptoms cannot be differentiated from those caused by other HIV-associated conditions. HIV-infected children are at increased risk of developing active disease after TB exposure/infection, which justifies the use of INH preventive therapy once active TB has been excluded.[9] HIV-infected children should also receive appropriate supportive care, including cotrimoxazole prophylaxis, and antiretroviral therapy, if indicated.[9] The management of children with TB/HIV infection could thus be vastly improved by better implementation of readily available interventions.

Multidrug-Resistant Tuberculosis

Primary resistance is resistance to anti-TB treatment in an individual who has no history of prior treatment. Secondary resistance involves the emergence of resistance during the course of ineffectual anti-TB therapy.

Risk factors for the development of primary drug resistance include patient contact with drug-resistant contagious TB, residence in areas with a high prevalence of drug-resistant *M. tuberculosis*, HIV infection, and the use of intravenous drugs. Secondary drug resistance reflects noncompliance to the regimen, inappropriate drug regimens, and/or interference with absorption of the drug.

The current guidelines are that if a child is at risk or has disease resistant to INH, at least two drugs to which the isolate is sensitive on culture should be administered. Another principle is to never add a single drug to an already failing regimen. The resistance pattern, toxicities of the drugs, and the patient's response to treatment should determine the duration and regimen selected.

The initial treatment regimen for patients with MDR-TB should include four drugs. At least two bactericidal drugs (e.g., INH, rifampin), pyrazinamide, and either streptomycin or another aminoglycoside (also bactericidal) or high-dose ethambutol (25 mg/kg/d) also should be incorporated into the regimen.

Six-month treatment regimens and intermittent therapy are not advocated for patients with strains resistant to INH or rifampin.

In isolated INH resistance, the four-drug, 6-month regimen is started initially for the treatment of pulmonary TB. INH is discontinued when resistance is documented, but pyrazinamide is continued for the entire 6-month course of treatment.

In the 9-month regimen, INH is discontinued upon the documentation of isolated INH resistance. If ethambutol was included in the initial regimen, treatment continues with rifampin and ethambutol for a minimum of 12 months. If ethambutol was not included, then sensitivity tests are repeated, INH is discontinued, and two new drugs (e.g., ethambutol and pyrazinamide) are added.

Resistance to both INH and rifampin is a complicated issue. The initial drug regimen is continued (with two drugs to which the organism is susceptible) until bacteriologic sputum conversion is documented, followed by at least 12 months of two-drug therapy. The role of new agents such as quinolone derivatives and amikacin in MDR cases remains unclear.

Default from treatment was observed to be a major challenge in the treatment of MDR-TB due to long duration and the expense of ATT.[36]

Monitoring for Side Effects

Adverse effects of INH (e.g., hepatitis) are rare in children; therefore, routine determination of serum aminotransferase levels is not necessary. Monthly monitoring of hepatic function tests may be done for patients with severe or disseminated TB, miliary TB, concurrent or recent hepatic disease, or clinical evidence of hepatotoxic effects, and for those receiving high daily doses of INH (10 mg/kg/d) in combination with rifampin, pyrazinamide, or both. In the rare case when the patient has symptoms of hepatitis, the regimen is discontinued and liver function is evaluated. If the tests are normal or return to normal, then a decision to restart the medications may be made. The drugs are reintroduced one by one.

Follow-up

A regular follow-up every 4–8 weeks is done to ensure compliance and to monitor the adverse effects of and response to the medications administered. The weight of the child is measured at each visit. The sclera is examined for any evidence of jaundice.

Follow-up ESR and chest x-ray (CXR) may be obtained after 2–3 months of therapy to observe the response to treatment in patients with pulmonary TB. However, hilar lymphadenopathy may take several years to resolve. Thus, a normal CXR is not required for termination of therapy.

Complications

Complications of Chest Tuberculosis

Complications of chest tuberculosis include:

- miliary tuberculosis;
- tubercular meningitis;
- pleural effusion;
- pneumothorax;
- complete obstruction of a bronchus if caseous material extrudes into the lumen;
- atelectasis;
- bronchiectasis;
- stenosis of the airways;
- broncho-oesophageal fistula; and
- endobronchial disease.

Complications of Abdominal Tuberculosis

Complications of abdominal tuberculosis include:

- subacute intestinal obstruction;
- adhesions;
- intestinal stricture;
- malabsorption; and
- short bowel syndrome.

Prevention

BCG vaccine is given at birth to all newborns in developing countries where tuberculosis is endemic.

The best method to prevent cases of paediatric tuberculosis is to find, diagnose, and treat cases of active tuberculosis among adults. Children do not usually contract tuberculosis from other children or transmit it themselves. Adults pass tuberculosis on to children. Improved contact investigations and use of directly observed therapy should increase the success rate of finding and treating adult cases of tuberculosis, therefore reducing the number of cases of paediatric tuberculosis.

Mothers infected with tuberculosis (but under regular treatment) should remain away from their babies until their sputum is negative. This is usually after 2 months of a four-drug regimen given to adults. During this period, mothers do not feed their babies directly, but the breast milk is expressed and then boiled before being fed to the baby, despite of the fact that this has the risk of destroying the nutrients. The baby is also given prophylactic INH therapy, 5 mg/kg daily for 6 months. The baby is immunised with INH-resistant BCG vaccine soon after birth.

Prognosis

The prognosis varies according to the clinical manifestation. A poor prognosis is associated with disseminated TB, miliary disease, and tubercular meningitis. Higher mortality rates (20%) occur in children <5 years of age.

Key Summary Points

The new WHO Stop TB Strategy, released in 2006, has identified six principal components to reduce the global burden of TB by 2015:

1. Pursue high-quality DOT expansion and enhancement.
2. Address TB/HIV, MDR-TB, and other challenges.
3. Contribute to health system strengthening.
4. Engage all care providers.
5. Empower patients and communities.
6. Enable and promote research.

References

1. Gupta DK, Sharma S. Abdominal tuberculosis. In: Bhave S, ed. Textbook of adolescent medicine. 1st ed. Jaypee Brothers, New Delhi, 2006; Chap 20.5; Pp 663–669.

2. Sharma S, Gupta DK. Abdominal tuberculosis. In: Gupta DK, ed. Pediatric surgery—diagnosis and management. Jaypee Brothers, New Delhi, 2008; Chap 57, Pp 646–658.

3. Gupta DK, Rohatgi M, Misra D. Abdominal tuberculosis in children. In: Seth V, ed. Indian Pediatrics, Indian Academy of Pediatrics, New Delhi, 1991; Chap 10, Pp 188–194.

4. Bhansali SK. Abdominal tuberculosis: experiences with 300 cases. Am J Gastroenterol 1977; 67:324–337.

5. Varma JK, Wiriyakitjar D, Nateniyom S, et al. Evaluating the potential impact of the new Global Plan to Stop TB: Thailand, 2004–2005. Bull World Health Organ 2007; 85(8):586–592.

6. Ridley R. Applying science to the diseases of poverty. Bull World Health Organ 2007; 85:509–510.

7. Sharma, Gupta DK. Tuberculosis in pediatric surgery. In: Gupta DK, ed. Pediatric surgery—diagnosis and management. Jaypee Brothers, New Delhi, 2008; Chap 41.

8. Friedland G, Harries A, Coetzee D. Implementation issues in tuberculosis/HIV program collaboration and integration: 3 case studies. J Infect Dis 2007; 15,196 Suppl 1: S114–123.

9. Marais BJ, Graham SM, Cotton MF, Beyers N. Diagnostic and management challenges for childhood tuberculosis in the era of HIV. J Infect Dis 2007; 15,196 Suppl 1: S76–85.

10. Nerli RB, Kamat GV, Alur SB, Koura A, Vikram P, Amarkhed SS. Genitourinary tuberculosis in pediatric urological practice. J Pediatr Urol 2008; 4(4):299–303.

11. Teegala R, Kumar P, Kale SS, Sharma BS. Craniovertebral junction tuberculosis: a new comprehensive therapeutic strategy. Neurosurgery 2008; 63(5):946–955.

12. Parthasarthy A, Sumathi N, Manohanan R, et al. Controversies in tuberculosis. Indian J Pediatr 1987; 54:779–784.

13. Acer T, Karnak I, Ekinci S, Talim B, Kiper N, Senocak ME. Multiple jejunoileal perforations because of intestinal involvement of miliary tuberculosis in an infant. J Pediatr Surg 2008; 43(9):17–21.

14. Vij JC, Malhotra V, Choudhary V, Jain, et al. A clinicopathological study of abdominal tuberculosis. Indian J Tuberc 1992; 39:213–220.

15. Güvenç BH, Ekingen G, Erkus B. Thoracoscopic assessment of mediastinal tuberculous lymphadenitis in a 4-month-old child. Surg Laparosc Endosc Percutan Tech 2008; 18:322–324.

16. Goussard P, Gie RP, Kling S, et al. The outcome of infants younger than 6 months requiring ventilation for pneumonia caused by Mycobacterium tuberculosis. Pediatr Pulmonol 2008; 43:505–510.

17. Sharma MP , Bhatia V. Abdominal tuberculosis. Indian J Med Res 2004; 120:305–315.

18. Tandon HD. The pathology of intestinal tuberculosis. Trop Gastroenterol 1981; 2:77–93.

19. Waqar SH, Malik ZI, Zahid MA. Isolated appendicular tuberculosis. J Ayub Med Coll Abbottabad 2005; 17:88–89.

20. Kapoor VK, Chatterjee TK, Sharma LK. Radiology of abdominal tuberculosis. Aust Radiol 1988, 32:365–367.

21. Sood R. Diagnosis of abdominal tuberculosis: role of imaging. J Indian Academy of Clinical Medicine 2001; 2:169–177.

22. Pombo F, Rodriguez E, Mato J, et al. Patterns of contrast enhancement of tuberculous lymph nodes demonstrated by computed tomography. Clin Radiol 1992; 46:13–17.

23. Pereira JM, Madureira AJ, Vieira A, Ramos I. Abdominal tuberculosis: imaging features. Eur J Radiol 2005; 55:173–180.

24. Zirinsky K, Auh YH, Kneeland JB, et al. Computed tomography, sonography and MR imaging of abdominal tuberculosis. JCAT 1985; 9:961–963.

25. Wilkins EGL. Tuberculous peritonitis: diagnostic value of the ascitic/blood glucose ratio. Tubercle 1984; 65:47–52.

26. Bhargava DK, Gupta M, Nijhawan S, Dasarathy S, Kushwaha AKS. Adenosine deaminase (ADA) in peritoneal tuberculosis: diagnostic value in ascites fluid and serum. Tubercle 1990; 71:121–126.

27. Wang YC, Lu JJ, Chen CH, Peng YJ, Yu MH. Peritoneal tuberculosis mimicking ovarian cancer can be diagnosed by polymerase chain reaction: a case report. Gynecol Oncol 2005; 97(3):961–963.

28. Shukla HS, Bhatia S, Nathani YP, et al. Peritoneal biopsy for diagnosis of abdominal tuberculosis. Postgrad Med J 1982; 58:226–228.

29. Anand BS, Schneider FE, El-Zaatari FA, et al. Diagnosis of intestinal tuberculosis by polymerase chain reaction on endoscopic biopsy specimens. Am J Gastroenterol 1994; 89:2248–2249.

30. Kalvaria I, Kottler RE, Max IN. The role of colonoscopy in the diagnosis of tuberculosis. J Clin Gastroenterol 1988, 10:516–523.

31. Immanuel C, Acharyulu GS, Kannapiran M, Segaran R, Sarma GR. Acute phase proteins in tuberculous patients. Indian J Chest Dis Allied Sci 1990; 32(1):15–23.

32. Bhargava DK, Shriniwas MD, Chopra P, Nijhawan S, DasarathyS, Kushwaha AK. Peritoneal tuberculosis: laparoscopic patterns and its diagnostic accuracy. Am J Gastroenterol 1992; 87:109–112.

33. Balasubramanian R, Nagarajan M, Balambal R, Tripathy SP, Sundararaman R, Venkatesan P. Randomised controlled clinical trial of short course chemotherapy in abdominal tuberculosis: a five-year report. Int J Tuberc Lung Dis 1997; 1:44–51.

34. Lorin MT, Katharine HKM, Jacob SC. Treatment of tuberculosis in children. Pediatr Clin North Am 1983; 30:333–348.

35. Ara C, Sogutlu G, Yildiz R, et al. Spontaneous small bowel perforations due to intestinal tuberculosis should not be repaired by simple closure. J Gastrointest Surg 2005; 9:514–517.

36. Dhingra VK, Rajpal S, Mittal A, Hanif M. Outcome of multi-drug resistant tuberculosis cases treated by individualized regimens at a tertiary level clinic. Indian J Tuberc 2008; 55:15–21.

CHAPTER 19
PYOMYOSITIS

John Chinda
Emmanuel A. Ameh
Lohfa B. Chirdan

Introduction

Pyomyositis is a primary acute bacterial infection of skeletal muscles associated with abscess formation. The use of the term "tropical pyomyositis" should be restricted to primary muscle abscess arising de novo. It should not be used to describe intermuscular abscess; abscess extending into muscles from adjoining tissues, such as bone or subcutaneous tissues; or abscess secondary to septicaemia.

Pyomyositis is predominantly experienced in the tropics and relatively low-income countries, but it can also occur in temperate and developed countries. Zur first described the condition in 1885 as an endemic disease in the tropics;[1] since then, there have been reports from tropical as well as temperate regions.[2-11]

Demographics

Pyomyositis is common among children in the tropics, accounting for 1–4% of all hospital admissions in some tropical countries[10,11] and 1 per 3,000 paediatric admissions in Southern Texas. In sub-Saharan Africa,[2] 70% of affected children are younger than 10 years of age and both sexes are equally affected. In another large report from sub-Saharan Africa,[3] 36% of all affected patients were children.

Although cases are seen throughout the year, maximum incidence has been noted during the rainy and wet monsoon season in India.[9]

Microbiology

Staphylococcus aureus is the most common primary causative pathogen. It is seen in up to 90% of cases in tropical areas and 75% of cases in temperate countries.[9,11] Group A streptococci account for another 1–5% of cases. Several other microorganisms implicated include streptococcus groups B, C, and G, *Pneumococcus, Salmonella, Escherichia coli, Neisseria, Haemophilus, Aeromonas, Serratia, Yersinia, Pseudomonas, Klebsiella, Citrobacter, Fusobacterium*, and *Mycobacterium*.

In tropical regions, pus cultures are sterile in 15–30% of cases[9] and 90–95% of patients also have sterile blood cultures, due largely to use of antibiotics before presentation. Blood cultures are positive in 20–30% of cases in temperate regions. Better microbiological culture techniques in the temperate regions may account for this difference.

Pathogenesis and Pathology

The precise pathogenesis of pyomyositis remains obscure. It is believed that staphylococcal bacteraemia and muscle damage are prerequisites for the clinical scenario. Skeletal muscle tissue is known to be intrinsically resistant to bacterial infection under normal circumstances, but it has been shown experimentally that if normal muscle is damaged, it becomes vulnerable to haematogenous invasion by bacteria, with subsequent abscess formation.[12]

A number of conditions predispose to skeletal muscle damage. These include trauma, nutritional deficiencies, immunosuppression, parasitic infestations, viral infections, and intravenous drug abuse.

In one report involving adults with pyomyositis,[13] serum immunoglobin M (IgM) level was found to be significantly lower, and mean levels of IgG and IgA significantly higher, than in controls.

Complement levels were normal. This prompted the proposition that defects of opsonising and complement fixing IgM antibodies against microorganisms are implicated in the aetiology of pyomyositis, at least in adults.

Human immunodeficiency virus (HIV) infection may have led to an increasing incidence of pyomyositis in areas with a high prevalence of HIV infection;[14,15] this is now thought to be an important predisposing factor in the aetiopathogenesis of pyomyositis.

Although the classical presentation is with muscle abscess, the hallmark of the disease is not an abscess but finding myositis in a biopsy specimen of involved muscle.

In the early stages of pyomyositis, muscles show oedematous separation of fibres, followed by patchy myocytolysis, progressing to complete disintegration. The fibres are surrounded by lymphocytes and plasma cells. Muscles fibres may heal without abscess formation or degenerate, progressing to suppuration with bacteria and polymorphonuclear leucocytes.

Clinical Presentation

The large muscles of the lower limbs and trunk are particularly prone to involvement, but small muscles, such as those of the orbit may rarely be involved. Commonly affected muscle groups are shown in Figure 19.1.[2]

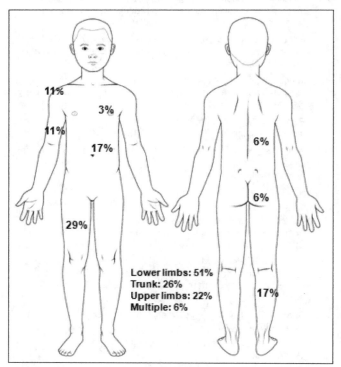

11%
3%
11%
17%
29%
6%
6%
17%

Lower limbs: 51%
Trunk: 26%
Upper limbs: 22%
Multiple: 6%

Source: Drawing of child taken from http://images.medscape.com/pi/features/ald/fb/fbc-ap.pdf.

Figure 19.1: Distribution of pyomyositis at 35 sites in African children.

Rarely, pyomyositis can present with acute fever and chills, also with toxic shock syndrome or pyrexia of unknown origin. It may present as an acute abdomen or spinal compression or compartment syndrome, depending on the anatomic location of the affected muscle. It has been reported that about 5% of patients present in this stage.[3]

In children younger than 5 years of age, when the lower limb is affected the main complaint on presentation may be that of an inability or refusal to walk.

In the tropics, the abscess is usually solitary,[9] but multiple abscesses may be seen in some patients. The clinical manifestations in both tropical and nontropical pyomyositis are similar and can be categorised in three stages: invasive, suppurative, and late or septic[3] (Table 19.1).

Table 19.1: Clinical stages of pyomyositis.

Clinical stage	Features
Invasive	Duration of symptoms <10 days
	Pain in affected muscle
	Low-grade fever
	Wooden or hard stiffness on palpation of muscle
	Mild leucocytosis
	Needle aspiration negative for pus
Suppurative	Duration of symptoms 10–21 days
	Oedema
	Marked tenderness of affected muscle
	Pyrexia
	Leucocytosis
	Needle aspiration yields pus
Late or septic	Duration of symptoms >21 days
	Fluctuant swelling in muscle
	High-grade fever
	Severely ill
	Septicaemia
	Leucocytosis
	Needle aspiration yields pus

Invasive Stage

The invasive stage is characterised by an insidious onset of dull cramping pain, with or without fever and anorexia. There is localised oedema, which is indurated or woody but usually causes little or no tenderness and lasts for about a week. Only about 2% of all patients (both adults and children) present in this stage.[3]

Suppurative Stage

The suppurative stage occurs when a deep collection of pus has developed in the muscle, usually from the second to the third week of the infection. The patient may complain of fever with chills. The overlying skin is mildly erythematous, and the swelling is fluctuant. Leucocytosis may be present, with elevated erythrocyte sedimentation rate (ESR) or C-reactive protein (CRP). A needle aspiration test is usually productive of pus. A little more than 90% of patients seen in sub-Saharan Africa[3] would typically present in this stage.

Late or Septic Stage

If the abscess remains untreated, dissemination of infection occurs. Bacteraemia, septicaemia, septic shock, multiple organ dysfunction syndrome, and metastatic abscesses are some of the complications.

Investigations

Needle Aspiration

When the diagnosis of pyomyositis is suspected, particularly for patients presenting in the suppurative or late stages, the swelling should be aspirated with a large-bore needle (not smaller than 18 gauge) to confirm the presence of pus. The aspirated pus is usually yellowish in colour but may be brownish or blood-stained.

Microbiology

Any aspirated and/or drained pus should be cultured (aerobic and anaerobic). A biopsy of the abscess wall and/or muscle taken at time of open drainage should also be cultured. The culture should help to identify the bacteria involved in the pathology. Blood should also be cultured to identify any septicaemic process. A sensitivity test would be helpful in the choice of antibiotics, but this should not delay institution of antibiotic therapy.

Imaging

Early radiological evaluation is a key to diagnosis of pyomyositis when a high index of suspicion exists. Ultrasonography should be used first because it is inexpensive and widely available, without the disadvantage of delivering a relatively high radiation dose to children. It has been shown that early application of sonography to any suspected lesson can help to establish early diagnosis of pyomyositis.[16,17]

Ultrasound features in the muscle include:[16]

- muscle swelling;
- hypoechoic areas in the muscle belly;
- heterogenous hypoechoic areas; and
- hyperechoic areas.

Other advanced imaging techniques, such as magnetic resonance imaging (MRI), computed tomography (CT) scan, and radionuclide scanning, if available, could help in identifying occult muscle abscesses or multifocal involvement. MRI, due to its excellent soft tissue resolution properties, is particularly useful, especially in deeply sited muscles that are not readily accessible to clinical examination. MRI features of pyomyositis include the following.[18]

- The affected muscle may appear swollen, with loss of architectural definition.
- Heterogenous areas of low intensity appear on T1-weighted images.
- In the early stage, the only finding may be oedema (area of high signal intensity on fluid-sensitive sequences).

It has been noted that MRI with gadolinium enhancement can increase the confidence of identifying or excluding the presence of abscess,[11,19] but this may give high-dose irradiation to the child.

Plain radiograph of the affected limb should always be done to exclude acute osteomyelitis, but it should always be remembered that, in the early stages, x-ray may not diagnose osteomyelitis. Clinical suggestion of complication by pneumonia, pleural effusion, and pyopericardium should warrant that a chest radiograph may need to be done serially. If the latter complication is suspected, an echocardiogram would be helpful.

Haematological Tests

A complete blood count should be done. Leucocytosis, neutrophilia, or eosinophilia may be present, and patients presenting late are often anaemic.

Excluding Underlying Disease

A serological test for HIV infection should be done, after appropriate counselling. Diabetes mellitus should also be excluded by ascertaining the blood sugar level.

Differential Diagnosis

The differential diagnoses are varied and include osteomylitis, septic arthritis, intermuscular abscess, muscle contusion, polymyositis, cellulitis, rhabdomyosarcoma, pyrexia of unknown origin, and appendix abscess. Pyomyositis of a limb may be difficult to differentiate from acute osteomyelitis at the early stage, and radiography may not be helpful in excluding osteomyelitis. As the latter is more serious and damaging, it is safer to make that diagnosis and institute appropriate treatment until proven otherwise.

Another area of clinical diagnostic difficulty is differentiating pyomyositis of the anterior abnormal wall from appendix abscess. Localisation of the abscess can be done easily by ultrasonography. Differentiating between pyomyositis and a rapidly growing rhabdomyosarcoma with erythema and tenderness of the overlying skin is extremely difficult in children and requires a high index of suspicion, especially when the history and site of the lesion are not entirely typical of pyomyositis.

Management

Early diagnosis and treatment are critical to survival and outcome. Diagnosis may be missed due to unfamiliarity with the disease, atypical presentation, a wide range of differential diagnoses, and lack of early specific signs. The treatment includes resuscitation, abscess drainage, antibiotics, analgesia, and rest of the affected limb.

Resuscitation

Patients may be anaemic, particularly those presenting late. Any severe anaemia may require correction by blood transfusion. Patients who are malnourished will require some form of nutritional support and rehabilitation.

Abscess Drainage

The definitive treatment of full-blown pyomyositis remains adequate drainage. Following this, the abscess cavity must be prevented from premature closure by any one of several methods, such as packing and daily dressing. EUSOL or honey[20] are effective, but sterile saline may serve the same purpose. Closure of the skin and drainage with a Penrose drain or other appropriate drain are also effective and obviate the need for daily dressing.

If properly drained, the abscess is unlikely to recur. In the very early stage of the disease, before an abscess has formed, antibiotic administration and resting the affected part may suffice.

Percutaneous drainage,[11] preferably under imaging guidance (ultrasonography), is also effective and avoids an incision and resulting scar, which would otherwise prolong the hospital stay.

Antibiotics

Appropriate antibiotics should always be given (initially intravenously). Before culture and antibiogram results are received, the choice of antibiotics should be based on the microbiological knowledge of commonly involved bacteria. Any antibiotic regime should include a potent antibiotic effective against *Staphylococcus aureus,* which is the most common bacteria involved.

In patients presenting early, treatment with antibiotics alone may control infection.[11] However, the duration of antibiotic therapy is often long (2–8 weeks).[11,19]

Analgesia

When pain is a prominent symptom, appropriate analgesics should be given to control it.

Rest of Affected Limb

When a limb muscle is affected, some form of splinting and resting of that limb helps to relieve pain. Elevation of the limb would be helpful in the presence of oedema and should help to prevent a compartment syndrome.

Prognosis and Outcome

Although mortality is low, morbidity could be high and hospital stay prolonged for several weeks. Extramuscular involvement, especially of the lung and heart, is life threatening and could lead to death, despite treatment.

In one report,[2] extraskeletal complications (pneumonia, pericarditis) occurred in 6.5% of patients. Complications with pericarditis resulted in the only mortality of 3% in that report. In one large series,[3] mortality in all patients (adults and children) was <1%.

Evidence-Based Research

Table 19.2 presents one of the few reports on pyomyositis in children in sub-Saharan Africa.

Table 19.2: Evidence-based research.

Title	Pyomyositis in children: analysis of 31 cases
Authors	Ameh EA
Institution	Paediatric Surgery Unit, Department of Surgery, Ahmadu Bello University Teaching Hospital, Zaria, Nigeria
Reference	Ann Trop Paediatr 1999; 19:263–265
Problem	Pyomyositis in children.
Intervention	Open drainage, local dressing of abscess cavity, antibiotics.
Results	Thirty-one children were treated for 35 instances of pyomyositis in Nigeria. Most (71%) were younger than 10 years of age, and the lower limb (51%) and trunk (26%) muscles were mostly afflicted. Patients presented after a symptom duration of 2–12 days (mean, 6 days) and a preceding history of trauma was obtained only in one patient. A pure culture of *Staphylococcus aureus* was obtained in 75% of cultured specimens, but mixed growth of staphylococci and streptococci and sterile growth were also obtained in a few patients.
Outcome/ effect	Recurrence of abscess occurred in one abscess (3%) after 3 days of open drainage. The hospital stay for survivors was long, at an average of 20 days (range, 12–30 days). Two patients (6.5%) developed extramuscular complications (pneumonia, pneumonia and pericarditis), resulting in mortality in one patient (3.2%) from pericarditis.
Historical significance/ comments	This is only one of the few reports of pyomyositis in children from sub-Saharan Africa. It characterises the clinical profile of the disease in African children and shows that life-threatening complications, although uncommon, can occur and even result in mortality.

Key Summary Points

1. Pyomyositis could be encountered in children in Africa.

2. A high index of suspicion is needed to make early diagnosis.

3. Symptoms are usually nonspecific; pain of the affected muscle, swelling, and pyrexia of more than a week may indicate the presence of the disease.

4. Intravenous antibiotics followed by oral administration for 3–6 weeks should be started early.

5. In established abscesses, adequate incision and drainage must be done.

References

1. Zur SJB. Aetiologic der myositis ocuta. Deutsche Zeit Chir 1885; 22:497–502.

2. Ameh EA. Pyomyositis in children. Analysis of 31 cases. Ann Trop Pediatr 1999; 19:263–265.

3. Chidozie LC. Pyomyositis: review of 205 cases in 112 patients. Am J Surg 1979; 137:255–259.

4. Chacha PB. Muscle abscesses in children. Clin Orthop 1970; 70:174–180.

5. Foster WD. The bacteriology of tropical pyomyositis in Uganda. J Hyg 1965; 63:517–524.

6. Ladipo GO, Dupunle YF. Tropical pyomyositis in the Nigerian savanna. Trop Geo Med 1977; 29:223–228.

7. Horn CV, Master S. Pyomyositis tropicans in Uganda. East Afr Med J 1968; 45:463–467.

8. Madziga AG, Na'aya UH, Gali BM. Pyomyositis in north-eastern Nigeria: a 10-year review. Niger J Surg Res 2004; 6:17–20.

9. Shija JK. Pyomyositis. In: Adeloye A, ed. Davey's Companion to Surgery in Africa. Churchill Livingstone, 1987, Pp 140–146.

10. Gibson RK, Rosenthal SJ, Lukert BP. Pyomyositis: increasing recognition in temperate climates. Am J Med 1984; 77:768–772.

11. Mitsionis GI, Manaudis GN, Lykissas MG, et al. Pyomyositis in children: early diagnosis and treatment. J Pediatr Surg 2009; 44:2173–2178.

12. Miyake H, Zur B. Kenntnis der soggennenta myositis inserctiosa (English abstract). Mitt Grenzgeb Med Chir 1904; 13:155.

13. Giasuddin ASM, Idoko JA, Lawande RV. Tropical pyomyositis: is it an immunodeficiency disease? Am J Trop Med Hyg 1986; 35:1231–1234.

14. Ansaloni L, Acaye GL, Re MC. High HIV seroprevalence among patients with pyomyositis in northern Uganda. Trop Med Int Health 1996; 1: 210–212.

15. Belec L, Di Costanzo B, Georges AJ, Gherardi R. HIV infection in African patients with tropical pyomyositis. AIDS 1991; 5:234.

16. Royston DD, Cremin BJ. The ultrasonic evaluation of psoas abscess (tropical pyomyositis in children). Paediatr Radiol 1994; 24:481–483.

17. Chaitow J, Martin AC, Knight P, Buchanan N. Pyomyositis tropica: a diagnostic dilemma. Med J Aust 1980; 2:512–513.

18. Yu JS, Habib P. MR imaging of urgent inflammatory and infectious conditions affecting the soft tissues of the musculoskeletal system. Emerg Radiol 2009; 16:267–276.

19. Gubbay AJ, Isaacs D. Pyomyositis in children. Pediatr Infect Dis J 2000; 19:1009–1013.

20. Okeniyi JAO, Olubanjo OO, Ogunlesi TA, Oyelami OA. Comparison of healing of incised abscess wounds with honey and EUSOL dressing. J Alternative Compl Med 2005; 11:511–513.

CHAPTER 20
OMPHALITIS

Mairo Adamu Bugaje   Emmanuel A. Ameh
Merrill McHoney   Kokila Lakhoo

Introduction

Omphalitis is defined as infection of the umbilicus—in particular, the umbilical stump in the newborn. It primarily affects neonates, in whom the combination of the umbilical stump and decreased immunity presents an opportunity for infection. It is rarely reported outside the neonatal period. Varieties of congenital conditions predispose to infection of the umbilical stump and are also among the differential diagnoses to consider for the presentation.

Omphalitis may extend into the portal vein and result in various acute complications requiring medical as well as surgical interventions. Although this condition is uncommon in developed countries, it remains a significant cause of morbidity and mortality in Africa and other parts of the world where health care is less readily available. Umbilical cord infection contributes significantly to newborn infection and neonatal mortality in Africa, especially for infants delivered at home without skilled birth attendants and under unhygienic conditions.[1]

Demographics

Omphalitis is uncommon in developed countries, with an incidence of 0.2–0.7%.[1] The incidence in developing countries has been quoted to be between 2 and 7 in every 100 live births.[2,3] However, the incidence is even higher in communities that practise application of nonsterile home remedies to the cord. In one study of neonates admitted to an African general paediatric ward, omphalitis accounted for 28% of neonatal admissions.[4] Hospital-based studies estimate that 2–54 babies per 1000 births will develop omphalitis.[5] However, one report from Tanzania[6] found a rate of 1.7% among babies of 3,262 women.

Although there is a male preponderance, there does not appear to be a racial or ethnic predilection to developing omphalitis. The mean age of onset is usually 3–5 days for preterm infants and 5–9 days for term infants. For those with complications, the age at presentation is 5–75 days (median, 33 days), according to one report.[7]

Unhygienic cord practices have been implicated as the main factor responsible for the high incidence of omphalitis in Africa. Risk factors include inappropriate cord handling (e.g., cultural application of substances such as engine oil, cow dung, talc powder, or palm oil to the cord); septic delivery secondary to prolonged rupture of membranes or maternal infection; nonsterile delivery; prematurity; and low birth weight. One report[1] cited use of old instruments to cut the cord, mother not bathing (washing the perineum with water and soap) or shaving before delivery, and application of substances on the umbilical cord to be independently associated with the risk of developing omphalitis. Other risk factors include neonates with weakened or deficient immune systems or who are hospitalised and subjected to invasive procedures such as umbilical catheterisation. Genetic defects in contractile proteins have been implicated, and in some, immunological factors such as leukocyte adhesion deficiency (LAD) syndrome and neutrophil mobility may play a role.

Aetiology/Pathophysiology

The umbilical cord presents a unique substrate for bacterial colonisation. It is relatively rich in substrate, without the normal barrier of skin

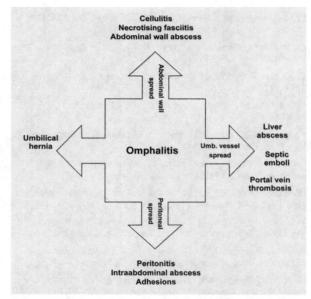

Figure 20.1: Pathophysiology of surgical complications of omphalitis.

defences, and it undergoes ischaemia and degradation as the umbilical stump dries and falls off. Normally, the cord area becomes colonised with potential bacterial pathogens intrapartum or immediately postnatal. Bacteria have the potential to invade the umbilical stump, leading to omphalitis. The pathophysiology of complications of omphalitis is closely related to the anatomy of the umbilicus. The infection can spread along the umbilical artery, umbilical veins, abdominal wall lymphatics and vessels, and by direct spread to contiguous areas (Figure 20.1).

The bacteriological spectrum of omphalitis is undergoing change, in light of the changes in cord care, antibiotic use, bacterial resistance profiles, and local practices. A single organism is causative in most cases. More often, aerobic organisms are causative. Common organisms include:

- *Staphylococcus aureus* (most common)
- Group A streptococcus
- *Escherichia coli*
- *Klebsiella*
- *Proteus*

Up to one-third of cases of omphalitis are associated with anaerobic infection caused by:

- *Bacteroides fragilis*
- *Peptostreptococcus*
- *Clostridium perfringens*

Clinical Presentation

Local signs of omphalitis include purulent or foul-smelling discharge from the umbilicus/umbilical stump, periumbilical erythema, oedaema, and tenderness. Systemic signs include fever (temperature >38°C) or hypothermia (temperature <36°C), unstable temperature, or jaundice. Other systemic manifestations may include tachycardia (heart rate >180/min), hypotension and delayed capillary refill, tachypnoea (respiratory rate >60/min), signs of respiratory distress or apnoea, or abdominal distention with absent bowel sounds. Central nervous system involvement may manifest as irritability, lethargy, poor suckling, hypotonia, or hypertonia. A history of delayed cord separation may be present in LAD syndrome.

In advanced cases, the infant may present with septic shock or necrotising fasciitis (NF). NF is a severe complication of omphalitis that should be considered if the local signs have progressed to include a peau d'orange appearance, discolouration or bruising of the skin, skin necrosis, and crepitation.

Differential Diagnoses

The differential diagnoses of omphalitis (and specific features of each) include:

- umbilical granuloma (visible granuloma at the umbilicus);

- patent vitello-intestinal duct remnants (cystic swelling or fistulous opening with feculent matter discharging);

- patent urachus (fistulous opening with urine discharging) or urachal cyst;

- necrotising enterocolitis (abdominal distention, bilious vomiting, bloody stools);

- general sepsis; and

- rarely, appendiculo-omphalic anomalies.

Investigations

A microbiological swab of the umbilicus should be sent for aerobic and anaerobic cultures. A blood culture should be included when appropriate. A blood count with differential for white cell counts may show a neutrohilia (or occasionally a neutropaenia).

Other investigations are necessary either to rule out other differential diagnoses or to diagnose complications. Diagnostics may include the following:

- A plain abdominal radiograph is useful if necrotising enterocolitis is suspected. In addition, it may reveal intraperitoneal gas in those with peritonitis (caused by gas-producing bacteria). Multiple fluid levels may suggest adhesion obstruction but may also be present in simple ileus. Gas may be present within the subcutaneous tissue of the abdominal wall when clostridial infection is involved.

- Abdominal ultrasonography is useful in imaging the abdominal wall if a cyst is suspected It is helpful in the diagnosis of intraperitoneal, retroperitoneal, and hepatic abscesses.

- Dopplar ultrasonography is helpful if portal vein thrombosis is suspected.

- A fistulogram is indicated if a fistulous connection to the umbilicus is discovered. This will help define the anatomy of a vitello-intestinal or urachal remnant.

- Rarely, magnetic resonance imaging (MRI) or a computed tomography (CT) scan may be useful in assessing or ruling out congenital tracts or fistulas. Also rarely, a CT scan may be necessary to adequately localise intraabdominal abscesses in difficult diagnostic cases.

Medical Treatment

Treatment of uncomplicated cases requires prompt antibiotic therapy. Antibiotics are the mainstay of medical treatment of omphalitis. Antibiotics specifically active against *Staphylococcus aureus* and an aminoglycoside to cover for both gram-positive and gram-negative organisms are used. The local antibiotic susceptibility patterns need to be considered in the initial therapy. Examples include ampiclox, cloxacillin, flucloxacillin, and methicillin in combination with gentamycin. Metronidazole may be added when anaerobes are suspected. Duration of treatment is typically for 10–14 days with initial parenteral therapy for complicated cases. A short antibiotic therapy of 7 days is adequate for simple uncomplicated omphalitis.

Complications such as respiratory failure, hypotension, and disseminated intravascular coagulation (DIC) arising from infection may require supportive care in the form of intravenous fluids, fresh whole blood, fresh frozen plasma, platelets, or cryoprecipitate.

Treatment of Surgical Complications

The surgical complications of omphalitis could be acute/early or long term/late and tend to be associated with significant morbidity and mortality. In addition to medical treatment for ongoing/active omphalitis, the surgical treatment is handled according to the surgical complication.

Necrotising Fasciitis

Necrotising fasciitis is one of the most commonly reported serious complications of omphalitis,[1,8–12] occurring in 26% of patients with major complications, according to one report.[6] It has been noted to occur in 13.5% of neonates with omphalitis.[8] The condition starts initially as periumbilical cellulitis, which, without treatment, progresses rapidly to necrosis of the skin and subcutaneous tissue (Figures 20.2 and 20.3), and in some instances,

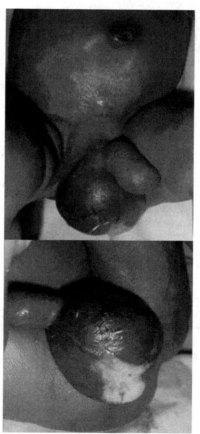

Figure 20.2: Periumbilical cellulitis with early necrosis of scrotal skin.

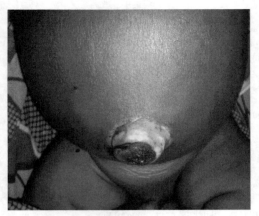

Figure 20.3: Early necrotising fasciitis beginning at the umbilicus.

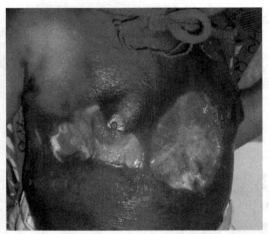

Figure 20.4: Advanced necrotising fasciitis involving upper abdominal and lower chest wall.

myonecrosis. The scrotum is the most commonly affected by NF,[7] but the abdominal wall may also be involved (Figure 20.4). If treated early, peri-umbilical cellulitis can be controlled by use of parenteral broad-spectrum antibiotics. The antibiotic regime should always include an antianaerobe (e.g., metronidazole).

NF should be treated by prompt debridement, removing all dead and dying tissues, followed by daily dressing of the wound. If the baby is too ill for a general anaesthetic, the debridement can be performed by the bedside (using parenteral paracetamol or rectal paracetamol for analgesia). The resulting wound will later require secondary closure (or skin grafting if the defect is large). However, scrotal wounds may heal well without secondary closure or skin grafting.[13]

Evisceration

Intestinal evisceration is another frequently reported serious complication (Figure 20.5).[7] The eviscerated intestine is usually loops of small intestine, but large intestine may be involved. Rarely, presentation may be late, and the eviscerated intestine may be gangrenous.[7]

The eviscerated intestine should be covered by clean moist gauze, and placed in an intestinal bag (a transparent plastic bag will do if there is no intestinal bag available). Care should be taken to ensure that the intestine is not twisted.

Under general anaesthetic, the eviscerated intestine is cleaned and returned to the peritoneal cavity and the umbilicus repaired. If the umbilical defect is narrow, it may require extension in the transverse plane. In the presence of features of peritonitis or intestinal gangrene, a formal laparotomy needs to be done to drain any abscesses and clean the peritoneal cavity. Gangrenous intestine needs to be resected and intestinal continuity restored.

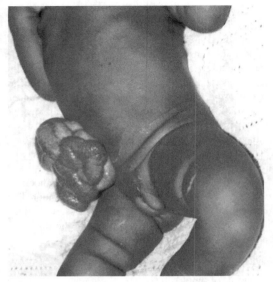

Figure 20.5: Intestinal evisceration from omphalitis.

Peritonitis

Peritonitis may occur with or without intraperitoneal abscess collection. In the absence of an abscess, the infection could resolve with use of broad-spectrum intravenous antibiotics alone, and surgery is usually not required.

If an intraperitoneal abscess is confirmed by ultrasound, or there is no facility for ultrasonography, then laparotomy is required. Any abscess is drained and the peritoneal cavity thoroughly cleaned.

Abscesses

Abscesses may develop at various sites, but are frequently intraab-dominal. Intraperitoneal abscess is drained at laparotomy. Retroperitoneal abscess[14] is best drained by an extraperitoneal approach, but if located ante-riorly in the retroperitoneal, an intraperitoneal approach may be required. Hepatic abscess should be properly localised by ultrasonography or CT scan. The abscess is aspirated by a wide-bore needle under imaging guid-ance, and the abscess cavity is irrigated with normal saline. This can be repeated once more if it recollects. In difficult cases, or in recurrence after needle aspiration, open drainage may be required. If the abscess is multiple, parenteral antibiotics alone may suffice, and aspiration/drainage reserved for persistent cases. Abscesses may be located in the anterior abdominal wall or in other superficial locations. These would require drainage.

Late Complications

Late complications occur several weeks, months, or years after ompha-litis in the neonatal period.

Portal Vein Thrombosis

Portal vein thrombosis (PVT) is a complication with serious conse-quences. Although an early complication, the major consequences produced are in the long term. In one report of 200 patients undergoing portosystemic shunt for portal hypertension due to PVT,[15] 15% of the PVT was suspected to be the result of neonatal omphalitis. The throm-bosis may produce a carvernoma, which can cause biliary obstruction.[16]

A portosystemic shunt may be required if portal hypertension develops.[15] Biliary obstruction is treated on its merit.

Umbilical Hernia

Umbilical hernia is a common problem in children in Africa, and several are the result of weakening of the umbilical cicatrix from neonatal omphalitis. The management of these hernias is discussed in Chapter 57.

Peritoneal Adhesions

Peritoneal adhesions are the result of previous subclinical or treated peritonitis from omphalitis. The adhesions may produce intestinal obstruction, which usually is not amenable to nonoperative measures. Laparotomy and lysis/excision of the adhesions are usually required. Any ischaemic intestinal segment needs to be resected.

Prognosis and Outcome

Promptly treated uncomplicated omphalitis usually resolves without serious morbidity. However, when presentation and treatment are delayed, mortality could be high, reaching 7–15%.[1,7,13,17]

Serious morbidity and mortality may occur from complications such as NF, peritonitis, and evisceration.[6] Portal vein thrombosis may be fatal.[18] Mortality may reach 38–87% following NF and myonecrosis.[1,19,20] Also, certain risk factors such as prematurity, small size for gestational age, male sex, and septic delivery are associated with poor prognosis.

Prevention

The incidence of omphalitis is low in well-resourced countries and for those born in hospital. For these, there is probably little benefit of prophylactic measures to reduce the incidence. In developing countries, and especially after home birth, however, the incidence is high enough to consider prophylaxis to prevent the morbidity and mortality associated with late presentation of the disease. Access to proper maternity and delivery services helps reduce the incidence.

Teaching safe cord-care practice to mothers as well as using traditional birth attendants and primary-care workers are of utmost importance in the prevention of omphalitis in Africa. Vigilance is also important to identify major complications and refer patients early for prompt intervention. In most African hospital settings, methylated spirit and gentian violet are commonly used for cord care. In other parts of the world, betadine, bacitracin, silver sulfadiazine, or triple dye is recommended. Currently, not using any medicinal washes on the cord but just simply allowing the cord to dry and fall off is being advocated in developed parts of the world. There is little data to support any one cord care or lack thereof over the other.

In one report, a simple clean delivery kit produced by the United Nations Population Fund (UNFPA) was found to reduce cord infections.1 Babies of mothers who did not use the kit were 13 times more likely to develop cord infection than babies of mothers who used the kit. The same report also noted that babies of mothers who did not bathe before delivery were 3.9 times more likely to develop cord infection than babies of mothers who bathed.

Evidence-Based Research

Table 20.1 presents an overview of an evidence-based study on early antisepsis with chlorhexidine.

Table 20.1: Evidence-based research.

Title	Topical applications of chlorhexidine to the umbilical cord for prevention of omphalitis and neonatal mortality in southern Nepal: a community-based, cluster-randomised trial
Authors	Mullany LC, Darmstadt GL, Khatry SK, Katz J, LeClerq SC, Shrestha S, Adhikari R, Tielsch JM
Institution	Johns Hopkins Bloomberg School of Public Health, Baltimore, Maryland, USA
Reference [21]	Lancet 2006; 367(9514):910–918
Problem	Omphalitis contributes to neonatal morbidity and mortality in developing countries. Umbilical cord cleansing with antiseptics might reduce infection and mortality risk, but has not been rigorously investigated.
Intervention	In this community-based, cluster-randomised trial, 413 communities in Sarlahi, Nepal, were randomly assigned to one of three cord-care regimens: 4,934 infants were assigned to 4.0% chlorhexidine, 5,107 to cleansing with soap and water, and 5,082 to dry cord care.
Comparison/ control (quality of evidence)	Cluster-randomised control study
Outcome/effect	The frequency of omphalitis was reduced significantly in the chlorhexidine group. Severe omphalitis in chlorhexidine clusters was reduced by 75% (incidence rate ratio, 0.25, 95% CI 0.12-0.53; 13 infections/4839 neonatal periods) compared with dry cord-care clusters (52/4930). Neonatal mortality was 24% lower in the chlorhexidine group (relative risk, 0.76 [95% CI 0.55-1.04]) than in the dry cord-care group. Within the first 24 hours, mortality was significantly reduced by 34% in the chlorhexidine group (0.66 [0.46-0.95])
Historical significance/ comments	Early antisepsis with chlorhexidine of the umbilical cord reduces local cord infections and overall neonatal mortality

Key Summary Points

1. Omphalitis is a common problem in resource-limited settings and is related to unhygienic cord practices.

2. Although a simple infection, life-threatening complications may occur if presentation and treatment are delayed.

3. Prompt recognition of complications and treatment is necessary to avoid morbidity and mortality.

4. Omphalitis is easily preventable by clean and safe delivery and cord-care practices.

References

1. Gallagher PG, Shah SS. Omphalitis: Overview. Available at http://emedicine.medscape.com/article/975422-overview (accessed 15 December 2008).

2. Sawardekar KP. Changing spectrum of neonatal omphalitis. Pediatr Infect Dis J 2004; 23:22–26.

3. Mullany LC, Darmstadt GL, Katz J, et al. Risk factors for umbilical cord infection among newborns of southern Nepal. Am J Epidemiol 2007; 165:203–211.

4. Simiyu DE. Morbidity and mortality of neonates admitted in general paediatric wards at Kenyatta National Hospital. East Afr Med J 2003; 80:611–616.

5. McClure EM, Goldenberg RL, Brandes N, Darmstadt GL, Wright LL. The use of chlorheidene to reduce maternal and neonatal mortality and morbidity in low-income settings. Int J Gynaecol Obstet 2007; 97:89–94.

6. Winani S, Wood S, Coffey P, Chirwa T, Mosha F, Changalucha J. Use of clean delivery kit and factors associated with cord infection and puerperal sepsis in Mwanza, Tanzania. J Midwifery Womens Health 2007; 52:37–43.

7. Ameh EA, Nmadu PT. Major complications of omphalitis in neonates and infants. Pediatr Surg Int 2002; 18:413–416.

8. Moss RL, Musemeche CA, Kosloske AM. Necrotizing fasciitis in children: prompt recognition and aggressive therapy improve survival. J Pediatr Surg 1996; 31:1142–1146.

9. Samuel M, Freeman V, Vaishnav A, Sajwany MJ, Nyar MP. Necrotizing fasciitis: a serious complication of omphalitis in neonates. J Pediatr Surg 1994; 29:1414–1416.

10. Lally KP, Atkinson JB, Woolley MM, Mahour GH. Necrotizing fasciitis: a serious sequel of omphalitis in the newborn. Am Surg 1984; 199:101–103.

11. Kosloske AM, Cushing AH, Borden TA, et al. Cellulitis and necrotizing fasciitis of the abdominal wall in paediatric patients. J Pediatr Surg 1981; 16:246–251.

12. Owa JA, Oyelami OA, Adejuyigbe O. Periumbilical cellulitis in Nigerian neonates. Cent Afr J Med 1992; 38:40–43.

13. Ameh EA, Dauda MM, Sabiu L, Mshelbwala PM, Mbibu HN, Nmadu PT. Fournier's gangrene in neonates and infants. Eur J Pediatr Surg 2004; 14:418–421.

14. Feo CF, Dessanti A, Franco B, Ganau A, Iannaccelli M. Retroperitoneal abscess and omphalitits in young infants. Acta Paediatr 2003; 92:122–125.

15. Orloff MJ, Orloff MS, Girard B, Orloff SL. Bleeding esophageal varices from extrahepatic portal hypertension: 40 years experience with portal-systemic shunt. J Am Coll Surg 2002; 194:717–730.

16. Perlemuter G, Bejanin H, Fritsch J, et al. Biliary obstruction caused by portal cavernoma: a study of 8 cases. J Hepatol 1996; 25:58–63.

17. Güvenc H, Güvene M, Yenioğlu H, Ayata A, Kokabay K, Bektas S. Neonatal omphalitis is still common in Eastern Turkey. Scand J Infect Dis 1991; 23:613–616.

18. Debes NM, Dahl M, Jonso F. Omphalitis with fatal outcome in new-born baby boy [abstract]. Ugeskr Laeger 2008; 170:158.

19. Airede AI. Pathogens in neonatal omphalitis. J Trop Pediatr 1992; 38:129–131.

20. Fraser N, Davies BW, Cusack J. Neonatal omphalitis: a review of its serious complications. Acta Paediatr 2006; 95:519–522.

CHAPTER 21
NECROTISING FASCIITIS

Jacob N. Legbo
Emmanuel A. Ameh

Introduction

The term necrotising fasciitis (NF) was first coined in 1952 by Wilson[1] to describe a rapidly progressive inflammation and necrosis of subcutaneous tissues and the deep layer of superficial fascia with sparing of the deep fascia and muscle. It had previously been described variously as haemolytic gangrene, acute streptococcal gangrene, gangrenous erysipelas, necrotising erysipelas, suppurative fasciitis, and hospital gangrene, among other names.[2,3] However, the term necrotising fasciitis is now used in a generic sense to include all diffuse necrotising soft tissue infections except gas gangrene (clostridial myonecrosis).[4] Diffuse necrotising soft tissue infections include classic gas gangrene, Meleney's haemolytic streptococcal gangrene, necrotising fasciitis as described by Wilson, and the gram-negative synergistic necrotising cellulitis of Stone. Generally, one condition cannot be distinguished from another at the time of diagnosis. Today, the orofacial form of NF is called cancrum oris (noma),[5] and the perineal form is called Fournier's gangrene. Idiopathic scrotal gangrene, however, is different in aetiology, extent, and clinical presentation from Fournier's gangrene.[4]

NF poses a serious surgical challenge not only because of its rapid and progressive nature, but also because of its attending high morbidity and mortality.[6,7]

Demographics

There is a general paucity of literature, particularly in Africa, on the exact incidence of NF, although one hospital-based report suggests two to three children are seen in most major tertiary health institutions every year; that report, however, excluded cancrum oris and Fournier's gangrene.[8] There had been reports of cases in Europe and North America, especially during World War II, but more recent reports are from the developing countries of Africa, Asia, and South America.[6,8–11] There is no gender or age preference, but studies would suggest that the trunk and the head and neck are more frequently involved in children.[8,12]

Pathology

Aetiology

Although NF may start spontaneously in apparently normal children, it is most often associated with pathological conditions related to impaired host response leading to lowered immunity.[3–8,13] Some recognised predisposing factors include:

1. *Debilitating state*, such as anaemia and malnutrition, for which protein and vitamin B deficiencies appear predominant in importance. Other conditions, such as obesity (Figure 21.1), diabetes mellitus, and cancer, play greater roles in adults than children. In recent years, human immunodeficiency virus/ acquired immune deficiency syndrome (HIV/ AIDS) is becoming increasingly significant.

2. *Trauma (or specific infection)*, such as needle pricks, skin abrasions, punctures, lacerations, or friction on cheek mucosa by an abnormally positioned tooth, could sometimes be trivial and go unnoticed. Occasionally, the trauma could be severe, such as those following road traffic accidents. NF can complicate such surgical procedures as colostomy (Figure 21.2), appendectomy, herniotomy,

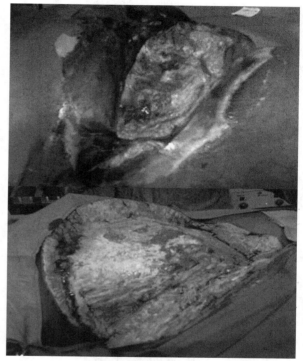

Figure 21.1: NF involving the anterolateral trunk and thigh in a 14-year-old obese but otherwise previously normal girl (before and after the first debridement). Note the relatively unaffected abdominal wall muscles.

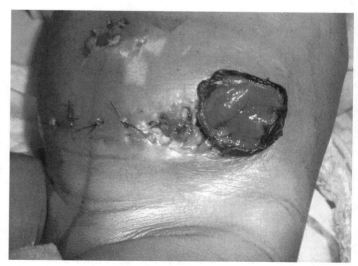

Figure 21.2: Necrotising fasciitis following colostomy.

Table 21.1: Clinical (pathophysiological) stages and features of NF.

Clinical stage	Pathology	Clinical features
I	Acute inflammation	Pain and tenderness in affected area
		Oedema and shininess (hyeraemia in light-skinned) of affected area
		Systemic features (fever, anaemia)
II	Progressive necrosis of skin and subcutaneous tissue	Discharge of infected fluid/pus (may be offensive)
		Necrosis and sloughing of affected area, resulting in tissue defects
		Systemic features may appear
III	Healing and tissue repair	Disappearance of acute inflammatory features
		Appearance of granulation tissue
		Gradual healing of affected area
IV	Maturation and contraction of scar	Contractures
		Disfigurement

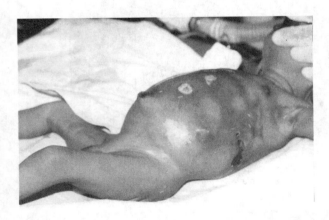

Figure 21.3: Inflammatory phase of necrotising fasciitis.

laparotomy, or dental extraction; or it can follow infections such as chicken pox, gingivitis, boil, or perineal abscess.[9,13–15]

3. General illness could be in the form of malaria or measles, especially in developing countries.

Microbiology

Necrotising fasciitis could result from a variety of microorganisms, particularly bacteria and occasionally fungi. Initially thought to be caused mainly by non-group-A beta-haemolytic streptococci, there is now enough evidence that NF results mostly from synergy between gram-positive cocci (such as non-group-A beta-haemolytic streptococci and staphylococci) and gram-negative organisms such as *Bacteroides fragilis,* peptostreptococci, *Proteus* sp., *Pseudomonas* sp., or *Enterobacter* sp.[3,4,16,17] Much less common is a pure group-A streptococcal infection. Anaerobic bacteria may also be involved, although

often not cultured. Vincent's organisms and bacteroides are commonly isolated in noma. Recently described are new varieties of NF caused by *Photobacterium damsela;*[18] halophilic marine vibrios, especially *Vibrio fulnificus;*[19,20] and phycomycoses, especially *Rhizopus arrhizus*[21] and *Cryptococcus neophormans.*[22] Approximately 70–80% of NF is polymicrobial.

Pathophysiology

Aerobic pathogens are usually the primary tissue invaders. They destroy tissues and create an anaerobic environment conducive for anaerobic or microaerophilic organisms, which are secondary invaders.[2,3,7,13] The primary pathogens produce exotoxins, such as streptolysin, streptodornase, streptokinase, and many other proteases and cholagenases, which result in extensive tissue destruction and necrosis. The infection is commonly polymicrobial and synergistic, and the resultant damage is usually more extensive than that attributable to any individual pathogen.[2,3] Most bacteria, especially facultative gram-negative rods such as *E. coli,* produce insoluble gases whenever subjected to anaerobic metabolism.[4] Because human tissue cannot survive in an anaerobic environment, gas associated with infection implies the presence of dead tissues.

Streptococcal NF associated with toxic shock syndrome (StrepTSS) has been on the increase in the past two decades and is observed in previously normal children. Caused by a highly invasive strain of group-A streptococcus, the pathogenesis is related to streptococcal pyrogenic exotoxins (SPE) produced by specific strains of *Streptococcus pyogenes.*[23]

Natural History (Clinical Stages)

The different pathophysiological stages observed (Table 21.1) include inflammation (stage I), necrosis (stage II), repair (stage III), and sequelae (stage IV).[2,3,7,13]

Inflammation (stage I)

The prominent feature of NF is the stage of acute inflammation and results from the effects of the exotoxins, which lead to the release of cytokines, with local and systemic effects.[4,23] The local features are mainly those of hyperaemia (or shiny skin), oedema (Figure 21.3) and pain. Systemic toxaemia commonly results in death if appropriate resuscitative measures are not put in place. The process can be arrested at this stage if appropriate antibiotics are given early.

Necrosis (stage II)

Tissue destruction results either from the direct effect of the enzymes or from vascular thrombosis involving the nutrient vessels serving the area. There is enough evidence to suggest that stages I and II may occur simultaneously in most cases.[2,3] In addition, tissue oedema that results from inflammation could increase the pressure within the tight fascial compartment, further reducing blood supply to the tissues in the area. This destruction is rapidly progressive and could occur within 3–5 days. Extensive subcutaneous/fascial necrosis may proceed with minimal skin involvement, giving rise to significant undermining. Although rare in NF, true muscle necrosis occurs in patients with StrepTSS.[23] This condition, known as gangrenous streptococcal myositis, is similar to clostridial myonecrosis (gas gangrene) but differs from it in the absence of gas in the tissues.[4]

Repair (stage III)

Healing takes place by rejection of the slough, appearance of healthy granulation tissue, and, subsequently, scar tissue formation.

Sequelae (stage IV)

Disfigurement, contractures and trismus may result from tissue loss and scar formation after months to years if no appropriate preventive measures are taken.

Complications

Common complications that may be encountered include:

1. compartment syndrome, leading to Volkmann's ischaemia, Volkmann's ischaemic contracture, or gangrene;

2. septic arthritis or osteomyelitis;

3. septicaemia and multiple organ failure syndrome;

4. herniation of intraabdominal organs;

5. joint stiffness; and

6. contractures and trismus.

Clinical Presentation

A high index of suspicion is required to ensure prompt recognition and early treatment of NF. In the past, a significant number of affected children died at home at the stage of inflammation as a result of toxaemia, before getting to the hospital. With the advent of antibiotics, a significant number of these children are now seen in hospitals (Figure 21.4). Most studies report a slight male preponderance, but any age group can be affected, including neonates and older children. In some studies, up to 40% of these children have malnutrition.[8,13]

The clinical presentation depends on the stage of NF at the time of presentation (see Table 21.1). The commonly encountered symptoms include pain, swelling, and fever. Although severe local pain that is out of proportion to the size and type of wound is a hallmark of NF in older children, this might be difficult to elucidate in neonates.

At the initial stages of cellulitis (inflammation), examination will reveal features of toxaemia, including elevated temperature (or hypothermia in neonates), oedema, hyperaemia, crepitus, tachycardia, and hypotension. Blebs and blisters may precede the appearance of dark skin patches (Figures 21.1, 21.4, and 21.5) that signify tissue necrosis, usually with severe undermining. Late presentation is common in Africa, and some patients are seen when the necrotic part of the skin, subcutaneous tissues, and fascia come out together as a complete cast from a limb (Figure 21.5). This exposes the underlying muscle(s), tendon(s), or teeth and oral cavity in the case of the cheek. Occasionally, some children are seen with structural deformities as a result of improper management of the earlier stages of the disease.

The clinical presentation of *Vibrio* NF is similar to classical NF and even more similar to streptococcal gangrene, which occurs in children with minor wounds exposed to seawater or sustained while cleaning seafood. In contrast, the clinical presentation of mycotic NF is insidious. On the other extreme are patients with StrepTSS, who present with rapid progression of the disease due to the high virulence of the offending organisms.[23]

Investigations

The diagnosis of NF is mainly clinical, but the following investigations are relevant.

Microbiologic Cultures

Any discharge or swab from the wound should be cultured (aerobic and anaerobic) to help in identifying the bacteria profile of the disease. Culture of tissue taken from the wound may provide a better yield, especially for anaerobes.

In patients with systemic features, blood culture should also be done.

Imaging

It is important to emphasize that imaging studies should be undertaken only in children in whom the diagnosis of NF is not clear cut, as they may delay surgical intervention and frequently provide conflicting information.[4]

Plain radiographs may show gas within the tissues at the initial stages of the disease, but they are rarely necessary.

Magnetic resonance imaging (MRI), where readily available, could assist in defining tissue planes and the presence of microabscesses.

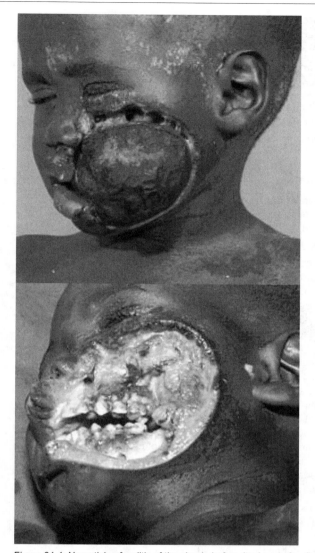

Figure 21.4: Necrotising fasciitis of the cheek, before (top) and after (bottom) removal of necrotic soft tissues.

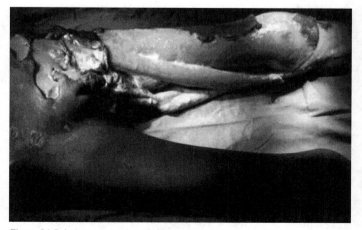

Figure 21.5: Late presentation of NF in a 9-year-old boy. Here, the necrotic skin, subcutaneous fat, and fascia came off like a full cast, exposing the underlying muscles, which are relatively uninvolved.

Complete Blood Count

A haemogram should be ascertained; white cell count may indicate leucocytosis.

Exclusion of Underlying Illness

Any underlying or predisposing illness should be excluded; often, this may involve HIV testing, blood film for malaria parasites, haemoglobin electrophoresis for sickle cell disease, and blood sugar to exclude diabetes mellitus. Doing any of these tests should be guided by clinical suspicion.

Treatment

Resuscitation

Correction of depletion

It is important to correct any existing physiological derangements, such as fluid and electrolyte imbalance. Blood transfusion may be necessary to correct anaemia.

Antibiotics and antimicrobials

The initial choice of parenteral antibiotics should take cognizance of the polymicrobial nature of the disease, previous knowledge of the microbiology of NF, and local sensitivity patterns.[24] This should be broad-based and must take control of gram-negative, gram-positive, aerobic, and anaerobic microorganisms. Combinations of penicillins, aminoglycosides, and metronidazole (or cephalosporins with metronidazole) have been found useful in most studies.[2-4,6-12] Some reports have found the use of quinolones equally effective in the treatment of NF;[25] others, however, have avoided it because of the potential effect on the growth plate of bones in young children, although this risk is now considered quite minimal.[8]

In severe cases with systemic toxaemia, as in StrepTSS, intravenous human immunoglobulin has been found useful in neutralising the exotoxin already present in the system. Intravenous amphotericin B may be administered if the presence of hyphae on gram stain or on histologic section suggests phycomycotic NF.[4]

Analgesia

In the early stage and when pain is a prominent symptom, appropriate analgesics should be given. This will facilitate wound care and also help in preventing later joint stiffness.

Tetanus prophylaxis

Tetanus immunisation (both active and passive) will be necessary in most African settings.

Nutritional support

Appropriate nutritional support should be provided, especially for those patients who are malnourished.

Surgical Intervention

Fasciotomy

Even in the absence of obvious tissue necrosis, fasciotomy in the form of single or multiple linear incision(s) over the affected area may be necessary to achieve adequate compartmental decompression. Thorough wound irrigation with antiseptics such as hydrogen peroxide or cetrimide and warm normal saline, then gentle packing with gauze in EUSOL (hypochlorite solution) or natural honey helps to control local infection and halts progression of the disease. At the time of fasciotomy, partial wound approximation could be effected without tension by using sutures, rubber bands, or special devices. About 5–7 days after fasciotomy, when oedema would have subsided and infection is reasonably controlled, skin closure could be achieved directly or by skin grafting.

Debridement

Prompt, adequate and sequential debridement of all necrotic tissues (see Figure 21.1) is of utmost importance in arresting progression of tissue necrosis in NF.[2-4,6-12] Adequate arrangements for possible blood transfusion should be made during such necrosectomies, as this exercise may be attended by blood loss that could be significant to the child, especially the neonate.

Debridement may be done by the bedside in very ill patients who are poor anaesthetic risks, especially neonates.

Wound resurfacing

Significant wound contraction could occur following adequate wound care, especially on the face, trunk, and perineum; the final mode of wound closure also depends on the initial size, however. Smaller wounds may contract adequately to heal by secondary intention or require direct suturing, whereas larger but granulating wounds will require skin grafting. In the event of three-dimensional tissue loss (such as check, lip, nose), or exposure of bare surfaces (tendon, bone, nerve, or blood vessels), local, regional, or distant flap reconstruction will be required.[6,8,12,26]

Rehabilitation

Rehabilitation efforts are directed at preserving the child's physical function and supporting the child emotionally through the use of activity. The pain of the local infection may cause the patient to voluntarily immobilise affected areas of the body, so both passive and active movements should be encouraged as soon as pain and other preconditions allow.

As the wounds heal, prevention of deformity by minimising the effects of joint stiffness or scar contracture should take priority. Accordingly, appropriate splint(s) should be applied when and where indicated. The goal is to attain a position that opposes the forces of contracture, provide safe joint alignment, and maintain tendon balance without causing stretch or pressure injuries to the peripheral nerves or skin.

Role of Hyperbaric Oxygen

As in clostridial myonecrosis (gas gangrene), the use of hyperbaric oxygen in NF is still controversial. Although experimental results in animals appear promising, its usefulness is less specific in NF than gas gangrene following clinical trials in humans.[4]

Treatment of Underlying Condition

Any identified underlying or predisposing condition should be treated appropriately. This treatment must be simultaneous with treatment of the NF to avoid relentless progression of the latter.

Prognosis and Outcome

Factors that may affect outcome and prognosis are the following:

- age (neonates fare poorly);
- overall general condition of the patient at presentation;
- pre- or co-morbid conditions;
- virulence of the offending organisms versus host immunity; and
- promptness/aggressiveness of resuscitative, surgical, and supportive forms of therapy.

Despite the aggressive use of antibiotics and surgical intervention, morbidity and mortality following NF remain very high.[2-4,6-12] Mortality rates range from 20% to 80%, but are frequently between 60% and 80%. Death results commonly from overwhelming infection and multiple organ failure. Those who survive are faced with a prolonged hospital stay and multiple surgical and reconstructive procedures, with their anaesthetic and socioeconomic implications.[26]

Prevention

Necrotising fasciitis is largely a preventable disease,[26,27] but prevention will involve a multidisciplinary commitment and action by individuals, health personnel, and policy makers. Preventive measures involve:

- good oral and general body hygiene;

- prevention and control of malnutrition;

- prevention of all childhood immunisable diseases, such as measles, through national mass immunisation programmes; and

- education on early recognition and treatment of NF.

Evidence-Based Research

Table 21.2 presents a study of treatment of necrotising fasciitis in children in Africa during a four-year period. Table 21.3 presents a study of the advantages of early recognition and prompt treatment of NF in children.

Table 21.2: Evidence-based research.

Title	Necrotising fasciitis: experience with 32 children
Authors	Legbo JN, Shehu BB
Institution	Department of Surgery, Usmanu Danfodiyo University Teaching Hospital, Sokoto, Nigeria
Reference	Ann Trop Paediatr 2005; 25:183–189
Problem	Presentation and outcome of treatment of NF in children.
Intervention	Wound debridement, direct wound suturing, skin grafting, local flap reconstruction, antibiotics.
Comparison/ control (quality of evidence)	In the four-year period of this study, 32 of 56 patients (57.1%) treated with NF were children aged 6 days to 12 years (mean, 2 years). The common presenting features were pain (84.4%), fever (78.1%), irritability (40.6%), and tissue necrosis with undermining and surrounding cellulitis/oedema (100%). Three patients (9.4%) presented with moderate to severe jaundice, and 13 (40.6%) were malnourished according to clinical, anthropometric, and laboratory measures. Precipitating factors included pustules/boils in 12 (37.5%) patients, intravenous scalp cannulation in 3 (9.4%), trauma in 2 (6.3%), and colostomy in 1 (3.2%). In 14 patients (43.8%), no factors could be identified. Duration of symptoms ranged from 3 to 19 days (mean, 6.4 days). The involved body surface area ranged from 2% to 16% (mean, 5.9%). The trunk was the most frequently involved (50%), followed by the head/neck (28.1%), upper limbs (21.9%), lower limbs (6.3%), and perineum (6.3%). Bacteria identified by aerobic culture included Staphylococcus aureus in 23 (71.9%) patients, streptococci in 19 (59.4%), Escherichia coli in 15 (46.9%), Pseudomonas aeruginosa in 12 (37.5%), and Klebsiella pneumoniae in 8 (25%). In 21 (65.6%) patients, infection was polymicrobial, and in 3 (9.4%), no organism was cultured. Anaerobic and fungal cultures were not undertaken routinely. Routine HIV screening (enzyme-linked immunosorbent assay, or ELISA) of all patients was negative.
Outcome/ effect	Septicaemia was the commonest complication, occurring in 71.9%, and mortality was 9.4%. Hospital stay was long, at a mean of 27.6 days (range, 14–96 days).
Historical significance/ comments	This is one of the occasional reports of NF in children in Africa including a large number of patients. The exclusion of children with cancrum oris and Fournier's gangrene means that the number could have been even higher. The study has shown that although NF is thought to be rare in children, it is more common than expected in the sub-Saharan African setting and carries a high morbidity and mortality. This report provides a good insight into the clinical profile of this condition in the African setting.

Table 21.3: Evidence-based research.

Title	Necrotising fasciitis in children: prompt recognition and aggressive therapy improve survival
Authors	Moss LR, Musemeche CA, Kosloske AM
Institution	University of New Mexico, School of Medicine, Albuquerque, New Mexico, USA; Ohio State University School of Medicine, Columbus, Ohio, USA
Reference	J Pediatr Surg 1996; 31:1142–1146
Problem	Recognition and treatment of NF in children.
Intervention	Surgical debridement, below-knee amputation, colostomy, primary wound closure, split skin grafting.
Result	A total of 20 children with NF were treated over a period of 18 years. The disease was observed in a wide variety of clinical settings covering the entire paediatric age range. Characteristics suggestive of diagnosis included marked tissue oedema, which was uniformly present, and almost all sites had a characteristic peau d'orange appearance. Bulla, petechiae, skin necrosis, and crepitus are strongly suggestive of NF, but these were present in only a few cases. Nineteen of the 20 patients were healthy before onset of the illness. White blood cell counts were not sensitive or specific in establishing diagnosis. Bacteriology was variable, as both aerobic and anaerobic bacteria were isolated. An average of 3.8 surgical debridements were required for each patient (range, 1–15). The surgical findings were typical. The subcutaneous tissue was grey and nonbleeding, with a watery discharge. The fascia ranged from viable to necrotic, depending on the severity of infection. The skin was viable early in the course of these cases. Skin necrosis was a late sign. Failure to gain local control of the infection before systemic organ failure from sepsis proved uniformly fatal. All patients who had positive blood cultures, renal failure, adult respiratory distress syndrome, or disseminated intravascular coagulation died.
Outcome/ effect	Mortality was 25%. The 15 survivors all underwent aggressive surgical debridement within 3 hours of admission, whereas the 5 who died all had inadequate initial management.
Historical significance/ comments	This report has shown that early recognition and prompt institution of treatment gives good survival in this rapidly progressive disease. It also emphasizes the differences between NF in children as compared to adults.

Key Summary Points

1. NF is generally not common but does appear more common in children in sub-Saharan Africa than previously thought.

2. NF is frequently polymicrobial.

3. Presentation varies widely from simple cellulitis to toxic shock.

4. Success in treatment depends on prompt resuscitation, adequate surgical debridement(s), and adequate supportive therapy.

5. NF is associated with high morbidity (complications, multiple surgeries, prolonged hospital stay) and high mortality.

References

1. Wilson B. Necrotizing fasciitis. Am Surg 1952; 18:416.

2. Howard R J, Pesa M E, Brennaman B H, Ramphal R. Necrotizing soft tissue infections caused by marine vibrios. Surgery 1985; 98:126.

3. Archampong EQ. Microbial infections in surgery. In: Badoe EA, Archampong EQ, da Rocha-Afodu JT, eds. Principles and Practice of Surgery Including Pathology in the Tropics. Assemblies of God Literature Centre, 2000, Pp 11–40.

4. Lewis RT. Soft tissue infections. World J Surg 1998; 22:146–151.

5. Enwonwu CO, Falkler WA, Idigbe EO, Savage KO. Noma (cancrum oris): questions and answers. Oral Dis 1999; 5:144–149.

6. Ogundiron TO, Akutte OO, Oluwatosin OO. Necrotizing fasciitis. Trop Doct 2004; 34:175–178.

7. Moss RL, Musemeche CA, Kosloske AM. Necrotizing fasciitis in children: prompt recognition and aggressive therapy improve survival. J Pediatr Surg 1996; 31:1142–1146.

8. Legbo JN, Shehu BB. Necrotizing fasciitis: experience with 32 children. Ann Trop Paediatr 2005; 25:183–189.

9. Mshelbwala PM, Sabiu L, Ameh EA. Necrotizing fasciitis of the perineum complicating ischiorectal abscess in childhood. Ann Trop Paediatr 2002; 23:227–228.

10. Adigun IA, Abdulrahman LO. Necrotizing fasciitis in a plastic surgery unit: a report of ten patients from Ilorin. Niger J Surg Res 2004; 6:21–24.

11. Sachdev A, Seth S. Necrotizing fasciitis. Indian Pediatr 2004; 41:623.

12. Legbo JN, Shehu BB. Necrotizing fasciitis: a comparative analysis of 56 cases. J Natl Med Assoc 2005; 97:1692–1697.

13. Enwonwu CO, Falkler WA, Idigbe EO, Afolabi BM, Ibrahim M, Onwujekwe D, Savage O, Meeks VI. Pathogenesis of cancrum oris (noma): confounding interactions of malnutrition with infection. Am J Med Med Hyg 1999; 60:223–232.

14. Vijaykumar, Rao PS, Bhat N, Chattopadhyay A, Nagendhar MY. Necrotizing fasciitis with chickenpox. Indian J Pediatr 2003; 70:961–963.

15. Waldhusen JHT, Holterman MJ, Sawin RS. Surgical implications of necrotizing fasciitis in children with chickenpox. J Pediatr Surg 1996; 31:1138–1141.

16. Schwartz B, Facklam RR, Brieman RF. Changing epidemiology of group A streptococcal infection in the USA. Lancet 1990; 336:1167.

17. Giuliano A, Lewis F, Hadley K, Blaisdell FW. Bacteriology of necrotizing fasciitis. Am J Surg 1977; 134:52.

18. Yamane K, Asato J, Kawade N, Takahashi H, Kimura B, Arakawa Y. Two causes of fatal necrotizing fasciitis caused by Photobacterium damsela in Japan. J Clin Microbiol 2004; 42:1370–1372.

19. Fujioka M, Nishimura G, Miyazato O, Yamamoto T, Okamoto F, Tsunenori K. Necrotizing fasciitis and myositis that originated from gastrointestinal bacterial infection: two fatal cases. Scand J Plast Reconstr Surg Hand Surg 2003; 37:239–242.

20. Gamez JM, Fajardo R, Patino JF, Arias CA. Necrotizing fasciitis due to Vibrio alginolyticus in an immunocompetent patient. J Clin Microbiol 2003; 41:3427–3429.

21. Patino JF, Castro D, Valencia A, Morales P. Necrotizing soft-tissue lesions after a volcanic catalysm. World J Surg 1991; 15:240.

22. Basaran O, Emiroglu R, Arikan U, Karakayali H, Haberal M. Cryptococcal necrotizing fasciitis with multiple sites of involvement in the lower extremities. Dermatol Surg 2003; 29:1158–1160.

23. Stevens DL, Tanner MH, Winship J, Swartz R, Ries KM, Schlievert PM, et al. Severe group A streptococcal infections associated with a toxic-like syndrome and scarlet fever toxin A. N Engl J Med 1989; 321:1.

24. Legbo JN, Legbo JF. Bacterial isolates from necrotizing fasciitis: a clinico-pathological perspective. Niger J Med 2007; 16:143–147.

25. Khan AT, Tahmeedullah O. Treatment of necrotizing fasciitis with quinolones. J Coll Physicians Surg Pak 2003; 13:649–652.

26. Bos K, Marck K, ed. The surgical treatment of noma. Vitgeverij Belvedere/Medidact 2006; 1–125.

27. Rouse TM, Malangoni MA, Schulte WJ. Necrotizing fasciitis: a preventable disaster. Surgery 1982; 92:765.

CHAPTER 22
HAEMATOGENOUS OSTEOMYELITIS AND SEPTIC ARTHRITIS

Donald E. Meier
Bankole S. Rouma

Haematogenous Osteomyelitis

Haematogenous osteomyelitis (HO) is a common and devastating problem for children in less developed areas of the world[1] due to its frequent association with sickle cell disease (23–44%), delayed presentation, misdiagnosis, and undertreatment.[1-5] Sixty to eighty percent of children do not initially present until they have reached the stage of chronic osteomyelitis.[1-4] In more medically advanced areas, the spectrum of HO has changed significantly in the past few decades with decreased prevalence, earlier presentation, better nourished children, increased awareness of HO, improved diagnostic modalities for confirmation, precise laboratory techniques for microbial identification, and advanced antimicrobial agents for successful eradication of the infection. In locations without advanced technology (LWATs), however, little has changed in the past half century in the presentation or management of children with HO. Most children in advanced areas undergo successful *nonoperative* eradication of HO, many with nothing more invasive than a blood culture or bone aspiration.[6-8] Most current Western literature concerning HO—which concentrates on whether diagnostic aspiration of the bone marrow is really necessary and whether one powerful antibiotic is better than another in the eradication of HO—therefore has little relevance to practitioners in LWATs who are fortunate if they have materials for a gram stain and enough antibiotics for a week of oral treatment before the family runs out of funds. The purpose of this chapter is to provide a functional and practical approach to the classification and treatment of HO in children, taking into consideration the economic and technologic restraints that are inherent in any medical practice in LWATs.

Demographics

The exact incidence of osteomyelitis in Africa is unknown, but in reported series, children with osteomyelitis represent 7–20% of hospitalised children.[1-3] Data from the United Kingdom have shown an annual incidence of 2.9 per 100,000,[9] with boys affected more than girls, and half of osteomyelitis cases occurring in the first 5 years of life. In Africa, 56% of affected children are between 8 and 11 years of age.[1] In Cote d'Ivoire, the median age is 7.2 years.[2]

Aetiology/Pathology

Haematogenous osteomyelitis begins with entry of bacteria through a break in the skin or mucosa from otitis, pharyngitis, respiratory tract infections, or urinary tract infections. Most often the bacteria are *Staphylococcus*, but in sickle-cell children, both *Salmonella* and *Staphylococcus* are implicated. The bacteria are haematogenously disseminated and deposited in the trabecular bone or marrow, usually in the metaphysis of the proximal tibia or distal femur (Figure 22.1(A)). Sluggish blood flow in the metaphysis provides an ideal milieu for bacterial replication. Increasing pressure from the progressive, intramedullary purulent process results in destruction of the endosteal blood supply to the cortex. The pus under pressure escapes outward through Volkmann and Haversian canals (Figure 22.1(B)) and then spreads subperiosteally, stripping the cortex of its periosteal blood supply (Figure 22.1(C)). Without either endosteal or periosteal blood supply, the cortex becomes nonviable bone called sequestrum (Figure 22.1(D)). As the exudate

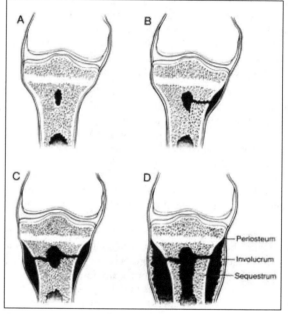

Figure 22.1: Pathologic development of haematogenous osteomyelitis.

increases in volume, it takes the path of least resistance. Sometimes, this involves circumferential stripping of the periosteum from one metaphysis to the other, resulting in a giant sequestrum consisting of the diaphysis and both metaphyses. At other times, the periosteum perforates under pressure, resulting in the spread of pus into muscles and along fascial planes. At this point, it is often confused with primary pyomyositis, and the bony origin is overlooked, resulting in inadequate decompression of the medullary canal. As the devascularised cortex is being absorbed, the inner surface of the periosteum produces new bone, called involucrum. The multiple areas of subperiosteal involucrum formation coalesce to form new bone on the inner surface of the periosteum but on the outside of the sequestrum. If the sequestrum totally resorbs, the patient may recover without a problem, but this rarely occurs. The nonviable, unresorbed sequestrum usually serves as a nidus for recurrent abscesses or chronically draining sinuses.

Clinical Presentation

Children may present with symptoms and signs of systemic sepsis, including fever, irritability, lethargy, or convulsions. Local symptoms include pain over the affected bone, which can be acute and overwhelming or insidious in onset, and unwillingness to use the affected extremity. The history may include a recent episode of impetigo, otitis, pharyngitis, or respiratory infection. Characteristically, there is tenderness, swelling, redness, or shininess over the affected bone. The adjacent joint usually appears normal.

Most laboratory values are nonspecific. The white blood count (WBC) may be elevated or normal. The erythrocyte sedimentation rate (ESR) is elevated in 80–90% of cases, and the C-reactive protein (CRP) is elevated in 98% of cases. Blood cultures are often positive in children presenting with systemic sepsis. None of these tests, however, are specific for HO, and therefore must be used only to supplement the history and physical examination. Indeed, many African hospitals will not have these laboratory tests available. The most accurate method for determining whether osteomyelitis is present is a bone marrow aspiration with stains and cultures to determine the infecting organism.

Plain radiography, early in the clinical course, may show soft tissue swelling and obliteration of tissue planes. After 10–14 days from onset of the symptoms, bone resorption is demonstrated by irregular patches of radiolucency in the metaphysis, and periosteal elevation is demonstrated by an outside rim of reactive new bone formation. In chronic osteomyelitis, plain radiographs may demonstrate lytic areas of the bone, sequestrum formation, or pathologic fractures. The TA technetium 99m bone scan is a sensitive (84–100%) and specific (70–90%) test for acute osteomyelitis, and magnetic resonance imaging (MRI) is the best special imaging study. However these studies are not available in most African health care facilities.

Classification

Traditionally, the stages of HO have been described as: (1) acute, (2) chronic, and (3) subacute. This traditional classification, however, is not very practical for use in LWATs. As a result, African practitioners have developed alternative classification systems.[10–11] The classification system shown in Table 22.1 was developed in a Nigerian general medical practice hospital in 1993.[12]

This simplified and functional system classifies children at the time of initial diagnosis of HO into one of four stages based on symptoms, signs, and x-ray findings. In stage 1 HO (acute), there is pus in the medullary canal and perhaps subperiosteally. There are usually local and systemic signs, but no significant x-ray changes that would demonstrate bone destruction or the presence of sequestra. Bone destruction and sequestra formation do not usually result in significant x-ray changes for at least 2 weeks into the HO process. Therefore, stage 2 HO (acute with x-ray changes) begins around 2 weeks into the process and indicates that significant bone destruction has already taken place. Children with stage 3 HO (chronic localised) have usually suffered an acute bout of HO that has drained spontaneously or has been operatively drained at a health care facility. However the sequestrum, which has not resorbed nor been surgically removed, serves as a nidus for chronic draining sinuses or recurrent abscesses (Figure 22.2). If a significant abscess occurs around the sequestrum and does not spontaneously drain, the child becomes systemically septic and reaches stage 4 HO (chronic systemic). This Nigerian staging system will be used throughout this chapter due to its practicality in areas with limited diagnostic and therapeutic resources.

Differential Diagnosis

Bone infarction can be difficult to differentiate from infection in a child with sickle cell disease. In both situations, children present with fever and bone pain and have elevated inflammatory markers. Biopsy and culture of affected bone is often necessary to establish the diagnosis. Cellulitis of soft tissues may restrict movement and cause the child to limp, but in most cases swelling and erythema of the skin are obvious. A fracture also causes swelling, pain, tenderness, and increased warmth of an extremity and may be differentiated from HO only by the history (although most children with HO also have a history of trauma) and more definitively by an x-ray. Neoplasms, especially leukaemia and Ewing's sarcoma, may be confused with osteomyelitis and may require a biopsy for the correct diagnosis.

Treatment

All African hospitals are not equal. Many, particularly university hospitals in major African cities, have state-of-the-art facilities comparable to those in Western hospitals. As a result, in African hospitals with

Table 22.1: Classification and treatment system for haematogenous osteomyelitis in developing world children.

Classification	Characteristics	Treatment
Stage 1 Acute	Local and systemic signs. No bone changes on x-ray (less than 2-week history).	Incision and drainage. Antibiotics for 2–6 weeks.
Stage 2 Acute with x-ray changes	Undrained acute osteomyelitis (2–8 week history). Local and maybe systemic signs with bone destruction on x-ray and no clear sequestrum.	Surgical drainage and debridement of obviously dead bone only. Perioperative antibiotics.
Stage 3 Chronic localised	Long history of osteomyelitis, usually with persistent spontaneous drainage. No systemic symptoms.	Wide drainage and removal of sequestra. Antibiotics not required.
Stage 4 Chronic systemic	Chronic osteomyelitis with systemic manifestations.	Urgent wide drainage, removal of sequestra, and administration of antibiotics until systemic manifestations resolve.

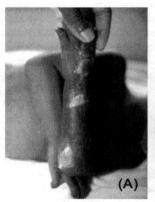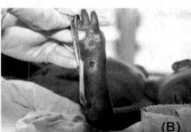

Figure 22.2: Neglected HO resulting in (A) chronic draining sinuses secondary to (B) a large sequestrum.

advanced technology, treatment for children with osteomyelitis is similar to that in Western hospitals. Early acute osteomyelitis is managed nonoperatively with a culture of the medullary contents and prolonged organism-appropriate intravenous antibiotics until the infection has been totally eradicated. Many other hospitals in Africa, however, are resource poor, and this section on treatment is directed more towards these hospitals.

Appropriate treatment, particularly in LWATs, depends on the stage of HO when the child presents and the resources (antibiotics, operative capabilities) physically and economically accessible in the particular location where the child presents. The best microbiological study available may be a gram stain. Surgical instruments, if available at all, are usually quite basic. Appropriate antistaphylococcal antibiotics may be totally unavailable or may be so expensive that parents are faced with the difficult decision of providing antibiotics for one child for a week or feeding the rest of the children in the family for the next several months. Health providers must therefore consider these painfully realistic socioeconomic factors in recommending appropriate practical treatment for a particular child with HO. The basic components of optimal treatment for HO are: (1) drainage of the pus under pressure, (2) acute antibiotics to treat systemic sepsis, (3) removal of nonviable bone, (4) sterilisation of the medullary contents with local or systemic techniques, and (5) wound closure. Unlike the current nonoperative treatment of HO in locations with advanced technology, operation is the essential modality in the treatment of all stages of osteomyelitis in LWATs.

Stage 1 HO is the most important stage for expeditious treatment, which may result in cure of the acute process and also prevent progression to chronic osteomyelitis. In acute HO, the operative goal is to decompress all pus under pressure. This involves decompression of both subperiosteal and intramedullary pus. Decompression must be adequate enough to prevent reaccumulation. Antibiotics are highly recommended in the initial treatment of stage 1 HO to manage the systemic sepsis. Antibiotics are also recommended for a 2–6 week period of treatment to prevent progression to chronic osteomyelitis.

Whenever HO has progressed to stage 2, x-ray changes already indicate nonviable bone while systemic and local sepsis remains. Treatment for stage 2 also involves prompt decompression and antibiotics to treat the systemic sepsis. Usually, the sequestrum is not well developed, and extensive debridement should be avoided because it is very difficult to differentiate viable from nonviable bone at this time. There is no documentation that prolonged antibiotics in stage 2 will prevent progression to chronic HO, but if antibiotics are available, they should be used for at least 2 weeks after resolution of the acute process.

Most children in LWATs present in stage 3 or 4. When HO has reached stage 3, antibiotics have little role in treatment. An x-ray serves as a "road map" (Figure 22.3) and is essential in planning proper treatment for both stages 3 and 4. With adequate debridement of sequestra, there is a chance of eventual healing of stage 3 HO even without antibiotics (Figures 22.4 and 22.5). The treatment for stage 4 HO (Figure 22.6) differs from the treatment for stage 3 only in the need for short-term antibiotics until the systemic sepsis has been controlled. Prolonged systemic antibiotic administration after total debridement of sequestra has not been proven effective in preventing further episodes of chronic HO.

Operative Techniques

This section considers in more detail the operative techniques used in the treatment of all stages of HO. An optimal basic instrument tray consists of the following instruments: soft tissue basic instruments (haemostat, scalpel, tissue forceps, needle holder, scissors); soft tissue

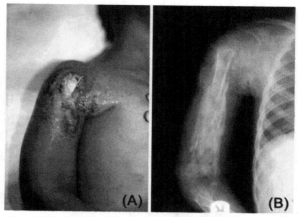

Figure 22.3: Stage 3 HO of the humerus in a 5-year-old child with (A) spontaneous extruding sequestrum, as seen on (B) a "road map" x-ray.

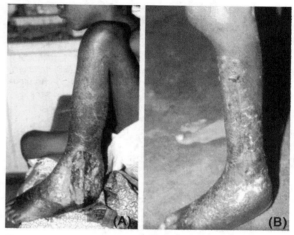

Figure 22.4: Stage 3 HO of the fibula with (A) spontaneous extrusion of the sequestrum. (B) After sequestrectomy, complete healing is achieved without antibiotics.

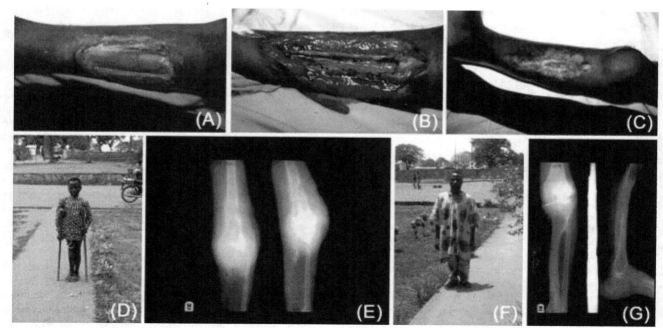

Figure 22.5: Stage 3 HO of the tibia in a 7-year-old male: (A) initial presentation; (B) tibia after removing a cortical trough, which showed that the tibial shaft was completely nonviable; (C) appearance after giant sequestrectomy and healing by secondary intention without using antibiotics; (D) child at time of discharge; (E) x-ray at time of discharge; (F) same patient 15 years later; (G) x-ray 15 years later.

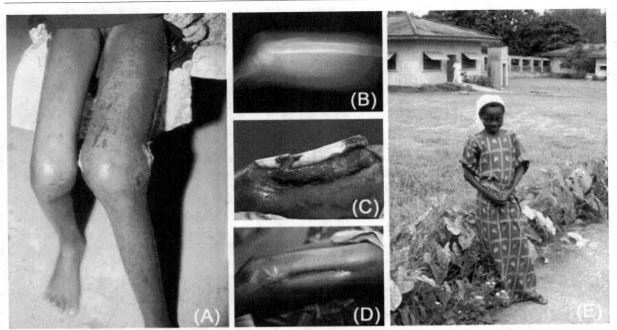

Figure 22.6: Stage 4 HO in a 12-year-old female with sickle-cell (SS) haemoglobin: (A) initial presentation with large abscess of left thigh, (B) x-ray showing giant sequestrum of femur, (C) drainage of abscess and sequestrectomy performed through a lateral thigh incision, (D) thigh wound, (E) child after complete healing by secondary intention with antibiotics used only to control the systemic sepsis.

retractors (self-retaining Gelpis are ideal); periosteal elevator; bone curette; bone rongeur; and bone drill. True orthopaedic bone drills are very expensive and justification of the cost is difficult for hospitals in LWATs. However, simple carpenter drills and bits can be used for orthopaedic purposes if proper sterilisation capabilities (ethylene oxide or formalin gas) are available. Cordless electric drills, commercially available in hardware stores, are relatively inexpensive and also can be effectively used for orthopaedic procedures if properly sterilised. They must, however, be used on a low speed because a high-speed mode will burn the bone. An orthopaedic exposure book[13] is a valuable asset in determining the safest approach for draining and debriding bones affected by HO. The cost of such books is prohibitive in most LWATs, however, and a basic anatomy book can be substituted to determine appropriate approaches to bones and joints in the least potentially destructive manner. The low-cost *Primary Surgery* textbook[14] presents good exposure techniques for the more commonly affected bones and joints. Ketamine anaesthesia is a very effective and safe technique in the operative management of children with HO in LWATs.[15] Using an extremity tourniquet significantly decreases the operative blood loss, but tourniquets should not be used in children with SS or SC haemoglobinopathies because this may precipitate a sickling crisis.

Treatment of acute HO (stages 1 and 2) begins with the soft tissue approach to the bone. The recommended approach to the proximal tibia (the most commonly affected bone) is from the medial or lateral aspect of the tibia so that there will be soft tissue remaining to cover the affected bone. For the health care provider unaccustomed to approaching the tibia in this manner, however, it is acceptable to incise the soft tissue directly over the tibia with as small a soft tissue incision as necessary. Usually the periosteum has already been elevated from the bone and needs to be incised longitudinally to drain the pus under pressure. If microbiological techniques (gram stain, culture) are available, a sample is taken. A periosteal elevator should not be used for this classic presentation because the increasing subperiosteal pressure has already stripped the periosteum from the cortex, and further periosteal elevation may impair blood flow to the remaining bone. After the periosteum is incised, a drill is used to enter the metaphyseal medullary canal. Usually pus drains from the drill hole. If so, other drill

holes are placed in the area and a curette and bone rongeur are used to remove a 2-cm cortical window. This window serves to decompress the medullary canal and allows for irrigation of the canal. The medullary canal in acute HO should not be curetted for fear of damaging the precarious endosteal blood supply. The wound is left open and the patient brought back daily for irrigation of the medullary canal using ketamine anaesthesia. When there is no more purulent drainage, an attempt can be made to close the incision (this is often unsuccessful), or it can simply be left open to heal by secondary intention.

The treatment of chronic HO (stages 3 and 4) often requires a more extensive operative approach. There is rarely a total cure for chronic HO, but very long periods of remission can be achieved if all of the nonviable bone is removed. Sometimes the child with chronic HO has been neglected for so long that the sequestrum begins to spontaneously extrude (see Figures 22.3 and 22.4). When this happens, the child can be appropriately treated by simply removing the sequestrum, curetting the inner surface of the involucrum, and irrigating the medullary canal to remove any remaining smaller pieces of the sequestrum. Sometimes the sequestra are incarcerated by the involucrum, and removal requires a cortical trough to adequately visualise and remove all of the sequestra (Figure 22.7(A)). After the removal of the sequestra, advanced techniques for closure are available, including muscle and fascio-cutaneous flaps. Placement of antibiotic-impregnated beads can be used to decrease the number of relapses for chronic HO. Most of these advanced procedures are not commonly used in LWATs since in such locations the incidence of HO is so common as to be overwhelming for the resources of the hospital. In these instances, the large wounds can be left completely open, and they eventually will heal by secondary intention as long as all of the nonviable bone has been removed (Figure 22.7(B)).

Parents can manage the wounds with daily water irrigation and coverage with a bandage made from scrap cloth. In hospitals with adequate health care personnel and facilities, the wounds can be managed in a wound care clinic, but hospitals without such facilities can provide alternatives. For example, the Baptist Medical Center in Ogbomoso, Nigeria, provides a water hose so each day children and parents can use the handheld shower apparatus to wash any debris

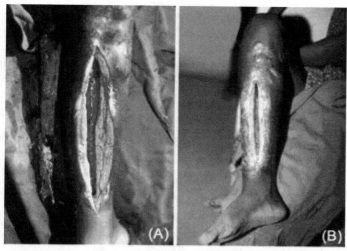

Figure 22.7: Stage 3 chronic HO of the tibia: (A) extensive sequestrectomy performed through a long cortical trough; (B) wound healing by secondary intention without antibiotics.

out of the cortical trough. It is not painful for the children, and the wound can be managed solely by a parent without using the services of hospital personnel.

The proper procedure is controversial for management of chronic osteomyelitis when the total bone from metaphysis to metaphysis has sequestered and there is not yet enough new involucrum to provide stability to the bone. Some surgeons prefer to proceed with removal of the giant sequestrum and splinting of the extremity to allow the involucrum to grow in a clean environment without the infected sequestrum interfering (Figure 22.5). Other practitioners believe that the best splint for the affected extremity is the sequestrum itself and that it should be left in situ until the involucrum has coalesced. There are obviously no prospective randomised studies to support either course of action.

Complications

Risk factors for development of complications of HO include delay in diagnosis, misdiagnosis, short duration of therapy, and a younger age at the time of initial illness. Recurrent bone infection is the most common complication after treatment for osteomyelitis followed by disturbance in bone growth, limb-length discrepancies, axial displacement of the limb, pathologic fractures, and abnormal gait.

Septic Arthritis

Pathogenesis

Although septic arthritis can be caused by joint trauma or extension of osteomyelitis into a joint, the most common aetiology in African children is haematogenous dissemination of *Staphylococcus* from an open skin or mucosal wound. Other offending organisms include *Streptococcus*, *Haemophilus influenza* (particularly in newborns), and *Salmonella* and *Escherichia coli* in sickle-cell children. Bacteria have an affinity for cartilage and directly attach to the chondral surface. An acute inflammatory response follows, resulting in migration of polymorphonuclear cells, production of proteolytic enzymes, and cytokine secretion by chondrocytes. Degradation of articular cartilage begins within 8 hours of onset of infection. The most commonly infected joints are the knee (41%), hip (20%), ankle (14%), elbow (12%), wrist (4%), and shoulder (4%).

Clinical Presentation

Any child with fever and reluctance to move an extremity should be considered to have osteomyelitis or septic arthritis until proven otherwise. The history should include any factors that may make the child more susceptible to the development of bacteraemia: recent systemic illness (chicken pox), respiratory or urinary infections, otitis media, indwelling intravenous catheters, immunosuppressive disorders, or sickle cell disease.[16] There is often the history of a traumatic event preceding the pain.

On examination, there is usually swelling and warmth over the joint, pain with mobilisation of the joint, and restricted range of motion of the joint. Tenderness over the metaphysis of a bone is more characteristic of osteomyelitis, whereas tenderness directly over a joint or pain with slight movement of a joint is characteristic of septic arthritis. The patient should also be evaluated for pharyngitis, rash, heart murmur, hepatosplenomegaly, and evidence of involvement of other bones or joints.

Diagnosis

Diagnosis must be made promptly to prevent damage to the articular cartilage. Blood and joint fluid should be obtained for cultures, and a gram stain and cell count should be performed on the joint fluid. A WBC count of 50,000/cu mm or greater with a predominance of polymorphonuclear cells is consistent with bacterial infection. Plain radiographs may show joint space widening, effusion, soft tissue swelling, or subluxation/dislocation of the joint. Radiographs are useful to rule out fracture, malignancy, or osteomyelitis as the cause of pain. Ultrasound is useful in determining whether fluid is present in the joint and is useful in guiding aspiration, but it cannot differentiate infected from noninfected fluid. The definitive diagnosis is made by either joint aspiration or operative identification of a purulent effusion.

Treatment

The three main therapeutic interventions are: (1) joint decompression and debridement, (2) antibiotics and initial joint immobilisation to decrease local irritation, followed by (3) mobilisation to decrease the development of fibrous adhesions and improve cartilage nutrition. Intravenous antibiotics (choice depends on availability in a given locale) should be started after the arthrocentesis and continued for 1–2 weeks, after which oral antibiotics are continued for another 2–6 weeks. Septic arthritis is a surgical emergency because prolonged elevated intracapsular pressure in the hip can tamponade blood flow to the femoral head and increase the possibility of developing avascular necrosis. A safe anatomical approach to the joint should be conducted.[13,14] The joint is opened and the pus drained. The joint is irrigated copiously with normal saline. After the effluent is clear, the joint is digitally palpated to determine how much of the cartilage has already been destroyed. If it is a superficial joint (knee), a drain is not necessary. For deeper joints (hip, shoulder), however, a Penrose or glove drain can be inserted to maintain the drainage tract between irrigations. The patient is placed at joint rest for at least 2 weeks. The joint undergoes repeat irrigation daily under anaesthesia until there is no more purulent drainage. It is important, particularly in joints with extensive cartilage destruction, that the joint be placed in a functional position because otherwise ankylosis may occur. If ankylosis does occur, reconstructive surgery will probably not be available in LWATs, and even if available, it will not be nearly as effective in providing function as would be a programme of splinting joints in a position of function before ankylosis. After the period of posterior plaster immobilisation, the joint is progressively mobilised to minimise ankylosis.

Key Summary Points

1. Haematogenous osteomyelitis (HO) is a common and devastating problem for children in developing countries.

2. Operation is the mainstay of treatment for HO in developing world children.

3. Acute stages of HO are best managed with subperiosteal and intramedullary decompression and antibiotics.

4. Chronic stages are best treated with extensive debridement to remove all sequestra, with antibiotics used to treat systemic sepsis.

5. In the absence of discharging sinuses the diagnosis of chronic osteomyelitis should be confirmed or excluded by biopsy.

6. Septic arthritis should be diagnosed and treated as an emergency because the longer intraarticular pus remains under pressure, the more likely there will be permanent destruction.

7. The African surgeon must be acquainted with a safe operative approach to all bones and joints commonly affected with osteomyelitis and pyarthrosis.

References

1. Tekou H, Foly A, Akue B. Oe profil actuel des osteomyelites hematogenes de l'enfant au Centre Hospitalier de Toioin, Lome, Togo a propos de 145 cas. Medecine Tropicale 2000; 60(4):365–368.

2. Kouame DB, Dick KR, Ouattara O, Gouli JC, Odehouri KT, Coulibaly C. Traitement des osteomyelites compliquees de l'enfant au CHU de Yopougon, Abidjan (Cote d'Ivoire). Cahiers Sante 2005; 15(2):99–104.

3. Nacoulma SI, Ouedraogo DD, Nacoulma EWC, Korsaga A, Drabo JY. Osteomyelite chroniques au CHU de Ouagadougou (Burkina Faso). Etude retrospective de 102 cas (1996-2000). Bull Soc Pathol Exot 2007; 100(4):264–268.

4. Oguachuba H. Mismanagement of acute haematogenous osteomyelitis by traditional medicine men (native doctors) in the Eastern and Northern Regions of Nigeria. Unfallchirurg 1985; 88:363–372.

5. Wong AL, Sakamoto KM, Johson EE. Differentiating osteomyelitis from bone infarction in sickle cell disease. Ped Emer Care 2001; 17(1):60–63.

6. Song KM, Sloboda JF. Acute haematogenous osteomyelitis in children. J Am Acad Orthop Surg 2001; 9(3);166–175.

7. Stanitski CL. Changes in pediatric acute haematogenous osteomyelitis management. J Pediatr Orthop 2004; 24(4):444–445.

8. Darville T, Jacobs RF. Management of acute haematogenous osteomyelitis in children. Pediatr Infect Dis J 2004; 23(3):255–258.

9. Marietta V. Osteomyelitis in children. Current Opinion in Ped 2002; 14:112–115.

10. Solagberu BA. A new classification of osteomyelitis for developing countries. East African Medical Journal 2003; 80(7):373–378.

11. Lauschke FH, Frey CT. Haematogenous osteomyelitis in infants and children in the northwestern region of Namibia: management and two-year results. J Bone Joint Surg Am 1994; 76(4):502–510.

12. Meier DE, Tarpley JL, OlaOlorun DA, Howard CR, Price CT. Haematogenous osteomyelitis in the developing world: a practical approach to classification and treatment with limited resources. Contemp Orthopaed 1993; 26(5):495–502.

13. Hoppenfeld S, de Boer P, eds. Surgical exposures in orthopaedics: the anatomic approach. Lippincott Williams & Wilkins, Philadelphia; 2003.

14. King M, Bewes PC, Cairns J, Thornton J, eds. Primary surgery, volume 1, non-trauma. Oxford University Press, Oxford, UK; 1993, Pp 83–103.

15. Meier DE, OlaOlorun DA, Nkor SK, Aasa D, Tarpley JL. Ketamine—a safe and effective anesthetic agent for children in the developing world. Pedi Surg Int 1996; 11:370–373.

16. Gutierrez K. Bone and joint infections in children. Ped Clin N Am 2005; 52:779–794.

CHAPTER 23
PARASITIC INFESTATIONS OF SURGICAL IMPORTANCE IN CHILDREN

Iftikhar Ahmad Jan

Usang E. Usang

Kokila Lakhoo

Introduction

The term "parasitic infestation" is used to refer to those infections caused by protozoa, helminthes, and arthropods. They are a major cause of morbidity and mortality in infants and children. However, parasitic infestations have received relatively little attention compared with infections due to viral, bacterial, and fungal agents.

Parasitic infestations are a worldwide problem in children, the prevalence and variety of organisms being greatest in areas with a warm, moist climate and in communities where standards of hygiene are low. But parasitic diseases are now occurring more frequently in developed countries due to immigration and increased foreign travel. This cosmopolitan distribution, in addition to the complications that often attend these infestations, make this subject an important surgical problem.

Of the parasitic diseases, those of surgical interest in children are:

1. Protozoan infections
- Amoebiasis

2. Helminthic infections
- *Ascaris lumbricoides* – Intestinal nematode
- Dracontiasis (Dracunculiasis) – Tissue nematode
- Malayan and Bancroftian filariae – Tissue nematode
- *Schistosomiasis* (Blood fluke) – Trematode

3. Arthropodal infections
- Myiasis – Tissue-invading arthropods
- Chigoe (jigger) – *Tunga penetrans*

4. Hydatid disease

Amoebiasis

Amoebiasis is a human intestinal infectious disease caused by the protozoan parasite *Entamoeba histolytica*. It is a ubiquitous parasitic infection affecting approximately 10% of the world's population and is the third most common cause of death from parasitic infections, the first two being malaria and schistosomiasis.

Demographics

Amoebic infections were previously reported as uncommon among children by the World Health Organization (WHO), which described *shigella* species as the most common and most important cause of dysentery in this age group. However, recent studies from Africa have shown that this condition is endemic, both in its invasive and noninvasive (carrier) states; it may affect any age group and has no gender preference in children. The reasons thought to be responsible for the endemism include poverty, malnutrition, and poor sanitation, among others. Amoebiasis is not uncommon even in some Western countries, however, as a result of immigration and increased foreign travel.

Aetiology/Pathophysiology

Amoebiasis is caused by the pathogenic *Entamoeba histolytica*, commonly transmitted via the faeco-oral route when water or food contaminated by faeces are consumed. Humans are the only reservoir and there are no intermediate hosts.

Upon ingestion of contaminated food or water, the cysts travel to the small intestine, where trophozoites are released (encystation). In 90% of patients, the trophozoites re-encyst and produce asymptomatic infection, which usually spontaneously resolves within 12 months. In the remaining 10% of patients who are infected, the parasite causes symptomatic amoebiasis.

E. histolytica causes its primary lesion in the colon, where the caecum and rectosigmoid are areas of predilection. The incubation period varies from 2 days to 4 months. Invasive disease begins with the adherence of *E histolytica* to colonic mucins, epithelial cells, and leukocytes mediated by a galactose-inhibitable adherence lectin. Following adherence, trophozoites invade the colonic epithelium to produce the ulcerative lesions typical of intestinal amoebiasis. The trophozoites of *E. histolytica* lyse the target cells by using lectin to bind to the target cells' membranes and the parasite's ionophore-like protein to induce a leak of ions (i.e., Na^+, K^+, Ca^{2+}) from the target cells' cytoplasm. Numerous haemolysins, encoded by plasmid (ribosomal) DNA (rDNA) and cytotoxic to the intestinal mucosal cells, have been described in *E. histolytica*. An extracellular cysteine kinase causes proteolytic destruction of tissue, producing flask-shaped ulcers. Phorbol esters and protein kinase C activators augment the cytolytic activity of the parasite.

Liver abscesses due to amoebiasis are 10 times more frequent in adults than in children. Amoebic liver abscess, however, is equally common in both sexes among prepubertal children, probably, in agreement with the equal distribution of intestinal disease in both sexes in children. Spread of amoebiasis to the liver occurs via the portal blood, after the pathogenic organisms have evaded the complement-mediated lysis in the bloodstream. Trophozoites ascend the portal veins to produce liver abscesses filled with acellular proteinaceous debris (so-called anchovy paste). The trophozoites of *E. histolytica* lyse the hepatocytes and the neutrophils. This explains the paucity of inflammatory cells within the liver abscesses. The neutrophil toxins may contribute to hepatocyte necrosis.

Clinical Presentation

The clinical presentation of amoebiasis is variable. It ranges from asymptomatic cyst passage to amoebic colitis, amoebic dysentery, amoeboma, and extraintestinal disease. *E. histolytica* infection is asymptomatic in about 90% of cases; invasive disease occurs in the remaining 10%. Severe disease is more common in children, especially if malnourished. Extraintestinal disease usually involves only the liver, but rare extraintestinal manifestations include amoebic brain abscess, pleuropulmonary disease, ulcerative skin, and genitourinary lesions.

Amoebic Colitis

Amoebic colitis affects all age groups, but its incidence is strikingly high in children 1–5 years of age. The clinical features depend upon the transmural as well as the longitudinal extent of the disease. The onset may be insidious, with nonspecific dysenteric symptoms, and is often confused with gastroenteritis or herbal intoxication. Severe amoebic colitis in infants and young children tends to be rapidly progressive with frequent extraintestinal involvement and high mortality rates. Rectal loss of blood and mucus is a frequent but not constant finding and may raise suspicion of intussusception or typhoid. The association between progressive disease and clinically overt malnutrition is striking, and the relationship may be provocative. The passage of large volumes of malodourous stools with slough from the mucosa in a child with preexisting malnutrition suggests amoebic colitis. Occasionally, amoebic dysentery is associated with sudden onset of fever, chills, and severe diarrhoea, which may result in dehydration and electrolyte disturbances.

Progressive disease in children is manifested by increasing abdominal distention with discomfort, tenderness, and toxaemia. Classical signs of peritonitis may develop very late, if at all, due to omental wrap.

Amoebic Liver Abscess

Amoebic liver abscess, a serious manifestation of disseminated infection, is uncommon in children, although some cases have been reported. Although diffuse liver enlargement has been associated with intestinal amoebiasis, liver abscess occurs in <1% of infected individuals and may appear in patients with no clear history of intestinal disease. This contrasts with the high incidence of cases of amoebic liver abscess (61%) seen in the surgical ward in Natal, South Africa, which occurred in association with active amoebic colitis.

Numerous small abscesses may coalesce to form large abscesses, which expand towards the surface and may rupture, giving rise to amoebic peritonitis. Amoebic liver abscess may occur months to years after exposure, so a high index of suspicion is very important. In children, fever is the hallmark of amoebic liver abscess and is frequently associated with abdominal pain, distention, and enlargement and tenderness of the liver. Changes at the base of the right lung, such as elevation of the diaphragm and atelectasis or effusion, may also occur.

Investigations

Stool examination

Light microscopy examination of a fresh stool smear for trophozoites that contain ingested red blood cells (RBCs) is rather insensitive. It is positive in 10% of patients, showing the presence of haematogenous amoebae. It cannot distinguish other species of *Entamoeba* from *E. histolytica*. Fulminant amoebic colitis or its complications may exist with a negative stool parasitology if treatment has started prior to referral. Stools for examination must be fresh when examined or be preserved in polyvinyl alcohol for later microscopy. Material from rectal scrapings has also proved most helpful. An enzyme immunoassay kit to specifically detect *E. histolytica* in fresh stool specimens is now commercially available in specialised centres.

Serologic studies

Serum antibodies against amoebae are present in 70–90% of individuals with symptomatic intestinal *E. histolytica* infection. Antiamoebic antibodies are present in as many as 99% of individuals with liver abscess who have been symptomatic for longer than a week. However, serologic tests do not distinguish new from past infection because the seropositivity persists for years after an acute infection. Several methods, such as indirect haemoagglutination antibody (IHA), enzyme-linked immunosorbent assay (EIA), and immunodiffusion (ID) tests are now commercially available in specialised centres.

Imaging studies

- *Chest radiography* may reveal an elevated right hemidiaphragm and a right-sided pleural effusion in patients with amoebic liver abscess.

- *Ultrasonography* is preferred for the evaluation of amoebic liver abscess due to its low cost, rapidity, and lack of adverse effects. A single lesion is usually seen in the posterosuperior aspect of the right lobe of the liver. Multiple abscesses may occur in some patients.

- *Computed tomography* (CT) and *magnetic resonance imaging* (MRI) may be done in selected cases.

Other tests

- Leucocytosis without oesinophilia is observed is 80% of cases.

- Mild anaemia may be noted.

- Liver function tests reveal elevated alkaline phosphatase levels (in 80% of patients), elevated transaminase levels, mild elevation of serum bilirubin level, and reduced albumin levels.

- The erythrocyte sedimentation rate is elevated.

Medical Treatment

Asymptomatic infections are not treated in endemic areas. However, in nonendemic areas asymptomatic infection should be treated because of its potential to progress to invasive disease. Luminal agents that are minimally absorbed by the gastrointestinal (GI) tract (e.g., paromomycin) are best suited for such therapy.

Metronidazole is the mainstay of therapy for invasive amoebiasis. Tinidazole is being used for intestinal or extraintestinal amoebiasis. Nitroimidazole therapy leads to clinical response in approximately 90% of patients with mild to moderate colitis. Chloroquine has also been used for patients with hepatic amoebiasis. Intraluminal parasites are not affected by nitroimidazole therapy. Therefore, nitroimidazole therapy should be followed by treatment with a luminal agent such as paromomycin to prevent a relapse.

Broad-spectrum antibiotics may be added to treat bacterial superinfection in a case of fulminant amoebic colitis and suspected perforation. Bacterial coinfection with amoebic liver abscess has occasionally been observed (both before and as a complication of drainage), and adding antibiotics to the treatment regime is reasonable in the absence of a prompt response to nitroimidazole therapy.

Surgical Treatment

Surgical intervention is required for acute abdomen due to perforated amoebic colitis, massive GI bleeding, or toxic megacolon. Toxic megacolon is rare, however. Surgical attempts to correct amoebic bowel perforation or peritonitis should be avoided, although some patients may benefit from peritoneal lavage.

Unlike pyogenic liver abscess, amoebic liver abscess generally responds to medical therapy alone, and drainage is seldom necessary. When necessary, imaging guided percutaneous treatment (needle aspiration or catheter drainage) has replaced surgical intervention as the procedure of choice for reducing the size of an abscess. The indications for drainage of amoebic liver abscess include the presence of left-lobe abscess (>10 cm in diameter), and impending rupture and abscess that does not respond to medical therapy within 3 to 5 days.

Ascariasis

Ascariasis is the parasitic infestation by the largest intestinal nematode of man, which is found worldwide. It is now a significant public health problem in many parts of the world. The organism maintains an ideal host-parasite relationship without any observable harm in the vast majority of individuals, but heavy parasitisation of the intestinal tract by *Ascaris lumbricoides* may be associated with nutritional disturbances and, more important, intestinal obstruction or perforation.

Demographics

Ascariasis is a common problem in the tropics and subtropics, where the moist humid climates of alternating dry season and rainy season permit all-year embryonation of the ova of *Ascaris lumbricoides*. This is further aggravated by the poor environmental standards, improper disposal of sewage, and low socioeconomic conditions prevailing in most cities in Africa.

Although it occurs at all ages, ascariasis is most common in children 2 to 10 years of age; the prevalence decreases after the age of 15 years. The incidence is higher in males than females, probably because they are more exposed to outdoor activities. Infants may be infested soon after birth, the mother transmitting the ova with her dirty fingers. In developing counties with poor sanitary conditions, more than 70% of children are infested, and globally more than 1.5 billion people are infested with *Ascaris lumbricoides*.

Aetiology/Pathophysiology

Ascariasis is caused by *Ascaris lumbricoides*, a large lumen-dwelling nematode contracted by the consumption of its eggs. Transmission occurs mainly via ingestion of water or food contaminated with these eggs from human faeces and occasionally via inhalation of polluted dust. Children playing in contaminated soil may acquire the parasite from their dirty hands. Transplacental migration of larvae has also occasionally been reported.

The eggs reach the small intestine, where the larvae are liberated. The larvae penetrate the small intestinal wall and migrate through the lymphatics and bloodstream to the liver, and then to the lungs, where they enter the alveoli. There they pause for at least 2–3 weeks and molt, giving rise to allergic bronchopneumonia in previously infected and sensitised individuals. Later, they wander up the bronchi and trachea, giving rise to bronchitis with bronchospasm and urticaria and occasionally larvae in the sputum. Most larvae are swallowed and grow to adulthood in the small intestine. Adult worms do not multiply in the human host, so the number of adult worms per infested person relates to the degree of continued exposure to infectious eggs over time.

The adult worms give rise to mechanical problems due to their size and the smaller diameter of the lumen of the bowel of children. Also, due to their large number and mass, they lead to a severe nutritional drain in these patients. A temperature elevation to 39°C, certain drugs, such as antihelminthic, and some unknown influences cause the worms to congregate, sometimes resulting in intestinal obstruction (Figure 23.1) and migration out of the gut into the bile duct, oesophagus, mouth, pancreatic duct, or appendix, and occasionally the liver. Adult worms may perforate the gut, leading to peritonitis. Sometimes, the presence and activity of large numbers of worms alone may be associated with vomiting, fever, and abdominal pain. By far, small intestinal obstruction (whether simple occlusive, intussusception, or volvulus) accounts for many of the serious pathologic effects attributed to this worm.

Clinical Presentation

The presentation of ascariasis may be straightforward. Early symptoms may be related to the larval migration in the lung. In established cases, the child may be malnourished. Worms may have been vomited out or passed rectally. The difficulty, however, is in clinching the diagnosis of intestinal obstruction as a result of ascaris worms. There is, therefore, need for a high index of suspicion in all cases of intestinal obstruction in children. A history of a recent purgative will be important, since these have been known to precipitate obstructions.

Among other presentations, pyrexia of moderate degree may be observed; colicky central abdominal pain may be the chief complaint; vomiting may be frequent, either due to the activity of the worms or as a result of actual obstruction; the abdomen may be generally tender; and in half the cases, an abdominal mass that is ill-defined, mobile, and sometimes multiple and commonly situated in the umbilical region may be palpable.

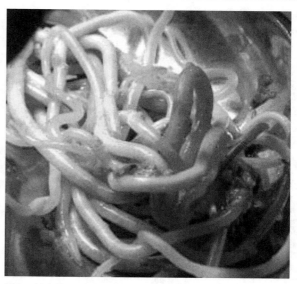

Figure 23.1: Exceptional ascaris burden causing acute intestinal obstruction.

Eosinophilia is present in the early phases of infestation, but due to the mixture of parasitic infestations present at the same time, it is not diagnostic.

Investigations

Erect plain abdominal x-ray

Radiographs are useful in heavily infested children where the worms appear radiolucent. A mass of worms may contrast against the gas in the bowel, typically producing a "whirlpool" effect. The radiographs also show features of intestinal obstruction, such as abdominal distention, dilated bowel loops, and multiple air fluid levels and free gas under the diaphragm in cases with intestinal perforation.

Ultrasonography

Ultrasonography may be helpful, with the round worm appearing sonographically as a thick echogenic strip with a central anechoic tube or multiple long, linear, parallel echogenic strips without acoustic shadowing. Curling movements of the worms may be observed on prolonged scanning.

Stool examination for ova

This is not helpful where infestation rates are high.

Treatment

Children with uncomplicated ascariasis are managed as paediatric outpatients and rarely referred to the surgeon. However, following intestinal obstruction due to ascariasis, the various options in management are as follows:

Conservative approach

Various authors have recorded a high success rate with a conservative approach. They observed that, unlike other mechanical causes of intestinal obstruction, most cases of acute intestinal obstruction due to ascariasis can be managed conservatively. This approach is, however, most suitable for mild cases with partial obstruction; it entails decompression of the bowel, intravenous fluid replacement, antispasmodics, and anthelmintic administered after the attack has subsided.

Surgical approach

Complete obstruction should be relieved surgically after resuscitation of the patient by any of the following methods:

- *Milking:* The bolus of worms is broken up and massaged into the larger diameter caecum and ascending colon.

- *Enterostomy:* The antimesenteric border of the bowel is opened, through which the worms are carefully extracted and the resulting opening repaired transversely in two layers.

- *Resection:* The affected bowel segment is surgically removed with the contained worms and an end-to-end anastomosis is performed. This is indicated in those cases for which the mass of worms is very tightly packed, causing partial necrosis of the gut, and stretching the gut wall may threaten its viability.

Prevention

- Mass treatments with single-dose mebendazole or albendazole for all preschool and school-age children every three to four months have been used in some communities.

- Encourage proper and safe methods of sewage disposal.

- Protect food from dirt and soil.

- Thoroughly washing raw food materials is good practice.

- Encourage proper hand-washing habits and other sanitary measures.

Dracontiasis

Dracontiasis is a disease caused by the adult female *Dracunculus medinensis*, the oldest human parasite. It is more commonly known as guinea worm disease (GWD), after the Europeans who first saw the disease on the Guinea Coast of West Africa in the 17th century.

Currently, transmission occurs in only 10 countries of the world, all in sub-Saharan Africa. Other countries are either certified free of transmission or are presently in the precertification period. The goal is for dracontiasis to be the first parasitic disease to be eradicated and the first disease in history eradicated through behaviour change, without use of vaccines or cure.

Demographics

Dracontiasis is essentially a disease affecting rural communities. Whilst the occurrence of cases is possible in urban environments, such cases usually have been "imported" and were contracted elsewhere. At present, the disease is endemic mainly in West Africa, the site of 9 of the 10 countries where transmission occurs: Benin, Burkina Faso, Côte d'Ivoire, Ghana, Niger, Nigeria, Mali, Mauritania, and Togo. The tenth country is Ethiopia in East Africa.

Dracontiasis rarely occurs in children younger than the age of 3 years because the babies are generally breast-fed, and the long period of incubation delays the first emergence of the worm to one year after weaning. The incidence of the disease increases significantly after 5 years and is maximal between 15 and 45 years of age. The incidence is high in active adults who, because of their farming activities, drink larger quantities of water and use water from unsafe sources such as nontreated ponds far from the village and close to the farming field.

The disease usually shows no significant gender difference in prevalence of infection. However, in some communities, such as in northern Nigeria, the rate of infection appears to be higher in males. This is observed in populations in which women do not participate in farming activities, and thus are less exposed to drinking water from unsafe sources.

Aetiology/Pathophysiology

GWD is acquired by the ingestion of the water flea, cyclops, in drinking water. It is the only disease transmitted exclusively through drinking water. The guinea worm requires a host (man) and an intermediate host (cyclops) for its full development. The larvae mature in the cyclops found in standing dirty water (e.g., puddles, ponds, and dams). When such water is consumed, the infected cyclops is digested in the gastric hydrochloric acid, thus liberating the larvae. The larvae, male and female, burrow through the intestine to enter the circulation. The males, only 2–3 cm long, die after fertilising the females.

The female then matures in the connective tissue to measure 550–800 cm long by 1.7–2.00 mm in diameter at 10–14 months after infection, before it emerges from the subcutaneous tissue, mainly of the lower leg around the ankle (Figure 23.2). However, it can emerge at any part of the

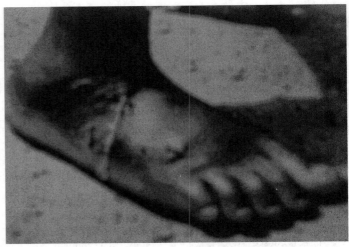

Figure 23.2: Dracontiasis in a child (note the worm emerging from the ankle).

body, including the trunk, arms and hands, buttocks, thigh, knee joint, genital area, and, rarely, the neck. At this stage, the female body is mostly occupied by a distended uterus containing millions of larvae. A substance secreted by the gravid female causes a blister to form in the skin of the host around the anterior extremity of the female worm. When in contact with water, as occurs during swimming, washing, bathing, or wading, the blister ruptures; the worm protrudes and discharges hundreds of thousands of larvae into the water. The larvae are then ingested by the cyclops and mature in about 3 weeks, thus completing the life cycle of the parasite.

Generally, two types of lesions are produced in man: vesicles, which ulcerate, and subcutaneous or deep abscesses around dead adult worms. Calcification of worms, which sometimes occurs in tissues, may induce local manifestations: pulmonary, cardiovascular, abdominal, urogenital, or gyn-obstetrical.

Secondary bacterial superinfection at the point of emergence of the worm is rather common when nursing is not available, and may lead to an aggravation of the condition and complications such as septicaemia and tetanus. Severe arthritis and ankylosis may be due to either the release of *D. medinensis* embryos inside the joint (aseptic arthritis) or the bacterial infection of the tunnel of the worm (septic arthritis). Such complications may lead to physical deformity and limitation of mobility.

Clinical Presentation

- GWD is rare in children <3 years old, but increases significantly after 5 years of age. Both sexes are equally affected.

- Symptoms arise when a live worm reaches the skin at the site of emergence.

- A cutaneous blister erupts with an intense burning sensation locally. A few hours before the development of the local lesion, the symptoms are exacerbated and may include erythema, urticarial rash, intense pruritus, nausea and vomiting, diarrhoea, dyspnoea, giddiness, and syncope.

- The lesion develops within a few hours in the form of a papule centred by a veside and surrounded by a local induration. On contact with water, the blister bursts and the anterior part of the worm emerges and discharges larvae and internal fluids. At this stage, the pain and the burning sensation are reduced and the other symptoms also tend to decrease.

- The worm can emerge at any place of the body, but most commonly at the lower part of the leg around the ankles.

- Calcified worms, which remain asymptomatic, have been discovered by chance on x-ray or during a surgical intervention.

- Secondary bacterial superinfection, septicaemia, tetanus, severe arthritis, and ankylosis may be additional clinical manifestations of GWD.

Treatment

The main treatment is extraction of the worm by cautious winding around a matchstick and gentle traction applied daily until it is removed. Wet compresses are applied to the ulcer daily until the discharge from the worm ceases.

Application of a topical antibiotic to the lesion prevents secondary bacterial infection and complications. The use of niridazole (Ambilhar®) (25 mg/kg in two divided doses given orally daily for 10 days), thiabendazole (50 mg/kg daily for three days), or metronidazole (10 mg/kg per dose at 8-hour doses daily for 10–20 days), can help to lessen the intense tissue reaction, make extraction easier, and relieve the pain.

The worm may be removed intact before it breaks through the skin. Preoperatively, an antihistamine is given to prevent untoward allergic reaction.

Prevention

Measures are directed to three different areas:

1. Providing a safe drinking water supply

- Providing piped water or drilled boreholes equipped with hand pumps are appropriate, although they are expensive to maintain.

- Improving the existing water system, such as protecting open wells or using concrete or stone masonry parapets, is a sustainable intervention. Small dams and ponds can be equipped with infiltration galleries to prevent people from wading into the water and therefore preventing infestation of the water sources by the parasite larvae.

2. Filtering drinking water

- When safe drinking water is not available, transmission can be interrupted by using filters made from fine mesh (100 microns).

- Ordinary cloth filters can be used at the household level, with the water boiled and aerated to restore taste.

- A monofilament nylon cloth filter is more robust and has the ability to remove the vector of the disease from drinking water.

3. Chemically treating pond water

- The application of temephos (Abate®) to surface water sources, mainly ponds, is an effective measure to prevent transmission by killing the vector. Treatment of the drinking water sources should be conducted monthly throughout the transmission season.

Schistosomiasis

Schistosomiasis is a group of diseases caused by trematodes (blood flukes) of the genus *Schistosoma*, the important species being *S. haematobium*, *S. mansoni*, and *S. japonicum*. It is also named bilharziasis in honour of Theodor Bilharz, a young German pathologist who discovered the aetiological agent for *S. haematobium* in Egypt in 1851. After malaria, schistosomiasis is the second most prevalent and most important parasitic disease in the world, with profound economic and public health consequences.

Demographics

Schistosomiasis remains a global health problem in the 21st century with an estimated 200 million people in 74 countries infected, of whom 85% are living in sub-Saharan Africa; the remainder live in South and Central America, the Caribbean, and the Far and Middle East. Travelers to endemic areas (particularly Africa) are at high risk of infection, and with increasing immigration globally, the chances of importing this disease to nonendemic areas are greatly increased.

The occurrence of species of schistosomiasis are highly variable from one country to another. *S. mansoni* is the most widespread, with *S. haematobium* concentrated in Africa and the Middle East, and *S. japonicum* primarily found in Asia. On the whole, school-aged children are more often and more heavily infected than adults because of their play habits and hygiene. Also, both the prevalence and intensity of infection have been found to be higher among males than females in many surveys. Like other parasitic diseases, poverty, ignorance, poor living conditions, inadequate sanitation, inadequate or total lack of public health facilities, and lack of safe water supplies, as well as deplorable personal and environmental hygiene characteristic of many developing Third World countries, are identified as important factors contributing to the increasing transmission of schistosomiasis.

Life Cycle of the Parasite

Of the different *Schistosoma* species that can infect humans, *S. haematobium*, *S. mansoni*, and *S. japonicum* are the most important because they cause the vast majority of infections.

Man is the definitive host of these parasites; *S. japonicum*, however, can live in other animals such as dogs, cats, cows, pigs, and rats. The intermediate host is the snail—bulinus for *S. haematobium*, biomphalaria and australorbis for *S. mansoni*, and oncomelania for *S. japonicum*.

For transmission to occur, there must be humans (or in the case of *S. japonicum*, animals) and snails living in close proximity and moving through the same aqueous environments. Additionally, infected humans must excrete their faeces or urine into or nearby the snail-infested water. When these conditions necessary to maintain the multistage life cycle are met, humans become infected when they come into contact with the cercariae during swimming, bathing, washing, or wading in infested water, or ingesting water from snail-infested sources. The cercariae penetrate the skin or mucous membrane to enter the body. They travel via the bloodstream, lung, and liver, and finally lodge within 30 days in the venules of the portal system, where they mature into adult worms. The adult males then move against the flow of blood, carrying the females in their gynaecophoric canal to the vesicular veins (in case of *S. haematobium*) or the mesenteric veins (in the case of *S. mansoni* and *S. japonicum*) in order to produce eggs.

Fertilised eggs or ova are released by the female parasites within the vasculature, then they cross the endothelium and basement membrane of the vein by means of a lytic substance they secrete, and enter the basement membrane and epithelium of the bladder or intestines, depending on the species involved. As a result, many eggs enter the lumen and are released from the body in urine or in the stool, but many are held up in the wall and die after 3 weeks; it is these dead ova that provoke the various pathological reactions. Those that are released from the body perish in 8 hours unless they come into contact with fresh water. The next phase of the flukes' life cycle takes place when humans urinate or defaecate into or near fresh water.

The eggs liberate their larvae or miracidia, which must enter the liver of the appropriate snail within 48 hours or die. In the snail, the miracidium forms a sporocyst that divides several times, forming daughter sporocysts containing cercariae. The sporocyst matures in 9 weeks and ruptures, releasing many cercariae excreted by the snails into the water. The tailed cercariae swim in the water until they come into contact with a human and the cycle is restarted. They die within 48 to 72 hours if no such contact is made. The life cycle takes 12–14 weeks.

Pathology

The pathological changes depend on the intensity and frequency of infection and the duration of exposure. The earliest reaction is papular dermatitis at the sites of entry of the cercariae, followed by pulmonary inflammatory reaction as the cercariae pass through the lungs. These changes may not be clinically apparent, especially in people normally resident in the endemic areas.

In the established infection, the basic pathological reaction is provoked by dead ova and consists of the formation of foreign body granulomata and fibrosis. The granuloma is made up of an ovum surrounded by epithelioid cells, plasma cells, lymphocytes, eosinophils, giant cells, and fibroblasts.

In *S. haematobium* infection, the lesions are most marked in the bladder and lower part of the ureters. The bladder often contains focal polypoid mucosal lesions or plaques of large masses of eggs. Eggs of *S. haematobium* in the bladder and ureteral walls appear to have a tendency to calcify, giving a "sand" appearance to these focal lesions and making them visible radiologically. Late effects are fibrous contraction of the bladder.

Ureteral polyps, strictures, and obstruction may lead to pyelonephritis and hydronephrosis. Cystitis with squamous metaplasia and ulceration leading to haematuria are common findings throughout the course of *S. haematobium* infection. Carcinomas of the bladder, of which half are squamous cell and almost half transitional with a few adenocarcinomas, are late complications.

The changes are more marked in *S. japonicum* infection compared to *S. mansoni* because a lot more ova are produced. The mucosa of the large bowel is hyperaemic and studded with pseudotubercles and shallow ulcers. Sessile or pedunculated polyps from coalescence of granulomata and epithelial hyperplasia are often present. Fibrosis leads to rigidity and consequent narrowing of the bowel.

The liver is also affected, especially in *S. japonicum*. It can be small, enlarged, or normal in size and nodular. The initial granulomata result in fibrosis around the terminals of the portal vein with ova embedded in them. These changes lead to portal hypertension with splenomegaly, ascites, and oesophageal varices.

Clinical Manifestation

Symptoms start after age 5 years but are marked in the second decade of life, and without treatment are severe in the third decade. Soon after penetration of the cercariae, there is a pricking sensation followed by papular dermatitis at the sites of penetration. This lasts for 2–3 days. About 4 weeks later, as a result of allergy to the developing flukes, the patient experiences intermittent fever, malaise, urticaria, and cough. These symptoms last about 2–8 weeks. Like the initial symptoms, these are mild, transient, or absent in infection by *S. haematobium*, especially in patients resident in endemic areas. In *S. mansoni* and *S. japonicum* infections, an allergic reaction to schistosomules in the liver results in pyrexia; malaise; painful, tender, and enlarged liver; splenomegaly; and at times jaundice and urticaria. From 6 to 24 months after the initial infection, symptoms develop due to the excretion of ova and the reaction to dead ova, the severity depending on the intensity of infection and the number of eggs produced.

Intermittent terminal haematuria after strenuous exercise is the main symptom of urinary schistosomiasis (*S. haematobium* infection). It occurs in about 50% of patients and is initially caused by damage of the mucosa by escaping ova and later by granulomatous ulcers or bilharzioma. Other symptoms are frequency of urination and burning sensation.

Investigations

The cornerstone of diagnosis of schistosomiasis is the detection of schistosome eggs in urine or faeces observed in saline. The characteristics of the respective ova aid their identification and diagnosis.

- *X-ray of the pelvis:* There may be calcification of the bladder wall and the lower end of the ureters in advanced cases.

- *Abdomino-pelvic ultrasound scan:* Ultrasound assessment of the changes in the urinary system are also promising. Ultrasound is still useful for early identification of periportal fibrosis and for assessment of hepatosplenomegaly.

- *Cystoscopy:* When examination of the urine and faeces is negative or there are marked bladder symptoms, cystoscopy is performed. Tubercles, sandy patches, granulomatous ulcers, or bilharzioma may be evident; biopsy of the lesion provides histological confirmation.

- *Rectal biopsy:* Ova are seen in snips of rectal mucosa.

- *Excretion urography:* Origraphy may demonstrate hydronephrosis, hydroureter, or multiple filling defects in the bladder due to bilharzioma.

- *Serological test:* Several serological tests may be done. Some of these may be used for screening of large populations.

- *Additional tests:* Tests such as sigmoidoscopy, liver biopsy, and barium swallow/oesophagogastroscopy may be indicated in intestinal schistosomiasis.

Strategies for Control

The four main foci for control of schistosomiasis are: (1) large-scale population-based chemotherapy, (2) vaccines, (3) molluscicides, and (4) environmental interventions. Various combinations of these strategies have resulted in remarkable progress toward reducing schistosomiasis. Sub-Saharan Africa, however, has had very little schistosomiasis control activity in the recent past. WHO is now rolling out initiatives to address this deficit. Current WHO initiatives target school-age children, with a goal of treating 75% of children at risk of schistosomiasis-related morbidity by 2010.

Medical Treatment

- *Praziquantel* is effective against all three species of schistomiasis. It may be given as a single oral dose of 50 mg/kg or 20 mg/kg three times at 4-hour intervals. Side effects are transient nausea, epigastric pain, pruritus or skin eruptions, headache, and dizziness. The cure rate is 80%.

- *Niridazole (Ambilhar)* is the drug of first choice for all the species of schistomiasis. The dose is 25 mg/kg (maximum 1.5 g) orally in two divided doses for 7–10 days. Side effects include confusion, depression, mania, epilepsy, slurred speech, and dark brown urine.

- *Metrifonate* is effective against *S. haematobrium* with a cure rate of 50–90%. It is given orally in a dose of 10 mg/kg repeated fortnightly for three doses.

- *Oxamniquine (Mansil®, Vansil®)* is effective against *S. mansoni* as a single oral dose of 30 mg/kg, but a second dose may be repeated in a few weeks. Fever, headache, and dizziness may occur.

Surgical Treatment

Surgical treatment may be necessary in later life. It is indicated for fibrous contracture or carcinoma of the bladder, stenosis of the ureter, hydronephrosis, portal hypertension and stenosis of the bowel.

Myiasis

Myiasis is a condition in which fly larvae (maggots) invade living tissue. They can be cutaneous, arterial, intestinal, or urinary in normal tissue or in preexisting wounds. Their importance lies in the fact that they are easily misdiagnosed, can cause mechanical damage, and cutaneous myiasis may require surgical removal of burrowed larvae.

Demographics

Myiasis is a parasitic infestation caused by the larvae of several fly species, such as *Cordylobia anthropophagi* (Tumbu fly), which is endemic in Tropical Africa and is known to have been widely distributed in the West African subregion for more than 130 years. Other fly species that produce larvae that cause myiasis are *Cordylobia rhodaini* (Lund fly), found in the rainforest areas of Tropical Africa, and *Dermatobia homonis* (human botfly), which is endemic in Central and South America.

Aetiology/Pathophysiology

Myiasis could result from a breach in healthy skin by the fly larvae themselves or through abrasions and wounds in which the respective flies deposit their eggs or larvae. The larvae can burrow through healthy tissue by using their cuticular spines aided by proteolytic enzymes.

The larvae arise from eggs deposited by the fly species on soil polluted with animal excrement, or clothing saturated with perspiration, or soiled diapers. After hatching, the larvae can stay alive for 7–20 days while attached to contaminated articles and clothing or the soil. They are activated by the warm body of the host and penetrate the skin and develop in the subcutaneous tissue in 12 days. Dogs and small rodents are a particularly important reservoir for the parasite; humans are infected accidentally. Children, because of their daily habits and liking for pets, are especially prone to developing the disease. Under normal circumstances, the fly larvae that have penetrated the skin remain in the subcutaneous tissue below the skin orifice until they reach maturity without migrating to deeper structures. However, there have been two reports of fatal cases of cerebral infestation caused by migration of the larvae through the open fontanelles in children.

Ultimately, the larvae emerge from the swellings, which may be situated on the forearm, scrotum, and other parts of the body (Figure 23.3) and fall to the ground to pupate in 36 hours.

Clinical Presentation

The clinical presentation is usually simple and includes swelling of the part of the body involved, pain, and itching. The history may suggest recent handling of infested pests from which similar larvae may have been extracted. The child may be unkempt.

A boil-like lesion may be seen with a tiny opening at the top from which the motile tip of the larva may be observed. Application of water on the lesion activates the indwelling larva, making the diagnosis obvious.

Investigation

Diagnosis is clinical. However, the extracted larva should be submitted for parasitological identification (Figure 23.4).

Treatment

The larvae may spontaneously exit from the lesion, which then subsides unless secondarily infected. Alternatively, obstructing the cutaneous orifice by pouring water, oil, or liquid paraffin suffocates the larva, which wriggles out and can be squeezed out gently with the gloved hands. Topical antibiotic creams may be applied to prevent secondary infection. Rarely, larvae that have burrowed through the subcutaneous or deeper tissues may require surgical removal.

Hydatid Disease

Hydatid disease is a common problem in the developing countries. The cause of the disease in human beings is the hydatid cyst, which is a larval form of *Echinococci*. There are three species of *Echinococci* that may cause hydatid disease: *E. granularis*, *E. multilocularis*, and *E. olgiettas*. The clinical presentation and management of various forms of hydatid disease are similar with only minor differences. Hydatid cyst is the most common cestodes infection in the world, with cosmopolitan distribution. It is especially prevalent in sheep- and cattle-raising areas where canines such as dogs, wolves, jackals, and foxes are present.

Pathophysiology

The adult echinococcus is a small tapeworm, 3–6 mm long. It has a life-span of about 5 months. Canines (dogs, wolves, jackals, and foxes) are the definitive hosts. It resides in the upper small intestine of the host and lays eggs that are passed in the faeces of the canine and infect soil, water, and the bodies of the dogs and other animals. Cattle, sheep, and other animals get infected by ingesting these eggs and are intermediate hosts. Humans get infected by ingesting raw vegetables and water, and by close association with dogs. After ingestion, either by human beings or an intermediate host, the embryo is liberated in the small intestine, which then penetrates the intestinal mucosa to reach the portal circulation. It may settle in the liver and form a hydatid cyst. The embryo may pass the portal circulation and enter into the general circulation, where it can form a hydatid cyst in virtually any organ and tissue of the body, such as the lung, brain, and bones.

The hydatid cyst is the larval form of *Echinococcus* and consists of an inner germinal layer and outer laminated membrane. Compressed host connective tissue forms the false capsule around the cyst. The germinal layer forms bulblike projections in the lumen called brood capsules. Inside the brood capsules, small invaginations occur that form the scolices, which are the future heads of the mature worms. These

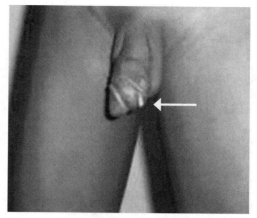

Figure 23.3: Penile myiasis (arrow) with fly larva exiting lesion after it was squeezed out with gloved hands (courtesy of Dr UE Usang, Calabar, Nigeria).

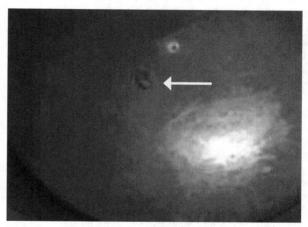

Figure 23.4: Fly larva of Cordylobia anthropophaga extracted from a 12-year-old child with penile myiasis (courtesy of Dr UE Usang, Calabar, Nigeria).

scolices have a sucker and hooklet and are infective. Multiloculated cysts are formed by infestation with *E. multilocularis*. After the death of the animal in the wild or the feeding of infected organs to the dogs by butchers, dogs and other canines ingest hydatid cyst-infested tissue. The scolices, using their hooks, settle in the proximal small intestine and grow into mature worms. Human beings are accidental hosts and do not complete the life cycle. In endemic areas, the parasite may cause infection in early childhood, but it takes a long time before the child may become symptomatic. Sometimes the disease may manifest 20–30 years after initial infection.

Epidemiology

Hydatid disease has a worldwide presence. It is seen in the countryside where cattle, sheep, dogs, and humans live in close association. In rural areas, especially in developing countries, animals are slaughtered in open areas and the infected tissue is fed to the street dogs, which may get infected and may also transmit the disease to humans. In adults, the liver and lungs are involved in 90% of the cases, and liver hydatid is seen in nearly 75% of the cases. In children, lung hydatid is more common.

Clinical Presentations

In humans, hydatid disease manifests as a hydatid cyst. Usually there is a single hydatid cyst, but there may be multiple cysts. The organs of predilection are the liver and lung, but it may involve virtually any tissues or organs of the body, such as bones, brain, spleen, heart, and peritoneum. The clinical presentation of a hydatid cyst depends on the organ involved and is either by its presence in the organ, its local pressure effects, antigenic reaction, or rupture. The cyst may remain silent for a long time and regress without causing any symptoms. Patients usually have nonspecific symptoms such as cough, abdominal discomfort, low-grade fever, and malaise. In liver hydatid, the patient may present with abdominal discomfort, painful abdomen, palpable mass, and sometimes jaundice due to compression of the biliary ductal system. In the lungs, the hydatid cyst manifests as coughing, haemoptysis, and passage of white flakes in sputum, or incidental findings on a chest x-ray. Bone hydatid cysts present with bone pains and pathological fractures. Hydatid cysts in the brain usually present with features of a space-occupying lesion in the brain.

The rupture of a hydatid cyst may occur secondary to infections or trauma and can cause serious allergic reactions and even anaphylactic shock. The rupture of an untreated hydatid cyst can cause seedling and formation of multiple daughter cysts, especially in wide cavities such as the peritoneum and pleural cavities.

Diagnosis

In the endemic areas the diagnosis is often easy due to the prevalence of the disease. Patients with hapatomegaly should be properly investigated. Ultrasound evaluation is a useful tool in differentiating solid and cystic masses and can make a confident diagnosis in liver hydatid cysts. Simple liver cysts and abscesses are not uncommon in developing countries; the ultrasound evaluation can easy differentiate internal membrane and floating hydatid sand (scolices). In a ruptured hydatid cyst, the laminated membrane floats on the fluid surface and can be detected by ultrasound. A multilocular hydatid cyst can be diagnosed by its classic ultrasound appearance but may be confused with cystic tumours. In these cases a CT scan may be helpful in making a diagnosis. A lung hydatid cyst is suggested by the well-circumscribed homogenous opacity in the lung (Figure 23.5). A ruptured pulmonary hydatid cyst shows as a rounded cavity with air fluid level and floating laminated membrane and may give the appearance of the so-called "water lily" sign. Patients with hydatid cysts have moderate eosinophilia, and their immunoglobulin levels are elevated. The diagnosis may be confirmed by serological tests. Countercurrent immunoelectrophoresis (CIE) for scolex antigen and enzyme-linked immunosorbent assay (ELISA) can confirm the diagnosis in most cases. The Casoni test is performed by intradermal injection of crude sterile hydatid fluid, but it is not a reliable test.

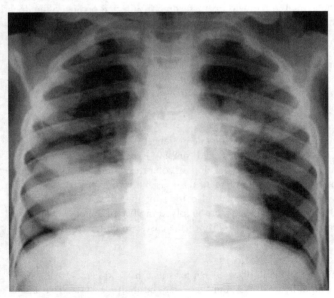

Figure 23.5: X-ray of hydatid disease of the lung.

Treatment

Management of patients with hydatid disease has changed significantly over the past few decades. Initially, surgery was considered the only option for hydatid cysts, but now medical management is useful in many cases. The drugs of choice are albendazole (12–15 mg/kg/day for 28 days) and praziquantel (50 mg/kg/day for 6-8 weeks). Mebendazole (200 mg/kg/day in 3 divided doses for 16 weeks) is also effective. Although primary surgery can eradicate hydatid cyst in most cases, there is always fear of daughter cyst formations. Furthermore, treatment with long-term albendazole can cure hydatid cyst in more than half the cases. The general consensus now is that patients with multiple hydatid cysts and having cysts less than 6 cm in diameter shall be treated medically, and any residual cysts may be tackled with surgery. In the case of a solitary cyst larger than 6 cm, surgery should be planned. Adjuvant medical therapy in these patients should be done to avoid recurrence of cysts and seedlings in adjacent tissue. PAIR (percutaneous aspiration, instillation [of hypertonic saline], and re-aspiration [after 15 minutes]) is another technique of treating hydatid cysts of the liver and lungs. These patients should also be treated with albendazole to avoid any recurrence. Recently, laparoscopic-assisted drainage of hydatid cysts has been performed with good results, but its advantage over PAIR and other procedures needs to be evaluated by long-term studies.

Evidence-Based Research

Table 23.1 presents an evidence-based study of intestinal parasitic infection among children in Karachi, Pakistan.

Table 23.1: Evidence-based research.

Title	Prevalence and factors associated with intestinal parasitic infection among children in an urban slum in Karachi
Authors	Mehraj V, Hatcher J, Akhtar S, Rafique G, Beg MA
Institution	Department of Pathology & Microbiology, Aga Khan University, Karachi, Pakistan. Awolowo University, Ile-Ife, Ilesa, Nigeria.
Reference	PLoS ONE 2008; 3(11):e3680.
Problem	Intestinal parasitic infections are endemic worldwide and have been described as constituting the greatest single worldwide cause of illness and disease. Poverty, illiteracy, poor hygiene, lack of access to potable water, and a hot and humid tropical climate are the factors associated with intestinal parasitic infections.
Intervention	The study aimed to estimate the prevalence and identify factors associated with intestinal parasitic infections among 1- to 5-year-old children residing in an urban slum of Karachi, Pakistan.
Comparison/ control (quality of evidence)	A cross-sectional survey was conducted from February to June 2006 in Ghosia Colony, Gulshan Town, Karachi, Pakistan. A simple random sample of 350 children aged 1–5 years was collected. The study used a structured pretested questionnaire, anthropometric tools, and stool tests to obtain epidemiological and disease data. Data were analyzed by using appropriate descriptive, univariate, and multivariable logistic regression methods. The mean age of participants was 2.8 years, and 53% were male. The proportions of wasted, stunted, and underweight children were 10.4%, 58.9%, and 32.7%, respectively. The prevalence of intestinal parasitic infections was estimated to be 52.8% (95% CI: 46.1; 59.4). Giardia lamblia was the most common parasite, followed by Ascaris lumbricoides, Blastocystis hominis, and Hymenolepis nana. About 43% of the children were infected with a single parasite, and 10% with multiple parasites. Age {Adjusted Odds Ratio (aOR) = 1.5; 95% CI: 1.1; 1.9}, living in rented households (aOR = 2.0; 95% CI: 1.0; 3.9) and a history of excessive crying (aOR = 1.9; 95% CI: 1.0; 3.4) were significantly associated with intestinal parasitic infections.
Outcome/ effect	Intestinal parasites are highly prevalent in this setting, and poverty was implicated as an important risk factor for infection. Effective poverty reduction programmes and promotion of deworming could reduce intestinal parasite carriage. There is a need for mass campaigns to create awareness about health and hygiene.

Historical significance/ comments

School-based health education for the control of soil-transmitted helminthiases in Kanchanaburi province, Thailand Anantaphruti MT, Waikagul J, Maipanich W, et al. T Ann Trop Med Parasitol 2008;102(6):521–528.

Department of Helminthology, Faculty of Tropical Medicine, Mahidol University, 420/6 Ratchawithi Road, Bangkok 10400, Thailand

Soil-transmitted helminthiases (STHs) are major parasitic diseases that cause health problems worldwide. School-based health education is one of several basic interventions currently recommended by the World Health Organization for the control of these infections. A 3-year programme of health education for the control of STHs has recently been completed in four primary schools in the Hauykayeng subdistrict of Thong Pha Phum district, in the Kanchanaburi province of Thailand.

Overall, the percentage of the schoolchildren infected with STH increased between the start of year 1 of the intervention (16.6%) and the end of year 2 (23.8%), but showed signs of falling by the end of year 3 (19.4%). Although none of these year-on-year changes in overall prevalence was statistically significant, some significant trends were detected when the six school grades (i.e., age groups) were considered separately. The grade showing the highest prevalence of STH infection changed, from grade 6 (representing the oldest children investigated) at the start of year 1 (when grade 1 children were excluded from the survey) to grade 1 (representing the youngest children) at the ends of years 2 and 3. By the end of year 3, the children in grades 5 and 6 had significantly lower prevalences of infection than the grade 1 subjects. The prevalence of STH infection in the grade 1 children was significantly higher than that in any of the older grades at the end of year 2 and significantly higher than that in grades 3–6 at the end of year 3.

These results indicate that health education had a greater impact on the children in the higher grades (who, presumably had better levels of understanding and practised better personal infection prevention) than on the younger children. Although school-based interventions can serve as a useful entry point for parasite control, more effort, including anthelminthic treatment, may be required among the youngest children. The activities need to be sustainable and supported by appropriate school health policies.

Key Summary Points

1. Parasitic infestations are a tropical disease with huge public health implications.

2. Parasitic infestations are associated with poor sanitation, low socioeconomic communities, and lack of primary health care.

3. The surgical relevance is the treatment of the complication of the disease (i.e., abscess formation, acute abdomen, and bowel obstruction).

4. A combination of medical and surgical treatment is pertinent; however, the focus for this disease should be on prevention.

Suggested Reading

Akinbode OA, Uduuebho OM, Akinrinmade JF, Abatan MO. Human amoebiasis: epidemiological studies at two hospitals in Ibadan, Nigeria. Int J Zoonoses 1986; 13(3):202–205.

Barry M. The tail end of guinea worm—Global eradication without a drug or a vaccine. New Engl J Med 2007; 356(25):2561–2564.

Behrman RE, Kleigman RM, Jenson HB. Nelson text book of pediatrics. Saunders, Philadelphia, 2000; Pp 1079–1081.

Cooney RM, Flanagan KP, Zehyle E. Review of surgical management of cystic hydatid disease in a resource limited setting: Turkana, Kenya. Eur J Gastroenterol Hepatol 2004; 16(11):1233–1236.

Frenkel JK, Taraschewski H, Voigt WP. Important pathologic effects of parasitic infections of man: ascariasis. In: Mehlhom H, ed. Parasitology in focus: facts and trends, 1st ed. Springer–Verlag, Berlin, Heidelberg, 1988; Pp 577–578.

Hadley GP, Mickel RE. Fulminating amoebic colitis in infants and children. J Roy Coll Surg Ed 1984; 29:370–372.

Karam M, Tayeh A. Dracunculiasis eradication. Bull Soc Pathol Exot 2006; 99(5):377–385.

Mavridis G, Livaditi E, Christopoulos-Geroulanos G. Management of hydatidosis in children: twenty-one year experience. Eur J Pediatr Surg 2007; 17(6):400–403.

Millar AJW, Bass DH, Van Der Merwe P. Parasitic infestation in Cape Town children: a random study of 101 patients. S Afr Med J 1989; 76:197–198.

Okyay P, Ertug S, Gultekin B, Owen O, Beser E. Intestinal parasites prevalence and related factors in school children, a Western city sample—Turkey. BMC Public Health 2004; 4:64–66.

Stanley SL Jr. Amoebiasis. Lancet 2003; 361(9362):1025–1034.

Strategies for the control of schistosomiasis. WHO Bulletin 2002; 80:235–243.

Veraldi S, Brusasco A. Cutaneous myiasis caused by larvae of Cordylobia anthropophagi. (Blanchard) Int J Dermat 1993; 32: 182–184.

Vilamizar E, Mendez M, Bonilla E, Varon H, de Onatra S. Ascaris lumbricoides infestation as a cause of intestinal obstruction in children: experience with 87 cases. J Pediatr Surg 1996; 31:201–205.

World Health Organization. The treatment of diarrhea: a manual for physicians and other health workers. WHO/CDD/95.3: 1995.

CHAPTER 24
HIV/AIDS AND THE PAEDIATRIC SURGEON

Lary Hadley

Kokila Lakhoo

Introduction

Three of every four HIV-positive people in the world live in sub-Saharan Africa.[1] This disease dominates our every activity as doctors, and intrudes into the practice of paediatric surgery in Africa as much as into every other sphere of human endeavour.

AIDS became recognised as a disease entity in the early 1980s, when an increase in the incidence of opportunistic infections was seen in Kinshasa and there were clusters of affected homosexuals in Los Angeles and San Francisco.[2] In Africa, HIV/AIDS has nothing to do with homosexuality, but may be related to heterosexual promiscuity.[3] HIV-1 was defined as the cause of the clinical syndrome called AIDS by French workers in 1983.[4] In 1985, a new human retrovirus, HIV-2, was identified in AIDS patients in West Africa.[5]

It is likely that HIV infection originated in tropical Africa in the 1930s, making the transition from a simian infection to a human pathogen.[6] It is a retrovirus that infects the CD4+ lymphocyte and monocyte, destroying them, reducing their absolute numbers and global function, thereby exposing the patient to the risks of impaired cellular immunity. There is no cure for the infection, but antiviral therapy has the potential to suppress the virus and restore immune function.

Demographics and History

By 2001, 20 million HIV-infected people lived in sub-Saharan Africa, of whom only a trivial number were receiving effective treatment. In 2007, 1.6 million people in Africa died of AIDS; more than 11 million children have been orphaned by the disease.[7] Figures 24.1 and 24.2 show the prevalence of HIV in Southern Africa and in West and Central Africa, respectively. Effective treatment against these retroviruses was known in the last decade, but proved to be too expensive for developing countries that were struggling with other important health issues and lacked the infrastructure to deliver the treatment in a sustainable fashion.[8]

In the face of these difficulties, the South African government initially denied any association between HIV and AIDS,[9] but later sought to parallel import generic antiviral drugs. Drug manufacturers were keen to protect their profits and intellectual capital, but the scale of the humanitarian disaster precluded the continuation of this precept, and at the World Trade Organisation (WTO) meeting in Doha in 2001, a resolution of the impasse was negotiated.[10]

In 2001, the Global Fund to Fight AIDS, Tuberculosis and Malaria was established, and in 2003, President Bush's President's Emergency Plan for AIDS Relief (PEPFAR), as well as private agencies such as the Bill and Melinda Gates Foundation, increased the money available to counter the scourge and to support necessary infrastructure development.[8] In 2004, antiretroviral drugs became available in South Africa, and currently, about 28% of the patients in need are on treatment.[7] Prior to 2004, there was little point in testing for HIV, as all that could be offered was symptomatic treatment, and such palliation did not require formal diagnosis.

Concomitant with the HIV pandemic are the TB pandemic[11], the lymphoma pandemic[12], the Kaposi pandemic,[13] the orphan pandemic,[14] and myriad evil social, ethical, and economic consequences, all of which complicate management decisions.

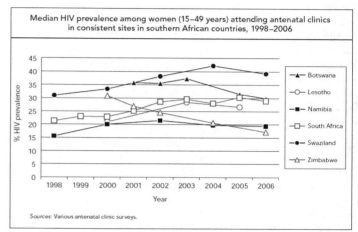

Source: Reproduced by permission from UNAID.

Figure 24.1: HIV prevalence in Southern Africa.[20]

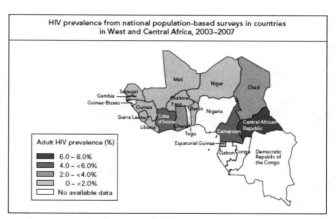

Source: Reproduced by permission from UNAID.

Figure 24.2: HIV prevalence in West and Central Africa.[20]

It should be emphasized that whilst some aspects of HIV/AIDS, such as the prevention of vertical transmission and the impact of breast-feeding, have been well studied,[15,16] and entire libraries of reports have been compiled on epidemiological studies and papers attempting to define and alter African sexual traditions,[3,17,18] paediatric surgeons have been slow to formally study the impact of this disease on their practices.[19] Much is not known.

Route of Infection

Most children become infected during gestation or delivery. The rate of transmission can be reduced from around 35% to less than 10% by offering perinatal nevirapine to the mother and child and may be further reduced by dual therapy with zidovudine and nevirapine.[21].Elective Caesarean section may even further reduce the transmission rate to around 2%.[21,22]

Confirmation of HIV infection in babies can be difficult because routine antibody tests may detect a maternally derived antibody that can persist for up to 18 months in the absence of active viral disease, and therefore polymerase chain reaction (PCR) testing is necessary.[23]

In many countries, blood transfusion remains a hazard due to inadequate screening of donors, and children requiring multiple transfusions of blood or blood products (e.g., haemophiliacs or sicklers), are at particular risk.[24, 25]

In addition, a myth that HIV can be cured by having sex with young girls has increased the spread of the virus through rape and other sexual abuse.[26]

Risk to Health Workers

Occupational infection with HIV is rare amongst health care workers. Certain categories of health workers (e.g., surgeons, dentists, and operating theatre staff) are at greater risk, but even following documented needle stick injury and exposure to blood from HIV positive patients this risk is small.[27] This is not to say that sensible precautions should not be taken. The risk of seroconversion can be minimised by postexposure prophylaxis with zidovudine.[27] Employers are required to provide adequate protection to employees, and all staff should be aware of the local policy for postexposure prophylaxis and report all injuries.[28]

Stages of the Disease

Like many malignant diseases the principles of management depend upon the stage of disease. In HIV/AIDS, the stage of disease is determined by CD4+ counts, the percentage of the total lymphocyte count represented by CD4+ cells, the viral load, and, most important, the general condition of the patient.[29] It must be remembered that children normally have higher CD4+ counts than adults, but this count declines with age, making absolute numbers difficult to interpret;[30] thus, the count is usually expressed as a percentage of the total lymphocyte count.[31] HIV-infected children may be identified by a low CD4+ count and decreasing percentage count as early as 3 months after birth.[31]

The formal diagnosis of AIDS requires the application of criteria established by the World Health Organization (WHO; see Table 24.1) or the Centers for Disease Control and Prevention (CDC). In children, unfortunately, these criteria are neither precise nor predictive,[32] and they are constantly being revised to include both clinical and laboratory parameters. Resources for the laboratory confirmation of HIV infection are not universal in developing countries, however, so a clinical approach is more generally useful, although difficult to quantify.

Table 24.1: World Health Organization temporary definition of AIDS in developing countries (the Bangui definition).

Major criteria	Minor criteria
Weight loss or slow weight gain	Generalised lymphadenopathy
Chronic diarrhoea (more than 1 month)	Oro-pharyngeal candidiasis
	Repeated common infections (e.g., otitis)
Fever (more than 1 month)	Persistent cough
	Pruritic dermatitis
	Confirmed maternal HIV infection

Surgical Approach

The paediatric surgeon may encounter HIV positive patients in a number of scenarios:

1. The patient may present with an unrelated pathology such as inguinal hernia, and may be coincidentally HIV infected. The immediate management of the patient will depend upon the stage of the HIV disease.

2. The patient may present, unaware of his or her HIV status, for management of a disorder that is likely to be HIV related, such as tuberculosis or fasciitis. Such patients should be offered serological testing so that antiviral therapy can be provided if necessary.

3. The patient may be referred for assistance in diagnosis of lymph node enlargement, particularly the differentiation between lymphoma and tuberculosis in an HIV-infected individual.

4. The patient may present de novo with an AIDS-defining pathology, such as spontaneous rectovaginal fistula,[33,34] or neonatal CMV enteritis,[35] among others.

5. The patient may be a neonate with an emergency condition, born to an HIV-infected mother, in whom the HIV status cannot be rapidly determined, or may be an older child with an emergency in whom the status cannot be determined.

The merit of the dictum that all patients, irrespective of age or clinical diagnosis, should be regarded as HIV positive is clear, and "universal precautions" against needle-stick and contact with body fluids should become routine.

It is apparent that asymptomatic HIV-infected individuals carry no greater surgical risk than noninfected patients, either in the general ward or the intensive care unit (ICU).[36] Other than referral for subsequent antiviral treatment no modification of surgical protocol is required.

In symptomatic patients, it is important to remember that it is the patient who requires treatment, not merely his surgical pathology. Any treatment plan must be modified according to the clinical and haematological status of the patient, but it is the clinical status of the patient that should determine the management approach, not the patient's HIV status. Patients in a poor clinical condition should not undergo elective surgery, no matter what their HIV status. Patients who are well should be offered surgery as needed, no matter what their HIV status.

Symptomatic HIV-infected patients exhibit a spectrum of clinical conditions from apparently well to moribund. Generally speaking, the least possible surgical intervention should be performed that "buys time" for the patient's general condition to be improved by medical interventions. Surgeons have been making these determinations for generations, long before the HIV pandemic arose; however, a new critical factor in management decisions is the availability of antiviral therapy for the patient. Untreated AIDS remains a lethal disease.

Thus, an asymptomatic HIV-infected individual with an uncomplicated inguinal hernia would be a candidate for an immediate herniotomy. A similar patient who has AIDS, severe wasting, candidiasis, encephalopathy, and any other comorbidity might be better served by a period of medical treatment that may include antiviral treatment.

Antiviral Treatment

Antiviral treatment is not without hazard, which is why it should be offered only within a structured programme that includes long-term follow-up and continued supervision. It should be remembered that HIV treatment is lifelong; this fact must be emphasized to caregivers who tend to discontinue treatment when wellness has been achieved. Failure to continue with treatment may increase the incidence of viral resistance to therapy, and this fear forms the basis for the strict criteria with which patients must comply before starting therapy.[37]

Each of the commonly used antiviral drugs has a specific toxicity profile, and continued surveillance for toxic effects is mandatory. Initiation of treatment may also result in clinical deterioration due to the immune reconstitution inflammatory syndrome (IRIS).[38] Whilst the exact pathogenesis of IRIS is unknown, it is clearly related to the severity of immunosuppression at the time of the initiation of antiviral therapy.[38] As the patient's immune function is restored, the CD4+ count rises, the viral load falls, and there is restoration of pathogen-specific immunity. This may recognise viable organisms, particularly tuberculosis, but also other pathogens, and in some patients an associated inflammatory response results in rapid clinical deterioration and, in some cases, death.[39] This condition was well recognised by physicians managing patients with disseminated tuberculosis in the pre-AIDS era, but appears to be more common in HIV-infected individuals. In HIV-infected patients with tuberculosis, it is recommended that antiviral therapy be delayed for several weeks after initiation of tuberculosis treatment in order to minimise the risk of IRIS particularly for those at greatest risk.[40]

Surgical Prophylaxis

Evidence suggests that male circumcision offers some protection against infection with HIV-1,[41] although this evidence is far from being incontrovertible.[42] All agree, however, that circumcision alone is insufficient to prevent transmission of the disease, and circumcised men must still be advised to engage only in safe sexual practices, including condom use. The acceptability of this form of potential partial preventative measure by individuals as well as to populations has yet to be determined.

Ethical Issues

The considerable stigma associated with HIV may stem from its original recognition in male homosexuals, as well as in the personal nature of human sexuality.[43] The stoning to death of Gugu Dlamini by members of her own community in South Africa after she had announced that she was HIV-infected was an extreme example of the stigmatisation of this disease.[43] Certainly at some point HIV became treated differently from other sexually transmitted diseases, presumably, amongst other reasons, due to the inability of governments to offer treatment and the dated perception that the condition was inevitably lethal. Clearly, patient confidentiality is paramount, but the singling out of HIV as a disease apart from all others adds to the stigmatisation that patients experience.

Every patient has a right to know his or her HIV status, and testing should be offered to all who are unaware.[44]

Key Summary Points

1. HIV is a retrovirus that infects and destroys the CD4+ lymphocyte and monocyte, exposing the patient to risks of immune deficiency.

2. Incidence of HIV/AIDS is high in Africa.

3. Most children become infected during gestation or delivery, and this risk may be reduced by perinatal antiviral therapy.

4. In asymptomatic neonates, PCR testing is more accurate than routine antibody testing.

5. The occupational HIV risk to health care workers is low, and is further reduced with universal precautions and postexposure prophylaxis with antiviral therapy.

6. There is no difference in the surgical risk for asymptomatic HIV-infected patients and noninfected patients.

7. In symptomatic patients, the clinical status—and not the HIV status—dictates the management of the patient.

8. The toxic effects of antiviral treatment dictate its use within a structured programme.

9. Circumcision alone is not an adequate prophylaxis for HIV.

References

1. de Cock KM, Mbori-Ngacha D, Marum E. Shadow on the continent: public health and HIV/AIDS in Africa in the 21st century. Lancet 2002; 360(9326):67–72.

2. Fauci AS. HIV and AIDS; 20 years of science. Nature Med 2003; 9(7):839–843.

3. Pettifor AE, Rees HV, Kleinschmidt I, Steffenson AE, MacPhail C, Hlongwa-Madikizela L, et al. Young people's sexual health in South Africa: HIV prevalence and sexual behaviours from a nationally representative household survey. AIDS 2005; 19(14):1525–1534.

4. Montagnier L. Historical essay: a history of HIV discovery. Science 2002; 298:1727–1728.

5. Clavel F, Guétard D, Brun-Vézinet F, Chamaret S, Rey MA, Santos-Ferreira MO, et al. Isolation of a new human retrovirus from West African patients with AIDS. Science 1986; 233:343–346.

6. Gao F, Bailes E, Robertson DL, Chen Y, Rodenburg CM, Michael SF, et al. Origin of HIV-1 in the chimpanzee Pan troglodytes troglodytes. Nature 1999; 397:436–441.

7. www.avert.org/aafrica.htm.

8. Harries AD, Nyangulu DS, Hargreaves NJ, Kaluna O, Salaiponi FM. Preventing antiretroviral anarchy in sub-Saharan Africa. Lancet 2001; 358(9279):410–414.

9. Fassin F, Schneider H. The politics of AIDs in South Africa: beyond the controversies. Brit Med J 2003; 326(7387):495–497.

10. Wohlgemut JP. AIDS, Africa and indifference: a confession. Can Med Assoc J 2002; 167(5):485–487.

11. Gandhi NR, Moll A, Sturm AW, Pawinski R, Govender T, Lalloo U, et al. Extensively drug-resistant tuberculosis as a cause of death in patients co-infected with tuberculosis and HIV in a rural area of South Africa. Lancet 2006; 368(9547):1575–1580.

12. Lazzi S, Ferrari F, Nyongo A, Palummo N, de Milito A, Zazzi M, et al. HIV-associated malignant lymphoma in Kenya (Equatorial Africa). Human Path 1999; 30(10):1269–1270.

13. Sitas H, Pacella-Norman R, Carra RA, Patel M, Ruff P, Sur R, et al. The spectrum of HIV-1 related cancers in South Africa. Int J Cancer 2000; 88(3):489–492.

14. Ansell N, Young L. Enabling households to support successful migration of AIDS orphans in southern Africa. AIDS Care 2004; 16(1):3–10.

15. Dabis F, Msellati P, Meda N, Welffens-Ekra C, You B, Manigart O, et al. 6-month efficacy, tolerance, and acceptability of a short regimen of oral zidovudine to reduce vertical transmission of HIV in breastfed children in Côte d'Ivoire and Burkina Faso: a double blind placebo controlled multicentre trial. Lancet 1999; 353:786–791.

16. Embree J, Njenga S, Datta P, Nagelkerke N, Ndinya-Achola JO, Mohammed Z, et al. Risk factors for post-natal mother-child transmission of HIV-1. AIDS 2000; 14(16):2535–2541.

17. Campbell C. Migrancy, masculine identities and AIDS; the psychosocial context of HIV transmission on the South African gold mines. Soc Sci and Med 1997; 45(2):273–281.

18. Leclerc-Madlala S. Infect one, infect all: Zulu youth response to the AIDS epidemic in South Africa. Med Anthrop 1997; 17(4):363–380.

19. Bowley DM, Rogers TN, Meyers T, Pitcher G. Surgeons are failing to recognize children with HIV infection. J Pediatr Surg 2007; 42(2):431–434.

20. Joint United Nations Programme on (HIV/AIDS) and World Health Organisation (WHO) UNAIDS/08.O8E/JC1526E (English original March 2008). 2008.

21. Andiman WA. Transmission of HIV-1 from mother to infant. Curr Opin Pediatr 2002; 14:78–85.

22. Kind C, Rudin C, Siegrist C-A, Wyler C-A, Biedermann K, Lauper U, et al. Prevention of vertical HIV transmission: additive protective effect of elective cesarean section and zidovudine prophylaxis. AIDS 1998; 12(2):205–210.

23. Praharaj AK. Problems in diagnosis of HIV infection in babies. Med J Armed Forces of India 2006; 62:363–366.

24. Moore A, Herrera G, Nyamongo J, Lackritz E, Granade T, Nahlen B, et al. Estimated risk of HIV transmission by blood transfusion in Kenya. Lancet 2001; 358(9282):657–660.

25. Fleming AF. HIV and blood transfusion in sub-Saharan Africa. Transfus Sci 1997; 18(2):167–179.

26. Bowley DM, Pitcher GJ, Beale PG, Joseph C, Davies MR. Child rape in South Africa—an open letter to the Minister of Health. S Afr Med J 2002; 92(10):744.

27. Cardo DM, Culver DH, Cieielski CA, Srivastava PU, Marcus R, Abiteboul D, et al. A case-control study of HIV seroconversion in health care workers after percutaneous exposure. New Eng J Med 1997; 337(21):1485–1490.

28. Puro V, Cicalini S, De Carli G, Soldani F, Antunes F, Balslev U, et al. Post exposure prophylaxis of HIV infection in healthcare workers: recommendations for the European setting. Euro J Epidem 2004; 19(6):577–584.

29. Greenberg AE, Coulibaly IM, Kadio A, Coulibaly D, Kassim S, Sassan-Morokro M, et al. Impact of the 1994 expanded World Health Organization case definition on AIDS surveillance in university hospitals and tuberculosis centers in Côte d'Ivoire. AIDS 1997; 11(15):1881–1882.

30. Denny T, Yogev R, Gelman R, Skuza J, Oleske E, Chadwick S, et al. Lymphocyte subsets in healthy children in the first 5 years of life. JAMA 1992; 267(11):1484–1488.

31. Embree J, Bwayo J, Nagelkerke N, Njenga S, Nyange P, Ndinya-Achola J, et al. Lymphocyte subsets in human immunodeficiency virus Type 1-infected and uninfected children in Nairobi. Pediat Infect Dis J 2001; 20(4):397–403.

32. Keou FX, Bélec L, Esunge PM, Cancre N, Gresenguet G. World Health Organization clinical case definition for AIDS in Africa: an analysis of evaluations. East Afr Med J 1992; 69(10):550–553.

33. Oliver M. Acquired recto-vaginal fistula. Archiv Dis Childhood 1995; 72(3):275.

34. Uba AF, Chirdan LB, Ardill W, Ramyil VM, Kidmas AT. Acquired rectovaginal fistula in human immunodeficiency virus-positive children: a causal or casual relationship. Pediatr Surg Int 2004; 20(11-12):898–901.

35. Cheong JLY, Cowan FM, Modi N. Gastrointestinal manifestation of postnatal cytomegalovirus infection in infants admitted to a neonatal intensive care unit over a five year period. Archiv Dis Childhood (Fetal and Neonatal ed) 2004;89 (4):F367–F369.

36. Muckart DJ, Bhagwanjee S, Jeena PM, Moodley P. Does HIV status influence the outcome of patients admitted to a surgical intensive care unit? A prospective double blind study. Brit Med J 1997; 314(7087):1077–1081.

37. Clavel F, Hance AJ. HIV drug resistance. New Eng J Med 2004; 350(10):1023–1035

38. Michailidis C, Pozniak AL, Mandalia S, Basnayake S, Nelson MR, Gazzard BC. Clinical characteristics of IRIS syndrome in patients with HIV and tuberculosis. Antivir Ther 2005; 10:417–422.

39. Dhasmana DJ, Dheda K, Ravn P, Wilkinson RJ, Meintjies G. Immune reconstitution inflammatory syndrome in HIV-infected patients receiving antiretroviral therapy: pathogenesis, clinical manifestations and management. Drugs 2008; 68(2):191–208.

40. Schiffer JT, Sterling TR. Timing of antiretroviral therapy initiation in tuberculosis patients with AIDS: a decision analysis. J Acq Immun Defic Synd 2007; 46(1):121–123.

41. Weiss HA, Quigley MA, Hayes RJ. Male circumcision and the risk of HIV infection in sub-Saharan Africa: a systematic review and meta-analysis. AIDS 2000; 14(15):2361–2379.

42. Dowsett GW, Couch M. Roundtable: male circumcision and HIV prevention. Is there really enough of the right kind of evidence? Reprod Health Matters 2007; 15(29):33–44.

43. Morrell R. Silence, sexuality and HIV/AIDS in South African schools. Austral Edu Res 2003; 30(1):41–62.

44. Heywood M. The routine offer of HIV counseling and testing: a human right. HIV/AIDS Pol Law Rev 2005; 8(2):13–19.

TRAUMA

CHAPTER 25
PAEDIATRIC TRAUMA: EPIDEMIOLOGY, PREVENTION, AND CONTROL

Francis A. Abantanga
Charles N. Mock

Introduction

Trauma is the leading cause of disability, death, and hospitalisation among children and adolescents globally. It constitutes an enormous financial burden on society in particular and governments in general. The impact of injury in developing nations has not been as extensively studied as in industrialised countries, and therefore often is not fully appreciated. Traditionally, infectious diseases and malnutrition have predominated as causes of morbidity and mortality in developing countries. All the same, injury is a major health problem among children of all ages worldwide.

For most parts of the African subregion, there are no trauma registries, and as such, it is difficult to know how much trauma contributes to injuries and death. Accurate data on the extent and nature of injuries are required to formulate effective policies targeted at reducing the burden of injury and in particular to compare the contribution to morbidity and mortality due to injuries with that due to infectious diseases and malnutrition. Most of the studies on injuries in the subregion are hospital-based; given the limited access to hospital care and emergency transport in low-income countries, these studies are unlikely to be truly representative of what is happening in the communities.

By the estimates of the World Health Organization (WHO) and the World Bank, injury is likely to account for 20% of all disability-adjusted life year (DALY) losses for the world's population by 2020. Road traffic injuries alone are the third leading cause of DALY losses. In spite of this, very little attention is paid to injury as a major health problem globally, particularly in the developing world.

The care of trauma patients is a continuous process and involves the initial first aid, the in-hospital care for the acute phase, and finally rehabilitation. For this to be successful, a trauma system must be put in place involving hospitals, trained personnel, and public agencies such as the ambulance services and the Red Cross, among others. Such a trauma system will require communication capabilities to be able to triage and rapidly transport injured children from the field of injury to a suitable facility for immediate treatment and rehabilitation. Frankly, the focus in the African subregion should be on injury prevention because treating injuries is very expensive and the costs of injuries to society are enormous.

Epidemiology of Injury in Children

Knowledge of the epidemiology of injury will help with prevention methods. Epidemiology is the study of the factors determining and influencing the frequency and distribution of disease, injury, and other health-related events, as well as their causes in a defined human population. Epidemiology of injury involves the collection of data concerning the time, the place, the mechanism, and the victim of injury. The purpose of studying injury and its causes is to establish programmes to prevent and control its development and spread. Injury is known to be a leading threat to the health of children in Africa, with unintentional injuries being the leading cause of morbidity and mortality.

Injuries are subdivided into life threatening and non–life threatening. Life-threatening injuries may be intentional or unintentional. Such injuries occur when a child is exposed to mechanical, electrical, or thermal energy. Childhood injuries can be penetrating or nonpenetrating, with blunt injuries predominating; but many penetrating injuries can be disturbing and life threatening.

Injuries should not be considered as random events or accidents. They have an association with many predictable factors, such as age, sex, geographic location, and socioeconomic status. Risk for serious injury is highly age-related. There are also developmental-related vulnerabilities. Young infants are at higher risk of inflicted trauma due to their small size and inability to protect themselves. Risks for teenagers are higher as a result of increased exposure to hazards and risk-taking behaviours. In other words, the range of causes of injury and the character of the injuries seen in children vary with age. For example, transport-related injuries are common in all age groups but are found to be more common in teenagers and adolescents, with resultant high morbidity and mortality rates in these age groups. Also, burn injuries are more rampant in children younger than 4 years of age than in older children. In developing countries, falls are usually the most common cause of injury seen in hospitals, affecting the age group of 5–9 years more than other age groups.

Overall, injury rates are higher in socioeconomically less-endowed communities than in more affluent societies. In addition, boys are more likely than girls to be harmed by unintentional injuries. Various research studies have demonstrated this fact and have concluded that male sex is a risk for all types of injury death, with the ratio of male deaths to female deaths varying by injury mechanism.

Unintentional Injuries

The mechanisms of unintentional injuries in children include transportation accidents, falls, burns, insect or animal stings and bites, agricultural injuries, drownings and submersions, poisonings, suffocations, and gunshot wounds.

Transport-related injuries

Transport-related injuries are considered in many studies (mostly hospital-based in the subregion) to be the leading cause of injuries, sometimes fatal, in children. Transport-related mechanisms of injury include motor vehicle crashes, pedestrian knockdowns, motorcycle crashes, bicyclists either falling off their bicycles or being hit by motorised vehicles, and injuries related to tractors, among others. Motor vehicle crashes predominate in low-income and middle-income countries. Road traffic injuries lead to serious head, chest, abdominal, and limb injuries with resultant severe permanent disability or even death. From two hospital-based studies in Ghana and Nigeria, for example, road traffic crashes were the most common cause of injuries to children; over 81% and 90% of children, respectively, in the two reports were pedestrians knocked down by automobiles and motorcycles. Table 25.1 illustrates the problem associated with pedestrian knockdowns, which is partly a result of rapid urbanisation and increased motorisation all over Africa in recent years. The table shows that a vast majority of road traffic injuries involve child pedestrians who have been knocked down by moving vehicles. Any prevention efforts should therefore target this mechanism of injury directly.

Table 25.1: Childhood road traffic injuries with emphasis on pedestrian knockdowns in sub-Saharan Africa.

Source*	Country	Age bracket (years)	Number of road traffic injuries	Number of pedestrian injuries**
Kibel SM, et al., 1990	South Africa	0–12	1311	927 (70.7)
Abantanga FA, et al., 1998	Ghana	0–14	271	219 (80.8)
Lerer LB, et al., 1997	South Africa	0–14	150	123 (82.0)
Roux P, et al., 1992	South Africa		100	91 (91.0)
Archibong EO, et al.,1996	Nigeria	0–14	17	12 (68.6)
Adejuyigbe O, et al., 1992	Nigeria	0–15	16	9 (56.3)
Adesunkanmi ARK, et al., 1998	Nigeria	0–15	324	292 (90.0)
Solagberu BA, 2000		0–15	169	109 (64.5)

*See Suggested Reading at the end of the chapter.
**Numbers in parentheses show pedestrian injuries as a percentage of road traffic injuries.

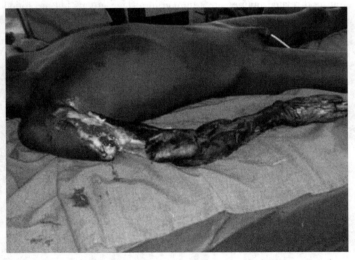

Figure 25.1: Injury sustained by an 8-year-old boy who climbed a carpenter's work table to pluck mangoes from a mango tree. He fell off the table, and in the process fractured his radius and ulna. He was treated by a traditional bonesetter who applied herbal concoctions. This is the end result of his fall. Treatment in hospital was by above-elbow amputation of the right upper limb. He survived the ordeal, but he will be permanently disabled.

Falls

Unintentional falls are usually the most common cause of nonfatal injury leading to a hospital visit in children younger than 15 years of age in developing countries. Accident and emergency (A&E) departments and outpatient surveillance systems show that falls are one of the most common mechanisms of injuries that require medical care and the most common nonfatal injury that at times needs hospitalisation. As many as 60% of all visits to the emergency department due to unintentional injuries in children younger than 1 year of age are due to falls. The combination of inquisitiveness, immature motor skills, and lack of judgment renders infants and toddlers particularly susceptible to falling. Most studies identify young age (0 to 6 years), male sex, and low socioeconomic status as consistent risk factors for fall injuries. In children younger than

4 years of age, most fall-related injuries occur at home; in those aged 5 to 15 years, approximately half of the falls occur at home and about a quarter at school on playgrounds during sports and recreational activities. Studies have shown that infants are at risk of falling from furniture or stairs, toddlers are at risk of falling from windows and beds, and older children are at risk of falling from playground equipment, especially climbing equipment and trees. Fall injuries range from very minor (bump or bruise) to severe, depending on the height of the fall, and may result in fractures, cuts, head injury, or even death.

The following ways children fall and injure themselves is by no means exhaustive. Falls can occur on level ground while playing or running, or from a height. Falls may occur either at home or in school. Locations for unintentional falls include playgrounds (from equipment such as climbing apparatus, trampolines, seesaws, tree houses, swings and so on); football fields; or from trees (especially fruit trees). Other fall scenarios are from multistorey buildings, down the stairs, from cots or beds, in the bathroom (due to water and slippery surfaces), or from objects or collapsing walls falling on children. Falls from the back or arms of caregivers/attendants also can cause injury.

Fall injuries can be blunt or penetrating, with the possibility of permanent disability, loss of an organ or part of it (Figure 25.1), or even death.

Burns

Paediatric burn injuries in sub-Saharan African are rampant and often lead to permanent disfigurement or death. The majority of fire deaths occur in homes, and most victims die from smoke and toxic gases rather than from the actual burns. Factors cited that may lead to an increase in burn injury include: poverty, illiteracy, cooking with open fires, and smoking. It is difficult to infer the rate of paediatric burns in communities in Africa because there are not many community-based studies available. Most of what we know about burns is largely from hospital-based studies. Available literature about paediatric burns treated per annum in Africa reveals the following:

• Luanda, Angola – 1,407

• Ashanti Region, Ghana – 1,300

• Abidjan, Cote d'Ivoire – 195

• Enugu, Nigeria – 107

• Harare, Zimbabwe – 104

It is estimated that in the Red Cross Children's Hospital in Cape Town, South Africa, about 650 to 900 paediatric burns are admitted per year. In the African literature, children aged less than 5 years are at the greatest risk of sustaining burn injuries; more young boys than girls are burned—a ratio of about 2:1.

The most common causes of paediatric burns in Africa are flames, hot liquids, and chemicals, with regional variations. For example, the most common cause of burns in Ghana is hot water, contact with hot objects, and flame burns, whereas in Southeastern Nigeria, it is hot liquids, followed by flames, petrol, kerosene explosions, and chemical burns. A vast majority of the burns in children occur in those younger than 6 years old, mostly at home and in the mornings when, for example, hot water is boiled to bathe the children.

Burn injuries are also due to electricity, caustic soda used in households for making soap, acid from vehicle batteries, and friction (e.g., from being dragged along a rough surface or tarred road). Explosions from kerosene or petrol are also reported among burn injuries.

Bites

Bites are also a cause of injury in children in sub-Saharan Africa, even though not much has been written about these injuries in the available literature. The most common causes are bites by dogs and other animals, envenomation by poisonous snakes (when children go to the bush alone or with adults to hunt for bush meat and put their hands into holes to retrieve animals such as rats), and stings by scorpions. Human bites do occur, especially among quarrelling children. These are usually intentional, however, or as a means of defence.

Animal bites (e.g., dogs or snakes), insect stings, or injury sustained from a farm animal, such as goring of shepherds (mainly boys) by cattle, are sources of injury.

Agricultural injuries

Agricultural injuries occur when children either accompany parents or go alone to the farm to help or to cut firewood. The children use implements such as hoes, cutlasses, machetes, and other sharp instruments to work. In the process, they injure their hands, legs, or feet. The most common activity on the farm is weeding or clearing the land in preparation for sowing and planting, or harvesting the crops; because this labour is not mechanised, serious injuries do not occur very often. Most farm injuries are unintentional and nonfatal in the African subregion but do lead to severe morbidity. There is the need for community education and public advocacy in relation to agricultural injury prevention in children.

Agricultural injuries include lacerations of various parts of the body, piercing of the sole of the foot by thorns or other objects, and falls from trees when harvesting fruits or cutting firewood on the farm.

Submersion or drowning

Drowning is a process resulting in primary respiratory impairment from submersion or immersion in a liquid medium. The victim may live or die after this process. The victim can be rescued at any time during the drowning process, thus interrupting the progression.

In the United States, drowning is the second cause of death from unintentional injuries in children aged 1–14 years. For sub-Saharan African countries, there is lack of information on drowning or near-drowning among children. However, WHO data show that Africa has the highest rates of drowning in the world for all ages considered together. The rate of death for drowning for the entire world (all ages) is 6.8 deaths per 100,000 people per year; for Africa, it is 14.2 deaths per 100,000 people per year.

According to figures from the United States regarding near-drowning, for every child who drowns, at least five receive emergency department care for nonfatal submersion injuries. The multiple causes of drowning are age and location related. Children younger than 1 year of age most often drown in bathtubs, buckets, or toilets. Drowning in bathtubs or water tanks or containers usually results from inadequate supervision. Children aged 1 to 4 years are likely to drown in swimming pools, ponds, and wells; this usually also happens when they are left unsupervised. Older children, in contrast, are likely to drown in fast-flowing streams, rivers, canals, and lakes; in such instances, alcohol use has been cited to be involved with 25–50% of adolescent drownings associated with water recreation. Male children are consistently more represented in drowning incidents than females.

Poisoning

A majority of unintentional poisoning injuries occur among children younger than 6 years old, and almost all exposures occur at home. Such children commonly ingest household products, such as cleaning substances, foreign bodies, drugs, and other substances (e.g., caustic soda used in manufacturing local soap). About half of the poisonings among teenagers, however, may be considered as intentional suicide attempts.

Others

Other unintentional injuries include suffocation and gunshot wounds on hunting expeditions from stray bullets or from children playing with guns.

Intentional Injuries

A big burden of injury-related disability and death in both high-income and less-developed countries is from self-inflicted injuries and interpersonal violence. These include violence against children, suicide, homicide, gunshot wounds, and war.

Assaults

Assault can take many forms: blunt or sharp instruments, rape or sexual abuse, and human bites, among others. Assault injuries can take the form of an adult molesting a child or a child maltreating another child. There is not much written in the literature about injuries as a result of assault in children in sub-Saharan Africa. Injuries as a result of assaults are known to occur with the use of sharp objects (knives, machetes, cutlasses, nails, glass or broken bottles, pens and pencils, scissors) or blunt objects (sticks, stones, rocks). Boys are more involved in assault injuries than girls.

Violence

The WHO defines violence as the intentional use of physical force or power, threatened or actual, against oneself, another person, or against a group or community that either results in or has a high likelihood of resulting in injury, death, psychological harm, maldevelopment or deprivation. Types of violence include self-directed, interpersonal, and collective. Such violence can take the form of child abuse or assault. Child abuse takes various forms, such as child labour, sexual abuse (vaginal, anal, oral, or even poking the finger or objects into the anal or vaginal orifice of children); or burning a child.

A child may be burned as a disciplinary measure for one reason or another. This takes the form of putting the child's hands in an open fire or on burning charcoal, or the use of a hot metal (e.g., a pressing iron) or a burning stick to press on the child's body with the purpose of causing harm. A child also may be burned to bring it out of a state of convulsion or any catatonic state. In the latter case, the hands or feet of a child who has convulsed for one reason or another are dipped into hot water to get the child out of that state.

Injury Prevention and Control

Injuries are a global problem in all countries of the world. Data on the extent and characteristics of injuries have to be collected in every country, especially in sub-Saharan African countries, to allow better targeting of interventions and assessment of their success. It will be difficult to design a meaningful injury prevention system without data on injuries and formal injury surveillance systems in place. Some less-developed countries have some system of collecting information on injuries, but these are usually unreliable and often underreported. Surveillance systems in sub-Saharan African countries should aim at upgrading preexisting systems such as police reports of injuries, hospital discharge data on injuries, and vital registries, and not seek to create entirely new data collection mechanisms.

Prevention efforts should tackle the various mechanisms of injury in children. These will include prevention or reduction of road traffic injuries, falls, burns, and drownings, among other injuries.

There is often a misperception that injuries are just due to random chance and little can be done to prevent them. However, much can be done by using the same scientific approach as with any other disease. This includes: (1) better understanding the extent and nature of the problem through surveillance and research, (2) identifying risk factors, (3) designing prevention programmes that target these risk factors, and (4) rigorously assessing the results of these prevention programmes to determine which are succeeding (and hence should be continued and expanded) and which are not succeeding (so that they can be discontinued or modified).

A useful tool to assist with designing and carrying out injury prevention strategies is the Haddon matrix. William Haddon proposed this classic matrix more than 30 years ago to determine ways to intervene to decrease morbidity and mortality from traffic injuries. Since then, the matrix has been used as a tool to help in developing ideas for preventing injuries of different types. The Haddon matrix is a grid with four columns (components) and three rows (phases of time). The rows represent different phases of an injury (pre-event, event, and post-event), and the columns represent different influencing factors (host, agent or vehicle of injury, physical environment, and social environment). If a fall from a mango tree is considered, then the pre-event is before the child climbs the mango tree to plug mangos, the event is the fall from the tree, and the post-event is what happens following the fall, which includes the first aid and/or treatment the child might (or might not) receive. One should identify, when using the Haddon matrix, the host, agent, and environmental factors that determine whether the event or injuries, along with their particular level of severity, occur during different points in time. Successful intervention in injury prevention should take all elements of the matrix into account. If these factors are understood, then appropriate intervention strategies can be developed.

Injury prevention strategies should be supported by successful interventions that include environmental changes, engineering, enforcement of legislation, and education (known as the four E's). Environmental changes are designed to reduce risk of injury; an example is well-designed roads, which can reduce the risk of head-on collisions. Engineering changes include the design of vehicles with air bags and antilock brake systems that reduce the risk of injury. Enforcement of laws requiring the nonuse of alcoholic drinks while driving, the use of seat belts for all occupants of a vehicle, and the observance of speed limits will reduce the incidence of road traffic injuries. A broad-based safety education campaign involving adults, children, and stakeholders (and supported by governments and nongovernmental organisations, or NGOs) will produce a safer environment for children.

Injury prevention strategies can also be considered as active or passive. Active interventions rely on actions taken by the child or caregiver (e.g., teaching the child not to climb or jump from high walls or tables). Passive interventions do not rely on efforts by the individual to be successful (e.g., child safety caps on medications). Most injury prevention interventions will have both active and passive elements, and the likelihood that an intervention will be successful in preventing injury is generally inversely related to the amount of individual effort required.

We next examine how these general principles of injury prevention can be applied in the circumstances of road safety and other types of injury prevention.

Road Safety

Prevention strategies for motor vehicle injuries are a complex problem and require political will to address them. Possible interventions include development of safe road infrastructure, enforcement of speed limits on all roads (both rural and urban), and enforcement of the use of restraints and protective gear such as seat belts and helmets. Specific interventions include placing children in the back seat of cars, adults serving as positive role models for children by always wearing their seat belts and obeying traffic safety regulations and laws, enforcing the use of hands-free mobile phones, and enacting laws (and rigorously implementing them) against driving under the influence of alcohol. To prevent pedestrian injuries, there is the need to modify the roads and environment to decrease motor vehicle speeds and increase the number and frequency of "zebra" crossings on busy roads that children are likely to use in going to or from school. To be most effective, such crossings can be augmented with traffic lights and crossing guards during peak times when children are crossing the roads. Measures to slow vehicle speeds can include roadway modification (such as speed bumps) and better police enforcement of speed limits.

Note that many of the strategies that have been successful are based on high-income country experiences. Some of these may be of use in the African context, but some may require considerable modification, and some completely new strategies may need to be developed. A major difference in emphasis in prevention efforts is needed, given the different aetiologies of traffic-related injuries. In high-income countries, most children who are injured are occupants in private vehicles that crash, so promoting better use of seat belts and car seats or booster seats for younger children is an important strategy. In sub-Saharan Africa, however, most children who are injured are pedestrians, so efforts to promote pedestrian safety should especially be emphasised.

Prevention for Other Types of Injuries

Prevention of falls, which in the African subregion includes also falls from trees, will consist of advising children to use methods of harvesting fruits from trees other than climbing them, and to be supervised by adults. No child should be left alone unsupervised on the playground, in school, or places where the child is likely to fall and be injured. Playground equipment should be safe and the surface covering soft to firm to permit safe play and well-cushioned "falls". Most falls occur at home, so supervision by parents or caregivers while the child is playing will go a long way to reducing serious falls that may lead to major injury and hospital visits for either outpatient treatment or admission.

In the case of burns, strategies for prevention include never leaving children alone around open flames, stoves, and candles; keeping matches, all flammable products, and hot liquids (especially hot water for bathing) away from children; and, as much as possible, restraining children from the kitchen when cooking.

Prevention strategies for submersion or drowning include constant supervision of children around water bodies, not allowing children to cross rivers alone for whatever purpose (e.g., attending school or going to the farm); emptying water containers or using water containers with childproof lids that cannot be easily pried open by an inquisitive child; and using a fence to separate swimming pools and other water bodies from children. The use of environmental barriers has been advocated by the WHO as the most effective method to prevent submersion deaths in all countries, irrespective of the level of income. It is also advisable to start swimming exercises for children of all ages, especially after the age of 5 years. Teenagers should be discouraged from drinking and swimming.

Eliminating agricultural injuries will require that children not be used on farms for either individual or commercial purposes. Child

Table 25.2: Examples of the interactions of phases and influencing factors within the Haddon matrix.

Phase	Human/host	Vector/vehicle	Environment: social and physical
Pre-event	Driver intoxication	Condition of brakes, tyres. Window bars to prevent falls	Speed limits and related enforcement. Highway design (road curvature, intersections, road conditions)
Event	Use of safety belts and child restraints (e.g., car seats and booster seats)	Airbags Side impact protection	Highway design (guard rails, breakaway poles)
Post-event	Age	Integrity of fuel system/ fireproof gasoline tanks	Trauma care systems

labour needs to be eliminated totally; if there is still the need to employ children, measures should be taken to ensure that they use protective clothing, gloves, and footwear, and they also should be coached on how to use agricultural implements properly and safely. All hazardous agricultural chemicals should be properly stored away from children, and children should be prevented from touching them for any purpose.

In the African subregion, most children are poisoned when they inadvertently take drugs that are not properly stored out of reach, or when chemicals such as caustic soda (used in the manufacturing of soap) are placed in such a way that toddlers can gain access to them and drink them. To prevent such occurrences, all potentially poisonous household products and substances should be stored safely out of the reach of children or disposed of carefully if they are no longer needed.

It is necessary to teach children to respect stray animals, especially dogs, and prevent children from playing with stray animals, which may lead to bites or other forms of injury. Children should be discouraged from going out to the bush to hunt—either alone or even in the company of adults. The risk is high of being bitten by snakes or insects, or even holding poisonous plants or twigs, which may result in various degrees of injury.

For many of the types of injuries discussed here, we have an inadequate understanding of causative factors and there is very little experience with prevention programmes oriented for the African context. This lack of data points out the need for better research into the extent and nature of the problem, causes and risk factors, and pilot prevention programmes.

What Can Be Done? The Role of the Surgeon

To confront the growing problem of childhood injury in Africa, a range of activities are needed, as shown in Table 25.2. This includes activities to provide better information on injuries through surveillance; promote road safety, for which there are a number of well-developed strategies; undertake research to better understand the causes of other types of injuries, such as burns, drownings, and falls, in the African context; and promote better organisation and planning for trauma care services. Table 25.2 identifies factors that can lead to injuries and indicates factors that can be controlled to prevent injuries.

This book and this chapter are primarily oriented for surgeons. Although many of the needed activities noted above may be done by others, there are numerous ways in which surgeons can become involved and help to move the process along. These include, among others:

1. *Surveillance:* Promote better data gathering in hospitals so that the extent of the problem of child injury can be better understood.

2. *Prevention:* Directly counsel injured children and their parents on safe behaviours that could prevent similar injuries from occurring. There are also opportunities for surgeons to become involved with other, broader injury prevention campaigns.

3. *Research:* Collaborate with others or be the main person conducting research on causes of childhood injury.

4. *Advocacy:* Provide facts and figures on the extent and nature of the child injury problem and bear witness to the horrible toll of suffering that such injuries cause. Probably the biggest role that surgeons can play is through advocacy. This advocacy can then lead to greater societal and political commitment to injury prevention.

For all of the above activities, there is much that surgeons can do alone. There is even more that can be done by forming alliances and working in partnership with others committed to the same goal of lowering rates of child injury. As just one example of how this can be done, in Ghana, the Building and Roads Research Institute (BRRI), the branch of the government involved with gathering crash statistics and recommending safety measures for dangerous sections of the roadways, has worked closely with surgeons at the Komfo Anokye Teaching Hospital (KATH) for several years. This has involved many activities, including collaborative research on the extent and nature of the injury problem, identification of opportunities to improve injury surveillance, and advocacy. The BRRI already had statistics from police crash reports, and KATH surgeons were also able to provide data from research done at their hospital on the economic costs of injury. Such economic figures showed a huge loss to the government and the economy from road traffic crashes. These data were highlighted together by both the BRRI and KATH, which resulted in greater governmental support for finally fixing dangerous sections of the roadway that the BRRI had previously identified, but which, for lack of such governmental support, had not yet been corrected.

In conclusion, the old adage that "prevention is better than cure" is certainly the case with child injury, as with any other disease or health problem. There is much that surgeons who care for the injured child can do to help make such prevention a reality, and thus to prevent the needless suffering caused by child injuries.

Evidence-Based Research

Table 25.3 presents a review of the problem of children's injuries in low-income countries. Table 25.4 presents research that examined the characteristics of childhood burns in Ghana.

Table 25.3: Evidence-based research.

Title	The problem of children's injuries in low-income countries: a review
Author	Bartlett S
Institution	Children's Environments Research Group, City University, New York, New York, USA
Reference	Health Policy and Planning 2002; 17(1):1–13
Problem	The absence of quality data on the issue of injuries in children in developing countries and the tendency to see injuries as random events leads to unpredictability and uncontrollability.
Intervention	An urgent need for research to guide the development of effective prevention measures.
Comparison/ control (quality of evidence)	The author has shown by this review that existing research from the developing world on injuries/trauma in children is scanty and largely hospital-based and therefore cannot present a comprehensive picture of either causes or outcome.
Outcome/ effect	There is an urgent need for more community-based and population-based studies that can contribute to effective analysis of the situation, increase awareness, and lead to the formulation of practical and well-targeted prevention measures.
Historical significance/ comments	This is a review that should spur researchers in the field of child health to not only concentrate on communicable diseases and nutritional problems, but spread out and research into childhood injury and its prevention—a field that is not well developed in sub-Saharan Africa.

Table 25.4: Evidence-based research.

Title	Childhood burns in Ghana: epidemiological characteristics and home-based treatment
Authors	Fordjuoh SN, Guyer B, Smith GS
Institution	Department of Maternal and Child Health and Injury Prevention Center, Johns Hopkins School of Hygiene and Public Health, Baltimore, Maryland, USA
Reference	Burns 1995; 21(1):24–28
Problem	Examination of epidemiological characteristics of childhood burns in the Ashanti Region of Ghana.
Intervention	A community-based, multisite survey was used for the study, and caretakers were interviewed by means of standard questionnaires.
Comparison/ control (quality of evidence)	The quality of the evidence gathered in this study is high and the analysis concentrated on children aged 0 to 5 years—the major age group that suffers burns.
Outcome/ effect	Prevention implication of the study—intensification of mass education on first-aid management of burns with special emphasis on alternatives to traditional preparations used to apply on fresh burns and the need to provide play areas for children to prevent them from playing with fire.
Historical significance/ comments	This study showed that a vast majority of children with burns are not seen in hospitals, and the health implications can only be imagined.

Key Summary Points

1. Surveillance: Develop and promote standards for injury surveillance systems in the subregion so that efforts to improve injury prevention and treatment can be based on solid facts and can be monitored.

2. Infrastructure/road engineering: Promote greater safety features in road design. Promote more prompt identification and correction of "black spots" (dangerous sections of roadways where many crashes occur). These factors should especially apply to speed-calming measures to reduce pedestrian injuries, the single greatest source of fatal traffic injuries to children.

3. Vehicle engineering and maintenance: Promote greater emphasis on safety-related vehicle maintenance, such as meaningful inspections by road safety authorities at the time that roadworthy certificates are issued, especially for commercial vehicles and heavy goods vehicles.

4. Driver behavior: Promote greater emphasis on decreasing overspeeding and alcohol-impaired driving, through both social marketing strategies and law enforcement.

5. Other unintentional injury: Conduct research into causative risk factors and undertake pilot prevention programmes for the many types of child injury that have not yet been well addressed, including burns, drownings, falls, and poisonings.

6. Injury treatment: Promote better organisation and planning for trauma care services, especially with regard to children, including all phases of trauma care, such as prehospital, emergency department, hospital-based care, and rehabilitation.

Suggested Reading

Abantanga FA, Mock CN. Childhood injuries in an urban area of Ghana: a hospital-based study of 677 cases. Pediatr Surg Int 1998; 13:515–518.

Adejuyigbe O, Aderounmu AO, Adelusola KA. Abdominal injuries in Nigerian children. J Royal Coll Surg Edinb 1992; 37(1): 29–33.

Adesunkanmi ARK, Oginni LM, Oyelami AO, Badru OS. Epidemiology of childhood injury. J Trauma 1998; 44(3):506–511.

Albertyn R, Bickler SW, Rode H. Paediatric burn injuries in Sub Saharan Africa—an overview. Burns 2006; 32:605–612.

Archibong AE, Onuba O. Fractures in children in south eastern Nigeria. Central Afr J Med 1996; 42(12):340–343.

Archibong AE, Anita UE, Udosen J. Childhood burns in south eastern Nigeria. East Afr M J 1997; 74(6):382–384.

Bartlet SN. The problem of children's injuries in low-income countries: a review. Health Policy and Planning 2002; 17(1):1–13.

Burd A, Yuen C. A global study of hospitalized paediatric burn patients. Burns 2005; 31:432–438.

Dowd MD, Keenan HT, Bratton SL. Epidemiology and prevention of childhood injuries. Critical Care Medicine 2002; 30(11):S385–S392.

Durkin MS, Laraque D, Lubman I, Barlow B. Epidemiology and prevention of traffic injuries to urban children and adolescents. Pediatrics 1999; 103:e74.

Falcone RA Jr, Brown RL, Garcia VF. The epidemiology of infant injuries and alarming health disparities. J Pediatr Surg 2007; 42:172–177.

Forjuoh SN, Guyer B, Smith GS. Childhood burns in Ghana: epidemiological characeristics and home-based treatment. Burns 1995; 21(1):24–28.

Hudson DA, Duminy F. Hot water burns in Cape Town. Burns 1995; 21(1):54–56.

Hyder AA, Labinjo M, Muzaffer SSF. A new challenge to child and adolescent survival in urban Africa: an increasing burden of road traffic injuries. Traffic Injury Prevention 2006; 7(4):381–388.

Hyder AA, Sugerman D, Ameratunga S, Callagan JA. Falls among children in the developing world: a gap in child health burden estimations? Acta Paediatrica 2007; 96:1394–1398.

Idris AH, Berg RA, Bierens J, et al. Recommended guidelines for uniform reporting of data from drowning: the "Utstein Style". Circulation 2003; 108:2565–2574.

Jaiswal AK, Aggarwal H, Solanki P, Lubana PS, Mathur RK, Odiya S. Epidemiological and socio-cultural study of burn patients in M. Y. Hospital, Indore, India. Indian J Plast Surg 2007; 40(2):158–163.

Khambalia A, Jashi P, Brussoni M, Raina P, Morrongiello B, Macarthur C. Risk factors for unintentional injuries due to falls in children aged 0–6 years: a systematic review. Inj Prev 2006; 12:378–385.

Lalor K. Child sexual abuse in sub-Saharan Africa: a literature review. Child Abuse & Neglect 2004; 28:439–460.

Lin T-M, Wang K-H, Lai C-H, Lin S-D. Epidemiology of pediatric burn in southern Taiwan. Burns 2005; 31:182–187.

London J, Mock C, Abantanga FA, Quansah RE, Boateng KA. Using mortuary statistics in the development of an injury surveillance system in Ghana. Bulletin of WHO 2002; 80:357–364.

Mock C, Quansah R, Krishnan R, Arreola-Risa C, Rivara F. Strengthening the prevention and care of injuries worldwide. Lancet 2004; 363:2172–2179.

Mock CN, Abantanga F, Cummings P, Koepsell TD. Incidence and outcome of injury in Ghana: a community-based survey. Bulletin of WHO 1999; 77(12):955–964.

Mock CN, Adzotor KE, Conklin E, Denno DN, Jurkovich GJ. Trauma outcomes in the rural developing world: comparison with an urban level I trauma center. J Trauma 1993; 36:518–523.

Rahman F ARSL. Potential of using existing injury information for injury surveillance at the local level in developing countries. Pub Health 2000; 114:133–136.

Rivara FP. Prevention of injuries to children and adolescents. Inj Prev 2002; 8:iv5–iv8.

Rivara FP, Mock C. The 1,000,000 lives campaign 2005: 321–323.

Roux P, Fisher RM. Chest injuries in children: an analysis of 100 cases of blunt chest trauma from motor vehicle accidents. J Pediatr Surg 1992; 27(5):551–555.

Solagberu BA. Trauma deaths in children: a preliminary report. Nig J Surg Res 2002; 4(3):98–102.

Spinks A, Turner C, McClure R, Nixon J. Community based prevention programs targeting all injuries for children. Inj Prev 2004; 10:180–185.

Suliman T, Ahmad AA. Falls from residential buidlings in the Tabuk area: review of 50 patients. Internet J Orthoped Surg 2006; 3.

van As AB, van Dijk J, Numanoglu A, Millar AJW. Assaults with a sharp object in small children: a 16-year review. Pediatr Surg Int 2008; 24:1037–1040.

Wesson DE. Trauma: epidemiology and prevention of childhood injury. In: Ziegler MM, Azizkhan RG, Weber TR, eds. Operative Pediatric Surgery. McGraw-Hill Professional, 2003, 1075–1079.

CHAPTER 26
PAEDIATRIC INJURY SCORING AND TRAUMA REGISTRY

Francis A. Abantanga
Erin A. Teeple
Benedict C. Nwomeh

Introduction

Injury scoring systems are designed to accurately assess injury severity, appropriately triage the injured, and develop and refine trauma patient care.[1] Trauma scores quantify the severity and extent of injury, aid with the prediction of survival and subsequent morbidity,[2] and allow health care providers to communicate in common terms. One disadvantage of injury scoring systems is that patient information is reduced to a simple score, and important details may be lost. To accurately estimate patient outcome, it is necessary to precisely assess the patient's anatomic and physiologic injury, as well as any preexisting medical conditions that can impair the patient's ability to respond to the stress of the injuries sustained.

Understanding and appropriate use of trauma scoring systems, along with the use of specific treatment guidelines, can significantly contribute to improvement in the prognosis of injured children. The majority of the injury scoring systems used in children today are extrapolations of the same systems used in adults but with some modifications.[3]

Injury scoring systems are divided into anatomic, physiologic, and combined categories.[2,3] Some of the scoring systems are discussed in further detail within the following sections, with demonstrations of their use where possible.

Anatomic Injury Scoring Systems

Anatomic injury scoring systems clearly characterise the degree of anatomic disruption but fail to delineate organ system derangements.[2] Examples of injury methods that evaluate anatomic status include the Abbreviated Injury Scale (AIS), Injury Severity Score (ISS), and Anatomical Profile (AP).[2] These injury scoring systems are based upon anatomic descriptions of identified injuries and are retrospectively used to analyse trauma populations.[1] In these systems, the site of the injury is important.

Abbreviated Injury Scale

The AIS was first introduced in 1969 as an anatomic scoring system to categorise automobile victims for epidemiological purposes.[5] It underwent revision in 1990, and body regions for the AIS were identified as follows: head, face, neck, thorax, abdomen and pelvic content, spine, upper extremities, lower extremities, and unspecified. In this revised version, external injuries are dispersed across body regions, and the AIS provides a reasonably accurate way of ranking the severity of injury by body regions.

With the AIS, injuries are ranked on an ordinal scale ranging from 1 to 6, with 1 being considered a minor injury or least severe, 5 being a severe injury or survival uncertain, and 6 being an unsurvivable injury[6] (Table 26.1). The AIS scores can be found in the AIS Dictionary Manual,[7] a compendium of more than 1200 injuries. An AIS score ≥3 is considered serious. The AIS correlates well with the degree of injury but suffers as a prognostic tool because it does not take physiologic derangements or chronic health into account. It is not intended to reflect patient outcomes, but only to score an individual injury. Its other limitation is that it does not provide a comprehensive measure of severity of injury because it focuses on singular but not combined injuries of the patient.

Table 26.1: The Abbreviated Injury Scale.

Type of injury	AIS score
Minor	1
Moderate	2
Severe, but not life-threatening	3
Severe, life-threatening, survival probable	4
Critical, survival uncertain	5
Not survivable/virtually unsurvivable	6

Injury Severity Score

The ISS, like the AIS, is an anatomic scoring system that provides an overall score for patients with multiple injuries.[8] Each injury must be assigned an AIS score, allocated to one of six body regions: head and neck, face, thorax, abdomen and visceral pelvis, extremities and bony pelvis, and external structures.[6] Injuries in each region are given an AIS score, and the highest AIS score in each body region is used. To generate the ISS, square the AIS score of each of the three most severely injured body regions (those with the highest AIS scores, including only one from each body region) and add the squares together.[6,8] The ISS has a good predictive power and correlates well with mortality, morbidity, length of hospital stay, and other measures of severity. The minimum score is 1 and the maximum possible score is 75, with higher scores reflecting an increased injury severity and mortality.[9] The ISS is not calculated when any single body region has an AIS value of 6; in such cases, an ISS value of 75 is automatically assigned.[6] Injury Severity Scores higher than 15 have been used as a proxy for injuries of sufficient magnitude to require hospital or trauma centre care.[4] However, it is inappropriate to use this as the sole criterion for triaging because it does not also measure alterations in the physiology of the trauma patient.

There are several disadvantages to using the ISS.[2] For example, the ISS cannot be used as an initial triage tool because detailed assessment, and in some cases surgical exploration, must be performed before a full description of the injuries can be obtained. Also, the patient's age and comorbidities are not taken into account. Furthermore, multiple injuries to the same body area are not weighted higher than a single injury to that area. Lastly, the ISS uses only three regions, so that injuries from the three remaining regions are not taken into account.

In spite of these limitations, the ISS has been validated as a predictor of trauma mortality, length of hospital stay, and length of intensive care unit stay, and it may have usefulness in predicting morbidity. It is currently the most widely used injury scoring system.[1,9] Automated ISS calculators are available to compute the value of the ISS once the AIS scores are entered. The ISS score can also be computed manually as follows:

$$ISS = \Sigma\ [(\text{AIS of most severe injury in ISS region})^2$$
$$+ (\text{AIS score of next most severe injury in another ISS region})^2$$
$$+ (\text{AIS score of most severe injury in any remaining ISS region})^2]$$

An illustration of how to calculate ISS is shown in Table 26.2.

The ISS score for the example in Table 26.2 is 50, which is a very severe injury requiring the patient to be admitted to a hospital for trauma care. Patients with ISS scores ≥15 should be cared for in a hospital or trauma centre with adequate resources and experience in trauma care.

The ISS calculations include spine injuries in the corresponding three ISS body regions: cervical in ISS head or neck, thoracic in ISS chest, and lumbar in ISS abdominal or pelvic contents.

New and Modified ISS

In 1997, a simple modification of ISS was formulated and referred to as the New ISS (NISS).[10] It is defined as the sum of the squares of the AIS of each of the patient's most severe AIS injuries irrespective of the body region in which they occur.[3,5,10] The NISS is reported to predict survival better[3] than the ISS by better predicting mortality in the more severely injured patients,[11] and it is simpler to calculate.

There is also a Modified ISS (MISS), specifically intended for paediatric trauma cases. This modification was made to account for the predominance of head injuries in paediatric trauma patients.[5] In the MISS, the number of body regions is reduced to four: face/neck, chest, abdomen/pelvic contents, and extremities/pelvis.[5] The MISS uses the Glasgow Coma Scale (GCS; see next section) value categories (Table 26.3) to determine the AIS head region scores and also assigns injuries of the skin/general category within any of the four body regions listed above. The MISS is calculated by summing the squared AIS values for the three most severely injured body regions. Several studies have validated the MISS in paediatric trauma and have shown it to accurately identify patients at high risk for mortality and long-term disability.[12] In spite of this, the MISS is not widely used because improvements have been made in the more recent versions of the AIS and ISS.

Anatomical Profile

The AP addresses some of the shortcomings of the ISS. It uses the AIS descriptors of anatomic injury, but includes only four body regions: A = head/brain and spinal cord; B = thorax/neck; C = all other serious injuries other than in the areas of A and B; and D = all nonserious injuries.[1,2] Injuries with an AIS value >2, which are defined as serious, are scored for the first three categories above.[1] All minor injuries, defined as AIS scores of ≤2, are classified as nonserious, regardless of their anatomic location.[2] The total AP score is the sum of the square roots of the sum of the squares of the AIS for all individual injuries within a region[1,2] (Table 26.4). This allows the second and third injuries occurring within a given region to be considered in the final AP score, preventing the loss of information that occurs with the ISS.[1] AP is most useful in an inpatient setting and has neither been widely used nor validated for paediatric trauma.[1,2]

Physiologic Injury Scoring Systems

Physiologic scoring systems attempt to measure multiorgan system derangements following trauma. These physiologic scoring systems are strong predictors of mortality and tend to focus on abnormalities of many systems, including respiratory, haematologic, and neurologic. They are especially valuable in triaging patients; hence, they are also referred to as triage scoring systems. They are also valuable in providing data on functional outcomes. Examples of physiologic scoring systems are: the Glasgow Coma Scale (GCS); the Trauma Score (TS) and Revised Trauma Score (RTS); Circulation, Respiration, Abdominal/Thoracic, Motor and Speech Scale (CRAMS); and the Acute Physiology and Chronic Health Evaluation (APACHE) scale.[2] These are mainly used for prehospital triage of patients,[4] with the exception of the APACHE scale, which is widely used in the intensive care unit (ICU) for assessing the severity of illness in acutely ill patients.

Glasgow Coma Scale

The GCS was developed as a means of assessing a patient's level of consciousness by assigning coded values for three behavioural respons-

Table 26.2: Sample calculation of ISS.

Body region	Description of injury	AIS score	Square of top three AIS scores
Head and neck	Cerebral contusion	3	9
Face	Minor injury	1	16
Chest	Unilateral flail chest	4	25
	Pneumothorax	3	
Abdomen	Minor contusion of bowel	2	
	Completely shattered spleen	5	
Extremity	Femoral shaft fracture	3	
Skin	Minor injury	1	
Injury Severity Score =			50

Table 26.3: The Modified Injury Severity Score (MISS).

Glasgow Coma Scale	Neurologic score
15	1: Minor
13–14	2: Moderate
9–12	3: Severe, not life-threatening
5–8	4: Severe, survival probable
3–4	5: Critical, survival uncertain

Table 26.4: Sample calculation of AP.

Component	Injury	AIS score
A	1. Head/brain	5
	2. Spinal cord	3
B	1. Thorax	4
	2. Front of neck	3
C	1. Liver laceration	4
	2. Above-knee amputation	4
D	1. All other injuries	1

$$AP = \sum[\sqrt{(5^2+3^2)} + \sqrt{(4^2+3^2)} + \sqrt{4^2+4^2}] = \sum[\sqrt{34} + \sqrt{25} + \sqrt{32}] = 5.8 + 5.0 + 5.7 = 16.5$$
The AP score = 16.5

es including eye opening, motor responses, and verbal responses. The GCS was first introduced in 1970. As shown in Table 26.5, the GCS has been modified for use in infants and children and is referred to as the paediatric GCS.[5,13] The GCS is scored between 3 and 15, with the worst score being 3 (indicating deep coma or death) and the best being 15 (indicating no neurologic deficit).

The GCS is easy to use even in the prehospital setting, and can be applied to the patient on multiple occasions throughout the postinjury period, following changes in level of consciousness over time. It has been found that the trend of multiple measures of GCS taken over time is a more sensitive predictor of outcome than a single, absolute value of the GCS. The ease of use of GCS makes it attractive to clinicians in the field, in the emergency department for triage, and by emergency physicians to document and communicate serial neurological

Table 26.5: Modified Glasgow Coma Scale for infants and children.

Area assessed	Infants	Children	GCS
Eye opening	Open spontaneously	Open spontaneously	E4
	Open in response to verbal stimuli	Open in response to verbal stimuli	E3
	Open in response to pain only	Open in response to pain only	E2
	No response	No response	E1
Verbal response	Alert, coos, and babbles	Oriented, appropriate	V5
	Spontaneous irritable cry	Confused	V4
	Cries in response to pain	Inappropriate words	V3
	Moans in response to pain	Incomprehensible words/sounds	V2
	No response to pain	No response	V1
Motor responses	Moves spontaneously and purposefully	Obeys commands	M6
	Withdraws to touch	Localises painful stimulus	M5
	Withdraws in response to pain	Withdraws in response to pain	M4
	Response to pain with decorticate posturing (abnormal flexion)	Abnormal flexion to pain	M3
	Response to pain with decerebrate posturing (abnormal extension)	Abnormal extension to pain	M2
	No response to pain	No response to pain	M1
Grimace component	Spontaneous normal facial/or motor activity (e.g., sucks tube, coughs)		G5
	Less than usual spontaneous ability or only responds to touch		G4
	Vigorous grimace to pain		G3
	Mild grimace or some change in facial expression to pain		G2
	No response to pain		G1

examinations. One major disadvantage of the GCS is the inability to obtain complete data from patients who are intubated and/or sedated.[14] This is usually signified by placing the letter "T" after the computed score (i.e., 3T indicates a patient with a GCS of 3 who is intubated).

The total GCS score is more meaningful when considered together with its components, that is: eye opening (E3), best verbal response (V3), and best motor response (M4). A GCS score ≤8 signifies coma or severe brain injury; a score of 9–12, moderate brain injury; and a score ≥13, mild or no brain injury.

Some workers add grimace to the GCS for adults and the modified GCS for infants and children, as shown in Table 26.5.[13]

The grimace component appears to be more reliable than the verbal component and may be useful in intubated and nonverbal patients when the verbal response is impossible to use.[14]

AVPU
During prehospital triage and primary assessment, the AVPU method may be used as a quick and simple tool to assess level of consciousness. The AVPU is a simple scale of whether a patient is responsive (Alert), responds to verbal stimuli (Verbal), responds to painful stimuli (Painful), or is unresponsive to any stimuli (Unresponsive). It provides a rough guide as to whether a patient needs airway protection. The AVPU method does not belong to any of the groupings mentioned above—physiologic, anatomic, or combined, and is not a scoring system as such.

Trauma Score
The TS is a physiologic measure based on information gathered in the prehospital setting, and capable of predicting patient outcome.[1,15] It assesses four physiologic components including respiratory rate (RR), degree of respiratory expansion/effort, systolic blood pressure (SBP), and capillary refill, in addition to the GCS (Table 26.6). These are all scored and added together to give the TS value, which ranges from 1 to 16. For each value, the probability of survival [$P(s)$] has been determined. If a patient has a TS value of 1, the associated $P(s)$ is 0, indicating a likely fatal process. A TS value of 16 is associated with a $P(s)$ of 99%.[1]

The advantages of the TS are that it uses parameters that are commonly measured in the prehospital and emergency department settings, it is easy to understand, it accurately predicts outcome, and it has a good interobserver (interrater) reliability.[1] The TS has also been validated for use in paediatric patients. Its limitations lie in its use of two subjective measurements, including respiratory expansion/effort and capillary refill, which can be difficult to gauge in the field. In addition, it is somewhat cumbersome, with five separate measures, and also underestimates the severity of head injury in patients who are in a stable cardiovascular state.[1] A TS value calculated in the field or emergency department will naturally underestimate severity in the trauma patient who becomes unstable later.[1]

Revised Trauma Score
In order to eliminate the subjectivity of TS, the degree of respiratory expansion/effort and capillary refill were removed, resulting in the Revised Trauma Score. The RTS is a physiologic scoring system with high interobserver reliability and demonstrated accuracy in predicting mortality.[1] It is frequently used to rapidly assess patients at the scene of an accident. The score consists of the patient's data from the GCS,

Table 26.6: Trauma Score

Clinical parameter	Parameter category	Coded value
Respiratory Rate (cycle/min)	10–24	4
	25–35	3
	>35	2
	<10	1
	0	0
Respiratory expansion/effort	Normal	1
	Abnormal	0
Systolic blood pressure (mm Hg)	>90	4
	70–90	3
	50–69	2
	<50	1
	0	0
Capillary refill	Normal	2
	Delayed	1
	Absent	0
Glasgow Coma Scale	14–15	5
	11–13	4
	8–10	3
	5–7	2
	3–4	1

Table 26.7: Revised Trauma Score.

Glasgow Coma Scale (GCS)	Systolic blood pressure (SBP)	Respiratory rate (RR)	Coded value (RTS)
13–15	>89	10–29	4
9–12	76–89	>29	3
6–8	50–75	6–9	2
4–5	1–49	1–5	1
3	0	0	0

SBP, and RR (Table 26.7).[16,17] These three elements of the RTS are considered reliable and were selected due to their statistical association with trauma mortality. Thus, the RTS is easier to use than the TS and is a highly sensitive and strong predictor of survival.[2,3] The RTS is calculated by multiplying each component score by a weighting factor and then summing the weighted scores by using the following formula:

RTS = (0.9368 × GCS value) + (0.7326 × SBP value) + (0.2908 × RR value).

RTS values range from 0.0 to 7.8408.[1] The RTS correlates well with survival, with higher values being more predictive of survival. However, the use of the RTS as the sole predictor of mortality in paediatric cases is not recommended. It is, however, the most widely used triage scoring system in the world trauma literature.[1]

The Triage-RTS (T-RTS), which is designed for prehospital use,[1] represents the sum of the values of the GCS, SBP, and RR, with the scores ranging from 0 to 12. A score of 0 represents the worst prognosis, with P(s) equalling 0. A score of 12 represents the best prognosis, with P(s) equalling 0.99.[1,2] It is recommended that injured patients with a T-RTS value ≤11 be admitted to a trauma centre for care.[1,17]

Circulation, Respiration, Abdomen, Motor, and Speech Scale
Another physiologic trauma scoring system is the CRAMS scale. It was developed in 1982 as a prehospital score to assist in trauma triage,[4] distinguishing those with major trauma from those with minor injuries. CRAMS scores five physiologic parameters and physical examination findings, including circulation, respiration, trauma to the abdomen and thorax, motor function, and speech on a scale ranging from 0 to 2 (Table 26.8). A score of 0 indicates severe injury or absence of the parameter, and a score of 2 signifies no deficit.[2] A value of 0 on the CRAMS scale indicates the worst prognosis or death, and a value of 10 indicates the best prognosis or lack of injury.[1] A CRAMS score ≤8 indicates a major trauma,[1] and a score ≥9 signifies a minor trauma.[2] CRAMS is cumbersome for field use and is limited by its reliance on subjective prehospital clinical components, such as capillary refill and respiratory effort. It is also often difficult to examine patients with thoracic and abdominal trauma in the field.[1]

The Apache Scale
The Acute Physiology and Chronic Health Evaluation scale is a more complex physiologic scoring system used predominantly later in the course of care to predict morbidity and mortality. The APACHE I was introduced in 1981 and had 34 physiological elements. This was revised in 1985, resulting in the APACHE II, which retained only 12 of the 34 physiological elements. The APACHE scale will not be discussed here. Readers interested in this scoring system should refer to the appropriate literature.

Combined Anatomic and Physiologic Injury Scoring Systems
Combined systems use anatomic and physiologic scoring to estimate morbidity and mortality risk for an individual patient as well as for trauma populations. These systems have an improved accuracy of both anatomic injuries caused by trauma and physiologic derangements caused by the patient's underlying chronic health state. As such, they are better predictors of survival than those systems based on anatomic or physiologic criteria alone.[2] However, they can be cumbersome. They are most often used in inpatient settings after the patient has been initially stabilised. Examples of this model are the Paediatric Trauma Score (PTS), Trauma and Injury Severity Score (TRISS), and A Severity Characterisation Of Trauma (ASCOT).[2] These are also known as outcome analysis systems.[1]

Paediatric Trauma Score
The PTS was devised specifically for the triage of paediatric trauma patients.[3] The PTS is calculated as the sum of individual scores from six clinical variables (Table 26.9). The variables include weight, airway, SBP, central nervous system (CNS) status (level of consciousness), presence of an open wound, and skeletal injuries.[1,3] Two of the clinical parameters, airway and CNS status, are somewhat subjective measures. Each of the six clinical parameters is assigned a score ranging from no injury to a major or life-threatening injury.[3] The PTS is calculated as the sum of individual scores, and its total values range from –6 to +12. A PTS ≤ 8 is recommended as an indication for prehospital triage of a patient to a trauma centre.[2] There are conflicting reports on the effectiveness of the PTS as a tool for assessing prognosis and in identifying those who will need a transfer to a paediatric trauma centre.[1,3,5,15,16]

Further refinements of the PTS include the Age-Specific PTS and the triage Age-Specific PTS. These scoring systems, however, have not yet been validated and are rarely used.

Trauma and ISS

The TRISS is a combination of the physiologic data in the RTS (and, less commonly, the TS) and anatomic data in the ISS to estimate the probability of survival for a given trauma patient.[2,3] The probability of survival [$P(s)$] for any one patient is determined by the formula.[1,2,3]

$$P(s) = 1/(1 + e^{-b}),$$

where $b = b_0 + b_1(\text{TS or RTS}) + b_2(\text{ISS}) + b_3(\text{age factor})$. The b coefficients (b_0, b_1, b_2, and b_3) are derived from logistic regression analysis of patients in the Major Trauma Outcome Study (MTOS) data base. These coefficients are different for blunt and penetrating trauma. The age factor (or age index, as used by other authors) is zero for all patients aged <55 years and 1 for all patients aged ≥55 years.[1] If the patient is younger than 15 years of age, the blunt index for b_3 is used regardless of mechanism. Values for $P(s)$ range from 0, for no survival expectation, to 1.00 for 100% survival expectation.[1] Generally, survivors have a $P(s)$ ≥ 0.5, and nonsurvivors have a $P(s)$ < 0.5. Trauma fatalities with a $P(s)$ < 0.5, by convention, are defined as expected outcomes, and fatalities with a $P(s)$ ≥ 0.5 are unexpected outcomes. This terminology is important for quality evaluation of trauma care. There is also the Paediatric Age-Adjusted TRISS, which simply uses the paediatric Age Specific PTS instead of the RTS, but this is not yet in wide use by investigators.[3]

The drawbacks of the TRISS are primarily related to the component scoring systems that form its basis: the RTS (or TS or PTS) and the ISS. It is also not easy to compute due to a complex logistic regression formula used to calculate $P(s)$.[2] Despite all these limitations, TRISS is the most validated and commonly used trauma mortality prediction model to date, and its methodology has been shown to perform reasonably well for both adult and paediatric trauma patients.[1]

ASCOT

The developers of ASCOT designed it as a mortality prediction model to improve on the limitations of the TRISS. ASCOT uses the AP instead of the ISS for the description of an anatomic injury.[1] It also uses separate algorithms for blunt and penetrating trauma. ASCOT takes into account each injury within a given body region by using the AP and, as such, better represents the increased mortality risk associated with multiple injuries.[1] The AP, as used in ASCOT, divides serious injuries (AIS > 2) into three categories—head, brain or spinal cord injuries; thorax or neck injuries; and all other serious injuries. Note that nonserious injuries (AIS of 1 or 2) are not significantly associated with mortality and are therefore dropped from ASCOT calculations.

Like the TRISS, ASCOT relies on the RTS to provide physiologic data but advocates the use of the individual components of the RTS rather than the total RTS score. It derives a measure of the probability of survival by combining values of the GCS, SBP, and RR as coded by the RTS, patient age (0 for all paediatric patients) and the AP.[3] $P(s)$ using ASCOT is calculated similarly to the TRISS by employing the following formula:[1,2]

$$P(s) = 1/(1 + e^{-k}),$$

where $k = k_1 + k_2(\text{RTS GCS value}) + k_3(\text{RTS SBP value}) + k_4(\text{RTS RR value}) + k_5(\text{AP head region value}) + k_6(\text{AP thorax region value}) + k_7(\text{AP other serious injury value}) + k_8(\text{age factor})$.

The k coefficients for blunt and penetrating injuries are all derived from the MTOS data base and can be found in the literature. ASCOT is more cumbersome to compute than the TRISS but appears to be more accurate at predicting trauma mortality, especially for penetrating injuries.[1]

Table 26.10 demonstrates example calculations of some of the trauma scores by using a single hypothetical case scenario: A 13-year-old boy, weighing 35 kilograms, was standing by the side of the road and was struck by a moving vehicle, hitting his head against the edge of a gutter. On arrival at the Accident and Emergency (A&E) department

Table 26.8: CRAMS scale.

Clinical parameter	Parameter category	Coded value
Circulation	Normal capillary refill, SBP >100 mm Hg	2
	Delayed capillary refill, SBP 85–100 mm Hg	1
	No capillary refill or SBP <85 mm Hg	0
Respiration	Normal	2
	Abnormal (laboured or shallow)	1
	Absent	0
Abdomen/thorax	Abdomen and thorax nontender	2
	Abdomen and thorax tender	1
	Abdomen and thorax rigid, flail chest, or penetrating trauma	0
Motor	Normal	2
	Responds only to pain (other than decerebrate)	1
	No response (or decerebrate)	0
Speech	Normal	2
	Confused	1
	No intelligible words	0

Table 26.9: Paediatric Trauma Score.

Clinical parameter	Severity category	Score value
Weight	≥ 20 kg	+2
	10–19 kg	+1
	<10 kg	-1
Airway	Normal	+2
	Maintainable	+1
	Unmaintainable	-1
Systolic blood pressure*	>90 mm Hg	+2
	50–90 mm Hg	+1
	<50 mm Hg	-1
Central nervous system	Awake	+2
	Obtunded/loss of consciousness	+1
	Coma/decerebrate	-1
Open wound	None	+2
	Minor	+1
	Major or penetrating	-1
Skeletal injury	None	+2
	Closed fracture	+1
	Open or multiple fractures	-1

*In the absence of a proper-sized blood pressure cuff, BP can be assessed by assigning the following values:[3] presence of palpable pulse at the wrist = +2; presence of a palpable pulse at the groin = +1; absence of pulse = –1.

Table 26.10: Examples of how to calculate some trauma scores for hypothetical scenarios.

Abbreviated Injury Score (AIS)

Head/Neck	Subdural haematoma	AIS score = 4
Face	Abrasions	AIS score = 1
Chest	Fracture of four ribs	AIS score = 4
Abdomen	Splenic laceration (Grade IV)	AIS score = 4
Extremity	Fracture right femur	AIS score = 3
Skin	Abrasions	AIS score = 1

Injury Severity Score (ISS)

ISS = $4^2 + 4^2 + 4^2 = 48$. This is a severe injury.

Paediatric Trauma Score (PTS)

Weight	35 kg	+2
Airway	Maintainable	+1
SBP	78 mm Hg	+1
CNS	Obtunded	+1
Open Wound	None	+2
Skeletal Fracture	Closed fracture	+1

PTS = 8. Such a patient should be triaged immediately to a paediatric trauma centre, where available.

Revised Trauma Score (RTS)

GCS = 10	Coded value = 3	Weight = 0.9368
SBP = 78	Coded value = 3	Weight = 0.7326
RR = 28	Coded value = 4	Weight = 0.2908

RTS = (0.9368 x 3) + (0.7326 x 3) + (0.2908) = 2.8104 + 2.1978 + 1.1632 = 6.1714

of the hospital, his GCS was found to be 10, with an RR of 28 cycles per minute and a SBP of 78 mm Hg. His airway was maintainable. A computed tomography (CT) scan revealed a right-sided parietal subdural haematoma. It was also revealed by CT scan that he had a grade IV laceration of the spleen. Radiography of the chest and right femur showed fractures of four ribs on the right and a femoral shaft fracture.

Paediatric trauma care has improved a great deal in the developed and industrialised countries as a result of standardisation of patient assessment and reporting. The various scoring systems, especially those combining anatomic and physiologic parameters, have helped to improve the care of trauma patients. A search of the African literature, especially by using African Journals Online (AJOL), did not reveal much activity in the use of these scoring systems. This deficiency needs to be rectified because some of these injury scoring systems are easily implemented without extra funding, yet may improve patient outcomes.

Trauma Registry

A trauma registry (TR) is an accurate and comprehensive collection of data on patients who receive hospital management for specified types of injuries. A TR provides an important and ongoing analytical tool to assess the management of patient care. The purposes[18-20] of any TR are

many and include the provision of data for injury surveillance, analysis, and prevention programmes; monitoring and evaluation of the outcome of care of trauma patients; support of quality assurance evaluation activities; provision of information for resource planning, system design, and management; provision of resources for research and education; and validation and evolution of scoring systems for improved management of trauma patients. The successful implementation of trauma care systems, including their quality assurance through trauma registries, has contributed to the decline in death and disability resulting from injuries. This is evidenced by a decline in projected road traffic deaths in high-income countries, whereas those in middle- to low-income countries continue to rise.[21,22] Improvement in trauma care in Africa will rely on further development of functioning prehospital and trauma care systems, as well as establishing local, regional, and national trauma registries. Conglomeration of multicentre data can then be used to further examine and improve trauma care in African countries.

A TR typically includes detailed information about injured patients, including prehospital data, resuscitation efforts, and outcome data. The actual data points may vary between registries, but it is important that they be detailed and consistently collected among patients.[23] Too few data points will lead to incomplete and ineffective data, and too many data points will be cumbersome and impossible to maintain.[24]

Unfortunately, a number of resources are needed to implement and maintain a TR. This begins with a well-defined patient population. Some registries record data only on the severely injured and those who arrive at the hospital alive. Some registries record data dependent on length of stay of the patient. Most registries derive some score of injury severity for all registered patients. Careful consideration must be given when defining the patient population because exclusion of certain patients may skew the data, altering the apparent severity of injury and affecting later conclusions based on the data.[25] Personnel must be adequately trained to collect and enter ongoing data. In the United States, a nationally recognised certification process has been initiated to ensure appropriately trained staff. The data must be collected by using reasonable and dependable software, with the ability to grow and expand as more patients are registered as well as the ability to protect patient privacy. Of course, ultimately, all of these resources require funding. Possible sources of funding to establish trauma registries throughout Africa include the ministry of health of each participating country, nongovernmental organisations (NGOs), and international development partners.

Barriers to the creation of trauma registries throughout Africa are many. The most prominent roadblock is that those tools that have been established and validated in other systems may not be applicable to the African population.[26-31] Also, the lack of a continuous power supply may limit the ability to record and maintain data. This may be surmounted by backing up data daily. Further barriers to the establishment of efficient TRs in developing countries are the following:[23]

• little or no prehospital care;

• nonavailability of (or inefficient) evacuation and transportation system;

• limited interhospital communication in the case of transfers;

• lack of standardised and uniform hospital data formats;

• limited availability of electronic data storage and retrieval facilities;

• inadequate funding;

• unfavourable government health policies;

• inadequate census and population data; and

• lack of awareness in the communities.

Despite these obstacles, existing trauma registries in developed countries can be used as initial guides to create a system that is applicable in resource-poor areas.

The implementation of the Kampala Trauma Score (KTS), a simplified system first introduced in Uganda, has fueled the hope that these barriers can be overcome. The KTS is a simplified conglomerate of the RTS and the ISS, resembling the TRISS.[32] Its validity and reliability have been demonstrated in both urban and rural settings in Uganda.[33–35] This hospital-based registry was initiated as the first step in an injury surveillance system.[34] Data were collected regarding demographics, injury causation, and outcomes by using a single-page form. The project was subsequently expanded to include five large hospitals in Kampala as well as Addis Ababa in Ethiopia.[35,36]

The organisation of a continent-wide paediatric trauma registry in Africa will require the participation of many hospitals in all countries.

Ideally, it would begin with the establishment of regional and state registries, followed by national registries. These can then be grouped into subregional registries, including North, East, South, and West African registries, which will eventually combine to form the African Trauma Registry Database (ATRD).

Evidence-Based Research

Table 26.11 presents a literature review of scoring systems for paediatric trauma, and Table 26.12 presents a report on the establishment of the first national Italian trauma registry.

Table 26.11: Evidence-based research.

Title	ABCs of scoring systems for pediatric trauma
Authors	Furnival RA, Schunk JE
Institution	Department of Pediatrics, Primary Children's Medical Center, University of Utah School of Medicine, Salt Lake City, Utah, USA
Reference	Pediatr Emerg Care 1999; 15(3):215–223
Problem	An overview of frequently used trauma scoring systems.
Intervention	Literature review.
Comparison/ control (quality of evidence)	This literature review does not compare patients, per se, but compares the effectiveness of various trauma scoring systems in the paediatric age group with or without modifications. The many existing trauma scoring systems are divided into triage scoring systems, injury scoring systems, and trauma outcome analysis systems, each with its advantages and limitations when used in children.
Outcome/ effect	The scoring systems are designed to enhance effective prehospital triage of trauma patients, organise and improve trauma system resource planning, allow accurate comparison of different trauma populations, and serve as quality assurance filters in trauma patient care.
Historical significance/ comments	This well-written article takes the reader through the historical development of some trauma scoring systems and provides a very good overview of frequently used systems. The authors even inform readers about an ideal scoring system: it should correlate well with the desired outcome (e.g., death, disability, costs, etc.); it should be reasonable to clinicians and correlate with their judgement; it should use available data; it should be reliable among different users; and it should be simple. This is, in fact, what all scoring systems should be.

Table 26.12: Evidence-based research.

Title	The first Italian trauma registry of national relevance: methodology and initial results
Authors	Bartolomeo SD, Nardi G, Sanson G, et al.
Institution	Unit of Hygiene and Epidemiology, DPMSC School of Medicine, University of Udine, Udine, Italy
Reference	Eur J Emerg Med 2006; 13:197–203
Problem	Endeavour to establish a multiregional trauma registry in Italy.
Comparison/ control (quality of evidence)	The evidence of success in Italy so far is good, and the goals of the project have been achieved.
Outcome/ effect	The possibility of using the data collected for future quality improvement and research appear great, and there are steps to link this registry to other European trauma registries. It is also envisaged that, considering its success, other hospitals in Italy will offer to participate in such a registry.
Historical significance/ comments	This is a beginning worth emulating in the African subregion if we want to build a recognisable trauma registry for Africa. Not all African countries have to start at the same time; the end result will be the same eventually, if we follow other people's examples.

Key Summary Points

1. Trauma scoring systems are grouped into three sections: anatomic, physiologic, and combined scoring systems.

2. Each system has its place of use and must be used appropriately.

3. Each system has its advantages and disadvantages, and these must be weighed carefully before a particular system is chosen for use in a clinical setting.

4. The system chosen must be reproducible, or at least should be reliable and simple.

5. The most widely used systems include the Revised Trauma Score (RTS), Paediatric Trauma Score (PTS), Abbreviated Injury Scale (AIS), Injury Severity Score (ISS) and its modifications, and the Trauma and Injury Severity Score (TRISS).

6. A trauma registry collects and maintains data on patients who have had injuries and is used for planning to develop newer methods of trauma care as well as quality assurance.

7. Trauma registry data are confidential and must be treated as such.

References

1. Furnival RA, Schunk JE. ABCs of scoring systems for pediatric trauma. Pediatr Emerg Care 1999; 15:215–223.

2. Fani-Salek MH, Totten VY, Terezakis SA. Trauma scoring systems explained. Emerg Med 1999; 11:155–166.

3. Gilbert JC, Arbesman MC. Pediatric injury scoring and triage methodology. In Ziegler MM, Azizkhan RG, Weber TR, Operative Pediatric Surgery. McGraw-Hill Professional, 2003, Pp 1089–1095.

4. Engum SA, Mitchell MK, Scherer LR, et al. Prehospital triage in the injured pediatric patient. J Pediatr Surg 2000; 35:82–87.

5. Marcin JP, Pollack MM.Triage scoring systems, severity of illness measures, and mortality prediction models in pediatric trauma. Crit Care Med 2002; 30:S457–S467.

6. Stevenson M, Segui-Gomez M, Lescohier I, Di Scala C, McDonald-Smith G. An overview of the injury severity score and the new injury severity score. Injury Prevention 2001; 7:10–13.

7. Gennarelli T, Wodzin E. AIS 2005: a contemporary injury scale. Injury 2005; 37(12):1083–1091.

8. Narci A, Solak O, Turhan-Haktanir N, et al. The prognostic importance of trauma scoring systems in pediatric patients. Pediatr Surg Int 2009; 25:25–30.

9. Rennie CP, Brady PC. Advances in injury severity scoring. J Emerg Nurs 2007; 33:179–181.

10. Osler T, Baker SP, Long W. A modification of the injury severity score that both improves accuracy and simplifies scoring. J Trauma 1997; 43:922–925.

11. Sullivan T, Haider A, DiRusso SM, et al. Prediction of mortality in pediatric trauma patients: new injury severity score outperforms injury severity score in the severely injured. J Trauma 2003; 55:1083–1088.

12. Sala D, Fernández E, Morant A, Gascó J, Barrios C. Epidemiologic aspects of pediatric multiple trauma in a Spanish urban population. J Pediatr Surg 2000; 35:1478–1481.

13. Tatman A, Warren A, Williams A, Powell JE, Whitehouse W. Development of a modified paediatric coma scale in intensive care clinical practice. Arch Dis Child 1997; 77:519–521.

14. Gabbe BJ, Cameron PA, Finch CF. The status of the Glasgow Coma Scale. Emerg Med 2003; 15:353–360.

15. Ott R, Krämer R, Martus P, et al. Prognostic value of trauma scores in pediatric patients with multiple injuries. J Trauma 2000; 49:729–736.

16. Beattie TF, Currie CE, Williams JM, Wright P. Measures of injury severity in childhood: a critical overview. Injury Prevention 1998; 4:228–231.

17. Pohlman, TH, Bjerke HS, Offner P. Trauma scoring system eMedicine. Available at: http://emedicine.medscape.com/article/434076-overview (accessed 21 January 2009).

18. Washington State Trauma Registry. Available at: http://www.doh.wa.gov/hsqa/emstrauma/traumareg.htm (accessed 16 January 2009).

19. Black N, Barker M. Cross sectional survey of multicentre clinical databases in the United Kingdom. Available at: http://bmj.com/cgi/content/full/328/7454/1478 (accessed 25 January 2009).

20. Bartolomeo SD, Nardi G, Sanson G, et al. The first Italian trauma registry of national relevance: methology and initial results. Eur J Emerg Med 2006; 13:197–203.

21. World Health Organization. 2004 World Report on road traffic injury prevention. Available at: http://www.who.int/world-health-day/2004/infomaterials/world_report/en/ (accessed 10 September 2006).

22. Murray CJ, Lopez AD. Alternative projections of mortality and disability by cause 1990–2020: Global Burden of Disease Study. Lancet 1997; 349(9064):1498–1504.

23. Nwomeh BC, Lowell W, Kable R, Haley K, Ameh EA. History and development of trauma registry: lessons from developed to developing countries. W Jour of Emerg Surg 2006; 1(32).

24. Rutledge R. The goals, development, and use of trauma registries and trauma data sources in decision making in injury. Surg Clinic North Am 1995; 75:305–326.

25. Bergeron E, et al. Paying the price of excluding patients from a trauma registry. J Trauma 2006; 60:300–304.

26. Gabbe BJ, Cameron PA, Wolfe R. TRISS: does it get better than this? Acad Emerg Med 2004; 11:181–186.

27. Zafar H, Rehmani R, Raja AJ, Ali A, Ahmed M. Registry based trauma outcome: perspective of a developing country. Emerg Med J 2002; 19:391–394.

28. Podang J, et al. Primary verification: is the TRISS appropriate for Thailand? Southeast Asian J Trop Med Public Health 2004; 35:188–194.

29. Murlidhar V, Roy N. Measuring trauma outcomes in India: an analysis based on TRISS methodology in a Mumbai university hospital. Injury 2004; 35:386–390.

30. Onwudike M, Olaloye OA, Oni OO. Teaching hospital perspective of the quality of trauma care in Lagos, Nigeria. World J Surg 2001; 25:112–115.

31. Talwar S, Jain S, Porwal R, Laddha BL, Prasad P. Trauma scoring in a developing country. Singapore Med J 1999; 40:386–388.

32. MacLeod JBA, et al. A comparison of the Kampala Trauma Score (KTS) with the Revised Trauma Score (RTS), Injury Severity Score (ISS) and the TRISS method in a Ugandan trauma registry: is equal performance achieved with fewer resources? Eur J Trauma 2003; 29:392–398.

33. Owor G, Kobusingye OC. Trauma registries as a tool for improved clinical assessment of trauma patients in an urban African hospital. East Central Afr J Surg 2001; 57–63.

34. Kobusingye OC, Lett RR. Hospital-based trauma registries in Uganda. J Trauma 2000; 48:498–502.

35. Kobusingye OC, Guwatudde D, Owor G, Lett RR. Citywide trauma experience in Kampala, Uganda: a call for intervention. Inj Prev 2002; 8:133–136.

36. Taye M, Munie T. Trauma registry in Tikur Anbessa Hospital, Addis Ababa, Ethiopia. Ethiop Med J 2003; 41:221–226.

CHAPTER 27
INITIAL ASSESSMENT AND RESUSCITATION OF THE TRAUMA PATIENT

Francis A. Abantanga
Sha-Ron Jackson
Jeffrey S. Upperman

Introduction

The initial evaluation and treatment of the paediatric trauma patient require an organised, thorough approach. All patients must be assumed to have multiple injuries until proven otherwise. Resuscitation efforts should be early and aggressive to avoid the onset of irreversible shock;[2,3] the ability to recognise and effectively treat shock is all that is required in the vast majority of injured patents in order to gain stability. Adequate assessment and management of the ABCs described in this chapter will provide adequate treatment of the patient's other injuries, leading to an overall improvement in morbidity and mortality. Thus, the ABCs play an essential role in the initial evaluation and treatment of the paediatric trauma patient.

Effective initial resuscitation can reduce mortality in most paediatric trauma patients. Guidelines have been developed to facilitate patient care in a systematic and productive manner. Advances have been made in both diagnostic and therapeutic methods. The evaluation and treatment of paediatric trauma patients will continue to engage paediatric surgeons as efforts in trauma prevention become more successful.

The initial evaluation and care of a paediatric trauma patient uses the same protocols and procedures employed in adult trauma patients, the exception being that children should not be considered as little adults.[4,5] In the same manner as in adults, the primary survey entails ABCDE: **A** is for Airway maintenance/access with control of the cervical spine (C-spine); **B** is for Breathing; **C** is for Circulation with external haemorrhage control; **D** is for Disability and neurological screening; and **E** is for Exposure/Environmental control with thorough examination.[6] This is followed by a thorough secondary survey, which examines the injured child from head to toe.

Guidelines in the Paediatric Advanced Life Support[7] and the Advanced Trauma Life Support (ATLS)[8] provide a consensus framework in which to manage the injured patient:

1. triage;

2. primary survey of the injured child;

3. resuscitation;

4. secondary survey of the injured child;

5. re-evaluation and monitoring the injured child after resuscitation; and

6. Definitive care.

In the prehospital care of the injured child, emphasis is placed on airway maintenance, ventilation, control of external bleeding and shock, immobilisation of the patient, and immediate transport of the child to the closest appropriately functioning (and equipped to handle the injured) trauma centre.[1,5,6] Every effort must be made to provide initial interventions for all life-threatening conditions to the extent possible at the scene of injury and to prevent delays in delivering the injured to such a facility.[6] Management of trauma patients involves a team—it is teamwork, and most of the assessment and resuscitation of the injured is done simultaneously by members of the team, with one of them acting as the leader.[9–10]

Triage

The most developed countries have designated centres where trauma patients, including children, are sent after being "sorted out" at the scene or field of injury. These centres are designated in levels.[10] The following discussion is from the perspective of the West African subregion, Ghana being a good example; but is also true for many other African countries. Most hospitals have an Accident and Emergency (A&E) Department or Emergency Department (ED), where the injured are rushed by various means—ambulances (rare), private vehicles, or any other means available at the time. It is usually in this form that injured children are received in the emergency departments of hospitals, and it is here that the sorting of the injured starts.

Triage is the sorting of patients based on the need for treatment and the available resources to provide that treatment.[8] Children with injuries are usually admitted and sorted for treatment regardless of availability of resources, and then those who cannot be treated in that particular hospital are resuscitated and stabilised before being referred to another hospital that can handle the situation (which may be several kilometres away).

Primary Survey

The primary survey identifies life-threatening injuries that compromise oxygenation and circulation.[6] The vital functions of the patient are assessed quickly and efficiently; this entails a rapid primary evaluation, resuscitation of the vital functions, and later a more detailed re-evaluation of the injured child. The evaluation of the child's ABCDEs is made the priority of the primary survey or initial phase.[11] **F** is sometimes added to ABCDE to signify Further interventions necessary to help manage the patient. It is during the primary survey that life-threatening conditions are identified and effectively managed simultaneously.[11] This initial assessment should not take long and should detect and manage all clinically evident, immediate threats to life. We expand on the ABCDEFs in the next subsections.

A: Airway Access/Maintenance and C-Spine Control

Management of the airway begins by assessing its patency, or assessing for potential obstruction.[12] Any impaired or obstructed airway is optimised by using the jaw thrust manoeuvre[1,11,13] or by looking for and removing foreign bodies and/or clearing the oropharynx of debris, as well as administering supplemental oxygen if required.[1,14] Visible gross debris is manually removed and the airway suctioned to maintain patency, if necessary. In the attempt to assess and manage the child's airway, it is necessary to control the C-spine to prevent its excessive movement. It is wise to always assume C-spine injury until proven otherwise by the necessary follow up investigations.[4] As such, the head and C-spine should always be appropriately immobilised with appropriate devices.

The child's breathing is carefully assessed again once a patent airway is established, and if there is the need to provide ventilatory support, this must be done immediately. A child has a large head relative to body size, a short neck and therefore a short trachea, a small and anterior larynx, a floppy U-shaped epiglottis (the narrowest part of the airway being the cricoid ring), and a small oral cavity with a relatively large tongue.[2,11,14] Knowledge of these facts will aid in the choice of equipment to maintain a patent airway (e.g., an oropharyngeal airway; a nasopharyngeal airway, provided a basal skull fracture has been ruled out; or an endotracheal tube).

Signs of impending or present respiratory failure include decreased breath sounds, tachypnoea, intercostal space retractions, cyanosis, stridor, grunting, nasal flaring, abnormal chest wall motion, noisy breathing, and paradoxical breathing. If such signs are detected, measures should be taken immediately to restore normal airway by positioning the patient and using the jaw thrust method without head tilt to create a patent airway, by suctioning or removing secretions, and by giving 100% oxygen via a paediatric mask. (Note that the head tilt/chin lift manoeuvre is not recommended because it may exacerbate a spinal injury.) Nasal prongs should not be used because, with them, oxygen concentration cannot be controlled.

B: Breathing

Once the airway is patent or secured, it is necessary to check whether the child is breathing adequately.[1] The respirations must be spontaneous, unlaboured, and at a rate that is normal for the age of the child (Table 27.1); chest expansion should be equal bilaterally; and if the child speaks, the speech should be normal. Look for the rise and fall of the chest and abdomen, listen at the child's nose and mouth for exhaled breath sounds, and feel for exhaled air flow from the child's mouth. If respiration is inadequate, then provide ventilatory assistance,[4,6] which may include supplemental oxygen, bag-mask ventilation, or even endotracheal intubation. If available, use pulse oximetry to monitor oxygen saturation. The indications for endotracheal intubation include the inability to ventilate the child by bag-mask or the need for prolonged airway management, respiratory failure, and shock unresponsive to volume resuscitation.

Table 27.1: Normal vital signs for infants and children.

Age	Heart rate (beats/min)	Systolic BP (mm Hg)	Respiratory rate (breaths/min)	Blood volume (ml/kg body weight)
Neonate	100–160	60–90	30–60	90
Infant	90–120	80–100	30–40	80
2–5 years	95–140	80–120	20–30	80
5–12 years	80–120	90–110	15–20	80
> 12 years	60–100	100–120	12–15	70

While ventilating the child, be sure the lungs are symmetrically auscultated to ensure air exchange in them;[14] the chest is also percussed to exclude pneumo- or haemothorax; and finally, the chest is inspected and palpated to exclude injuries to the wall that may compromise ventilation to some extent.

Note that adequate ventilation, combined with fluid resuscitation to maintain perfusion, is the basis for resuscitation in the paediatric trauma patient. Therefore, treat any life-threatening chest injuries immediately to alleviate any respiratory distress. Potentially life-threatening injuries include tension pneumothorax, open pneumothorax, flail chest, cardiac tamponade, airway obstruction, and massive haemothorax.[5] These injuries should be actively sought in an injured child and treated appropriately and immediately.

C: Circulation

For a positive outcome in paediatric trauma patients, it is necessary to recognise hypovolaemia.[6] An attempt should be made to stop any external bleeding, if present, by direct manual compression over the wound or proximal to the point of bleeding. It is known that children have an increased physiological reserve and manifest signs of hypovolaemic shock much later, with hypotension followed quickly by complete cardiovascular collapse.[1] It is not easy to diagnose the severity of shock in injured children. Tachycardia is usually the earliest and most reliable measurable response to hypovolaemia in children, but anxiety and pain can confound tachycardia as an indicator of hypovolaemic shock.[1] Clues to immediately recognising early signs of hypovolaemic shock in children include tachycardia; mental status change (level of consciousness); decreased pulse pressure; respiratory compromise; skin perfusion (cold peripheries/cool extremities, mottled skin); decreased urine output (minimum urine output for infants and children ranges from 1 to 2 ml/kg per hour); delayed capillary refill; hypothermia; and hypotension.[1,4,6] Hypotension is a late finding and occurs in profound shock. Hypotension must be treated immediately and aggressively if the child is to survive without any adverse consequences.[3,4] Children have an amazing cardiovascular reserve, so one should not be led into a sense of security with regard to the status of the child's circulating blood volume if the initial vital signs of an injured child are normal. Hypotension in a paediatric trauma patient is an indicator of uncompensated shock and occurs following the loss of more than 45% of the circulating blood volume,[8] estimated to be 80 ml/kg body weight (see Table 27.1).[6,11,14]

Vascular Access and Venous Cannulation

Once adequate ABCs have been established, the next priority is vascular access and venous cannulation. This can be difficult in the early stages of shock, and the largest bore cannula possible should be used. If necessary, two percutaneous intravenous (IV) cannulae should be placed in the upper extremities,[3] preferably in the veins on the dorsum of the hands. Generally, two to three attempts are made at cannulating a peripheral vein; if this fails in children younger than 6 years of age, an intraosseous (IO) access is established by using the anterior tibial plateau about 3 cm below the tibial tuberosity[1,4-6] (Figure 27.1) or the inferior one-third of the femur about 3 cm above the external condyle;[14] if a percutaneous line is established later on, the intraosseous line should be discontinued. There are special IO needles for this purpose; a 16 G or 18 G needle should be used. The chosen site of the bone is entered perpendicularly. Aspiration of marrow indicates that one is in the correct position.[15] An injured limb should never be used for IO cannulation.[11] The potential complications of IO infusions include infection, cellulitis, and osteomyelitis.[4,15]

Other options are saphenous vein cutdown at the ankle[6] (above the medial malleolus); median cephalic vein cutdown on the elbow (not to be performed on the injured limb); or central venous cannulation using the femoral, subclavian, or internal jugular veins.[1,12] Central venous lines should be used in the postresuscitation stabilisation phase for monitoring and should not be attempted by an inexperienced doctor.

Once venous access is established, blood samples are taken for the determination of full blood count, grouping and cross-matching, urea,

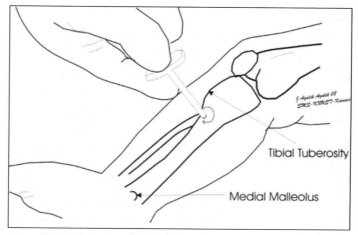

Figure 27.1: Method of setting up an intraosseous infusion.

creatinine and electrolytes, prothrombin time (PT), and amylase, after which volume replacement begins.

Initial fluid replacement will depend on the child's weight and should consist of warm isotonic crystalloids. Warm intravenous fluids will prevent hypothermia during the initial phase of resuscitation. As we know, hypothermia results in vasoconstriction, acidosis, and consumptive coagulopathy[6]—all deleterious to the injured child. The weight of a child (in kilograms), if unknown, can easily be estimated by using the following formula:

$$\text{Weight} = 2 \times (\text{age in years} + 4) \quad \text{or} \quad \text{Weight} = [5 \times (\text{age in years} + 3)]/2$$

Systolic blood pressure (SBP) and diastolic blood pressure (DBP) in children can be estimated by using the appropriate formula:

$$SBP = 80 + (2 \times \text{age in years})$$
$$DBP = 2/3 \times SBP$$

Resuscitation

The solutions to use for resuscitation include isotonic normal saline (NS) (0.9%) or Ringer's lactate (RL) at an initial bolus of 20 ml/kg body weight with a goal to achieving haemodynamic stability and improvement and restoring tissue perfusion as quickly as possible.[6,12] If there is no improvement in the haemodynamic status within 30–60 minutes, then another bolus of 20 ml/kg body weight of the same warm crystalloid solution should be given, for a total of 40–60 ml/kg;[12] in the case of children with evidence of haemorrhagic shock who fail to respond to fluid resuscitation, they should receive a transfusion of grouped and cross-matched packed red blood cells at a dose of 10 ml/kg body weight, or whole blood at a dose of 20 ml/kg body weight.[4,6,13] Of course, the source of bleeding should be identified and appropriately managed.

The algorithm in Figure 27.2 can be used for the initial assessment and resuscitation of a child admitted with trauma.

During resuscitation, it is prudent to have a urinary catheter in situ because urine output is an excellent indicator of volume status and can be used to guide resuscitation.[2] Aim to get about 2 ml/kg or more per hour of urine for children up to 1 year of age and about 1 ml/kg per hour for older children. If there is suspicion of a pelvic fracture with the possibility of injury to the urethra, then passage of a catheter is contraindicated (this is a relative contraindication).

Fluid resuscitation for children with isolated head injury should be considered carefully so as not to cause a rise in the intracranial pressure with too much fluid.[4]

D: Disability

A rapid neurological survey is performed to assess the level of consciousness, pupillary response, symmetry and size. The mnemonic AVPU is used to quickly assess the child's conscious level:[1] **A**lert, response to **V**erbal stimulus, response to **P**ainful stimulus, **U**nresponsive.

In using this rapid method of assessment, it is necessary to observe the ability of the child to follow simple commands and the quality and rapidity of the responses.[15] The pupils are briefly tested for size, equality, and bilateral reactivity. Both pupils should react briskly and positively.

The Glasgow Coma Scale (GCS) (see Chapter 26) can be used either during the primary survey or during the secondary survey for a more detailed neurological assessment of an injured child, especially after resuscitative efforts. There is evidence available to indicate that children who present with an initial GCS score of 6–8 in the presence of hypotension (SBP <90 mm Hg) have a significantly increased mortality rate;[12] therefore, it is important to prevent systemic hypotension during the initial efforts at resuscitation of the paediatric trauma patient, especially children with head injury.[12] A GCS score ≤ 8 is an indication for intubation of the child with head injury.[3] Administration of phenytoin (10–20 mg/kg body weight), diazepam (0.25 mg/kg body

weight) or phenobarbital (2–3 mg/kg body weight) may be given if traumatic brain injury is suspected.[12] Mannitol (0.5–1 gm/kg body weight) and furosemide (1 mg/kg body weight) should be used with care because they can exacerbate hypovolaemia in haemodynamically unstable patients.[12]

It is prudent to perform neurological assessment of the injured child frequently to detect any changes that might occur during the resuscitation period.

E: Exposure

Expose the child by completely cutting away clothing where necessary; it is also wise, however, to preserve evidence of torn clothing as well as to address patient modesty. The patient must be well exposed to aid thorough physical examination and to facilitate practical procedures.[1,4,15] Expose both front and back to ensure that no injuries are missed—for this, the child should be log rolled while maintaining C-spine immobilisation. The child is also assessed for signs of heat or chemical exposure to determine whether there is a need for irrigation of the affected area. Measures should be taken to prevent the child from losing heat and becoming hypothermic during exposure and examination in the A&E department.[13,15] The child is kept warm and intravenous fluids warmed before being administered. This may not be a requirement in our subregion where intravenous fluids are usually warm, except for blood and blood products. Lastly, signs of child abuse are assessed and carefully documented.[13] Nothing should be left out as being unimportant.

F: Further Interventions

Further interventions include:[13]

- the passage of a nasogastric tube to decompress the stomach since acute gastric dilatation may precipitate vomiting and aspiration; compress the inferior vena cava leading to diminished venous return to the heart and result in hypotension; splint the diaphragm leading to respiratory embarrassment.

- insertion of a urinary catheter in the urinary bladder; and

- managing pain relief by using the appropriate analgesics, such as morphine (0.1 mg/kg), once the primary survey is completed.

Other necessary confirmatory investigations can be done at this stage when the child is considered stable enough to be moved.

Secondary Survey

Once tachycardia, hypotension, hypoxia, and hypothermia have been managed, then a secondary survey with definitive treatment can be safely started.[6] The secondary survey begins when the primary survey is completed, resuscitation has been started, and the child is responsive or haemodynamically stable.

The secondary survey involves a more detailed systemic assessment of the patient than the initial evaluation (from head to toe, front and back) and initiation of relevant diagnostic investigations[3,6] (all the necessary radiographs and laboratory tests). It should never be started in a haemodynamically unstable patient. Attention should be paid to the history and signs and symptoms of the present injury. The history should be taken directly from the child (if the child is old enough and cooperative to do so), from family, and from bystanders, or other relevant persons. It should include the name, age, and what happened. It may sometimes be necessary to interview older children in the absence of caregivers if accurate information is to be obtained in areas such as child abuse, drug and alcohol use, and sexual abuse.

It is in the interest of both the child and the doctor to allow a parent to be by the child.[4] This will calm anxiety from both parent and patient and allow the physician to completely examine the child. Again, pain must be treated adequately, and all critically injured children must be admitted to an intensive care unit (preferably, a paediatric intensive care unit).

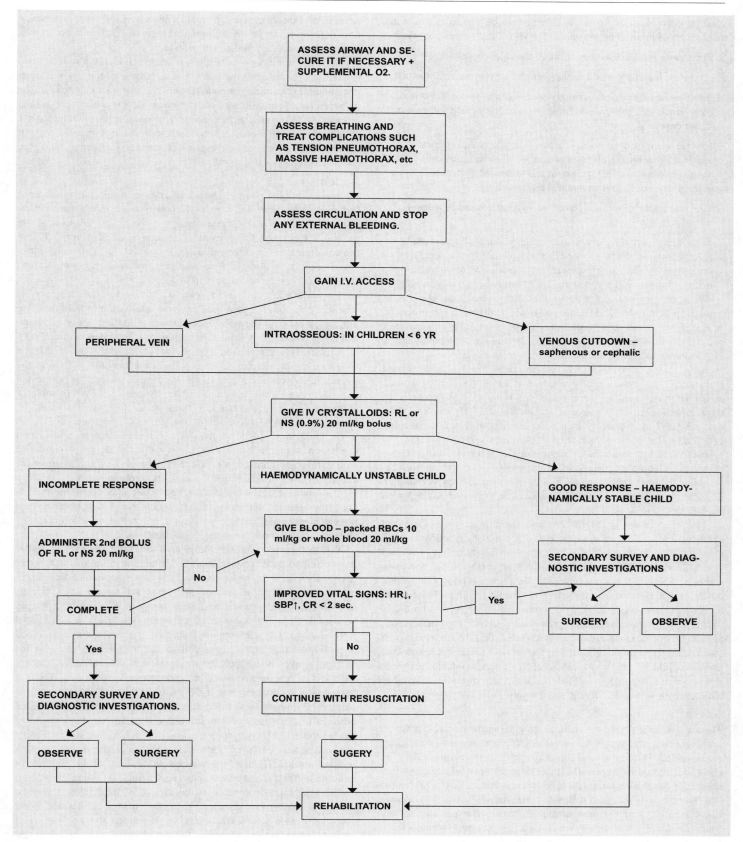

Figure 27.2: Algorithm for the initial assessment and resuscitation of a paediatric trauma patient.

A good and focused history is necessary to be able to ascertain the mechanism of injury. The mnemonic SAMPLE can be applied here.[1]

S: Signs and symptoms as they relate to the chief complaint;

A: Allergies, including medications, food, and environmental factors;

M: Medications the patient currently takes—over-the-counter drugs, compliance with prescribed dosing regimen, time, date and amount of last dose;

P: Past pertinent medical history, including medical and surgical problems, preexisting diseases or chronic illnesses, previous hospitalisations; for infants, a neonatal history of gestation, prematurity, congenital anomalies, and so on;

L: Last oral intake of liquids, food, and—for adolescent females—sexual activity;

E: Events related to the current injury, such as onset, duration, and precipitating factors, associated factors such as toxic inhalants, drugs, and alcohol; injury scenario and mechanism of injury; and treatment or first aid given at the site of injury or by caregivers.

When treating children with injuries, the clinician should bear in mind the possibility of child abuse and examine the child appropriately. A history not consistent with the injury or multiple injuries not consistent with what had happened should cause the clinician to have a high index of suspicion and try to exclude child abuse.[1,6]

After taking a good history, the patient is thoroughly examined from head to toe, including an evaluation of the child's vital signs, such as temperature, blood pressure, pulse, and respiration as compared to the normal for the child's age group (see Table 27.1). The goal is to recognise and appropriately treat potential life- and limb-threatening pathology. The body is examined region by region to identify the problem(s) and to assess the child for specific injuries to various organ systems.[1] A complete neurological examination is also performed, including the use of either the GCS or its modified version for children. The Paediatric Trauma Score (PTS) should be evaluated and recorded in the notes (see Chapter 26).

The head is examined for bruises, lacerations, contusions, and skull fractures. The eyes are examined for pupillary reaction to light, size, shape, equality, and the conjunctiva for haemorrhage. The face is examined for facial symmetry, epistaxis, rhinorrhoea, raccoon eyes, and bony fractures. Look for trauma to the gums and tongue in the oral cavity, as well as missing or broken teeth. The neck is immobilised until a cervical spine injury (a rare occurrence in children) is completely excluded by evaluating the appropriate radiographs.[4] If the radiographs are normal but the child still has neurological deficits or tenderness over the cervical spine, immobilisation of the cervical spine should continue until the child is seen by a neurosurgeon. Where available, magnetic resonance imaging (MRI) will aid the assessment of the spinal cord in children with suspected cervical spine injury.

Chest

The chest is re-inspected for changes from the initial primary survey to assess thoracic trauma. Both posterior and anterior walls of the chest are inspected. The contour and integrity of the chest wall are noted. The chest is inspected for hyperinflated hemithorax, open wounds, and flail chest. The ratio of inspiration to expiration is compared—a prolonged expiration usually indicates distress.[16] The chest is palpated to exclude rib, clavicular, scapular, and sternal fractures. The presence of rib fractures signifies that significant trauma has occurred. Where the rib fractures are multiple and segmental, then a flail chest may occur and paradoxical respiratory motion may be noticed.[8]

In the presence of contusions or haematomas on the thoracic wall, the examining physician should have in mind the possibility of occult injury to the chest. The lungs should be auscultated for the presence or absence of breath sounds and whether heart sounds are heard clearly or are muffled. Absent or reduced breath sounds may indicate the presence of a pneumothorax or haemothorax; distant or muffled heart sounds may be suggestive of cardiac tamponade.

Thus, in examining the chest of an injured child, the physician tries to exclude life-threatening injuries such as tension pneumothorax, open pneumothorax, cardiac tamponade, and massive haemothorax. In the management of children with chest trauma, a chest radiograph (supine or erect) will confirm the presence of a haemo- or pneumothorax. If a child is hypoxic after chest trauma, then suspect lung contusion and put the child on supplementary oxygen with chest physiotherapy, and give adequate analgesics to control pain.

Abdomen

Abdominal trauma patients should be assessed to decide which need further investigations and which will benefit from an immediate laparotomy because of an unstable condition. The abdomen of the stable patient is examined for tenderness, guarding, or distention.[1] If any intraabdominal solid organ injury is suspected, an abdominal ultrasound scan, in the form of focused abdominal sonography for trauma (FAST) in experienced hands, will be helpful.[5,6,12,17]

An abdominal ultrasound scan will visualise the presence or absence of fluid in the peritoneal cavity. Visualisation of fluid by using ultrasonography, in the right upper quadrant, the left upper quadrant, and the pelvis suggests solid organ injury or a mesenteric injury. FAST is particularly useful in the hypotensive child and is the evaluation of choice for the determination of significant amounts of fluid in the paediatric abdominal cavity.[12] It can also be used to diagnose pericardial tamponade. In a stable patient, however, the choice of investigation for abdominal trauma evaluation is a computed tomography (CT) scan.[1,6,18] It remains the gold standard for the accurate diagnostic evaluation of the child involved in trauma.[12] The CT scan provides a structural evaluation of organs better than an ultrasound scan, and if combined with intravenous contrast injection at the time of the scan, improves the clinician's ability to determine the severity of organ injury.[18]

The stable child with a suspected blunt abdominal injury that does not demand immediate surgery should be closely observed and re-evaluated several times, preferably by the same examiner. The abdominal symptoms can change over time.

Where the vital signs of the injured child are still unstable after proper and adequate resuscitation and after evaluation of the thoracic cavity, then it is in order to consider either an intraabdominal or pelvic injury and try to find out the cause and treat it appropriately. In such cases, a diagnostic peritoneal lavage (DPL) can occasionally be useful[12,19] in the absence of an ultrasound machine. DPL is a method of rapidly determining whether free intraperitoneal blood is present and is especially useful in the hypotensive child or the haemodynamically unstable trauma patient.[20] In experienced hands, DPL is fast and inexpensive, but more invasive than FAST, and it has a low complication rate. If DPL is to be performed in a child, the volume of fluid to be infused should be about 10 ml/kg of normal saline or Ringer's lactate.[1] The stomach and the urinary bladder should be decompressed by passing a nasogastric tube into the stomach and a urethral catheter into the bladder before the procedure is performed. A positive result is signified by microscopic findings of the presence of more than 100,000 red blood cells (RBCs)/ml, 500 white blood cells (WBCs)/ml, bile, or urine from the sample of fluid infused into the peritoneal cavity. The presence of organic matter or elevated WBC count indicates a hollow viscus has been disrupted.[12]

It is important to note that the presence of free blood in the peritoneal cavity of a child does not always mean a laparotomy is the next logical thing to do.[1] Such a child, if stable haemodynamically, can be managed nonoperatively provided there are no increasing signs of peritonitis, abdominal distention, and hypotension, which would indicate continued bleeding into the peritoneal cavity.

The abdominal examination is not complete if the perineum is not inspected and a digital rectal examination is not done. The perineum should be examined for bruises, haematoma, contusions, and lacerations. The rectum should be assessed for blood in the gastrointestinal tract, and the urethral meatus also should be inspected for blood. This will inform the physician as to the next line of action. For example, in the case of blood in the urethral meatus, the physician will think of a possible urethral tear and try to avoid unnecessary manipulations in passing a urethral catheter or, better still, inform the urologist to do that if there is the need for passing a bladder catheter.

Musculoskeletal Examination

The musculoskeletal system should be inspected. Here the four extremities (upper and lower) should be evaluated for pain, pallor, paresthesia, paralysis, and pulselessness. It is important to inspect the limbs for skin colour, ecchymoses, pallor or cyanosis, for symmetry and for length and position. Where there is suspicion of a fracture, the limb must be straightened and splinted or immobilised.[6] It is important to bear in mind the possibility of compartment syndrome when manipulating and splinting limb fractures. Remember to examine the child's pelvis for fractures.

Skin and Soft Tissues

Skin and soft tissues should be carefully examined, especially in the case of burns. Airway management is paramount in children with burns, especially if they involve the face, with the possibility of inhalation injury. The percentage of body surface area (BSA) burned should be assessed by using the Lund and Browder chart[21] and fluid resuscitation started using either RL or NS at 3–4 ml/kg body weight × % BSA burned, in addition to the maintenance fluid.[1] The calculated amount should be given over the next 24 hours, with half of it being given in the first 8 hours. Burns should be cleaned with normal saline and a nonocclusive dressing applied. The child should be transferred to a burn centre for further management. All the following burns in children should be managed in a burn centre or in a hospital if a centre does not exist: partial thickness burns of over 10% of the BSA; full thickness burns of over 5% of the BSA; burns on the face, neck, hands, genitalia, perineum, feet and over major joints; circumferential burns of any part of the body; electrical or chemical burns; and burns due to inhalation. All children with burns must have appropriate pharmacologic pain management, such as injection pethidine or oral morphine.

Neurological Examination

The neurological examination determines the mental status of the child, or the level of consciousness. The level of consciousness can be determined by using either the GCS or the modified GCS for infants. The size and reaction of the pupils to light are determined. Both pupils are examined for size, shape, equality, deviation, and reactivity to light—direct or consensual. Finally, all the limbs must be examined for spontaneous and purposeful movements, response to verbal commands, and sensory deficits or abnormalities. Where there is paralysis or paresis of a limb, injury to the spinal cord or peripheral nervous system should be suspected and the child immobilised with appropriate immobilisation devices until a spinal injury is ruled out.

Re-evaluation

Ongoing assessment or re-evaluation of the injured child is very critical to successful care and rehabilitation. Re-evaluation is usually performed following the detailed physical examination in the secondary survey. Repeated assessments are essential for the clinician to effectively maintain awareness of changes in the condition of the child. Repeated assessments should be performed every 5 minutes for the unstable child and every 15 or so minutes for the stable injured child.[16] Re-evaluation includes:

- standard respiratory monitoring (ventilatory rate, signs of impaired airway, breath sounds, etc.);
- standard cardiovascular monitoring (pulses, BP, heart sounds, etc.);
- standard neurological monitoring (GCS, pupils, motor and sensory changes, etc.);
- monitoring of temperature; and
- response to pain management.

Definitive care is carried out after the secondary survey. All problems found during the secondary survey are managed at this stage. All the essential investigations are also carried out during this stage of the child's care. The decision to manage the child's problems nonoperatively or surgically (with reference to the haemodynamically stable patient) is also made at this stage.

Conclusion

In conclusion, paediatric trauma patients undergo the same principles of management as for adult patients. Children should never be considered as little adults—their physiology, anatomy, and psychological needs differ from those of adults. The primary survey and initial phase of resuscitation of a paediatric trauma patient should address life-threatening injuries that compromise oxygenation and circulation. Control of the airway is the most important and first priority. The evaluation of the paediatric trauma patient's ABCs, disability, and exposure are made the priority of the initial phase. The aim is to stabilise the injured patient by thoroughly assessing for injuries and treating those injuries appropriately before transferring the patient to a trauma centre or to a facility or hospital where the injuries can be managed better.

After the primary survey, during which resuscitation of the patient is carried out at the same time, the patient then undergoes a secondary survey, in which a detailed history is taken and examination is performed; diagnostic investigations are carried out, and the appropriate treatment is instituted. At this stage, a decision should be made as to whether the injured child is to be managed in the present facility or be transferred to a more appropriate centre, provided, of course, that the patient's condition is stable.

Evidence-Based Research

Table 27.2 presents an example of holistic management of a case involving a 5-year-old child who sustained an injury in a traffic accident. Table 27.3 presents a study addressing the use of a CT scan to noninvasively evaluate and treat paediatric patients with head and abdominal injuries.

Table 27.2: Evidence-based research.

Title	Pediatric trauma—the care of Anthony
Authors	Lawton L
Institution	Accident and Emergency, The Radcliffe Hospital, Headington, Oxford, UK
Reference	Accident Emerg Nurs 1995; 3:172–176
Problem	The care of a paediatric trauma patient.
Intervention	The adaption of the ABCs of trauma care for a paediatric patient, taking into consideration the differences between adults and children.
Comparison/ control (quality of edvidence)	This is a practical example of how a 5-year-old child, who was involved in a road traffic injury, was managed holistically. The primary survey of the child and resuscitation started immediately when he was brought into the Accident and Emergency unit.
Outcome/ effect	This study reinforces the point that paediatric trauma care follows the same principles as for adult trauma with important differences such as the child's physiology, anatomy, and psychological needs, which should be taken into consideration if the child with trauma/injury is to survive. The trauma child should never be considered as a "little adult".
Historical significance/ comments	This study reinforces the point that paediatric trauma care follows the same principles as for adult trauma with important differences such as the child's physiology, anatomy, and psychological needs, which should be taken into consideration if the child with trauma/injury is to survive. The trauma child should never be considered as a "little adult".

Table 27.3: Evidence-based research.

Title	The efficacy of computed tomography in evaluating abdominal injuries in children with major head trauma
Authors	Beaver BL, Colombani PM, Fal A, et al
Institution	Department of Pediatric Surgery and Radiology, The Johns Hopkins University School of Medicine, Baltimore, Maryland, USA
Reference	J Pediatr Surg 1987; 22(12):1117–1122.
Problem	The efficacy of combined computed tomography of the head and abdomen in evaluating abdominal injury in a child with major head trauma and unreliable physical examination.
Intervention	Combined head and abdominal CT scans were performed on children with serious closed head trauma (GCS ≤ 10) and suspected abdominal injury at the same time.
Comparison/ control (quality of edvidence)	Of 65 children with GCS ≤ 10, 23% were found to have significant intraabdominal injury, but only two required laparotomy.
Outcome/ effect	All patients survived.
Historical significance/ comments	The significance of the study is that, based on the fact that nonoperative treatment of injuries to the spleen, liver, etc. have been carried out successfully, there is a need to find noninvasive methods of evaluating patients with suspected abdominal injury and concomitant severe head trauma without resorting to DPL. With this method, they avoided surgery in 13 children.

Key Summary Points

1. Start the management of the injured child with a primary survey (ABCDEF), which involves assessment, stabilisation, and management of all acute life-threatening conditions.

2. The primary assessment and resuscitation are performed simultaneously, which means there should be a paediatric trauma team in readiness for such an eventuality. There is always a leader of such a team who organises the members of the team to execute various functions.

3. It is necessary to reassess the injured child frequently with normal parameters of the child's age group in mind so as to take the appropriate action should these change for the worse. The proper sequence to bear in mind is: assessment of injured child, interventions and reassessment after each intervention.

4. Always keep the cervical spine immobilised until a neck injury is excluded.

5. Do not hesitate to consult other subspecialties, such as the neurosurgeon, urologist, trauma surgeon, and so forth.

6. Do the minimum radiologic and laboratory investigations necessary during the primary survey period. The rest can be done when the child is haemodynamically stable and a secondary survey has been performed to determine the need for more extensive investigations.

7. Do not hesitate to carry out a laparotomy (for damage control) if all efforts at resuscitating the child are not yielding the desired results, the patient's condition remains unstable, and an intraabdominal catastrophe is suspected.

8. Transfer only haemodynamically stable but severely injured children to the next competent facility. It is good practice to try to stabilise the injured child before transfer.

References

1. Arensman RM, Madonna MB. Initial management and stabilization of pediatric trauma patients. The Child's Doctor. J Children's Memorial Hospital, Chicago. Available at http://www.childsdoc.org/fall97/trauma/trauma.asp (accessed 17 November 2008).

2. Shafi S, Kauder DR. Fluid resuscitation and blood replacement in patients with polytrauma. Clin Orthopaed Related Res 2004; 422:37–42.

3. Vella AE, Wang VJ, McElderry C. Predictors of fluid resuscitation in pediatric trauma patients. J Emerg Med 2006; 31(2):151–155.

4. Lawton L. Paediatric trauma—the care of Anthony. Accident Emerg Nurs 1995; 3:172–176.

5. Schvartsman C, Carrera R, Abramovici S. Initial assessment and transportation of an injured child. J Pediatr (Rio J) 2005; 81(5 Suppl):S223–S229.

6. Alterman DM. Considerations in pediatric trauma. Available at http://www.emedicine.com/med/TOPIC3223.HTM (accessed 5 October 2008).

7. Zaritsky AL, Nadkarni VM, Hickey RW, et al., eds. Pediatric Advanced Life Support Provider Manual. American Heart Association, 2002.

8. American College of Surgeons. Advanced Trauma Life Support Course for Physicians. Student Manual, 1993.

9. Simon B, Gabor R, Letourneau P. Secondary triage of the injured pediatric patient within the trauma center: support for a selective resource-sparing two-stage system. Pediatr Emerg Care 2004; 20(1):5–11.

10. Harris BH, Barlow BA, Ballantine TV, et al. American Pediatric Surgical Association principles of pediatric trauma care. J Pediatr Surg 1992; 27(4):423–426.

11. Inaba AS, Boychuk RB. Case based pediatrics for medical students and residents. Available at: http://www.hawaii.edu/medicine/pediatrics/pedtext/s14c08.html (accessed 17 November 2008).

12. DeRoss AL, Vane DW. Early evaluation and resuscitation of the pediatric trauma patient. Seminars Pediatr Surg 2004; 13(2):74–79.

13. Lloyd F. Pediatric trauma. Available at http://www.physicianeducation.org/downloads/PDF%20Download%20for%20website/Pediatric%20Trauma.pdf (accessed 17 November 2008).

14. Lloyd-Thomas AR. Paediatric trauma: primary survey and resuscitation–I. BMJ 1990; 301(6747):334–336.

15. Lloyd-Thomas AR. Paediatric trauma: primary survey and resuscitation –II. BMJ 1990; 301(6747):380–382.

16. Illinois Emergency Medical Services for Children: Initial Pediatric Assessment Teaching Tool. Available at www.luhs.org/emsc.

17. Becker A, Lin G, McKenney MG, et al. Is the FAST exam reliable in severely injured patients? Injury 2009; doi:10.1016/j.injury.2009.10.054

18. Beaver BL, Colombani PM, Fal A, et al. The efficacy of computed tomography in evaluating abdominal injuries in children with major head trauma. J Pediatr Surg 1987; 22(12):1117–1122.

19. Ameh EA, Chirdan LB, Nmadu PT. Blunt abdominal trauma in children: epidemiology, management, and management problems in a developing country. Pediatr Surg Int 2000; 16:505–509.

20. Bjerke HS, Bjerke JS. Splenic rupture. Available at http://emedicine.medscape.com/article/432823 (accessed 12 January 2010).

21. Harvey JS, Watkins GM, Sherman RT. Emergent burn care. South Med J 1984; 77(2):204–214.

CHAPTER 28
THORACIC TRAUMA

AB (Sebastian) van As
Dorothy V. Rocourt
Benedict C. Nwomeh

Introduction

The physiological constitution of children differs substantially from that of adults. As a result, injured children often require specific management as compared to adults. This chapter focuses on the management of chest trauma.[1-3]

Chest injuries occur commonly in children and include damage to the chest wall, diaphragm, lungs, and mediastinal structures. The presence of chest injury often portends involvement of other organs, reflecting the transmission of substantial force to the child's compact body. The severity of chest trauma in children ranges from minor to rapidly fatal. It is therefore imperative to promptly diagnose and appropriately treat these injuries to ensure an optimal outcome.

Anatomic Considerations

The chest wall in children is elastic; therefore, energy can be transmitted to underlying organs without breaking the protective ribs. Severe pulmonary contusion or injuries to spleen and liver can occur without overlying rib fractures. Rib fractures and mediastinal injuries are distinctly uncommon in children, and when present they usually indicate the transfer of a massive amount of energy; multiple serious organ injuries should be suspected.[4] The mediastinum is highly mobile in children, and a tension pneumothorax can develop rapidly.[5]

Resuscitation

All resuscitations should strictly follow the general ABC pattern of basic life support, as discussed in Chapter 27.

Demographics

Chest injuries are the leading cause of childhood injury death. Approximately one million children globally die annually as a result of trauma. The most common cause of trauma is motor vehicle crashes. Thoracic trauma in children may be classified by mechanism, anatomical site, and severity (immediately or potentially life threatening). The vast majority of thoracic injuries result from blunt trauma, usually inflicted to a child pedestrian by a motor vehicle. Less than 5% are attributable to penetrating injuries.

Penetrating chest trauma in children, just as in adults, is often the result of knife stabs or gunshot wounds. These include BBs or pellets fired from recreational air guns that can produce life-threatening injuries. Other unusual causes of penetrating trauma seen in children 12 years of age or younger include impalement onto shards of broken glass or metal rods.

Most chest injuries occur as a part of multiple injuries, including head and abdominal injuries, and it is these associated injuries that expose these children to a high mortality. It is therefore crucial to assess the whole patient in the case of a chest injury. Paediatric trauma scores may help to identify mortality early in this patient population to facilitate and expedite treatment.

Clinical Presentations

Chest Wall Injuries

The elasticity and flexibility of a child's chest cage often protect the child from a serious injury. If rib fractures do occur, however, this is usually a sign of a major energy transfer to the child's chest and often indicative of a high-velocity injury. A flail segment is an unusual event in a child, and the underlying pulmonary contusion is much more important for the prognosis than the flail segment itself.

Rib fractures are extremely painful because immobilisation is practically impossible. Therefore, adequate analgesia is of the utmost importance to render the child pain-free and to ensure adequate breathing. Intravenous morphine is the drug of choice (as bolus: 0.1 mg/kg body weight). Oral analgesia is not often tolerated, and intramuscular (IM) or subcutaneous drugs often are poorly absorbed. Respiratory exercises are essential in the proper management. In the case of multiple rib fractures, admission to a specialised trauma unit with availability of continuous chest physiotherapy is preferred.

Traumatic Asphyxia

Traumatic asphyxia usually occurs as a result of major chest and sometimes abdominal trauma. The exact pathophysiology is not clearly understood, but the proposed mechanism is a closed glottis and tensed abdominal muscles, causing the force of the injury to be transferred to the superior vena cava and to the head and neck, with subsequent rupture of the superficial blood vessels. Usually, the child presents tachypnoeic with petechiae over the face, neck, and chest. Additionally, the face might be blue and swollen, and retinoscopy might reveal retinal haemorrhages.

Children suffering from traumatic asphyxia should be very carefully examined for underlying injuries of the vital organs. Treatment should be symptomatically; however, because these children are likely to develop respiratory insufficiency, they should be managed in a paediatric intensive care unit (PICU). Long-term follow-up of isolated traumatic asphyxia has proven to have an excellent prognosis.

Tracheobronchial Injuries

Like oesophageal injuries, tracheobronchial injuries are rare. Rupture of the trachea or bronchae is usually complete, associated with vascular and oesophageal injuries, and occurs mostly within 2.5 cm from the carina. Proper airway management takes priority; the injuries can usually be repaired primarily via a thoracotomy.

In the event of a tracheo-oesophageal injury, it is crucial to establish a muscular or pleura flap between the injuries to prevent a fistula.

Lung Injuries

Lung contusion is one of the most common childhood chest injuries, followed by infection and haematoma. It occurs in approximately two-thirds of all cases of chest trauma. Usually, it results from a rapid acceleration/deceleration injury (primarily motor vehicle collisions). Contusions occur within minutes after the injury, are mostly localised to a (lower) segment or lobe of the lung, and can be diagnosed on the initial chest radiograph.

Management is symptomatic, but intensive care is often required in the initial phase, where there is danger of respiratory collapse and ventilation might be indicated for adequate oxygenation. The prognosis is good if infection does not occur; healing can be expected within 1–2 weeks. Unfortunately, in two-thirds of these cases, infection occurs due to the extravasation of fluid and blood in interstitium and alveoli, which creates an excellent microbial culture medium. Ventilation efforts are often poor due to pain, and without active and passive chest physiotherapy, the prognosis is poor.

Pulmonary haematoma is rare. It is usually caused by an injury to a major blood vessel within the lung, creating a so-called coin-lesion in the lung tissue. Management is nonoperative, except in massive bleeds.

Simple Pneumothorax

Pneumothorax is a common occurrence in childhood chest injury. Collapse of the lung might be caused by a penetrating injury, a rupture of lung parenchyma, or a tear in the oesophagus or tracheobronchial tree.

Physical signs are diminished breath sounds, poor motion of the hemithorax, hyperresonance to percussion, subcutaneous emphysema, and deviation of the trachea to the ipsilateral site. Diagnosis is confirmed with an erect expiratory chest radiograph.

Treatment consists of a tube thoracostomy in the 4th intercostal space, in the anterior axillary line, under adequate analgesia. Care should be taken not to cause injury to the lung parenchyma or diaphragm during the insertion of the tube. An underwater seal should immediately be connected to the bottle. If the child is asymptomatic and can be closely monitored, aspiration or even observation of a simple pneumothorax may be appropriate, but the resources to rapidly insert a chest tube must be available in the event of any deterioration.[5]

Tension Pneumothorax

Progressive accumulation of air under pressure in the pleural space is usually due to a valve-effect tear in the lung parenchyma. It may lead to ipsilateral collapse of the lung and mediastinal shift, thereby compressing the (only properly ventilating) contralateral lung. This might result in severe impairment of ventilation as well as compromise the venous return to the heart, and is often a lethal condition if not acted upon rapidly.

Diagnosis should be made clinically. Decreased breathing sounds, a hyperinflated ipsilateral hemithorax, trachea deviation to the contralateral side, and a severely distressed patient all indicate that a fast needle-puncture of the anterior chest (2nd intercostal space, midclavicular line) will be life saving. The needle has to be replaced by a proper tube thoracostomy as soon as possible because blockage occurs frequently, and the excursions of an inflated lung will damage its visceral pleural surface against the sharp tip of the needle.

Haemothorax

Haemothorax is the accumulation of blood in the pleural space. Up to 40% of the blood volume can easily be lost in one pleural cavity. The blood loss usually arises from injury to a major artery, either from the chest wall or the lung, although this is not always the case. Persistent bleeding from an intercostal artery or a tear in the lung parenchyma can also produce major blood loss.

The diagnosis is made clinically and confirmed with an erect chest radiograph. Blood in the lower part of the pleural cavity often causes referred pain in the upper abdomen. Once the haemothorax is drained, the abdominal symptoms disappear.

Treatment consists of chest tube thoracostomy; only rarely is a thoracotomy indicated. The main indications for thoracotomy are ongoing active bleed while an intercostal drain is in place, or an infected haemothorax (usually 5–7 days after injury). On rare occasions, a massive haemothorax may lead to a tension haemothorax with deviation of the heart and mediastinum to the opposite side (Figure 28.1).

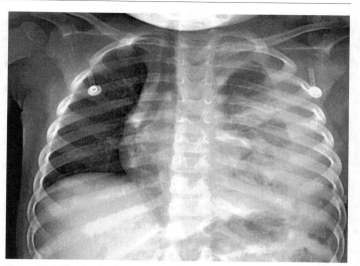

Figure 28.1: Chest radiograph of a ruptured left hemidiaphragm, with displacement of the heart and mediastinum to the right.

Oesophageal Injuries

Fortunately, due to the location of the oesophagus, injuries to it are rare. Transmitted pressure from the stomach may cause either Mallory-Weiss bleeding (if the lower oesophageal sphincter is closed) or the more sinister Boerhaave syndrome, characterised by perforation of the lower oesophagus into the left chest cavity (if the upper oesophageal sphincter is closed).

Penetrating injuries may cause oesophageal injuries if they are *transthoracic*. Radiographic contrast studies and/or endoscopies are strongly advocated in these cases. A nonionic contrast material should be used.

The management of the oesophageal injuries depends on the nature of the injury, the timing of presentation, and the location. With the exception of major (high-velocity) gunshot injuries, the majority can be repaired primarily within 24 hours of the injury. Beyond the first 24 hours, the operative strategy may include oesophageal diversion, exclusion, T-tube drainage, or even total oesophagectomy.

Cervical oesophageal injuries

Cervical oesophageal injuries rarely represent a large problem because leakage from a repair produces localised tissue infection or abscess, which can be drained externally.

Thoracic oesophageal injuries

Thoracic oesophageal injuries are notorious for the fast spread of saliva, food, and acid from the stomach through the injury into the chest, able to cause a rampant and usual lethal mediastinitis. Oesophageal diversion might be indicated in these cases.

Abdominal oesophageal injuries

Abdominal oesophageal injuries will usual present as an acute abdomen and will require a laparotomy for repair.

Diaphragmatic Injuries

Traumatic disruption of the diaphragm is usually caused by blunt trauma. It involves the left side in the majority of cases. The injury is high velocity in nature, such as from motor vehicle collisions and falls from a height. Because the force required to damage the diaphragm is considerable, associated injuries are common (about 80%) and include intrathoracic and intraabdominal as well as extratruncal injuries.

The clinical presentation varies according to the associated injuries; an isolated diaphragmatic rupture can easily be misdiagnosed. In children, the mechanism of injury might be slightly different from that in adults. Whereas in adults the typical injury involves the dome of

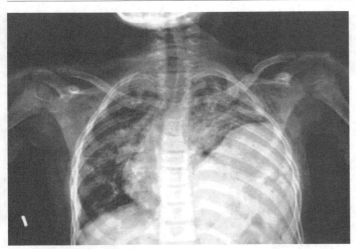

Figure 28.2: Chest radiograph of a ruptured left hemidiaphragm, with displacement of the heart and mediastinum to the right.

the diaphragm (as a blow-out), rupture in children seems to take place more often along the periphery of the diaphragm (probably due to the increased elasticity of the chest wall).

Diagnosis is made on an erect radiograph, which typically shows the nasogastric tube in the stomach above the diaphragm (Figure 28.2). However, herniation can involve nearly any intraabdominal organ, and the appearance of the stomach below the diaphragm does not exclude a diaphragmatic rupture.

Penetrating injuries in the lower half of the chest as well as the upper part of the abdomen can involve the diaphragm. In these cases, herniation will rarely occur in the acute phase, but an undiagnosed hole in the diaphragm can lead to complications on the long term. Repair should be performed via a laparotomy, during which the state of the intraabdominal organs also can be assessed.

Heart and Pericardium

Blunt chest trauma can produce several types of cardiac injuries, including contusions, concussions, and frank rupture of the myocardium, a valve, a septum, and—very rarely—a coronary artery. Pericardial tears leading to herniation of the heart often lead to diminished cardiac function and a low output state. Occult structural cardiac injuries (i.e., atrial or ventricular septal defects, valvular insufficiency, and ventricular aneurysm formation) may also occur and present without physiologic signs of injury. Often, these injuries are identified only after a new murmur is noted or a change in the electrocardiogram (ECG) occurs. Echocardiography, when available, can assist to confirm the diagnosis.

Myocardial contusion

The most common type of blunt cardiac injury is the myocardial contusion. Unlike myocardial concussions, myocardial contusions produce focal damage to the heart that can be demonstrated histologically. Patients with myocardial contusions often have an associated chest wall injury. Many tests have been proposed to diagnose a contusion (e.g., echocardiography, electrocardiography, enzyme determinations, and nuclear imaging), but still no definitive diagnostic test exists. A 12-lead ECG is the simplest test and may show reversible changes in the ST and T waves. Symptomatic myocardial contusions are diagnosed by echocardiography based on finding a reduced ejection fraction, localised systolic wall motion abnormalities, and an area of increased end-diastolic wall thickness and echogenicity.

Myocardial contusions may be silent and asymptomatic, can present with cardiovascular collapse from reduced cardiac output, or cause arrhythmias that may be life threatening.

The treatment of myocardial contusions remains supportive, with 12- to 24-hour electrocardiographic monitoring and inotropic support

as needed. Most authors recommend cardiac monitoring in an intensive care unit to identify arrhythmias. Patients with arrhythmias and obvious thoracic injuries should be monitored with ECG, serum cardiac enzymes, and echocardiogram as needed.

Myocardial rupture and valve injury

Traumatic rupture of any chamber of the heart usually results in rapid death. The most common cause of death from thoracic injury is myocardial rupture. The majority of these are due to high-energy impacts such as motor vehicle collisions or falls from great heights. The majority of these patients die at the scene. The right ventricle is the most commonly ruptured cardiac chamber. Children with myocardial rupture present *in extremis* with pericardial tamponade. Patients with traumatic atrial or ventricular septal defects may be clinically stable, with the only finding being that of a new murmur. Early diagnosis and repair is mandatory for survival from these lethal injuries.

Valvular injuries may occur following severe blunt chest trauma, but these are rare. The atrioventricular valves are most susceptible to injury, and the damage often occurs to the valve apparatus (i.e., annulus, ruptured chorda tendinae, or papillary muscle). These injuries in clinically stable patients may be repaired electively.

Pericardial tamponade

The accumulation of blood within the pericardial sac from blunt or penetrating trauma can produce pericardial tamponade. Although a range of clinical signs may be seen, the most common presentations are tachycardia; peripheral vasoconstriction; and the Beck's triad of jugular venous distention, persistent hypotension unresponsive to aggressive fluid resuscitation, and muffled heart sounds. In resource-poor environments, the tools needed to establish an accurate diagnosis, such as an ECG or focused abdominal sonography for trauma (FAST), often are not available. Although pericardiocentesis can be life saving, it should not be done by those without the proper training and skill.

Resuscitative Thoracotomy

Immediate resuscitative thoracotomy may be life saving when performed in children with penetrating trauma who arrive pulseless, but with myocardial electrical activity.[5] However, even when myocardial function is restored, survival ultimately requires additional operative procedures and intensive care, which are generally not available in resource-poor African subregions. Under these conditions, resuscitative thoracotomy becomes a futile exercise. In any case, such heroic measures are rarely effective following blunt trauma, which is far more common than penetrating trauma in children.[6]

Pitfalls in the Management of Paediatric Thoracic Trauma

Several pitfalls exist in the management of paediatric thoracic trauma, as outlined here.

- Underestimating the degree of chest injury at the initial survey because of little external evidence and performing only a supine chest radiograph.

- Administration of excess intravenous fluid during resuscitation, aggravating pulmonary contusion and oedema.

- Inadequate analgesia and chest physiotherapy, promoting retention of secretions, which leads to pulmonary infection.

- Iatrogenic damage through emergency (and faulty) procedures such as endotracheal intubation, chest drain insertion, and central line insertion.

Prevention of Thoracic Trauma

The top three causes of child mortality from unintentional injury are road traffic collisions (32%), drowning (17%), and burns (9%).[7] All of these causes are highly preventable.[2] Factors that influence injuries are supervision, particularly of small children; a single caregiver; a home with multiple siblings; and substance abuse by the caregiver and in large families. Although these risk factors are located within particular households, the larger context in which they operate cannot be ignored; child safety is ultimately a matter of crucial concern for all societies. Some studies have demonstrated the feasibility of interventions to reduce child mortality and morbidity from unintentional injury.

Risk factors for child abuse include the demographic characteristics of the child (e.g., younger age); caregiver characteristics (e.g., prior history of abuse); family structure and resources; and community factors (e.g., increased poverty, decreased social capital).[8–9]

Evidence-Based Research

Table 28.1 presents a retrospective review of paediatric blunt chest trauma.

Table 28.1: Evidence-based research.

Title	Blunt chest trauma in childhood
Authors	Inan M, Ayvaz S, Sut N, et al.
Institution	Departments of Pediatric Surgery and Biostatistics, Faculty of Medicine, Trakya University, Edirne, Turkey
Reference	ANZ J Surg 2007; 77:682–685
Problem	Evaluate the clinical features of children with blunt chest injury and investigate the predictive accuracy of their paediatric trauma scores.
Methods	Retrospective review evaluating children with blunt thoracic trauma.
Outcomes	Forty-four patients were identified, of which 27 were male and 17 were female. The mean paediatric trauma score was 7.6 ± 2.4. Causes of injury consisted of motor vehicle/pedestrian collisions, 19 cases; motor vehicle collisions, 11; falls, 8; and motor vehicle/bicycle or motorbike accidents, 6. Injuries included pulmonary contusions, 28; pneumothoraxes, 12; haemothoraxes, 10; rib fractures, 9; haemopneumothoraxes, 7; clavicle fractures, 5; flail chest, 2; diaphragmatic rupture, 1; and pneumatocele, 1. In this cohort, 27 patients were managed nonoperatively, 17 were treated with tube thoracostomy, and 2 required thoracotomy. Four patients (9.09%) had concomitant abdominal injuries.
Comments	Thoracic injuries are rare in children and are a predictor of severe and multiple—frequently fatal—injuries.
Historical significance/ comments	This well-written article takes the reader through the historical development of some trauma scoring systems and provides a very good overview of frequently used systems. The authors even inform readers about an ideal scoring system: it should correlate well with the desired outcome (e.g., death, disability, costs, etc.); it should be reasonable to clinicians and correlate with their judgement; it should use available data; it should be reliable among different users; and it should be simple. This is, in fact, what all scoring systems should be.

Key Summary Points

1. The majority of thoracic injuries can be diagnosed by a good clinical exam and a plain chest x-ray.

2. The majority of chest trauma in children can be treated nonoperatively, often with a well-placed chest tube.

3. Life-threatening injuries from thoracic trauma are relatively uncommon in children, and when they occur, they are related to associated head and abdominal injuries.

4. Optimum treatment and outcomes can be achieved only by having a thorough understanding of the unique anatomy and physiology of children.

5. Even the most severe of injuries requiring operative therapy can, if recognised early, be managed successfully.

References

1. Buntain WL, ed. Management of pediatric trauma. Saunders, 1995.

2. Eichelberger MR, ed. Pediatric trauma: prevention, acute care, rehabilitation. Mosby, 1993.

3. Mayer TA, ed. Emergency management of pediatric trauma. Saunders, 1985.

4. Nwomeh, BC. Peculiarities of the injured child. In: Ameh EA, Nwomeh BC, eds. Paediatric Trauma Care in Africa: A Practical Guide. Spectrum Books, 2006, Pp 12-24.

5. American College of Surgeons Committee on Trauma. Advanced Trauma Life Support for Doctors, 8th ed. American College of Surgeons, 2008.

6. Abdessalam SF, Keller A, Groner JI, Kable K, Krishnaswami S, Nwomeh BC. An analysis of children receiving cardiopulmonary resuscitation (CPR) following cardiac arrest with blunt trauma. J Am Coll Surg 2004; 199(3S):S53(abstract).

7. Peden M, Oyegbite K, Ozanne-Smith J, et al., eds. World Report on Child Injury Prevention. WHO and UNICEF, 2008.

8. Peden M, Hyder AA. Time to keep African kids safer. South Afr Med J 2009; 99:36–37.

9. van As S and Naidoo S, eds. Paediatric Trauma and Child Abuse. Oxford University Press, 2006.

CHAPTER 29
ABDOMINAL TRAUMA

Emmanuel A. Ameh   Iyore A. Otabor
Lohfa B. Chirdan   Benedict C. Nwomeh

Introduction

Abdominal trauma is common in children, accounting for about 5% of admissions to major paediatric centres.[1-5] Most injuries are blunt in nature, but the incidence of penetrating trauma injuries is increasing. Although most blunt trauma injuries result from traffic injuries, falls (frequently off fruit-bearing trees) are particularly important in sub-Saharan Africa and other developing countries.[1,3,6] Firearms, bicycles, sports, and injuries inflicted as a result of child abuse are becoming increasingly noticeable in developing countries.[7-8]

A number of factors make children particularly vulnerable to abdominal injury. The relatively thin abdominal wall and lower rib cage in children means that the liver, kidney, and pancreas lie in close proximity to the anterior abdominal wall and are prone to injury even if the cause of trauma is trivial. Besides, the liver and kidneys, which are normally protected by the rib cage in adults, lie relatively lower in the abdomen of the child, making them vulnerable to injury. The liver also occupies a proportionally larger percentage of the child's abdomen, further exposing it to increased risk of injury.

Abdominal trauma is frequently associated with other extraabdominal injuries, which should not be overlooked. A distended stomach and full bladder may interfere with the evaluation of the injured child, and may need to be promptly emptied. The initial assessment and resuscitation of the injured child is detailed in Chapter 27.

Blunt Abdominal Trauma

Blunt injury accounts for up to 86% of abdominal trauma.[3] In children, blunt abdominal trauma produces a spectrum of injuries that may pose diagnostic and treatment challenges in the African setting, with its limited diagnostic facilities.[4] Special attention should be directed at handlebar injuries (which cause focused liver, pancreatic, duodenal, and jejunal injuries); lap-belt injuries (which produce a triad of abdominal abrasion, intestinal perforation, and intestinal laceration), and child abuse (in which the face and head may be involved). Bowel injuries may also cause significant morbidity due to a delay in diagnosis.[6]

Clinical Evaluation

After the initial evaluation, resuscitation, and stabilisation, the child with blunt abdominal trauma is carefully and thoroughly evaluated. An additional history is obtained, paying particular attention to vomiting, haematemesis, or rectal bleeding, which may indicate rectal or proximal intestinal injury. A history of loss of consciousness should be sought, as this may indicate head injury.

The presence of pallor, abdominal distention, and pain on physical examination may be a pointer to intraabdominal bleeding. The pulse rate should be carefully monitored, as it is a more sensitive indicator than blood pressure of haemodynamic status in children. Careful examination of the abdomen is performed, with particular attention to abrasions, bruises, distention, and tenderness. Note that peritoneal signs are particularly difficult to discern in a child with lower rib fractures, contusion or abrasions of the abdominal wall, pelvic fractures, and distended bladder. Abdominal examination may be unreliable in patients with head injury or depressed sensorium, so repeated examination or other diagnostic tests are often necessary in such patients.

Decompression of the stomach with a nasogastric tube and the passage of a urethral catheter (except if there is blood at the external meatus or a floating prostrate) may be helpful when examining children with blunt abdominal trauma. Rectal examination should be done to look for perianal soilage with blood, tenderness, floating prostate, or a palpable rent in the rectum. The examining finger should be inspected for blood stain.

The chest, central nervous system and musculoskeletal system should be examined to exclude injury in these systems.

Investigations

Relevant investigations of a child with abdominal trauma would include the techniques discussed in the following subsections.

Abdominal Ultrasonography

Focused abdominal sonography for trauma (FAST) is directed at identifying intraperitoneal or pericardial fluid, which may result due to solid organ injuries (spleen, liver, kidneys, heart). When available, it could be used as a screening tool in the immediate assessment of blunt abdominal trauma. The FAST examination evaluates four areas:

1. right upper quadrant including the hepatorenal fossa;

2. left upper quadrant including the perisplenic region;

3. right and left paracolic gutters and the pelvis; and

4. intercostal or subdiaphragmatic view of the heart.

Note that the FAST examination does not always identify injured solid organs, and its sensitivity depends on the skills of the operator.

Diagnostic Peritoneal Lavage

The aim of diagnostic peritoneal lavage (DPL) is to detect bleeding or leakage of intestinal contents or pancreatic juice into the free peritoneal cavity. This investigation is used for the evaluation of a traumatised child who is unstable. It may require urgent laparotomy for deteriorating neurologic status or when the source of blood loss or clinical findings are in doubt. DPL may be very helpful in resource-poor settings, where advanced imaging modalities are not available, to select patients who need operative intervention.

DPL is performed by placing a catheter under direct vision into the peritoneal cavity. In infants with no previous surgery, a plastic-sheathed needle is passed obliquely into the lower quadrant. In older children without previous surgery, the catheter may be passed by using the Seldinger technique. A positive result is obtained when blood, intestinal contents (bile-stained fluid), or free peritoneal air is encountered. If free fluid is obtained, 15 ml/kg body weight of Ringer's lactate or normal saline is introduced into the abdominal cavity and the effluent is analysed for red blood cells (RBC) (> 50,000/ml), white blood cells (WBC) (>500/ml), and the presence of intestinal contents and amylase. In children, the presence of blood alone at DPL is not necessarily an indication for operation because it could be due to solid organ injuries that can be managed nonoperatively.

Erect Plain Abdominal Radiograph

An erect plain abdominal radiograph should include the chest and pelvis. The findings should be correlated with clinical findings to avoid unnecessary laparotomy. Findings may include free peritoneal air (Figure 29.1) in intestinal rupture, medially displaced gastric or colonic gas shadow in splenic rupture, or generalised ground-glass appearance of massive intraperitoneal or retroperitoneal haemorrhage. Rib and pelvic fractures may be seen.

Computed Tomography

The contrast-enhanced (intravenous (IV) or enteral) computed tomography (CT) scan is probably the most useful imaging modality to identify and characterise solid and hollow visceral injury. It provides clear and accurate imaging of the intraabdominal organs, including intestinal perforation and injuries to retroperitoneal structures. The CT scan may show a contrast blush—a well-circumscribed area of contrast extravasation that is hyperdense with respect to the surrounding parenchyma (Figure 29.2). The contrast blush is a specific marker of active bleeding associated with a higher rate of operative intervention in children. Notwithstanding whether a contrast blush is present, however, the decision to operate should be made on the basis of clinical response to resuscitation; clinically stable patients with a contrast blush can be successfully treated nonoperatively.[9] Although a CT scan is widely accepted and gives accurate results with few false-positive and false-negative interpretations, it may not be readily available in some centres in Africa.

Exploratory Laparoscopy and Laparotomy

When available, laparoscopy can be valuable in the diagnostic evaluation of patients who are haemodynamically stable but there is a strong suspicion of intraabdominal organ injury.

Laparotomy may be needed for definitive diagnosis and treatment. It is indicated in the patient who responds poorly to adequate resuscitation efforts consisting of greater than 40 ml/kg of crystalloids or one-half the child's blood volume within the first 24 hours after injury. Blood should be grouped, cross-matched, and stored for a transfusion, when necessary.

To summarise, the surgeon in Africa, and indeed elsewhere, must be proficient in the clinical evaluation of the traumatised child with suspected intraabdominal injuries, even with the availability of advanced imaging techniques.[10] The value of clinical examination was demonstrated in a study by Chirdan et al. showing a drastic reduction in the rate of laparotomy without compromising outcome in resource-poor settings when a simple management algorithm is used. The algorithm includes clinical examination and simple radiology and laboratory tests.[4]

Treatment

Liver and Spleen

The liver and spleen are the solid organs most frequently injured in blunt trauma.

Nonoperative management

Most injuries stop bleeding spontaneously and can be managed nonoperatively, but the child must be haemodynamically stable.[11] Nonoperative management entails admission into the intensive care unit, where available. The child is placed on strict bed rest, and then carefully and repeatedly monitored. Vital signs are recorded every half hour until stability is achieved. The abdomen is examined every 4 hours for increasing distention and tenderness. Increasing distention may indicate intraperitoneal haemorrhage or gaseous distention, and further evaluation should be done immediately to ascertain whether operative intervention is necessary. Supportive laboratory investigations are done regularly. Any anaemia or fluids and electrolyte derangements are treated promptly.

If nonoperative management is successful, the activity of the child, such as sports or heavy work at school or home, must be limited for about 4 weeks. In Western countries, follow-up imaging is often not needed because patients have easy access to trauma centres in the event of rebleeding. This is not the case, however, in the African setting,

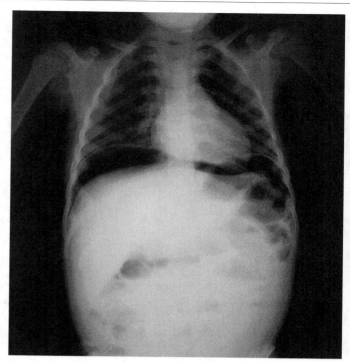

Figure 29.1: Free air in the peritoneal cavity due to intestinal perforation from blunt trauma.

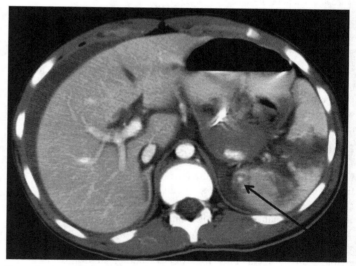

Source: Courtesy of Manuel Meza, MD, Children's Hospital of Pittsburgh, Pittsburgh, Pennsylvania, USA.

Figure 29.2: Contrast blush seen on CT scan in a patient with grade 4 splenic laceration (arrow), indicating active bleeding. Note the haemoperitoneum over the liver.

where a follow-up CT or abdominal ultrasound (US) scan done before discharge from hospital helps the surgeon decide whether further hospital stay is necessary.

The nonoperative management approach is not without hazards, such as missed hollow viscus injuries and rebleeding. In the following situations after blunt trauma, nonoperative management may not be possible, and operative treatment then becomes necessary:

1. haemodynamic instability;

2. transfusion requirement is greater than half of estimated blood volume (estimated blood volume is 70–80 ml/kg body weight);

3. presence of associated injuries requiring surgery;

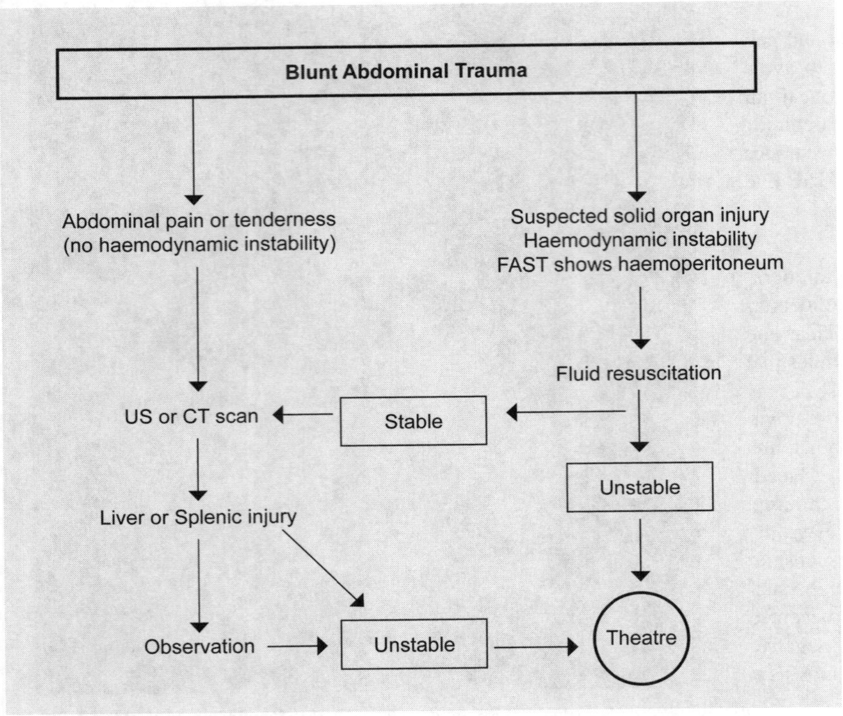

```
          ┌─────────────────────────────────────────┐
          │         Blunt Abdominal Trauma          │
          └─────────────────────────────────────────┘
```

Figure 29.3: Algorithm for the management of blunt splenic or liver injury when CT or US is available. FAST is used for the rapid detection of haemoperitoneum in unstable patients, whereas detailed US may be used for the evaluation of stable patients.

4. unsure of the nature and extent of intraabdominal injury;

5. evidence of hollow viscera injury; or

6. lack of appropriate imaging facilities for adequate evaluation and monitoring of intraabdominal injury (e.g., CT scan, US).

Operative treatment entails full laparotomy using a midline incision, which may be extended. If US or CT is available, we recommend the algorithm for the management of solid organ injury illustrated in Figure 29.3.

Operative Management

Liver

Once the peritoneal cavity is entered, large packs are placed around the liver posteriorly, inferiorly, and superiorly to control initial haemorrhage. The packs are removed one by one to assess the extent of injury. If packing is unable to control haemorrhage, the Pringle manoeuvre (occlusion of the porta between the thumb and forefinger or using a vascular clamp) is done. Some lacerations may need to be extended to enable proper assessment of the extent of injury. The following interventions could be done, depending on the degree of injury to the liver:

• simple repair;

• exploration of expanding haematomas;

• resectional debridement where there is much devitalised liver tissue; or

• rarely, lobectomy if hepatic damage is extensive.

Spleen

The guiding principle in the operative management of splenic injury is to avoid splenectomy as much as possible to prevent the complication of overwhelming postsplenectomy infection (OPSI).

The spleen can be preserved by the following procedures: (1) splenorrhaphy, in which simple repair of lacerations is done, or (2) segmental resection if a segment of the spleen is devitalised or the spleen is wrapped up with the omentum. Haemostatic agents such as haemacele could be used to stop bleeding from the spleen. Splenectomy may be necessary in the following situations:

• multiple abdominal injuries;

• haemodynamic instability;

• uncontrollable bleeding; or

• lack of experience on the part of the surgeon.

If splenectomy is performed, place the child on long-term prophylactic antimalarials using proguanil or pyrimethamine. Give vaccination against pneumococcal infection (Pnuemovac(R), if available). Educate the parents on the susceptibility of the child to infections, and the need to report any infections early. Treat any infection promptly.

Injury to other solid organs

Injuries to other solid organs should be handled on their own merit. The management of injuries to the kidneys is discussed in Chapter 31.

Hollow viscera injury

Hollow viscera injuries are less common than solid organ injuries. The most commonly injured hollow viscera are those of the gastrointestinal tract, and only these are discussed here. The various types of gastrointestinal injuries include:

• contusion;

• serosal lacerations;

• perforation; and

• transverse mesenteric tear.

These features may not be obvious at initial assessment. A high index of suspicion and repeated examination are essential for the diagnosis.

DPL, plain abdominal radiographs, and a CT scan may need to be repeated after 24 hours to reach a diagnosis. Indicators of gastrointestinal injury are listed below:

• fever;

• haematemesis or drainage of blood-stained effluent from nasogastric tube;

- increasing pulse rate;
- increasing abdominal distention and tenderness;
- loss of bowel function;
- presence of intestinal contents at DPL; and
- free intraperitoneal air on erect plain abdominal x-ray or CT scan.

When diagnosis is made, operative treatment is necessary. The operative options include repair of laceration and closure of perforation and resection with primary anastomosis for extensive laceration, multiple perforations, and intestinal gangrene from transverse mesenteric tear.

Injuries to the left colon may be repaired primarily with or without the creation of a proximal colostomy, or the injured colon may be exteriorised as a colostomy and mucous fistula.

Penetrating Abdominal Trauma

Penetrating abdominal trauma is less common than blunt trauma and accounts for approximately 14% of abdominal trauma in children. It is frequently due to a fall onto sharp objects, a cow gore, gunshot wound, and, rarely, a stab injury. Treatment depends on the penetration of the peritoneum. After adequate resuscitation and stabilisation, the wound is explored under general anaesthesia to identify peritoneal breach.

If the peritoneum is breached, a formal laparotomy is required, through a separate incision, to identify and treat organ injuries. If a peritoneal breach is not detected (or a breach is only suspected), DPL is done and a laparotomy is performed if it is positive.

Where available, a triple-contrast CT scan (oral, IV, plus bladder contrast) should be done. If the CT scan is negative, the patient is observed for 24–48 hours; if it is positive, a laparotomy should be done.

In stab injuries to the flank or back, a CT scan is done. If a CT scan is not available, a laparotomy is done to exclude injuries to retroperitoneal organs. DPL is usually not useful.

If there is obvious organ evisceration, the organ is covered with clean moist gauze and polythene to decrease desiccation, loss of fluid, and hypothermia.

Whenever laparotomy is performed, it must be thorough to avoid missing any injuries. Injuries to solid organs or the gastrointestinal tract are treated as in blunt trauma.

Tetanus prophylaxis should be given if the child is unimmunised or if the immunisation status is unknown.

Anorectal Injuries

Anorectal injuries are not common in children, but they may be associated with significant morbidity if not identified and treated properly.[12–13]

Most anorectal injuries are due to penetrating trauma, and the penetrating objects often are potentially contaminated and capable of introducing infections, particularly tetanus.

Presentation

There may be a history of falling onto a sharp object or falling astride an object. Motor vehicle crashes may also produce anorectal injury. The common symptoms include:

- rectal bleeding;
- vaginal bleeding;
- vaginal discharge; and
- abdominal pain and tenderness.

Fever, if present, is an indication of intraperitoneal involvement or late presentation. Careful abdominal examination should be done to exclude intraperitoneal involvement. Examination of the perineum and anorectum after trauma is usually limited due to pain and tenderness. As such, adequate evaluation should be done under general anaesthetic and good lighting.

Evaluation

Under general anaesthetic, careful and meticulous examination of the perineum, anorectum, and vagina should be done. The aim of this evaluation is to ascertain the nature and extent of injury. The examination begins with inspection of the vagina, with particular attention to the posterior vaginal wall, which is frequently injured in girls. Any laceration in the perineum is noted, and the depth is ascertained. The anorectum is then examined; this may require proctosigmoidoscopy. Once the evaluation is complete, the injury should be graded (Figure 29.4).

Treatment

The treatment of anorectal injuries is summarised in Figure 29.5. The wound should be carefully explored. All dead or devitalised tissue should be completely excised. The wound should be repaired if accessible. Adequate drainage of the wound (perirectal) may be necessary. Laparotomy is required if intraperitoneal rectal injury is present. A protective (proximal) colostomy may be necessary in some situations. Tetanus prophylaxis and broad-spectrum antibiotics should be given. Sphincteric function should be evaluated after wound healing is complete.

Evidence-Based Research

Table 29.1 presents a retrospective review of management protocol using ultrasonography in laparotomy.

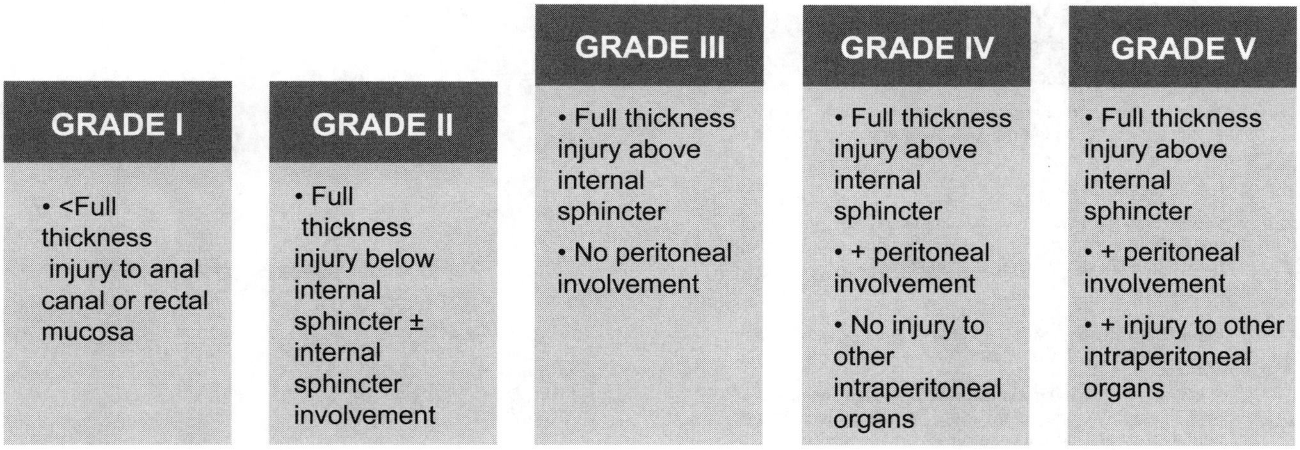

GRADE I	GRADE II	GRADE III	GRADE IV	GRADE V
• <Full thickness injury to anal canal or rectal mucosa	• Full thickness injury below internal sphincter ± internal sphincter involvement	• Full thickness injury above internal sphincter • No peritoneal involvement	• Full thickness injury above internal sphincter • + peritoneal involvement • No injury to other intraperitoneal organs	• Full thickness injury above internal sphincter • + peritoneal involvement • + injury to other intraperitoneal organs

Figure 29.4: Grading of anorectal injuries.

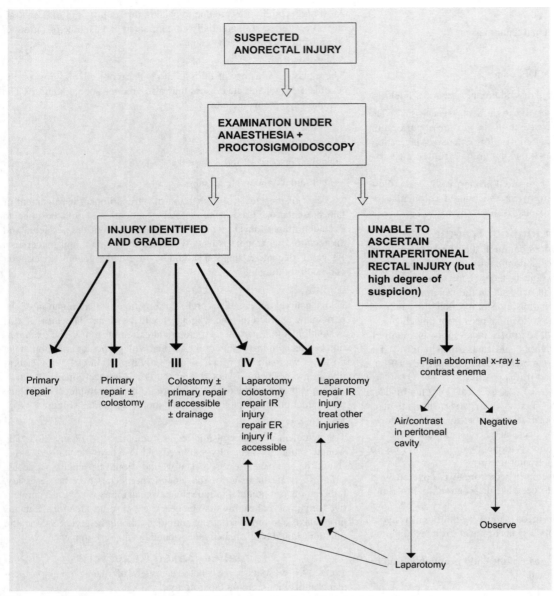

Figure 29.5: Treatment of anorectal injuries (IR: intraperitoneal rectum; ER: extraperitoneal rectum).

Table 29.1: Evidence-based research.

Title	Paediatric blunt abdominal trauma: challenges of management in a developing country
Authors	Chirdan LB, Uba AF, Yiltok SJ, Ramyil VM
Institution	Jos University Teaching Hospital, Jos, Nigeria
Reference	Eur J Pediatr Surg 2007; 17:90–95
Problem	To determine whether a simple protocol with ultrasonography significantly reduced the rate of laparotomy in countries with limited facilities.
Intervention	Retrospective review.
Comparison/ control (quality of evidence)	Laparotomy rates were compared between two groups, with and without a management protocol that included abdominal ultrasound (US) and plain abdominal films.
Outcome/ effect	Laparotomy rates were lower in the group in which the management protocol was followed.
Historical significance/ comments	Paediatric abdominal trauma in resource-poor settings can be successfully managed by using a simple protocol that depends on careful clinical assessment and simple radiologic tests.

Key Summary Points

1. Abdominal trauma in children is mostly due to blunt injuries.

2. Clinical evaluation is the most vital tool in diagnostic assessment.

3. When available, FAST, DPL, abdominal CT scan, or diagnostic laparoscopy are useful diagnostic adjuncts.

4. Laparotomy may be needed for definitive diagnosis and treatment.

5. Most solid abdominal organ injuries can be managed nonoperatively, but the child must be carefully monitored for signs of deterioration that will require laparotomy.

6. A high index of suspicion must be maintained to avoid missing hollow viscera injuries.

7. Patients undergoing splenectomy are at risk of overwhelming postsplenectomy infection (OPSI), and the child should be placed on long-term prophylactic antimalarials (proguanil or pyrimethamine) and receive vaccination against pneumococcal infection.

8. Anorectal injuries are associated with significant morbidity and should be promptly evaluated and treated.

References

1. Ameh EA, Chirdan LB, Nmadu PT. Blunt abdominal trauma in children: epidemiology, management and management problems in a developing country. Pediatr Surg Int 2000; 16:505–509.

2. Adesunkanmi ARK, Oginni LM, Oyelami OA, Badru OS. Road traffic accidents to African children: assessment of severity using the injury severity score (ISS). Injury, Int J Care Injured 2000; 31:225–228.

3. Nakayama DN. Abdominal and genitourinary trauma. In: O'Neil JA, Grosfeld JL, Fonkalsrud EW, Coran AG, Caldamone AA, eds. Principles of Pediatric Surgery, 2nd ed. Mosby, 2004, Pp 159–175.

4. Chirdan LB, Uba AF, Yiltok SJ, Ramyil VM. Paediatric blunt abdominal trauma: challenges of management in a developing country. Eur J Pediatr Surg 2007; 17:90–95.

5. Snyder CL. Abdominal and genitourinary trauma. In: Ashcraft KW, Murphy JP, Sharp RJ, et al., eds. Pediatric Surgery. Sanders, 2000, P 204.

6. Chirdan LB, Uba AF, Chirdan OO. Gastrointestinal injuries in children. Niger J Clin Prac 2008; 11:250–253.

7. Bahebeck J, Atangana R, Mboudou E, Nonga BN, Sosso M, Malonga E. Incidence, case fatality rate and clinical pattern of firearm injuries in two cities where arm owning is forbidden. Injury, Int J Care Injured 2005; 36:714–717.

8. Fleggen AG, Wiemann M, Brown C, van As AB, Swingler GH, Peter JC Inhuman shields—children caught in the crossfire of domestic violence. S Afr Med J 2004; 94:293–236.

9. Nwomeh BC, Nadler EP, Meza MP, Bron K, Gaines BA, Ford HR. Contrast extravasation predicts the need for operative intervention in children with blunt splenic trauma. J Trauma 2004; 56(3):537–541.

10. Afifi RY. Blunt abdominal trauma: back to clinical judgement in the era of modern technology (editorial): Intl J Surg 2008; 6:91–95.

11. Landau A, van As AB, Numanoglu A, Millar AJW, Rode H. Liver injuries in children: the role of selective non-operative management. Injury, Int J Care Injured 2006; 37:66–71.

12. Ameh EA, Anorectal injuries in children. Pediatr Surg Int 2000; 16:388–391.

13. Reinberg O, Yazbeck S. Major perineal trauma in children. J Pediatr Surg 1989; 24:982–984.

CHAPTER 30
CRANIOCEREBRAL AND SPINAL TRAUMA

Bello B. Shehu
Mohammed R. Mahmud

Craniocerebral Trauma

Introduction
Paediatric cranial injuries constitute a major portion of paediatric admissions and are the cause of the greatest number of deaths and chronic disabilities among children. Brain injuries are responsible for 7,000 paediatric deaths per year in the United States.[1] The figures are quite a bit higher in Africa, with various figures being quoted in different regions. Paediatric cranial injuries are a challenge to manage, requiring difficult decisions in a setting of limited resources. As in the developed countries, the socioeconomic impacts of head injury are enormous, including school failure, social maladjustment, and public liability.

Epidemiology
Adult cranial injuries are primarily diseases of young men, with a male-to-female ratio of 3–4:1. The sex ratio disparity is less in children; in all age groups, including infants, the boy-to-girl ratio is about 2 to 1. The great majority of cranial injuries in children are mild (86%).[2] Severe injuries show a bimodal age distribution; first, in infancy, due to a higher incidence of nonaccidental injuries, and second, in adolescence, due to road traffic accidents.[3–5]

Aetiology/Classification
The cause of head injuries based on mechanism of injury is classified into blunt or penetrating.

Blunt
Falls are the most common cause of paediatric blunt cranial injuries. Low-height falls rarely cause significant neurological morbidity. Falls from heights greater than four feet (1.2 meters), and falls from a caretaker's arms, however, may be associated with severe injuries, including contusions and depressed skull fractures.

Although motor vehicle accidents may account for a smaller percentage of all paediatric head injuries, they outweigh all other causes of serious head injury. The trauma may involve children as passengers, or as pedestrians and cyclists being struck by motor vehicles.

Crush injuries usually occur at home from falling objects, such as collapsed buildings, falling tables, televisions, and so on. They are characterised by skull fractures.

Birth injuries occur during delivery. Neonates may suffer cranial injuries such as cephalhaematomas, skull fractures, intracranial haematomas, and even brain injuries.

Penetrating
Penetrating head injuries involve falls unto playing objects such as pencils, nails, or sticks. Increasingly, though, penetrating cranial injuries are being seen from assaults, stab wounds, and gunshot wounds (Figure 30.1). Animal bites and horses' hooves are also common causes.

Inflicted injuries
Inflicted injuries may occur from child abuse, which includes beating, excessive shaking, and striking the head against hard surfaces.

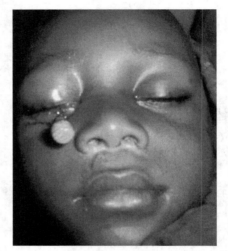
Figure 30.1: Penetrating orbitocranial foreign body.

Classification of Head Injury by Pathology
Head injuries may be focal or diffuse, but both actually coexist to some degree. In severe head injury, diffuse predominates, but focal lesions carry a higher mortality rate.

In a diffuse injury, the alteration of mental status is out of proportion to computed tomography (CT) findings. Rotational acceleration/deceleration forces are usually responsible. Examples include concussion with transient loss of consciousness and diffuse axonal injury characterised by shearing at grey-white matter interfaces.

In focal injuries, scalp lacerations are of special importance when associated with skull fractures because the child is at risk of developing meningitis.[6] Basal skull fractures are suspected in the presence of raccoon eyes, Battles sign, haemotympanum, otorrhea, or rhinorrhea.

Depressed skull fractures (Figure 30.2), also called pond fractures, are the results of focal impacts. Intracranial haematomas, which may include epidural subarachnoid, intraventricular, and intraparenchymal, are also prominent, depending on the severity of the impact energy.

Pathophysiology of Brain Injury

Normal homeostasis
Cerebral blood flow is normally maintained at a constant level via autoregulation. Autoregulation is effective between systolic blood pressures of 50 and 150 mm Hg. Autoregulation may be lost following head injury, making the brain prone to ischaemia. Thus, hypotension should be avoided.

Intracranial hypertension
Intracranial hypertension is the end result of multiple intracranial processes that can be seen in trauma and which impair the cerebral blood flow. Cardiorespiratory compensatory processes produce hypertension

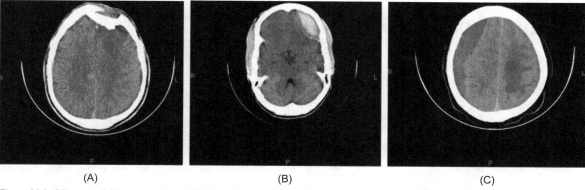

Figure 30.2: CT scans of (A) depressed skull fracture; (B) epidural haematoma; (C) chronic subdural haematoma.

and bradycardia, as well as irregular breathing—this is known as Cushing's triad. Therefore, in head injury, it is important to follow the cerebral blood flow (CBF). Because it is difficult to measure CBF directly, cerebral perfusion pressure (CPP) is used, which is calculated as: CPP = ICP − MAP, where ICP is intracranial pressure and MAP is the mean arterial pressure.[3,5]

Physiology of injury

Following the initial injury at impact, known as the primary injury, biochemical alterations occur, in particular, the release of glutamate, which is an excitatory neurotransmitter. This initiates a cascade of cytotoxic reactions, resulting in alterations in cellular energy metabolism, cerebral blood flow, transmembrane ion concentration gradients, free radical production, and cytokine release. Gross secondary changes, such as haematomas, cerebral oedema, hypotension, seizures, and hypoxia, further worsen the neurologic injury.

Clinical Features

History

Details of the mechanism of injury, such as distance of fall, the surface struck, and the velocity of striking objects, are important. In motor vehicular trauma, the speed of the vehicle and use of restraints should be determined. A careful history regarding immediate posttraumatic events, such as loss of consciousness, its duration, seizures, and vomiting, should be sought. In the older child, specific questions about neck pain, numbness, and weakness are asked. The possibility of child abuse should also be kept in mind.

Physical assessment

Observation of the mildly head injured child provides a great deal of information. The level of consciousness is determined. Examination of the head and scalp are done. Scalp abrasions, lacerations, and haematomas are carefully examined. The skull is palpated for areas of tenderness and fractures without inflicting pain. In older children with moderate to severe injuries, age-specific behavior is a great guide to neurological assessment. They may appropriately respond to noxious stimuli by grimacing, crying, or exhibiting a facial expression of distress. Palpation of an open fontanelle provides a good idea of intracranial pressure.

Assessment of injury severity

The Glasgow Coma Scale (GCS) is a good measure of acute injury severity and has been modified using age-appropriate parameters as indicated in Table 30.1. The table shows the best score achievable by a normal child for each parameter at various age groups.

Laboratory Assessment

Infants and small children can develop acute anaemia with relatively little blood loss. Haemogram and baseline serum electrolytes levels and blood gasses are assessed.

Radiological Assessment

Skull x-ray

A skull x-ray is useful as an initial assessment tool, particularly in Africa, where CT scans are not readily available. Skull fracture sites may herald potential intracranial pathologies. The x-ray may also show other pathologies, such as pneumocephalus (Figure 30.3), and linear fractures parallel to the slice plane, which may be missed by a CT scan.[7,8]

CT scan

A CT scan is the most useful tool for acute assessment of traumatic head injury. Bony and parenchymal lesions are usually well seen. Haematomas are clearly seen and can easily be categorised based on age.[9]

Magnetic resonance imaging

Magnetic resonance imaging (MRI) offers superior resolution in visualising small lesions, such as is seen in diffuse axonal injury, but is not as widely available and affordable as the CT scan. It is also not an investigation of choice in terms of skull fractures and intracranial haematomas.[10,11]

Cranial ultrasound

Cranial ultrasound (US) is usually a bedside technique used to monitor intracranial collections and ventricular size following trauma. This useful tool is underutilised for the child with an open fontanelle, largely as a result of lack of experience by radiologists and unavailability of US to the neurosurgeons.[10]

Management

Initial management

Adequate resuscitation and stabilisation must be given priority. The airway is the highest management priority. A child with severe head injury will require control of the airway with intubation. This helps to prevent secondary injury from hypoxia and hypercarbia.[12] The cervical spine must be assumed to be unstable until proven otherwise by plain radiographs later. Meanwhile, the breathing, circulation, and the stabilisation of vital signs are then attended to. It is the postresuscitation GCS score that is useful.

A focused neurological examination is performed to determine life-threatening intracranial pathology and assess the child's baseline neurological level; the papillary examination and the GCS score are most important for this purpose. Efforts are made to look for lateralising signs, such as hemiparesis, pupillary dilatation, facial nerve palsy, and so on. The next priority in a child who is unresponsive is to assess brainstem function by means of the corneal and gag reflexes. Corticosteroids and routine administration of anticonvulsants are not recommended.

Measures to treat raised intracranial pressure

Where ICP can be monitored, the treatment threshold for raised ICP is 20–25 mm Hg.[13]

Table 30.1: Paediatric (Adelaide) Scale.

Normal score at age	Normal eye opening	Score	Normal motor response	Score	Normal verbal response	Score	Total
0–6 months	Spontaneous	4	Flexion	3	Cries	2	9
6–12 months	Spontaneous	4	Localises	4	Vocalises	3	11
1–2 years	Spontaneous	4	Localises	4	Words	4	12
2–5 years	Spontaneous	4	Obeys	5	Words	4	13

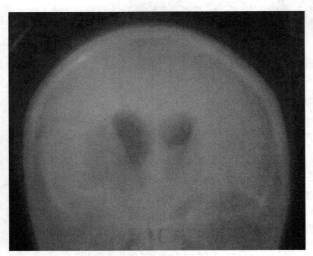

Figure 30.3: Skull x-ray showing intraventricular pneumocephalus.

Positioning
Elevation of the head of the bed to 15–30 degrees, when not contraindicated, optimises arterial flow and venous drainage.

Oxygenation
Oxygenation leads to improved cerebral oxygenation and a reduction in cerebral oedema.

Mannitol
Mannitol is very effective and can be life saving. It reduces blood viscosity and acts as an osmotic diuretic. It is given only after adequate volume resuscitation. The dose is 0.5–1g/kg body weight over 20 minutes (bolus). However, because of its rebound effect, it should be administered only when the patient is being prepared for an indicated surgery.

Controlled hyperventilation
Hyperventilation has a very rapid effect and is aimed at reducing the $PaCO_2$ to about 40 mm Hg. Lowering the $PaCO_2$ further is associated with a risk of cerebral vasoconstriction, leading to cerebral ischaemic injury.

Surgery
Intracranial haematomas in children are treated more aggressively.

Specific head injuries
Scalp injuries
In young children, blood loss from scalp laceration can lead to shock and should be promptly controlled. Scalp loss is managed with skin grafts or rotational flaps.[6]

Skull fractures
Linear, diastatic, and stellate fractures occur from focal contact forces. They may occur over a venous sinus with resultant tear haemorrhage. A CT scan is advised in the setting of stellate fractures due to the high incidence of underlying contusion.

Ping-pong fractures are managed most often nonoperatively because they often resolve spontaneously.

Depressed skull fractures are treated with elevation when indicated.

Fractures at the base of the skull are common in children, but cerebrospinal fluid (CSF) leaks often resolve spontaneously. Persistent leaks, however, require surgical intervention. Accompanying cranial nerve deficits may require surgical decompression and corticosteroid.

Growing skull fractures are peculiar and are characterised by a pulsatile scalp swelling overlying an enlarged bony defect with an associated underlying leptomeningeal cyst. They are repaired via cyst drainage, dura graft, and autologous skull graft.

Haematomas
Subgaleal haematomas can be very massive in children to the extent of inducing hypovolaemic shock.

Prompt recognition and evacuation of epidural haematomas via a craniotomy leads to a good and rapid neurological recovery.

Acute subdural haematomas carry a high mortality. The recommended surgery is craniotomy and evacuation. Chronic subdural haematomas are approached via burr-hole evacuation.

Intraparenchymal haemorrhage may be large enough to cause neurologic deficit or midline shift, and surgical evacuation is indicated in such children as they tend to recover from neurologic deficits.

Intraventricular haematoma is managed with external ventricular drainage.

Penetrating injuries
In the presence of a protruding penetrating foreign body, the offending object should not be removed instantaneously. Following clinical evaluation, a plain radiograph in two views and a brain CT scan should be requested. Appropriate consultation should be sought, such as from an ophthalmologist for orbitocranial injuries. Appropriate broad spectrum antibiotics and tetanus prophylaxis are to be instituted. The aim of surgery is removal of the foreign body in a controlled condition in the operating room.[14] In the absence of a retained foreign body, the goal of surgery is to debride the tract and repair the dura and bony defects.

Basic Neurosurgical Procedures

Burr-hole evacuation of chronic subdural haematoma

1. The patient is positioned supine, head turned laterally and elevated 15 degrees, with shoulder support.

2. The site of surgery is shaved and cleaned, and the patient is then draped.

3. A vertical incision is made over the site of the haematoma.

4. Usually, the first burr hole is temporal, 2.5 cm above the zygomatic arch, just anterior to the ear.

5. Scalp bleeding is controlled with cautery and self-retaining mastoid retractors.

6. The periosteum is incised and retracted.

7. A burr hole is made with a drill.

8. The dura is coagulated and incised in a cruciate fashion with a size 11 blade.

9. The haematoma is evacuated with gentle suction and irrigation, taking care not to injure any bridging vessels. Any bleeding point is controlled with bipolar cautery.

10. The subdural space is irrigated with normal saline.

11. A subdural drain may be left in place for 24–48 hours.

12. The incision is closed.

Craniotomy for trauma

1. The patient is positioned supine, head turned laterally, and elevated 15 degrees, with shoulder support.

2. A large trauma flap ("question mark") incision is made, starting anterior to the ear, above the tragus, extended rostrally above the pinna, turned posteriorly circling around the occipitoparietal area, and turning anteriorly to end frontally behind the hairline.

3. Haemostasis is secured by using Riney clips or artery forceps.

4. When necessary, the temporalis muscle is dissected by using monopolar diathermy after raising the scalp flap.

5. A series of burr holes are placed encircling the area of the haematoma, connected by using a foot plate on a power drill or a Gigli saw.

6. An epidural haematoma should now be exposed and is evacuated with gentle suction and irrigation; bleeding vessels are controlled with diathermy.

7. The dura is "tented" to prevent re-collection, and the bone flap is replaced.

8. The scalp flap is closed in layers over a closed drain.

9. In the case of acute subdural haematoma, the dura is incised, the haematoma evacuated, and haemostasis is controlled.

10. The bone flap is replaced immediately and postoperative measures instituted to control the brain swelling.

Postoperative Complications
Postoperative complications include re-collection, wound infection, and dehiscence. Re-collection of haematoma is managed by re-evacuation.

Prognosis and Outcome
Children have better outcomes compared to adults for the same type and severity of injury.[15] Mortality is age dependent—it is highest in infants and declines until about age 12 years, and then increases in the teens. In terms of morbidity, the youngest children have the worst outcome.[16] Factors that influence the prognosis include low GCS at 72 hours posttrauma, extracranial trauma, acute hypoxia, elevated raised intracranial pressure, and duration of coma.[17] The Glasgow Outcome Scale (GOS; Table 30.2) gives a reproducible outcome, which means different patients with similar GOS scores from different centres will have similar outcomes.

Table 30.2: The Glasgow Outcome Scale.

Score	Meaning
5	Good recovery
4	Moderate disability
3	Severe disability
2	Persisten vegetative state
1	Death

Complications of Head Injury

Intracranial haematoma
A majority of patients who die from head injury have an intracranial haematoma that has caused brain shift and compression. This complication may be present at the time of presentation or it may develop later. The haematoma may be in the epidural, subdural, or subarachnoid space. It may also be intraventricular or within the brain parenchyma. The patient presents with a deteriorating level of consciousness and localising signs or features of rising intracranial pressure. A brain CT scan or MRI will accurately localise the haematoma; it will also show the size of the clot and whether there is a midline shift. Evacuation of the clot through an appropriately sited burr hole or a craniotomy is life saving. A small haematoma can be managed nonoperatively.

Intracranial infections
Intracranial infections are associated with very high mortality and morbidity if not treated energetically. Meningitis can occur within a few days after head injury. The predisposing factors are open skull fractures, penetrating injuries, fractures into air sinuses, and skull base fractures with CSF otorrhoea or rhinorrhoea. The patient usually has a headache, restlessness, vomiting, photophobia, and seizures. There is high-grade fever, rigors, neck stiffness, and a positive Kernig's sign.

A CSF sample is taken through lumbar puncture for cultures and biochemical analysis. An empirical intravenous antibiotic is commenced. Intravenous (IV) benzyl penicillin (50-75 mg/kg every 6 hours) and IV chloramphenicol (1 gm every 6 hours) are effective. Cerebral abscess may develop following meningitis or when there is gross contamination from compound fractures. If the abscess is large, there may be features of raised intracranial pressure. Evacuation of the abscess with appropriate antibiotic cover is essential.

CSF leakage and fistula
The most common cause of CSF fistula is trauma. Skull fractures and associated arachnoid tears can lead to the development of CSF leakage and fistula. The incidence of posttraumatic rhinorrhea in closed head injury is 2–3%. CSF fistula occurs in 8.9% of penetrating head trauma. Posttraumatic CSF leaks are seen commonly in penetrating injuries and compound fractures of skull bones, paranasal sinuses, middle ear, and mastoid air cells. Basilar fractures are notorious for development of CSF fistula. Diagnosis is usually obvious with copious CSF leakage. A blotting paper test can be done by the bedside to show the double ring sign. A glucose test is positive in CSF as against mucus. β_2 transferin is specific to CSF. An x-ray usually shows a fracture at the base of the skull or opacity in the paranasal sinus. A CT scan is diagnostic. It may show associated pneumocephalus. In difficult cases, a dye test (metrizamide or Iohexol injected intrathecally) can be used to locate the site of the CSF leakage. Treatment is usually conservative. The use of an antibiotic is controversial unless when leakage. Treatment is usually conservative. The use of an antibiotic is controversial unless there are signs of meningitis. Most cases can be managed nonoperatively. Persistent fistulae are repaired via craniotomy.

Pneumocephalus
A fracture involving the paranasal sinuses could lead to intracranial gas collection, known as pneumocephalus. When the gas is under pressure, it is called tension pneumocephalus, which is a surgical emergency. The gas may collect in the epidural, subdural, or subarrhacnoid spaces. It may also be, within the brain parenchyma, or in the ventricular system. Intracranial infection with gas-forming organisms also cause pneumocephalus. The patient presents with headache, vomiting, dizziness, alteration in level of consciousness, and CSF leakage. An x-ray may show intracranial gas. A CT scan shows hypodense (very dark) areas. Treatment is conservative if the gas collection is small and there is no mass effect, as the gas will resolve with time. Tension pneumocephalus must be urgently evacuated. Craniotomy and repair are done for persistent CSF leakage.

Cranial nerve palsy
Any of the cranial nerves may be injured, depending on the magnitude and location of trauma. The most commonly affected nerves are olfactory, optic, oculomotor, trochlear, abducent, facial, and vestibulocochlear nerves. Healing is usually spontaneous after a variable period of time.

Posttraumatic hydrocephalus
Hydrocephalus occurs following trauma with associated subarachnoid haemorrhage. It is a communicating hydrocephalus; the patient may present with the triad of dementia, gait disturbance, and urinary incontinence. Lumbar puncture yields CSF under normal pressure. Diagnosis is made by CT or MRI. Symptoms can be remediated by CSF shunting.

Posttraumatic seizures

Seizures that occur in the first 7 days of injury are termed early post-traumatic seizures, and those that occur after 1 week are late post-traumatic seizures. The incidence of early posttraumatic seizures is 1–5%. It can precipitate adverse events as the result of an elevation of intracranial pressure, alteration in blood pressure, and changes in oxygenation. The estimated incidence of late posttraumatic seizure is 10–13% within 2 years after head injury. The risk of seizure is higher in patients with acute intracranial haematoma, open depressed skull fractures, parenchymal injury, seizures within the first 24 hours of injury, GCS <10, penetrating brain injury, history of significant alcohol abuse, and cortical haemorrhagic contusion on CT scan. Treatment with anticonvulsants is started early. IV phenobarbitone (5–10 mg/kg in 3 divided doses) or IV phenytoin (15 mg/kg loading dose; at a rate of 1-3 mg/kg per minute is given to control convulsion, and continued orally for 18-24 months).

Fat embolism

Fat embolism may occur especially in the presence of multiple injuries. Symptoms include drowsiness, confusion, epilepsy, and irritability. Dyspnoea, tachypnoea, and tachycardia may also occur. Petechial haemorrhage over the base of the neck and upper chest appears after 48–72 hours. Treatment is by measures aimed at protecting the brain from anoxia (i.e., proper care of the airway, tracheostomy, and oxygen therapy).

Posttraumatic (concussion) syndrome

This syndrome is a collection of symptoms that is considered as a sequel of a mild head injury. It can also be seen in patients recovering from severe head injury. The symptoms include headache, dizziness, lightheadedness, visual disturbances, and anosmia, as well as memory impairment, loss of intellectual ability, depression, anxiety, disruption of sleep/wake cycles, photophobia, and personality changes. The treatment of the condition is supportive. Recovery follows a variable course.

Carotico-cavernous fistula

This fistula is between the intracavernous part of the internal carotid artery and the cavernous sinus. The patient complains of noise in the head and has pulsating exophthalmos, which is usually unilateral. A continuous to-and-fro murmur is synchronous with the pulse and audible on auscultation of the eyeball. This murmur is abolished by compression of the carotid artery in the neck.

Posttraumatic headache

Posttraumatic headache is a common complaint. It may be caused by intracranial haemorrhage, increased intracranial pressure, skull fractures, CSF leaks, and infections. Treatment of the primary cause is essential; analgesics and bed rest are supportive.

Posttraumatic aneurysm

Posttraumatic aneurysms comprise less than 1% of intracranial aneurysms. Most are false aneurysms. They commonly arise from closed head injury and penetrating trauma. They present with delayed intracranial haemorrhage. The patient may present with recurrent epistaxis, progressive cranial nerve palsy, or severe headache. A CT scan shows intracerebral and subarrhacnoid haemorrhage. Angiography can demonstrate the site of the aneurysm. Although cases of spontaneous resolution have been reported, direct treatment is usually recommended by clipping, coiling, or trapping.

Posttraumatic hypopituitarism

Posttraumatic hypopituitarism follows penetrating trauma or closed head injury with or without a basilar skull fracture. The patient may have deficiency of the growth hormone, gonadotropin, corticotrophin, or reduced TSH. Some patients will develop diabetes insipidus.

Prevention

The greatest majority of paediatric head injuries are preventable. The mortality and morbidity from motor vehicle accidents could be reduced by 50% with proper use of child restraints and responsible driving. Enforcement of legislation for observation of speed limits, use of seat-belts and restraints, and wearing motorcycle helmets are said to have worked well in the developed world. Parental attitudes and sibling behavior influence a child's attitude immensely.

Children playing by the roadside, street hawking, and engaging in activities such as tree climbing to obtain a means of livelihood should be discouraged. Legislation should be enacted and enforced to contain child abuse.

Spinal Cord Injury

Introduction

Spinal cord injuries remain one of the most devastating of all survivable trauma. Paediatric spinal cord injury is relatively uncommon, accounting for 5–7% of all spinal injuries.[18,19] The peculiar developing anatomy and biomechanics of the child's spine make the management of spinal cord injury in children distinct. A good number of affected children will need supportive care for life. The availability of only a few specialised centres in Africa compounds the problem of adequate care for these children.

Epidemiology

Paediatric spinal injuries peak from June to September in the West due to extracurricular activities during the summer holidays. About 1–13% of spinal cord injuries occur in children 1–15 years of age, with 60–75% occurring in older children aged 10–15 years. The male-to-female ratio in paediatric spinal cord injury varies with age, being 1.1–1.3:1 for ages 0–9 years, to 2.3–2.5:1 for ages 15–17 years. Most spinal cord injuries occur in the cervical spine (42%), thoracic (31%), and lumbar (27%).[20] In children younger than 9 years of age, 67% of the cervical spine injuries occur between the occiput and C2 due to the higher level of the fulcrum for maximal flexion.

Aetiology

The cause of spinal cord injuries varies with age. Pedestrian-vehicle accidents and falls account for 75% of the injuries in the 0–9 year age range.[21] Motor vehicle accidents account for about 40%, and in the 15–17 year age group, motor vehicle accidents account for more than 70%. Other causes include sporting activities and motorcycle and bicycle accidents, which tend to occur in the older child.

Pathophysiology

The mechanisms of spinal cord injury in children are similar to those seen in adults. They include hyperflexion, rotation, hyperextension, axial loading, flexion rotation and shearing forces. The initial injury, either concussive or compressive, leads to immediate death of neural cell bodies in the local central grey matter. Subsequently, secondary damage occurs, initiated by the release of inflammatory mediators such as glutamate and free oxygen radicals. Oedema and spinal cord infarction result. Apoptotic changes in neurons and glial cells are now evident.[22]

Paediatric spinal traumas commonly cause ligamentous injury and facet capsule rupture. In the cervical region, there could be avulsion and epiphyseal separation of basal synchondrosis of the odontoid into the body of C2. There could be a split in the cartilaginous end plate, particularly of the growing zone. Fractures of the vertebral bodies and disc herniation are uncommon in children.[23]

Epidural, intradural, or intramedullary haematomas also occur following trauma.

Clinical Presentation

The area of spinal cord damage and nerve root involvement determine the clinical presentation. In complete spinal cord injuries, there is a loss of voluntary nervous function below the level of injury. There is an initial temporary phase of spinal shock, with loss of all reflexes below the injured segment that may last for minutes or days. About 3% of patients with complete injuries on initial examination will develop some recovery within 24 hours. In incomplete spinal cord injuries, some nervous function is present in the form of some muscle power or sensation below the level of injury; these injuries carry a better prognosis for recovery. Frankel grading is used to categorise spinal cord injuries, as shown in Table 30.3.

Table 30.3: Frankel grading of spinal cord injuries

Class	Functional status	Description
A	Complete	Total motor and sensory loss
B	Sensory only	Sensory sparing
C	Motor useless	Motor sparing of no functional value
D	Motor useful	Motor sparing of functional value
E	Recovery	No functional deficit

The various spinal cord syndromes include:

• *Anterior cord syndrome*: Damage to the spinothalamic and corticospinal tracts with resultant predominant motor weakness.

• *Brown–Sequard's syndrome*: Hemicord injury with ipsilateral motor weakness and loss of proprioception and contralateral loss of pain and temperature below the level of injury.

• *Central cord syndrome*: Injury to the central portions of the cervical spinal cord with resultant predominant motor affectation of the upper limb.

• *Conus medullaris syndrome*: Injury towards the end of the spinal cord results in a mixed upper motor neurone and lower motor neurone dysfunction.

Spinal cord injury without radiographic abnormality (SCIWORA) is a unique type of spinal cord injury common to children characterised by posttraumatic neurological deficits with normal plain radiographs or tomographs. It occurs mostly in children younger than 8–10 years of age. The mechanism of occurrence is thought to be vascular or ischaemic in origin, resulting in spinal cord infarction.

Investigations

Radiographic evaluation is done after adequate resuscitation. A lateral plain x-ray is the most informative and may show fractures, subluxation, or angulation of the spine. Soft tissue swellings may indicate ligamentous injury. In suspected odontoid fractures, an open mouth view can be done for the older child. In infants, a CT scan is recommended. At least 75% of patients with spinal cord injury have injury to the vertebral column and thus some degree of radiographic abnormalities. Therefore, initial plain films are indispensable.

Dynamic studies can be done to search for occult instability in the older cooperative child with neck pain but no neurologic deficit.

CT scans and MRI could further elucidate the extent of the injury (Figure 30.4).

Radiographic signs of cervical spine trauma include:

• soft tissue in retropharyngeal space >22 mm (child not crying);

• displaced prevertebral fat stripe;

• tracheal deviation and laryngeal dislocation;

• vertebral malalignment;

• loss of lordosis;

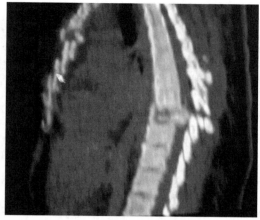

Figure 30.4: CT scan, saggital reconstruction. Slide shows retropulsed thoracic vertebra into spinal canal.

• acute kyphotic angulation;

• widened interspinous space;

• axial rotation of vertebra;

• discontinuity in contour lines;

• abnormal joints;

• atlanto-dental interval of more than 5 mm;

• narrow or widened disc space; and

• widening of apophyseal joints.

Management

The goal of management of spinal cord injuries is to prevent further injury and reduce neurological deficits.

Initial management and evaluation

Ideally, initial management and evaluation are commenced at the scene of the injury. In most African settings, however, prehospital management is not well established, and the initial management is usually commenced at the receiving hospital. The initial management includes resuscitation, immobilisation, constant monitoring, and assessment of the injured child.[24]

Resuscitation

The main causes of death of in a child with spinal cord injury are aspiration and shock, and so the "ABC" of life support is commenced. Early airway control with endotracheal intubation and oxygen administration may be indicated in respiratory insufficiency. Manual in-line immobilisation of the cervical spine is mandatory during intubation. Hypotension accompanied by bradycardia may be present due to autonomic paralysis. Therefore, adequate hydration with systolic blood pressure maintained at or above 90 mm Hg prevents shock.[25] Volume resuscitation suffices, but occasionally ionotropes such as ephedrine may be indicated.

Nasogastric tube decompression of the stomach is instituted because gastric distention can interfere with respiration or lead to gastric mucosal ulceration.

The loss of sympathetic tone may also lead to urinary retention and hypothermia. An indwelling urethral catheter is passed, and attention paid to the temperature of the child with constant monitoring.

Immobilisation

The entire spine of the child with suspected spinal injury should be immobilised. Whole-body braces usually are not readily available, so the cervical spine is immobilised with collars, particularly in the older child. Infants can be immobilised with sand bags or intravenous fluid bags secured at both sides of the head, with the head taped to the board.

Evaluation

Following resuscitation, a detailed history should be taken as soon as possible, including mechanism and time of injury, severity of injury, the first aid given, and mode of transportation. Examination should include all motor functions of the major muscle groups as well as a rectal examination to assess sphincteric tone. Sensory functions, reflexes, and motor functions of the diaphragm and intercostal muscles should be assessed.

Treatment

Medical

High-dose methylprednisolone administration within 8 hours of injury is said to be beneficial to long-term outcomes. The patient is given 30 mg/kg bolus over 15 minutes, followed by a 45-minute pause. Maintenance infusion of 5.4 mg/kg per hour over 23 or 47 hours is given. However, the efficacy has not been fully evaluated in children younger than 13 years of age. Gastric erosion is prevented by the use of H_2-receptor antagonists such as ranitidine.

Attention is paid to the prevention of pressure ulcers, chronic urinary tract infection, and contracture and deformities of the limbs.

Cervical injury

Besides collars, bracings immobilise the cervical spine (Table 30.4). Cervicothoracic orthosis (CTO) incorporates a body vest to immobilize the cervical spine and includes the Guilford brace, sterno-occipito-mandibular Immobilisation (SOMI), and Yale brace.

Table 30.4: Recommended bracing for various cervical spine injuries.

Condition	Recommended brace
Cervical strain	Philadelphia collar
Jefferson fracture stable unstable	Cervicothoracic orthosis Halo
Odontoid fracture type I types II & III	Cervicothoracic orthosis Halo
Hangman's fracture stable unstable	SOMI Halo
Flexion injuries mid cervical (C3-C5) low cervical (C5-T1)	SOMI, cervicothoracic orthosis Cervicothoracic orthosis
Extension injuries mid cervical (C3-C5) low cervical (C5-T1)	Halo, cervicothoracic orthosis Halo

Traction

Skull traction is aimed at reducing cervical fracture or dislocation, maintaining normal alignment, immobilising the spine, and decompressing the spinal cord and nerve roots. It also facilitates bone healing. Traction includes Crutchfield tongs, Gardner-Wells' tongs, or halo traction. The traction weight should be increased slowly under the guidance of an image intensifier to achieve reduction. Three pounds per cervical vertebral level is recommended (but not more than 10 pounds should be used in children younger than 14 years of age).

Thoracolumbar injury

Perhaps the most popular theory in terms of spinal stability is the three-column theory of Dennis. In this model, the anterior column includes the anterior longitudinal ligament, anterior portion of disc, and vertebra. The middle column incorporates the posterior portion of disc and vertebra, posterior longitudinal ligament, and the pedicle. The posterior column includes the posterior ligamentous complex and arch. The rib cage-sternum complex serves as a fourth column of support unique to the thoracic spine.

Damage to more than one column of the spine renders it unstable. Thoracolumbar spine instability can be categorised into (1) first-degree instability, which is mainly mechanical; (2) second-degree instability, in which there is neurological instability; and (3) third-degree instability, in which there is both neurological and mechanical instability. Those with stable and first-degree instability can be managed with bed rest for 1–6 weeks followed by ambulation in an orthosis (e.g., thoracolumbar sacral orthosis (TLSO) or Jewett brace) for 3 to 5 months. Second- and third-degree instability may require instrumentation.

Surgery

Operative management of spinal cord injury aims at decompression and stability. Emergency decompression has been associated with neurological deterioration, although it is indicated in incomplete lesions. Other indications are as follows:

• progressive neurological deterioration;

• complete spinal block (on MRI or myelogram);

• bone fragment within the spinal canal;

• cervical root compression;

• compound fracture or penetrating spinal trauma;

• acute anterior cord syndrome; and

• nonreducible, locked facet causing compression.

Complications of Spinal Cord Injury

Respiratory complications

Respiratory insufficiency is common in patients with injuries of the cervical cord. If the neurological lesion is complete, the patient will have paralysed intercostals muscles and will have to rely on diaphragmatic respiration. Partial diaphragmatic paralysis may also be present ab initio or after 24–48 hours if ascending posttraumatic oedema develops. In thoracic spine injuries, there may be associated rib fractures, haemopneumothorax, ventilation perfusion, mismatch, and so on.

Patients need to be nursed in the recumbent position even after spinal stabilisation to ensure that diaphragmatic excursion is not compromised. Regular chest physiotherapy and respiratory function monitoring should be done.

A patient whose respiratory function is initially satisfactory after injury but then deteriorates should regain satisfactory ventilatory capacity once spinal cord oedema subsides. Artificial ventilation should therefore not be withheld.

Cardiovascular complications

Haemorrhage from associated injuries is the most common cause of posttraumatic shock and must be treated vigorously. In traumatic quadriplegia, the thoracolumbar (T1–L2) sympathetic outflow paralysis gives rise to hypotension and bradycardia. Pharyngeal suction and tracheal intubation stimulate the vagus, and in high spinal cord injuries, these can produce bradycardia and cadiac arrest. Hence, atropine and glycopyrronium should be used before such procedures or when heart rates fall below 50 per minute.

Cardiac arrest from sudden hyperkalaemia following the use of depolarising agents such as suxamethonium is a risk in these patients between 3 days and 9 months after injury. Hence, nondepolarising agents are preferred.

Thromboembolism

Newly injured quadriplegics or paraplegics are at risk of thromboembolism. Antiembolism stockings and anticoagulants must be started immediately once medical contraindications and head injury are ruled out.

Bladder complications

After severe cord injury, the urinary bladder is initially acontractile, and if untreated this leads to acute urinary retention. A Foley catheter should be passed.

Gastrointestinal tract complications

Paralytic ileus is a common accompaniment of severe spinal cord injury and should be treated with intravenous fluids, nil per os (NPO), and nasogastric tube decompression. Uncommonly, ulceration, haemorrhage and perforation may occur. Therefore, proton pump inhibitors or H_2-receptor antagonists should be started immediately.

Skin and pressure areas
The patient must be turned every 2 hours manually or automatically, and all pressure areas must be padded to prevent pressure sores.[26]

Joints and limbs
Joints must be passively moved and splinted if necessary to prevent contractures.

Autonomic dysreflexia
Autonomic dysreflexia is seen particularly in patients with cervical injury above the sympathetic outflow. It occurs after spinal shock and usually is due to distended bladder or detrusor-sphincter dyssynergia. Distended bladder causes reflex sympathetic overactivity below the level of the spinal cord lesion, causing vasoconstriction and severe hypertension. The carotid and aortic baroreceptors respond via the vasomotor centre with increased vagal tone and bradycardia, but these stimuli cannot pass distally through the injured cord.

Patient suffers headache, profuse sweating, and flushing above the level of the cord lesion. Without prompt treatment, intracranial haemorrhage may occur.

Another cause of autonomic dysreflexia includes urinary tract infection.

Treatment is by removing the cause, sitting the patient up, and administering nifedipine or glycryl trinitrate; spinal or epidural anaesthetics are used occasionally.

Hyponatraemia
Hyponatraemia is usually caused by fluid overload, diuretic usage, and the sodium-depleting effect of some drugs such as carbamazepine and inappropriate ADH secretion. It is treated by treating sepsis, fluid restriction, and administration of frusamide with potassium supplements.

Hypercalcaemia
Hypercalcaemia is caused by prolonged immobility and manifests with constipation, abdominal pain, and headache. Treatment involves hydration, achieving diuresis, and the use of sodium etidronate or disodium pamidronate.

Para-articular heterotopic ossification
New bone is often deposited in soft tissue around paralysed joints. Best treatment is surgical excision after 18 months when the bone is matured.

Spasticity
Spasticity is seen only in patients with an upper motor neurone lesion whose intact spinal reflex arcs below the level of the lesion are isolated from the higher centres. It enhances the tendency to contractures.

Aggravating factors are detected and treated, pain is managed, and spastic muscles are passively stretched. Oral baclofen is usually helpful. In intractable cases, however, the use of butulinum toxin, motor point injection, intrathecal baclofen pump, tenotomy, neurectomy, or Intrathecal block may be employed.

Urologic complications
After spinal cord injury, dysfunctional voiding patterns may soon emerge. These are associated with serious sequelae. Therefore, as part of early management, intermittent catheterisation, tapping and expression, indwelling catheterisation, suprapubic cystostomy, or intermittent self-catheterisation can be used. Later management may involve augmentation cystoplasty, neuromodulation and sacral anterior root stimulation (SARS), or intermittent self-catheterisation (Mitrofanoff's technique).

Prognosis and Outcome
The neurological examination and age of the patient are the most critical prognostic factors for short- and long-term recovery. Children with complete lesions rarely improve, whereas those with incomplete but severe lesions improve with time but hardly regain normal function. Only children with mild to moderate deficits can hope for full recovery. Mortality in the acute setting is 20%.

Prevention
The majority of spinal cord injury is caused by pedestrian-motor vehicle accidents and falls. Enforcement of traffic rules cannot be overemphasized. Prevention of children from engaging in activities that are detrimental, such as climbing trees and unprotected heights or depths must be ensured.[27,28]

Ethical Issues
Those who survive spinal cord trauma develop life-long disabilities. Treatment is often not curative. The decision to operate must be carefully discussed with the family, and the prospective multidisplinary mode of subsequent management should be instituted.

Evidenced-Based Research
Table 30.5 is a review of paediatric severe head injuries that compares two age groups. Table 30.6 is a review of paediatric spine fractures that compares parameters of the injuries.

Table 30.5: Evidence-based research.

Title	Severe head injury in children: early prognosis and outcome
Authors	Zuccarello M, Facco E, Zaampieri P, Zanardi L, Andrioli GC
Institution	Department of Neurosurgery and Institute of Anesthesiology and Intensive Care, University Hospital, Padova, Italy
Reference	Child's Nervous System 1985; 1:158–162
Problem	Identifying indicators for early prognosis and outcome in children with severe head injury.
Intervention	Controlled hyperventilation and bolus infusion of hypertonic (20%) mannitol, surgical removal of any mass lesions.
Comparison/ control (quality of evidence)	Sixty-two children with severe head injury were divided into two groups: infants aged <36 months (24.2%) and children aged 36 months–14 years (75.8%). The study was limited to patients who remained in coma for at least 6 hours.
Outcome/ effect	The difference between good and poor results in patients with GCS 4 or less and those with score of 5 points or better was significant ($p < 0.001$). There was a correlation between the best motor response and outcome. Of flaccid patients, 85% did poorly or died, whereas 69% of those who withdrew in response to pain did well ($p<0.001$).
	The presence or absence of brainstem dysfunction (assessed on basis of pupil reaction and oculocephalic reflex) was statistically related to good or poor result but oculocephalic reflex was considered to be the most indicative ($p<0.001$).
	The necessity for assisted ventilation at admission was associated with a less favourable outcome ($p<0.001$). An intracranial haematoma was not associated with a worse outcome.
	The authors observed that recovery was almost complete when the duration of coma was less than 2 weeks, with 93% of patients moderately disabled or with a good recovery. There was high incidence of poor outcome in those with coma lasting >2 weeks ($p = 0.0002$).
	Overall mortality was 32%.
Historical significance/ comments	This study provides a useful insight into the early prognostic factor in children with severe head injury. Clinical features available soon after injury that are important indicators of treatment and outcome are identified.

Table 30.6: Evidence-based research.

Title	Pediatric spine fractures: a review of 137 hospital admissions
Authors	Carreon LY, Glassman ST, Campbell MJ
Institution	Leatherman Spine Center, Louisville, Kentucky, USA
Reference	J Spinal Disorders Techniques 2004; 17: 477–482
Problem	In children with spinal injury, prevention of further neurologic damage and deformity, as well as good potential for recovery, makes timely identification and appropriate treatment of the injury critical.
Intervention	Decompression, fusion, instrumentation.
Comparison/ control (quality of evidence)	The 137 patients were divided into three groups for analysis: 0–9 years of age (36 patients), 10–14 (49 patients) and 15–17 (52 patients). This allowed for comparison of age with mechanism of injury, injury pattern and level, incidence of cord injury, treatment, and outcomes.
Outcome/ effect	Thirty-six (1%) of 3,685 injured children aged 0–9 years sustained spine injury, compared to 49 (3%) of 1,609 injured children aged 10–14 years, and 52 (5%) of 921 injured children aged 15–17 years (p < 0.001). Motor vehicle accidents were the most common cause of injury across all ages, followed by falls, sports, and pedestrian accidents. The incidence of multilevel and noncontiguous injuries in the different age groups was not significantly different. Twenty-four patients (19%) had spinal cord injury; 21 (87%) were complete cord injuries, and 3 (13%) were incomplete. Cord injury was more common in the 0–9 year age group. Four of five patients with spinal cord injury without radiographic abnormality (SCIWORA) were in the 0–9 age group and had complete neurologic injuries. Young children with cervical injuries were more likely to die than older children. Fifty-three percent had associated injuries. Eighteen percent underwent decompression, fusion, and instrumentation. Two patients developed scoliosis. The complication rate in surgical patients was higher than in patients treated nonsurgically and in polytrauma patients.
Historical significance/ comments	This retrospective clinical case series has presented important and useful data from a large series of paediatric patients with spine injuries from a single regional trauma center.

Key Summary Points

Craniocerebral Trauma

1. Paediatric head injury is common in our environment.

2. Motor vehicle accidents cause the severest form of injury.

3. Child abuse is increasingly becoming recognised as a cause of paediatric head injury.

4. Prompt resuscitation and cervical spine protection are key to survival.

5. Scalp bleeding may easily cause anaemia because of small intravascular volume.

6. The postresuscitation GCS score is an important prognostic factor.

7. Intracranial haematomas are aggressively managed.

8. Education and enforcement of legislation on vehicle safety rules are important in preventive strategies.

Spinal Cord Injury

1. Paediatric spinal cord injury presents an enormous challenge, not only to the neurosurgeon but to the health and economic resources of any nation.

2. The care of the spinally disabled child is far from ideal in our environment.

3. Late presentation is the rule in most African settings, precluding those who would have benefitted from the institution of early treatment modalities.

4. Prompt resuscitation and optimal fluid administration limit further cord injury.

5. More personnel, facilities, and dedicated centres for spinal care are in arrears, needing urgent attention.

References

1. Winn HR, ed. Paediatric head injury In: Youman's Neurological Surgery, 5th ed. Saunders, 2004.

2. Tindall GT,Cooper PR, Barrow DL, eds. Head Injury in the Paediatric Patient. In: The Practice of Neurosurgery, Version 4.18.4; Williams and Wilkins, 1996.

3. Basso A, Previglioano I, Duarte,JM, Ferrari, N. Advances in Management of Neurosurgical Trauma in Different Continents. World J Surg 2001; 25:1174–1178.

4. Shokunbi MT, Solagberu BA. Mortality in Childhood Head Injury in Ibadan. Afri J Med Sci 1995; 24:159–163.

5. Solagberu BA, Adekanye AO, Ofoegbu CP, Udoffa US, Abdur-Rahman LO, Taiwo JO. Epidemiology of trauma deaths. West Afr J Med 2003; 22:177–181.

6. Legbo JN, Shehu BB. Managing scalp defects in Sub Saharan Africa. East Afri Med J 2004; 81:87–91.

7. Thanni L. Evaluation of guidelines for skull radiography in head injury. Niger Postgrad Med J 2003; 10:231–233.

8. Obisesan AA, Bohrer SP. The uses and abuses of skull x-ray in head injury. Niger Med J 1979; 9:65–69.

9. Nagy KK, Joseph KT, Krosner SM, et al. The utility of head computed tomography after minimal head injury. J Trauma 1999; 46:268–270.

10. Umerah B. Cerebral angiography in Central Africa. Diagn Imaging 1981; 50:225–228.

11. Otieno T, Woodfield JC, Bird P, et al. Trauma in rural Kenya. Injury 2004; 35:1228–1233.

12. Muhammad I. Management of head injuries at the ABU Hospital, Zaria. East Afr Med J 1990; 67:447–451.

13. Brain Trauma Foundation AAON. Guidelines for the acute medical management of severe traumatic brain injury in infants, children and adolescents. Paediatr Crit Care Med 2003; 4:S1–S75.

14. Bullock MR, Chestnut R, Ghajar J, et al. Guidelines for the surgical management of traumatic brain injury. Neurosurgery 2006; 58(3 Suppl.):S1–S60.

15. Shokunbi MT, Olurin OI. Childhood head injuries in Nigeria: causes, neurologic complications and outcome. West Afr Med J 1994; 13:38–42.

16. Mwang'ombe NJ, Kiboi J. Factors influencing the outcome of severe head injury at Kenyatta National Hospital. East Afr Med J 2001; 78:238–241.

17. Bahloul M, Chelly H, Ben Hmida MS, et al. Prognosis of traumatic head injury in south Tunisia: a multivariate analysis of 437 cases. J Trauma 2004; 57:255–561.

18. Winn HR, ed. Paediatric vertebral column and spinal cord injuries, In: Youman's Neurological Surgery, 5 ed. Saunders, 2004.

19. David P. Spinal cord injury in children. In: Principles and Practice of Paediatric Neurosurgery. Thieme, 1999, Pp. 955–969.

20. Brockmeyer DL. Spinal cord and spinal column injuries in children : current management options. In: Paediatric Neurosurgery for the General Neurosurgeon. Thieme, 2002, Pp. 36–48.

21. Hamilton MG, Myles ST. Paediatric spinal injury: review of 174 hospital admissions. J Neurosurg 1992; 77:700–704.

22. Rauzzino MJ, Grabb PA, Hadley MN. Paediatric vertebral column and spinal cord injuries. Persp Neurolog Surg 1997; 8:27–60.

23. Scher AT. Trauma of the spinal cord in children. S Afr Med J 1976; 50:2023–2025.

24. Adeolu AA, Shokunbi MT, Malomo AO, Komolafe EO, Adeloye EA. Cervical spine injury in children with head injury in Ibadan, Nigeria. Afr J Paediatr Surg 2005; 1:76–79.

25. Mayuri G, Maharajh J. Case report of cranio-cervical dislocation in a child. S Afr Radiographer 2006; 44(2):18

26. Chen Y, DeVivo MJ, Jackson AB. Pressure ulcer prevalence in people with spinal cord injury: age-period-duration effects. Arch Phys Med Rehabil 2005; 86:1208–1213.

27. Odeku EL, Richard DR. Peculiarities of spinal trauma in Nigeria. West Afr Med J 1971; 20:211–225.

28. Rhodes N. Focus on parents: teen's perceptions of parental safety messages. Workshop presentation at the 2007 Lifesavers Conference. Chicago, IL, March 2007.

CHAPTER 31
UROGENITAL AND PERINEAL TRAUMA

Lohfa B. Chirdan
Ronald S. Sutherland

Introduction

Trauma is a leading cause of death in children in developed countries.[1,2] In Africa, as in many developing countries where malnutrition and infectious diseases are leading causes of death in children, trauma may not be encountered as often by the surgeon. As developing countries improve the general health care of children with better nutrition and control of infectious disease vectors, however, trauma is becoming a leading cause of death in children in Africa. This is largely due to the rise of high-speed motor vehicle travel and increasing traffic congestion along poorly developed transportation routes. Most areas lack emergency response systems with trained personnel, adequate emergency transport vehicles, and avenues for medical evacuation to higher echelons of care, which are critical to the survival and decreased morbidity. Dilapidated vehicles traveling on these roads often add to the burden of trauma in these regions.[3] Many of these young trauma victims arrive to the surgeon a long time after injury, so the surgeon operating in developing countries must be prepared to quickly and accurately evaluate and manage these youngsters in order to save lives and decrease morbidity from urinary tract injuries.[4]

The urogenital tract is involved in up to 12% of children with abdominal and pelvic trauma.[1] The same mechanisms causing injury to the urinary and genital systems also frequently involve the perineum and challenge the surgeon who is attempting to evaluate the extent of injury. After conducting the primary survey and instituting resuscitative measures, the surgeon will need to employ diagnostic imaging studies to evaluate and identify the urological injuries that can be managed nonoperatively. Advances in radiological imaging have led to a greatly decreased number of unwarranted exploratory operations because some of these patients can be managed nonoperatively.[5] In settings with limited facilities, the use of a simple protocol in children with blunt abdominal trauma could lead to a reduction in laparotomy and mortality rates.[3]

Aetiology and Mechanism of Injury

Injury to the urogenital tract results from either blunt or penetrating trauma. Blunt trauma accounts for more than 98% of injuries to the urogenital tract, and penetrating trauma occurs in less than 2%.[1,2] There are many different mechanisms of injury to the urinary tract; in Africa, the majority of these injuries occur as a result of motor vehicular accidents. Most accidents occur on poorly maintained roads with minimal emergency response capability.[3] The aetiology of urogenital trauma can be divided into blunt and penetrating causes and regions of involvement (renal, ureteral, bladder, urethral, genital, and gonadal).

Blunt

Blunt injuries in Africa commonly are caused by motor vehicle and traffic accidents, falls from heights, and direct blows to the abdomen or perineum from child abuse, sports injuries, and straddle accidents.

Penetrating

Penetrating injuries in Africa are commonly due to gunshots, stab wounds from a knife or other sharp object, machete hacking, or foreign body insertion into the urethra. Medical procedure–related penetrating injuries include catheter trauma (i.e., urethral disruption from balloon inflation inside the urethra or creation of a false passage), penile surgery (especially circumcision), and surgeries of the retroperitoneum, pelvis, and anorectal area (e.g., posterior sagittal anorectoplasty).

With increasing violence in many parts of urban Africa, urogenital tract trauma from high-velocity gunshot wounds and use of sharp objects in children are likely to increase. The ability to provide early and rapid treatment to victims in war-torn regions may be severely limited due to the remote locations and transportation difficulties. Domestic violence also must be remembered as a significant cause of paediatric trauma, which may be from sexual abuse (usually penetrating injury) or use of blunt force.

Evaluation

To avoid serious long-term complications, significant urogenital tract injuries in children must be appropriately and promptly managed. Improper or inadequate treatment may have a long-term disabling effect on these children and condemn a child to lifelong urological disability. The initial approach to the child with any urogenital tract injury is identifying life-threatening conditions and applying the ABCDE's of resuscitation. These include identification and control of any airway obstruction, breathing problems, control of the circulatory system, management of other life-threatening (usually neurological) disabilities, and control of potentially lethal environmental threats (exposure). Once these priorities are addressed, then the assessment and subsequent management of the urogenital tract injuries follows.

History

A detailed history after resuscitation includes the description of the accident scene and mechanism of injury. One should strongly suspect urogenital tract involvement in any sudden deceleration accident with anuria, penetrating flank injury, urethral bleeding, or gross haematuria. In penetrating injuries, the type and calibre of the missile or weapon must be determined. It should be noted that, due to the kinetic properties of high-velocity injuries, one must suspect a much more extensive injury than appears on the surface.

The paediatric patient's medical history must also be known. Certain congenital or acquired conditions of the urinary tract are predisposed to injury. Congenital hydronephrosis from pelvi-ureteric or uretero-vesical junction obstruction may cause the kidney to rupture with a sudden deceleration accident. Urethral obstruction from posterior urethral valves or urethral stricture may result in bladder distention and increase the risk of bladder rupture after blunt force trauma. Other conditions, such as urinary tract calculi or a history of urinary infections (e.g., schistosomiasis/bilharziasis), may complicate the management of these patients.

Physical Findings

After the initial quick primary general assessment, the abdomen and genitalia are examined, looking for evidence of contusion or subcutaneous haematoma, which may point to serious internal injuries to the retroperitoneum or pelvic fractures. Several important points should be noted when examining a child with suspected urogenital tract injuries:

1. Abdominal flank tenderness or bruising and lower rib fractures may suggest renal injury (Figure 31.1), although one-quarter of children with severe renal injuries may not have abdominal examination findings; therefore, a high index of suspicion and further evaluation are needed to make an accurate diagnosis.[1,2]

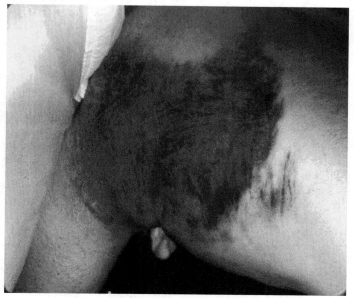

Figure 31.1: Patient with flank haematoma found to have fractured kidney.

2. Swelling or ecchymosis in the perineum as well as lacerations or bleeding are suggestive of urinary tract injuries, so a patient with any or a combination of the above should be further evaluated to determine the exact part of the urinary tract that is injured.

3. The presence of blood at the external urethral meatus may be the only indicator of a urethral injury. Another sinister sign is upward displacement of the prostate in boys on digital rectal examination. This physical finding may be very difficult to interpret in a child, but must be investigated further due to the risk of posterior urethral disruption.

Investigations

The suspicion of urinary tract injury on history and physical examination warrants additional investigations to accurately determine the site and extent of the injury for proper treatment and good outcome. These investigations are divided into laboratory studies and imaging studies.

Laboratory Studies

Laboratory studies supplement clinical history, good physical examination, and imaging techniques. The results of these studies, when interpreted well, would be very helpful to surgeons practicing in Africa because most of the advanced imaging techniques are unavailable in many centres, or even unaffordable in places where they are available. These investigations include a complete blood count; urinalysis; serum levels of electrolytes and urea, creatinine, and amylase; and liver function tests. The results of these laboratory investigations must be interpreted in line with the general condition of the patient. For instance, in a patient with intraperitoneal bladder rupture, the serum urea may be markedly elevated, whereas the creatinine may be normal due to the absorption of urea by the peritoneum.

Urethral catheterisation may be required to obtain an accurate urinalysis, and a clean, appropriate-sized urethral catheter should be passed gently into the bladder under aseptic conditions. This is done only when there is no blood at the urethral meatus, or gross haematuria. The presence of blood in the urine after passing the urethral catheter indicates urinary tract injury.

Imaging Studies

Abdominal and pelvic plain film x-ray

A plain film x-ray is done routinely for all abdominal and pelvic trauma, especially if intravenous contrast is to be given. This film should identify the presence and nature of bony injury, foreign bodies, and stones, and should strengthen the suspicion of bladder and urethral injury.

Abdominal/pelvic ultrasound

Ultrasound is readily available in many centres in Africa, is less expensive than many other imaging modalities, and can be readily used by the consulting surgeon. This can be done to evaluate injuries to the retroperitoneal organs, such as the kidney and bladder. It can also be a useful tool in assessing injuries to other organs in the abdomen and pelvis.

Urethrocystography

Urethrocystography is a very useful investigation, especially in Africa, because most radiological services are able to obtain plain film radiographs necessary for this investigation. It is done by the passage of a small-size catheter into the urethral meatus and held in place by inflating the balloon by with 1–2 ml of sterile water.

The patient is placed in the oblique position, and, if the patient is a male, the penis is placed on stretch. A water-soluble contrast is then injected and the retrograde urethrogram is done. This outlines the urethra, giving a diagnosis of the type of urethral trauma, if present. If the urethra is uninjured but a bladder injury is suspected, the catheter is advanced into the bladder and then filled with a water-soluble contrast. In children, the bladder should be filled to at least 50% of expected bladder capacity, calculated by

$$EBC \, (\text{ml}) = (age + 2) \times 30.$$

In adolescents or older children, fill with at least 350 to 400 ml for an adequate study to be done. If possible, have the patient void and capture an antegrade voiding view of the urethra. To be complete, a postvoid view of the bladder must be obtained. If the patient is unable to void, drain the bladder and take a second film.

Urethrocystoscopy

Paediatric-sized fibre-optic cystoscopes are becoming increasingly available in most tertiary centres in Africa, and these scopes can be used to diagnose and manage some urethral and bladder injuries. In certain types of urethral injuries, this may enable the surgeon to pass a wire beyond the injury and then place a catheter over the wire.

Intravenous urography

In intravenous urography (IVU), urografin, or other water-soluble contrast is given intravenously and serial abdominal films are taken at 30 seconds, and at 1, 5, and 10 minutes. If there is delay in uptake of the contrast by the kidneys, then delayed images should be obtained at 30, 60, 120, or 180 minutes, if necessary. In an urgent scenario, where the child is taken to the operating theater for exploratory laparotomy, an "on-the-table", two-shot IVU can be done by obtaining a plain film, followed by a 2-ml/kg bolus of intravenous contrast, and then imaging at 10 minutes. This evaluates renal and ureteral injuries. Bladder injuries also can be evaluated on the cystogram phase (although imprecise).

Computed tomography scan

Computed tomography (CT) is rapidly becoming available in most tertiary centres throughout Africa and is extremely useful in evaluating urinary tract injuries. Cost is a major drawback of this investigation, but as medical insurance becomes readily available to patients, CT scans are becoming more widely used. Another limitation of the use of CT in the paediatric population is the large amount of ionising radiation children receive if they require serial scanning. CT is the most accurate imaging modality for the evaluation of renal trauma and has several advantages over IVU by virtue of its three-dimensional imaging capability and exceptional anatomical clarity. CT cystography is a very reliable method for staging bladder injuries and can be used in place of plain film cystography. Obtain CT images before contrast is given, at bladder capacity, and after the bladder is drained.

Renal scintigraphy

Nuclear renography is not readily available in most centres across Africa because of the requirement for a radiation physicist and/or nuclear radiographic pharmacist. It has almost no role in the immediate evaluation of patients with urinary trauma. Nevertheless, nuclear scintigraphy can identify the presence or absence of a functional renal unit. Scanning a trauma patient is cumbersome and yields no additional anatomical details; therefore, CT scans are the preferred imaging modality in almost every case of acute trauma. In the chronic, posttraumatic recovery phase, it may have a role to monitor differential renal function or to assess the degree of obstruction if used with furosemide (diuretic renography).

Renal angiography and interventional radiography

This imaging modality is limited to institutions where an interventional radiologist is present and where digital, multiplanar fluoroscopy is available. Most developing countries do not have access to this complex and expensive technology. However, where present, it is very useful to determine the extent of renal vascular injury and also provide an opportunity for the interventional radiologist to access actively bleeding sites within the kidney and embolise them. Arteriography is useful in nonoperative management of major renal trauma because up to 25% of complex renal injuries may have delayed bleeding. Selective embolisation is 80% effective in treating posttraumatic arteriovenous malformations or pseudoaneurysms. Interventional radiologists can also percutaneously access and drain an obstructed kidney or abdominal/pelvic fluid collection.

Retrograde pyelography

Retrograde pyelography is done during urethrocystoscopy, when the ureteric orifices are catheterised and a soluble contrast injected. It is used to confirm ureteric injuries.

Kidney Trauma

Renal injuries account for 30–70% of all urogenital tract injuries in children.[1,2] There is a higher incidence of renal injuries in children compared to adults because of several anatomical reasons. The kidney in the child is proportionally larger and more mobile than that of the adult; the abdominal wall and retroperitoneal fat in the child give little or no protection to the kidney; and foetal lobulation may initiate cleavage planes after even minor trauma to the child's abdomen. Certain conditions predispose children to renal injury, including congenital hydronephrosis, multicystic kidney, renal tumours (e.g., Wilms' tumour), duplication or fusion anomalies of the kidney, and compensatory hypertrophy (solitary kidney).

Blunt trauma is responsible for up to 80% of the injuries.[2] Direct trauma crushes the kidneys against the lumbar spine or paravertebral muscles. Indirect acceleration-deceleration injury, when applied to the kidney, may disrupt the ureteropelvic junction.

Renal injury may be classified as minor, major, or complex.

1. Minor injuries account for 85% of renal injuries and include contusions, subcapsular haematoma, and superficial lacerations. There is parenchymal damage without capsular tears or pelvicalyceal system involvement.

2. Major injuries account for 10% of renal injuries. There is cortical laceration, deep parenchymal laceration involving the collecting system with limited extravasation.

3. Complex injuries account for 5% of renal injuries. They include rupture of a solitary or malformed kidney, kidney fragmentation, significant renal vascular injury, or rupture of the renal pelvis or ureter.

Management of Renal Injuries

The management of renal injuries in a child depends on the stability of the child and the extent of injury sustained by the child. It is, however, pertinent to define the goals of management of renal injuries in children. These goals are to preserve renal tissue and function and to minimise morbidity.

Following careful imaging and stratification of the renal injury, children are either managed nonoperatively (i.e., expectantly) or operatively. Whichever management option is chosen, it is important to bear in mind the goals of management stated above.

Minor Injuries

There is little controversy over the management of minor renal injuries. Most cases are managed nonoperatively with the expectation that complete renal tissue will be preserved and full renal function will return. Microscopic haematuria in a stable child with a renal contusion would not require hospitalisation of the child, but that child's activity should be restricted until the haematuria clears. Gross haematuria would, however, require strict bed rest in hospital. Ambulation starts when the haematuria clears. If the haematuria persists, then IVU or contrast enhanced CT is done and bed rest continued. If the bleeding is due to small-calibre renal vessels, angiography with embolisation is done if facilities are available. In Africa, where interventional radiology facilities for embolisation are not routinely available, expectant management is usually the preferred management.[4] If bleeding persists, however, then open laparotomy with direct repair of bleeding sites is done. A follow-up ultrasound or CT scan is then done 6–8 weeks later. Renal scintigraphy, where available, or IVU in many centres in Africa, is done to assess renal function. The blood pressure is monitored at each clinic follow-up.

Major Injuries

Children with major renal injuries pose a significant challenge to the surgeon in Africa. In children whose vital signs are stable, either immediate or delayed surgery is employed, depending on the circumstances.

Early or immediate surgery

As a general rule, if the vital signs of the child with major renal injury are unstable, an expanding flank mass is present, and the haematocrit is decreasing, then renal vascular injury is likely and immediate operative intervention should be carried out. The only absolute indication for early surgery is haemodynamic instability. Because most complex renal injuries in children are associated with hypotension, bleeding, and other organ injury, almost all require exploration if the goals of management are to be achieved. Early operation may also decrease the incidence of morbidity such as abscesses, sepsis, and intestinal ileus. Early operation also reduces the duration (and cost) of the hospital stay, which is important to practitioners in Africa, as a short hospital stay means there would be bed space available for other patients. Early operation also reduces the incidence of postoperative hypertension.

McAninch[6] has described a transabdominal approach to gain early access to the renal pedicle before mobilising the overlying colon laterally and entering the Gerota's fascia of the injured kidney. This method resulted in a higher renal salvage rate due to better vascular control and less bleeding. An incision is made through the posterior peritoneum and base of the mesentery immediately on top of the aorta; the inferior mesenteric vein is used to guide the surgeon to the site of incision on the aorta. Through this more medial incision, the renal vessels are readily identified (compared to a lateral approach through the bed of the injured kidney) and secured with a temporary Rommel tourniquet or bulldog clamp. The colon can then be reflected and Gerota's fascia entered in a more controlled fashion.

Nonoperative or delayed management

Proponents of nonoperative management of major renal injuries argue that no controlled trials have conclusively shown a benefit of early surgery.[5,6,7] In fact, with a delayed approach, the risk of early nephrectomy is avoided. However, delayed surgery is necessary in up to 13% of cases.[1,2] Nonoperative management is generally favoured in children with major blunt renal trauma, except in the presence of haemodynamic instability.[7,8] Central to the nonoperative management of renal and other solid organ trauma is the use of serial CT scanning. Operative management should not be overdelayed, however, due to the general unavailability of CT scanners in most hospitals in Africa.[4]

Penetrating Renal Injuries

Penetrating renal injuries should be explored immediately (Figure 31.2). This is especially true in children who sustain a gunshot wound to the flank in which there is a high incidence of associated intraabdominal injuries and complex renal injuries. Adequate debridement of devitalised tissues must be carried out.

Ureteric Injuries

Injuries to the ureters are not common in children.[1,2] Rapid deceleration accidents (falls or motor vehicle accidents) may result in severe hyperextension of the trunk and possible disruption of the pelviureteric junction by stretch-induced injury. In cases of isolated ureteral injury, one must have a high index of suspicion to make this diagnosis, as patients may present in a delayed fashion with fever, ileus, sepsis, and flank pain. Severe blunt trauma may be associated with fractures of ribs, spine, and pelvis, which can also injure the ureters, much like penetrating trauma. Penetrating trauma to the flank and abdomen may transect or destroy a significant segment of the ureter. The cavitation effect of high-velocity gunshot wounds can result in ureteral necrosis and require extensive reconstruction.

Once the diagnosis of pelviureteric junction disruption is made, the best course of action is to perform an immediate primary repair by using the dismembered pyeloplasty technique. If there is extensive loss of a portion of the ureter, one may need to perform one or more of the following procedures:

• For distal ureteral injuries, one may be able to excise and reimplant the ureter into the bladder.

• For lower-half ureteral injuries, a bladder Boari flap, with or without a psoas hitch technique, may be required.

• For more extensive injuries, the kidney may be mobilised and nephropexy may allow several additional centimetres of length.

• If just the upper ureter remains, a trans-uretero-ureterostomy can be performed.

• If there is significant damage to the renal pelvis and pelviureteric junction, a ureterocalicostomy may be employed with wide amputation of the inferior-most renal parenchyma and anastomosis of the ureter to the lower pole calyx.

• With complete loss of the ureter, one may be required to place a segment of tapered ileum as an interposition tube flap. The appendix has also been used as an interposition tube flap for midureteral injuries on the right side.[9] As a last resort, autotransplantation of the kidney to the iliac vessels can be performed.

Bladder Injury

The bladder is an intraabdominal organ in young children; therefore, it can be easily injured in trauma to the abdomen, regardless of whether it is full or empty. As the bony pelvis grows, the bladder becomes more protected from injury. Blunt trauma is responsible for most bladder injuries. Road traffic accidents and falls from heights are the most common causes of bladder injury in the paediatric age group in the African setting. Pelvic fractures cause injury near the bladder neck, whereas the dome of the bladder is usually affected by direct blow to the lower abdomen. Only a small number of patients with pelvic fractures sustain bladder injury. Patients who present with bladder injury are found to

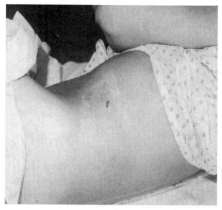

(A)

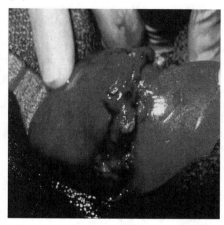

(B)

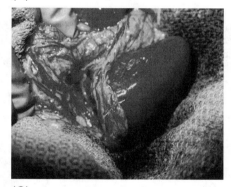

(C)

Figure 31.2: (A) Child who sustained a stab wound to left flank. (B) Renal exploration revealed laceration of the kidney. (C) Following repair of the renal laceration, omentum is placed into the wound to promote healing and prevent urine leakage.

have associated pelvic fractures in 75–90% of the cases. About one-half of bladder injuries in children are associated with other intraabdominal organ injuries.

Classification

Bladder injuries in children can be classified as blunt or penetrating.

Blunt trauma

In a contusion, there is a disruption in bladder muscularis without loss of continuity of the wall. With a rupture, there is complete disruption of the bladder wall.

The cystogram is the ideal radiographic study to diagnose intra- or extraperitoneal rupture. As previously mentioned, the bladder must be filled to at least one-half the expected capacity in a child, or more than 350 ml in the adolescent or adult. Three films should be obtained: the scout, or plain, film; an anteroposterior (AP) film; and a postdrainage film.

Penetrating injury

Penetrating bladder injuries may result from a pelvic fracture with boney penetration or laceration, gunshot wounds, a stabbing, falls onto sharp objects, surgical mishaps (e.g., trochar placement during laparoscopy), migration or erosion from drains, or manipulation of the umbilical artery catheter in neonates.

Management of Bladder Injuries

Contusion

Most cases of bladder contusion do not need treatment and they usually have an excellent outcome. Pelvic haematoma may cause difficulty in micturition, and in these patients, catheter drainage is all that is required.

Extraperitoneal rupture

An extraperitoneal rupture accounts for 80% of bladder injuries. Cystography often reveals a flame-shaped area of contrast extravasation that is confined within the pelvis. In one-fifth of patients, it is associated with urethral injury as well.

The preferred treatment is urethral catheterisation and drainage alone for a period of about 2 weeks. Tears usually heal completely, even if extensive extravasation has occurred. If laparotomy is done for associated intraabdominal injuries, the dome of the bladder is opened and the tear repaired without disturbing any pelvic retroperitoneal haematoma. If the bladder is opened, a temporary suprapubic bladder catheter should be left in place. Repeat cystography should be performed prior to removal of the urethral or suprapubic catheter.

Intraperitoneal rupture

An intraperitoneal rupture occurs mainly at the dome of the bladder and is usually due to a direct blow to the distended bladder or a sudden deceleration injury. Contrast may be seen within the peritoneal cavity outlining the intestines.

Intraperitoneal rupture occurs more commonly in children than adults. Thus, early operative repair is the treatment of choice for children because the presence of urine in the peritoneal cavity can lead to life-threatening metabolic and infectious problems.[10]

Operative Details

The bladder is approached through a lower abdominal incision. One must carefully inspect the ureteral orifices and bladder neck. Overlooking an injury in these areas may result in ureteral obstruction, sepsis, and/or incontinence. An extraperitoneal tear is closed from within the bladder by using absorbable sutures, taking care to avoid occlusion of the ureteric orifices. Suprapubic bladder drainage is maintained for 7–10 days and removed once the cystogram has shown resolution of the extravasation. The peritoneum is drained by using a closed suction drain. The drain is removed when the patient is voiding normally.

Penetrating Injuries

Penetrating injuries of the bladder are managed by laparotomy due to the high incidence of associated injury to other organs. These bladder injuries are often more extensive than seen on radiographic images. Meticulous debridement and dual layer closure of the bladder are key to a successful outcome. If there is also a bowel injury, a flap of omentum should be placed over the bladder repair to prevent formation of a fistula. After thorough debridement of the injury and bladder closure, a suprapubic bladder catheter is left in place and the perivesical area is drained by closed suction drain.

Urethral Injury

Urethral injuries in children can occur as a result of blunt or penetrating trauma to the abdomen, pelvis, and perineum. Blunt trauma with pelvic fracture accounts for most posterior urethral injuries in children. The mechanism of most of these types of injuries include motor vehicle accidents, falls from heights (commonly occurring during fruit har-

vesting season in Africa), crushing and straddle injuries, and sporting injuries. Instrumentation of the urinary tract with catheters, scopes, and sounds may also cause urethral injury, especially in the patient with underlying urethral stricture. Children with congenital anorectal malformations (high imperforate anus) or girls with disorders of sexual differentiation may require surgery that involves the urethra. Prepubertal girls who sustain a pelvic fracture are four times more likely than adult women to have a urethral injury.

Classification of Urethral Injuries

Urethral injuries are classified into four grades:

- *Grade I:* Contusion. Normal urethrogram.

- *Grade II:* Stretch injury. Elongation of urethra with extravasation of contrast on urethrogram, but with visualisation of the bladder. These are usually located in the anterior urethra (penile and bulbar portions). See Figure 31.3.

- *Grade III:* Partial disruption. Elongation without visualisation of bladder on urethrogram. These can occur in either the anterior or posterior urethra (prostatic and membranous portions).

- *Grade IV:* Complete disruption. Complete transection with separation or extension into the prostate or vagina. In children, complete disruption usually occurs in the posterior urethra between the prostatic and membranous portions of the urethra (Figure 31.4).

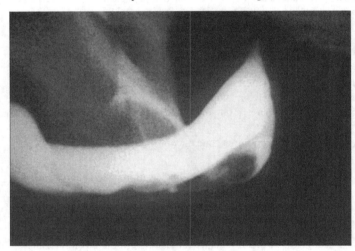

Figure 31.3: Retrograde urethrogram showing grade II urethral stretch injury with extravasation of contrast.

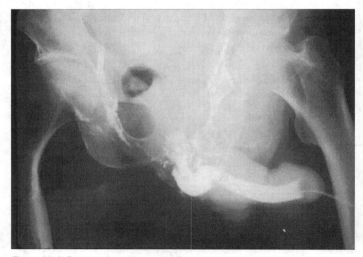

Figure 31.4: Retrograde urethrogram after pelvic fracture showing complete urethral disruption.

Diagnosis

Blood at the external urethral meatus, gross haematuria after trauma, and inability to void after trauma in the presence of the urge to micturate are physical findings in children with urethral injuries. Other findings that may indicate underlying urethral injury include a sensation of micturition without passing urine; swelling; or ecchymosis of the penis, scrotum, and perineum. The urethral tunics include the corpus spongiosum, Buck's fascia, and the outer layer, or Colle's fascia. Urethral rupture is usually confined by Colle's fascia, giving the classic finding of a perineal butterfly haematoma. A digital rectal examination should be done, and if upward displacement of the prostrate is encountered, one should suspect urethral disruption. In girls with blood at the introitus, careful inspection of the vagina should be done. Retrograde urethrography should be done in all children suspected of having urethral injury. This may reveal a filling defect cause by haematoma or contusion or extravasation of contrast.

Management

If a urethral injury is suspected from the history and physical examination of a child, no urethral catheterisation should be done until urethral rupture has been ruled out. An emergency retrograde urethrogram is done to ascertain the nature (grade) of the injury. If the urethrogram is not possible on an emergency basis, a suprapubic bladder catheter is inserted and urethrogram done the following day.

Grade I and II injuries are managed without surgery and without an indwelling urethral catheter.

For grade III injuries, a suprapubic bladder catheter usually is inserted. However, if the urethra is not completely transected and contrast is seen entering the posterior urethra and bladder, a Foley catheter (especially one with a coude-tip) can be inserted carefully under fluoroscopic guidance. Another option is to use a cystoscope to place a wire across the defect and then a council-tip catheter over the wire into the bladder. After 10–14 days, a cystourethrogram is performed. If there is no extravasation or stricture, the catheter is removed. Careful follow-up is necessary because a stricture may occur months or years later. The best results are obtained by ensuring the urethral lumen is patent, even if this requires open repair of the urethra tear within 10–14 days, before the tissues have become rigid.

For grade IV injuries, or complete disruption, a suprapubic catheter should be inserted. Usually, these patients are severely injured, and an attempt to reapproximate the disrupted bladder neck and prostatic urethra to the membranous urethra may provoke further bleeding from the pelvic haematoma and worsen the child's condition. The sooner the ends of the urethra are brought together, however, the better. This is usually facilitated by accurate reduction and fixation of the pelvic fractures. Once the child is stabilised, immediate (within 2 days) realignment of the urethra over a catheter can be attempted. If the child is unstable, delayed repair (2–14 days) can be attempted by using cystourethrography and limited suprapubic manipulation and downward displacement of the bladder. If the anterior urethra is completely blocked, perineal urethroscopy can be performed. In some situations, late repair (>3 months) must be done and may require extensive pelvic surgery, including transpubic urethroplasty or a combined suprapubic and perineal approach with or without pubectomy.[11,12] Long-term complications from complete urethral disruption may include erectile dysfunction and incontinence. Urethral injuries are rare in girls; however, in the presence of pelvic fracture and blood at the meatus/introitus, one must carefully inspect the vagina and retrograde urethrogram or cystoscopy for injury. Urethral injuries in girls may result in urethral stenosis, urethrovaginal fistula, urinary incontinence, and vaginal stenosis. Meticulous management is needed to avoid these serious complications.

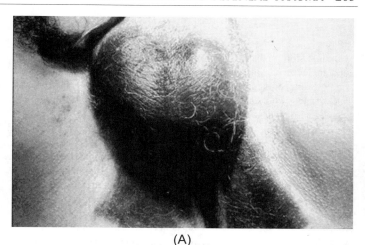

(A)

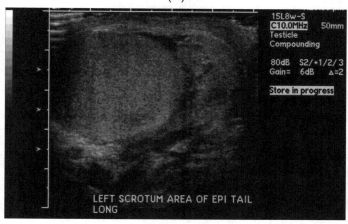

(B)

(C)

Figure 31.5: (A) Scrotal/perineal haematoma with (B) ultrasound showing disruption of the tunica albuginea. (C) Exploration reveals rupture of the inferior pole of the testis.

Genital and Scrotal Injuries

Boys

Circumcision mishap is the commonest cause of penile injury in boys and includes partial glans and/or meatal amputation or skin degloving.[13,14] The penis may also be injured in motor vehicle accidents, falls and straddle injuries, and animal or human bites. Penile injuries may also be associated with scrotal and testicular injuries.

Circumcision injuries should be immediately debrided and lacerations repaired. In cases of partial glans amputation, reattachment of the excised segment should be done immediately. Complete amputation in children is exceedingly rare. If significant skin loss has occurred, a split-thickness skin graft may be required.

Scrotal and testicular injuries occur from mechanisms similar to those for penile and urethral injuries. Trauma from sports is perhaps the most common form of blunt injury to the scrotum. If there is significant swelling of the scrotum and one cannot completely or adequately examine the testes, an ultrasound or CT scan should be immediately obtained. Ultrasound documentation of disruption of the tunica albuginea of the testis or the presence of a haematocele should prompt immediate exploration of the scrotum, given the high likelihood of testicular rupture (Figure 31.5). A drain should be placed into the scrotum following exploration and repair of testicular rupture.

Girls

Genital injuries in girls may result from sexual abuse or straddle injuries.[15] Types of injuries include lacerations or contusions of the perineal body, vagina, and labia. Adequate evaluation for abuse is necessary if this is suspected. Necrotic tissues should be debrided and lacerations repaired.

Evidence-Based Research

Table 31.1 presents a study to develop a prediction model for the need for exploration after renal trauma.[7]

Table 31.1: Evidence-based research.

Title	Development of a highly accurate nomogram for prediction of the need for exploration in patients with renal trauma
Authors	Shariat SF, Trinh QD, Morey AF, Stage KH, Roehrborn CG, Valiquette L, Karakiewicz PI
Institution	Department of Urology, University of Texas Southwestern Medical Center, Dallas, Texas, USA; Cancer Prognostics and Health Outcomes Unit, University of Montreal, Montreal, Quebec, Canada; Brooke Army Medical Center (AFM), Fort Sam Houston, Houston, Texas, USA
Reference	J Trauma Injury Infect Crit Care 2008; 64(6):1451–1458
Problem	To develop a highly accurate nomogram for predicting which patients would need exploration after renal trauma.
Comparison/control (quality of evidence)	Logistic regression models were used to develop a nomogram for prediction of the need for renal exploration after renal trauma. Internal (200 bootstrap resamples) and 50% split sample validations were performed.
Outcome/effect	Overall, 89 patients (21.2%) underwent renal exploration, from which 60.7% (54 of 89) underwent nephrectomy and 39.3% (35 of the 89) underwent renorrhaphy. Nine percent of patients with grade II injury underwent renal exploration, 16% with grade III injuries, 41% with grade IV injuries, and 100% of grade V injuries. The kidney injury scale, the mechanism of injury, the need for transfusion, blood urea nitrogen level, and serum creatinine represented the most informative predictors of the need for renal exploration, and were included in the nomogram. The split sample accuracy of the nomogram for prediction of the need for renal exploration was 96.9%. It significantly (p < 0.001) exceeded the accuracy of each of its components, including the American Association for the Surgery of Trauma kidney injury scale (87.7%).
Historical significance/comments	This article gives the scientific basis for predicting which patients with renal injury would need exploration, and whether it could be applied to children with renal injury. The nomogram generates highly accurate and reproducible predictions of the probability for renal exploration according to the authors' decision-making process. It could help standardise the management of patients with renal trauma (i.e., inclusion criteria for clinical trials) and serves as a proof-of-principle that predictive tools can be applied to the trauma setting. Its use may improve the management of renal trauma patients at institutions with limited trauma experience.

Key Summary Points

1. The urogenital tract is involved in up to 12% of children with injuries.

2. Perineal injuries are quite common in children.

3. Most urogenital and perineal injuries follow blunt trauma. Road traffic accidents are the most common. Child abuse should be suspected in unusual cases.

4. Due to advances in radiological imaging, evaluation and identification of most urological tract injuries in children can be made nonoperatively; the operation rate has therefore greatly decreased.

5. The aim of managing a child with renal trauma is the preservation of renal function.

References

1. Garcia VF, Sheldon C. Genitourinary tract trauma. In: O'Neil JA, Rowe MI, Grosfeld JA, Fonkalsrud EW, Coran AJ, eds. Pediatric Surgery, 1998, Pp 205–302.

2. Nakayama DN. Abdominal and genitourinary trauma. In: O'Neil JA, Grosfeld JL, Fonkalsrud EW, Coran AG, Caldamone AA, eds. Principles of Pediatric Surgery, 2nd ed. Mosby, 2004, Pp 159–175.

3. Chirdan LB, Uba AF, Yiltok SJ, Ramyil VM. Paediatric blunt abdominal trauma: challenges of management in a developing country. Eur J Pediatr Surg 2007; 17:1–6.

4. Chirdan LB, Mbibu HN. Urogenital trauma. In: Ameh EA, Nwomeh BC, eds. Paediatric Trauma Care in Africa: A Practical Guide. Spectrum Books Ltd, 2006, Pp 70–82.

5. Polsky EG, Smaldone MC, Gaines BA, Schneck FX, Bellinger MF, Docimo SG, Wu HY. Computerized tomography findings in pediatric renal trauma—indications for early intervention? J Urol 2008; 179:1529–1532.

6. McAninch J, Carroll PR. Renal exploration after trauma: indications and reconstructive techniques. Urol Clin North Am 1989; 16:203–212.

7. Shariat SF, Trinh QD, Morey AF, Stage KH, Roehrborn CG, Valiquette L, Karakiewicz PI. Development of a highly accurate nomogram for prediction of the need for exploration in patients with renal trauma. J Trauma 2008; 64:1451–1458.

8. Henderson CG, Sedberry-Ross S, Pickard R, Bulas DI, Duffy BJ, Tsung D, Eichelberger MR, Belman AB, Rushton HG. Management of high grade renal trauma: 20-year experience at a pediatric level I trauma center. J Urol 2007; 178:246–250.

9. Dagash H, Sen S, Chacko J, Karl S, Ghosh D, Parag P, Mackinnon AE. The appendix as ureteral substitute: a report of 10 cases. J Pediatr Urol 2008; 14:14–19.

10. Routh JC, Husmann DA. Long-term continence outcomes after immediate repair of pediatric bladder neck lacerations extending into the urethra J Urol 2007; 178:1816–1818.

11. Orabi S, Badawy H, Saad A, Youssef M, Hanno A. Post-traumatic posterior urethral stricture in children: how to achieve a successful repair. J Pediatr Urol 2008; 4:290–294.

12. Singla M, Jha MS, Muruganandam K, Srivastava A, Ansari MS, Mandhani A, Dubey D, Kapoor R. Posttraumatic posterior urethral strictures in children—management and intermediate-term follow-up in tertiary care center. Urology 2008; 72:540–544.

13. Ahmed A, Mbibu HN. Aetiology and management of injuries to male external genitalia in Nigeria. Injury 2008; 39:136.

14. Okeke LI, Asinobi AA, Ikuerowo AS. Epidemiology of complications of male circumcision in Ibadan, Nigeria. BMC Urology 2006; 6:21.

15. Abassiatai AM, Etuk SJ, Asuquo EE, Udoma EJ, Bassey EA. Reasons for gynaecological consultations in children in Calabar, South Eastern Nigeria. Trop Doct 2007; 37:90–92.

CHAPTER 32
MUSCULOSKELETAL TRAUMA

Jonathan I. Groner
Michael O. Ogirima

Introduction

Musculoskeletal trauma principally includes fractures of the bones of the extremities; however, ligamentous injuries, joint injuries, and soft tissue trauma involving muscle may also be placed in this category. This represents one of the major burdens of injury in children. In developed countries, many extremity fractures are of little consequence and are often regarded as a "badge of courage"; the child is immobilised in a plaster or fiberglass cast for a few weeks and then returns to normal activity. In the third world, however, extremity fractures and other musculoskeletal trauma can result in permanent disability and even life-threatening injuries. Perhaps the most serious complication of fracture management in Africa is "bonesetter's limbs" or "bonesetter's gangrene", which, if it does not kill the patient, can destroy all of the soft tissue of the affected limb, leaving only contractures or exposed bones.[1]

Demographics

Data from a large paediatric trauma centre in the United States indicate that fractures are the reason for more than half of all children's admissions to the hospital for injuries. The most common injury mechanism is a fall, and the most common fracture from this mechanism is a supracondylar humerus fracture. The most common bone fracture seen in victims of both motor vehicle crashes and child abuse is of the femur. The most common bone fracture in children up to age 10 years is to the humerus, and the most common bone fracture from age 11 to 15 years is to the tibia/fibula.

Data from other studies indicate that the most common paediatric long bone fracture occurs at the forearm, followed by the femur, and then the tibia. Approximately half of all tibia fractures occur in the distal third of the bone, and 70% of tibia fractures occur as isolated injuries.[2] Combined tibia/fibula fractures are most often the result of high energy trauma such as motor vehicle crashes.[2]

The incidence of paediatric musculoskeletal trauma in most African countries is unknown; however, fractures are quite common in childhood. Fractures were the second most common injury (after burns) among 798 injured children treated at Royal Victoria Hospital (RVH) in Banjul, The Gambia.[3] Motor vehicle crashes accounted for 50% of the fractures in one study.[4] Penetrating trauma can cause musculoskeletal trauma as well.

Aetiology/Pathophysiology

Most musculoskeletal trauma is caused by falls, motor vehicle crashes, and pedestrian/vehicle injuries. Child abuse is an extremely important cause of these injuries in infants and young children. One US study demonstrated that 67% of lower extremity injuries in patients younger than 18 months of age admitted to a trauma centre were due to child abuse.[5] There is virtually no literature, however, on child-abuse–associated musculoskeletal trauma in Africa. One of the rare studies of child abuse in Africa demonstrated that, of 916 paediatric autopsies for "unnatural deaths", 24 (2.6%) were attributed to child abuse.[6] By contrast, 30–50% of the paediatric fatalities at some paediatric trauma centres in the United States are due to abuse-related injuries.

Clinical Presentation

History

The history for most musculoskeletal injuries is obvious. Most children with tibia fractures, for example, will present with a history of a traumatic event. In addition, these children typically have pain, inability to bear weight, and swelling or deformity.[2]

However, injured patients younger than 3 years of age must be evaluated carefully, as 90% of child abuse cases occur in this age group.[5] These children are nonverbal, so the history must be provided by parents or caregivers. A history that changes over time or is told differently by different adults raises suspicion of an abusive injury. Likewise, a history that is not consistent with the child's developmental ability should also raise concerns. Although child-abuse–related fractures are seen daily in major paediatric trauma centres across the United States, this mechanism of injury in children is scarcely reported in the African literature.[6,7]

Physical Examination

Tenderness, pain, and swelling of an extremity or bony prominence are the hallmarks of musculoskeletal trauma. The majority of long bone fractures will have significant pain, tenderness at the fracture site, pain with passive motion, and inability to bear weight. Bruising is often not seen acutely but may develop later.

One major pitfall when examining a child for possible musculoskeletal trauma is the failure to recognise an open fracture. With some fracture mechanisms, a long bone fragment may transiently protrude through a break in the skin, only to retract when the extremity is returned to normal position. Therefore, any break in the skin in close proximity to the fracture site should be considered an open fracture.

Open fractures are categorised into three types:

- Type I: Wounds are smaller than 1 cm with minimal soft tissue damage or contamination.

- Type II: Wounds are greater than 1 cm but without extensive soft tissue damage.

- Type III: Extensive soft tissue injury can be subcategorised as having adequate soft tissue for coverage, inadequate coverage, or vascular injury requiring repair.

All patients with musculoskeletal injuries require a thorough neurovascular examination. It is critical to identify vascular injury early, so that limb loss can be prevented. The "5 P's" mnemonic is used to look for signs of vascular insufficiency in an injured limb:

1. *Pain* is the most sensitive sign. Note that this refers to pain in the distal extremity (i.e., hand or foot), not at the fracture site.

2. *Paraesthesias* is numbness as well as loss of proprioception (position sense).

3. *Pallor* is pale appearance of the hands or feet.

4. *Poikolothermia* is cold to the touch.

5. *Pulselessness* is a late sign. Permanent muscle damage has probably already occurred by the time pulses are lost.

The fractures most commonly associated with vascular injuries are supracondylar fracture of the humerus (brachial artery injury), posterior knee dislocation (popliteal artery injury), and distal femur fracture (distal femoral artery injury).

In most cases, fracture reduction is all that is required to relieve compression of the artery and restore circulation. If many hours have elapsed between injury and fracture reduction, however, fasciotomy may be required to restore adequate blood flow to the extremity. If the combination of fracture reduction and fasciotomy does not restore perfusion to the extremity (as evidenced by return of pulse, capillary refill, and sensation), it is likely that an arterial thrombosis is present. The choice at this point becomes vascular reconstruction or amputation if gangrene begins to set in and threatens life. Reconstruction can require an arteriogram, exploration of the arterial injury, a vein patch, or even a reverse autologous vein graft, which is not likely to be available in rural areas except in major teaching hospitals.

Even in the absence of the suspicion of a fracture, it is important to examine all soft tissue wounds for evidence of penetration into the muscle, dirt contamination, and the presence of other foreign bodies. Deep contaminated wounds are setups for serious infections. It is difficult to get children to cooperate with infiltration with local anaesthetics for exploration of wounds; therefore, the use of general anaesthetics is advocated for full exploration of deep wounds in most cases.

Investigations

Plain film radiography remains the standard diagnostic modality for most fractures. At least two images that are at right angles to each other should be obtained. In addition, plain films should also include the joint above and below (proximal and distal to) the fracture site. Not all fractures are immediately apparent on initial radiographs. Images should be repeated 1 to 2 weeks after injury if pain persists.

Plain film imaging, using lower energy "soft tissue" settings, can be useful for identifying imbedded foreign bodies or undisplaced subtle fractures (such as the fat pad sign seen in intraarticular fractures of the elbow). The presence of gas bubbles in the soft tissues on plain film imaging is an ominous sign of a potentially life-threatening anaerobic soft tissue infection. Plain film radiography is also useful for detecting dislocations in children.

Management

Stabilising the Patient at Presentation

A head-to-toe general examination of the fully undressed child should be carried out on presentation. First, the patient is assessed for associated injuries, particularly in injuries from high-energy mechanisms such as motor vehicle crashes. Thereafter, when other life-threatening injuries have been excluded, an examination of the injured limb is done. After the examination of the injured extremity is complete, including a thorough neurovascular examination, a splint is applied. Splinting the injured extremity reduces pain and discomfort, minimises further soft tissue trauma, preserves neurovascular function, prevents swelling of the soft tissue, and makes future repairs easier.

If bone is protruding through an open wound in the skin (an open fracture), thorough pulsatile irrigation with isotonic saline and coverage with sterile dressing soaked with the saline should be done. No attempt should be made to return the bone to the depths of the wound until debridement and cleansing have been achieved in an orthopaedic unit. Splints can be made out of virtually any rigid material; even folded magazines bound with loose mesh gauze can be used to splint a forearm fracture. Sling and swath is used for fractures of the humerus or the shoulder girdle. Femur fractures typically can be bound to the other thigh with a splint or traction may be used. All open fractures must be covered with parenteral third-generation cephalosporins and tetanus prophylaxis, and the patient should receive pain medication.

For seriously injured children, it is important to remember that no matter how severe the injured extremity, the patient's life has priority over the limb. In the initial hours after a child suffers a mangled extremity, the two most likely causes of death are hypovolaemia (from haemorrhage) and hypothermia. The standard Advanced Trauma Life Support (ATLS®) resuscitation protocol of the American College of Surgeons is designed to address these issues. Patients with complex open fractures or fractures requiring internal or external fixation will likely require transfer to an orthopaedic unit. Proper attention to these injuries will improve their outcome.

Wound Care, Damage Control, and Life-Saving Operations

Care of the soft tissue trauma in association with fractures takes precedence over the definitive treatment of the fracture. The bone needs an envelope of healthy soft tissue for optimal healing. Therefore wound cleaning and debridement are essential. Damaged muscle is an excellent growth media for bacteria. Copious irrigation with normal saline solution and manual debridement is probably as important as antibiotic coverage in preventing infection. This procedure may need to be repeated more than once to achieve a clean, healing wound. In the absence of intravenous antibiotics, deep wounds involving muscle should probably be left open with twice daily dressing changes. These wounds will gradually heal by secondary intention.

Damage control orthopaedics can be defined as an operation that corrects that underlying pathophysiology (hypothermia, wound contamination, vascular obstruction) without necessarily correcting the pathology (such as a long bone fracture). The damage control philosophy emphasizes (1) prevention of hypothermia; (2) removal of all foreign material and bacterial contamination from the wound; (3) reduction of fractures and traction, if necessary, to reduce vascular compromise; (4) sterile dressings; and (5) a planned return trip to the operating room to complete the definitive repair. Damage control orthopaedics can also be considered a "life over limb" approach, meaning that saving the child's life is given priority over definitive repair of the extremity injury. In a worst-case scenario, amputation of a potential viable extremity may be contemplated. The consideration for amputation should be based on weighing the condition of the patient, the condition of the extremity, and the resources available to treat the patient.

Treatment of Musculoskeletal Trauma

Management of musculoskeletal trauma can be divided into three phases:

1. reduction of fracture;

2. immobilisation; and

3. rehabilitation.

Reduction of fractures

The goals of fracture management are (1) satisfactory bone healing (return to full weight bearing), (2) full mobility of the limb, and (3) no limb-length discrepancy. To accomplish these goals, the fracture must first be reduced.

Nonoperative treatment

The closed method (or nonoperative treatment) of fracture reduction can be done under general or local anaesthesia. Local anaesthesia can be applied to the fracture haematoma for safe and effective fracture reduction. This is particularly useful in situations where general anaesthesia is not readily available. The use of longer-acting local anaesthetics will provide pain relief for several hours after the reduction. An injection of 0.5% bupivacaine with epinephrine (1:200,000) can be administered locally at a dose of 0.5 ml/kg body weight. For patients weighing less than 10 kg, 0.25% bupivacaine with epinephrine (1:200,000) can be used at 1 ml/kg body weight. Care must be taken to avoid intravascular injection, and the injection should be performed at least 30–40 minutes before the procedure to allow maximal effect. In children with fractures of both bones of the forearm, both sites must be anaesthetised for reduction.

Ideally, fractures should be reduced under an image intensifier (C-arm). When this is not possible, fractures should be reduced by palpation only, then postreduction plain films must be obtained immediately to verify the result. It is particularly important to correct rotation when reducing fractures; otherwise, a permanent deformity will result. Some degree of fracture overlap may be acceptable and beneficial due to the overgrowth phenomenon in skeletally immature bones.

This closed method of fracture reduction is applicable to even type I open fractures, with a resultant infection rate in some series of 2.5%.[8]

Operative treatment

Many closed fractures in the adolescent age group are managed operatively in the developed countries. Open fractures are generally considered orthopaedic emergencies. Most orthopaedic surgeons agree that type II and III open fractures require urgent operative management. The goal of operative management of type II and III open fractures is to prevent infection in or around the fracture site, which can lead to osteomyelitis. Infection prevention is accomplished by: (1) administration of antibiotics, (2) copious irrigation and removal of all foreign material, (3) debridement of all devitalised tissue, and (4) coverage of all exposed bones when possible. Irrigation is generally accomplished with several litres of warmed normal saline. Battery-powered pulse irrigation devices are available in the United States. A reasonable substitute is a 60-ml syringe attached to sterile intravenous (IV) tubing with a three-way stopcock. The IV tubing is attached to a bag of warm, sterile saline off the surgical field. The stopcock is rotated to allow rapid filling, then flushing of 60-ml aliquots of saline for cleansing the wound. The saline should be ejected with force to dislodge contaminants in the wound.

Immobilisation

Casts

Once closed reduction has been effected on fractures, casts could be used to immobilise it. Casts are bandages that contain chemicals that harden after water is applied. Plaster cast materials contain anhydrous calcium sulfate, which solidifies when water is added. An injured extremity must be covered with a layer of gauze or cotton padding (such as orthoban) before a cast can be applied. Additional padding should be applied to bony prominences. The cast material must be molded over bony prominences and joints. As a general rule, the joint proximal and distal to the fractured bone must be included in the cast to fully immobilise the fractured bone. However, fingertips or toes must be left exposed so that peripheral circulation can be evaluated.

The most serious complication of plaster cast application for fracture immobilisation is vascular insufficiency due to unrelieved swelling. This is the pathophysiology of bonesetter's gangrene, a serious and potentially life-threatening complication of the folk medicine practice of tightly splinting fractured extremities. The resulting vascular insufficiency leads to gangrene that is usually advanced by the time the patient seeks attention at a hospital. In one review of 35 major extremity amputations among children at a centre in Nigeria, 26 were due to trauma, and 24 of these patients had "simple, straightforward fractures" that were treated by traditional bonesetters.[9]

In the case of a cast, if unrelieved pain, sensory loss, or motor paralysis occurs, the cast must be opened immediately by splitting the cast down to the skin, allowing expansion and return of circulation. If the patient complains of localised pain, then a pressure point may be developing under the cast. The treatment of this condition is to cut a "window" into the cast, add more padding to the area, then cover the window with additional plaster.

Casts commonly used in children include the "short arm cast" for wrist fractures, which extends from just below the elbow to the metacarpo-phalangeal joints but leaves the thumb free. Forearm fractures require casting above the elbow (with the elbow at 90°).

A long leg cast extends from the proximal thigh to the metatarsophalangeal joints, and is used to treat tibia fractures. Immobilising the femur is particularly difficult because the hips must be stabilised, which requires a hip spica cast. This cast begins just below the nipples and extends to the thigh on the unaffected side and the ankle on the injured side. This is particularly useful for fractures in infants.

Traction

Traction, which is application of force along the axis of the injured bone, is used to overcome muscle spasm to reduce fractures in long bones. It is also used to immobilise long bone fractures. In other words, patients on traction do not require casts. There are two main types of traction: skin traction, where up to 5 kg of weight can be applied by attaching adhesive tapes to the skin; and skeletal traction, which requires a pin inserted transversely through a bone, taking care not to go through the growth plates to avoid premature epiphysiodesis and shortening of the bone. Traction can also be applied by gravity acting on the weight of the upper limb or a combination of traction and a cast. These are seen in distal fractures of the humerus with a hanging cast.

In children, skin traction can usually provide enough traction to overcome muscle tension and reduce most fractures. Russell's traction uses a weighted cord to elevate the knee and distract the lower leg, and is useful for fractures of the femoral shaft. In younger children and toddlers, Bryant's traction is used for femoral fractures: both feet and legs are suspended from the bed.

Traction is also useful to reduce an anterior shoulder dislocation, which typically occurs from a fall on an abducted arm. More than 90% of these dislocations can be reduced by having the patient lie prone on a table with the arm hanging down by the side. The dependent arm is weighted to increase the traction. Following reduction, the arm is immobilised to the body with the elbow at 90°.

Other methods

Fractures of the clavicle can be managed with a figure-of-eight splint that draws back and elevates the shoulders. This position applies traction on the distal clavicle and stabilises the fracture. These splints may occasionally cause swelling of the arms and hands.

After operative reduction of fractures, many hardware options are available to internally fix or immobilise the fractures, depending on the fracture configuration and proximity of fractures to the growth plates. This hardware includes smooth pins and wires, plates and screws, and external fixators (Figure 32.1). Intermedullary nails (interlocking or not) are not commonly used in children for fear of premature epiphysiodesis. Implants are available in most orthopaedic units in Africa, but tractions and casts are devices that are still handy in remote practice areas. The advantage of internal fixation is that it leads to earlier mobilisation. Any hardware used in children should be removed as soon as consolidation of the fracture sites are achieved; otherwise, growing bones could overgrow the implants and even mold onto the contours of the implants. This makes delayed removal difficult and sometimes impossible and abandoned. The development of biodegradable implants has solved these challenges.

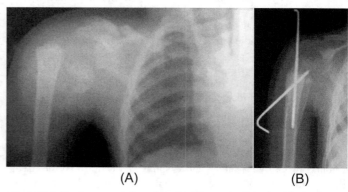

(A)   (B)

Figure 32.1: Fracture separation of proximal humeral epiphysis with shoulder dislocation (A) before treatment; (B) treated with smooth cross pin fixation.

The minimal access surgery with the aid of an image intensifier in the developed world is gradually being practiced in Nigeria and can be helpful in intraarticular fractures.

Postoperative Complications

Fortunately, nonunion of fractures is extremely rare in children. In addition, fairly significant fracture angulation will correct itself with the remodeling process that occurs during healing. Infection of an open fracture leading to osteomyelitis is a dreaded complication because it can be extremely difficult to treat, requiring long-term antibiotics and debridement of the bone to achieve control.

Prognosis and Outcomes

Fortunately, children have very resilient bones, and most fractures, including some with significant angulation, will heal without complication. Vitamin D deficiency and malnutrition can lead to delayed or poor wound healing. Lack of tetanus prophylaxis can be life-threatening following major soft tissue trauma, as the tetanus organism is common in the soil.

For open fractures, prognosis is directly affected by the availability of health care. Open fractures require treatment within 4 to 6 hours of injury. If open wounds at a fracture site are not treated by that time, the risk of infection increases markedly (Figure 32.2).

Dislocations, once promptly recognised and reduced, result in excellent outcome with a full range of movement and stable joint. Unfortunately, ignorance and cultural beliefs and (to a little extent) poverty in developing countries have led to late presentations, condemning many joints.

Prevention

Because there are very little continentwide or even countrywide paediatric trauma data, injury prevention is a difficult task in Africa. Clearly, motor vehicle usage is increasing, and motor vehicle crashes place children at high risk for major musculoskeletal injuries. Surgeons should advocate for children riding in the back seat, wearing proper restraint devices, and using car seats or booster seats where available. Children are far more likely to die when they are unrestrained and ride in the front passenger seat of the vehicle.

In urban environments, falls from heights, particularly from upper levels of multistorey buildings, are a significant cause of major injury and death. The placement of window guards, which prevent toddlers and small children from falling out of upper-storey windows, has been associated with a significant reduction in injury and death in densely populated urban neighborhoods in New York City. This pioneering work is an example of a paediatric surgeon advocating for the safety of children.[10]

In rural areas, many fractures are due to falls from economic trees. Better fruit harvesting techniques should be promoted.

Firearm trauma is also common in Africa, and more likely due to political (civil war or communal clashes) than criminal (robbery) reasons, compared to Western countries.[11,12] In a study from Nigeria, more than 40% of casualties involved noncombatants (mainly government workers and students), and the most common skeletal injury from gunfire was a femur fracture.[12] Firearm injury prevention in Africa is an enormous challenge due to political unrest and high levels of gun ownership.[11,12]

Finally, surgeons must advocate to limit or end the practise of traditional bonesetting (Figure 32.3). Complications of traditional bonesetting include nonunion or malunion (Figure 32.4) and wet gangrene, requiring amputation.[13] Nonunion or malunion typically requires open reduction and internal fixation. Death from sepsis has also occurred. Nevertheless, one recent study demonstrated that 14 of 46 patients admitted in a hospital with a known fracture opted for treatment by a bonesetter. The availability of health care facilities, the cultural environment, and the financial status of the patient were among

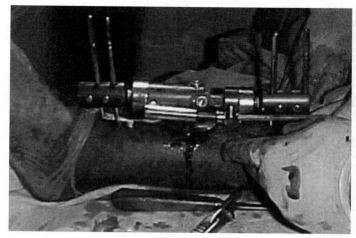

Figure 32.2: Orthofix in place to treat open infected fracture of the tibia.

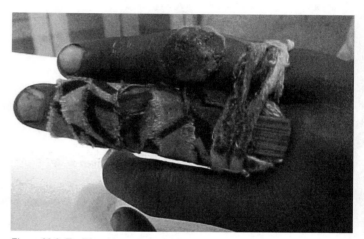

Figure 32.3: Traditional bonesetters' splints in use.

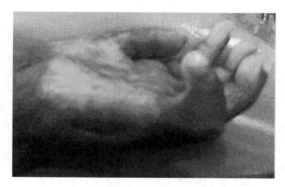

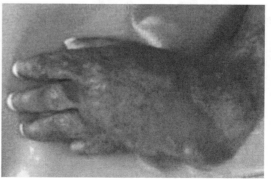

Figure 32.4: Volksmann's ischaemic contracture of the wrist from tight traditional bonesetter's splint.

the reasons patients sought alternative care.[14] Clearly, more specialists must be trained to manage these injuries, which will eliminate the menace of traditional bonesetters in the long run.

Perhaps it is possible that African paediatric surgeons could negotiate some form of peaceful coexistence with traditional healers, so that their methods, which are highly regarded in some communities, are supplemented by modern biomedical science to prevent catastrophes; this form of relationship has been successful with traditional birth attendants in reducing maternal mortality rates in Nigeria.

Ethical Issues

In the setting of major soft tissue infections, open wounds, or complex open fractures in African children, the decision to perform an amputation can be extremely difficult. Western countries have countless approaches to these complex injuries, including hyperbaric oxygen for soft tissue infections and microvascular tissue transfer for massive open wounds. However, these are extremely expensive procedures that require prolonged hospitalisations and frequent return trips to specialists. Due to the limitations in resources and transportation in Africa, it is possible that an early amputation will result in more rapid healing of wounds, less burden on the family, and a more rapid return to a stable home life. Limb loss may have consequences, however, when the child becomes an adult with a disability. Thus, the decision to amputate an extremity will weigh heavily on a surgeon.

Evidence-Based Research

Table 32.1 presents a retrospective case series involving nonoperative management of paediatric type I open fractures of the tibia. Table 32.2 presents a retrospective case series involving bonesetter's gangrene.

Table 32.1: Evidence-based research.

Title	Nonoperative management of pediatric type I open fractures
Authors	Iobst CA, Tidwell MA, King WF
Institution	Miami Children's Hospital, Miami, Florida, USA
Reference	J Pediatr Orthop 2005; 25(4):513–517
Problem	Open tibial fractures.
Intervention	Nonoperative management of type I open fractures using antibiotics, wound cleansing, sterile dressings, and fracture immobilisation.
Comparison/ control (quality of evidence)	Retrospective case series, no controls.
Outcome/effect	There was only 1 deep infection out of 40 patients treated with the nonoperative management protocol (2.5%).
Historical significance/ comments	The techniques described in this paper could be easily adapted to the care of open fractures in children in Africa.

Table 32.2: Evidence-based research.

Title	Bone setter's gangrene
Authors	Bickler SW, Sanno-Duanda B
Institution	Department of Surgery, Royal Victoria Hospital, Banjul, The Gambia; Division of Pediatric Surgery, Department of Surgery, University of California, San Diego Medical Center, San Diego, California, USA
Reference	J Pediatr Surgery 2000; 35(10):1431–1433
Problem	Bonesetter's gangrene.
Comparison/ control (quality of evidence)	Retrospective case series, no controls.
Outcome/effect	Nine children were treated for bonesetter's gangrene during a 29- month period, accounting for 0.5% of all paediatric surgical admissions. The average age of children with bonesetter's gangrene was 8.2 years (range, 5 to 14 years). There were 6 boys and 3 girls (male to female ratio, 2:1). The left upper extremity was most commonly involved (n = 54), followed by the right upper (n = 53) and left lower (n = 51). Eight of 9 children (89%) were from rural areas in which access to health care was limited.
Historical significance/ comments	Bonesetter's gangrene is a major public health problem for children in Africa.

Key Summary Points

1. Fractures are common among children in Africa.

2. Traditional bonesetters commonly treat fractures in rural areas. This treatment may result in nonunion, ischaemic contracture, gangrene of the effected extremity, and even death. Encouraging parents to seek professional orthopaedic care for their children should be a major public health priority in Africa.

3. Nonoperative fracture reduction with immobilisation is the mainstay of fracture management for rural African children. The majority of extremity fractures will have good results with these techniques, and most children will return to full function.

4. Simple (type I) open fractures can be treated with antibiotics, local wound cleansing, sterile dressings, and fracture immobilisation.

5. Deep wounds into the muscle, even in the absence of fractures, require inspection, foreign body removal, and cleansing to prevent infection.

6. It is important to remember the "life over limb" philosophy when a child with a mangled extremity is encountered. Resuscitation is the first priority. The principles of orthopaedic damage control should be followed. It is possible that an amputation will be necessary to save the child's life.

7. There is almost no literature on child abuse in Africa. However, it is a major cause of injury and death in the United States, suggesting that these cases likely also occur in Africa.

References

1. Bickler SW, Sanno-Duanda B. Bone setter's gangrene. J Pediatr Surg 2000; 35:1431–1433.

2. Setter KJ, Palomino KE. Pediatric tibia fractures: current concepts. Curr Opin Pediatr 2006; 18:30–35.

3. Shen C, Sanno-Duanda B, Bickler SW. Pediatric trauma at a government referral hospital in The Gambia. West Afr J Med 2003; 22:287–290.

4. Archibong AE, Onuba O. Fractures in children in south eastern Nigeria. Cent Afr J Med 1996; 42:340–343.

5. Coffey C, Haley K, Hayes J, Groner JI. The risk of child abuse in infants and toddlers with lower extremity injuries. J Pediatr Surg 2005; 40:120–123.

6. Phillips VM, Van Der Heyde Y. Oro-facial trauma in child abuse fatalities. S Afr Med J 2006; 96:213–215.

7. Saidi H, Odula P, Awori K. Child maltreatment at a violence recovery centre in Kenya. Trop Doct 2008; 38:87–89.

8. Iobst CA, Tidwell MA, King WF. Nonoperative management of pediatric type I open fractures. J Pediatr Orthop 2005; 25:513–517.

9. Akinyoola AL, Oginni LM, Adegbehingbe OO, Orimolade EA, Ogundele OJ. Causes of limb amputations in Nigerian children. West Afr J Med 2006; 25:273–275.

10. Pressley JC, Barlow B. Child and adolescent injury as a result of falls from buildings and structures. Inj Prev 2005; 1:267–273.

11. Aderounmu AO, Fadiora SO, Adesunkanmi AR, Agbakwuru EA, Oluwadiya KS, Adetunji OS. The pattern of gunshot injuries in a communal clash as seen in two Nigerian teaching hospitals. J Trauma 2003; 55:626–630.

12. Yinusa W, Ogirima M O. Extremity gunshot injuries in civilian practice: The National Orthopaedic Hospital Igbobi Experience. West Afr J Med 2000; 19:312–316.

13. Alonge TO, Dongo AE, Nottidge TE, Omololu AB, Ogunlade SO. Traditional bonesetters in south western Nigeria—friends or foes? West Afr J Med 2004; 23:81–84.

14. Aries MJ, Joosten H, Wegdam HH, van der Geest S. Fracture treatment by bonesetters in central Ghana: patients explain their choices and experiences. Trop Med Int Health 2007; 12:564–574.

CHAPTER 33
BURNS

Peter Nthumba
Renata Fabia

Introduction

A burn wound is a wound resulting from physical heat (thermal), chemical agents, or electric current applied to any part of the body. Burn injuries are common, complex injuries of cutaneous and underlying structures that are particularly difficult to manage in Africa due to inadequacies in infrastructure, resources, and staff. Factors such as poverty, illiteracy, urban migration, and the development of slums and shanty towns contribute to the high incidence of burn injuries in African children.

Burn injuries produce significant morbidity and mortality, particularly in children younger than 5 years of age. Prevention of burn injuries is of great importance because the consequences of burn injury in a child are scars that affect the child's life in a variety of ways.

Demographics

Although burn injuries are quite common, exact statistics are not available. Extrapolation from population-based studies suggests that the incidence of hospitalised paediatric burn patients is highest in Africa and lowest in the Americas, Europe, the Middle East, and Asia. However, hospital-based data vastly underestimate the true incidence of burn injuries because many children are seen in outpatient settings with minimal documentation.

Children younger than 5 years of age are at greatest risk of burn. Children younger than 2 years of age have more than twice the mortality rate of older children and adults with equivalent injuries.

Aetiology

Burn injuries may result from hot liquids (scalds), hot objects, flames, explosives, chemicals, friction, and electrical current. Scald burns are the most common, contributing up to 80% of burn injuries in some series. In comparison, in the United States, the leading burn injury mechanisms among children younger than 4 years of age are also scalds, followed by hot objects and outdoor fires. Kerosene is the most common source of flame burns in Africa.

Most paediatric burn injuries in Africa occur in the home environment, often while the child is under the care of a nonparental caregiver. In some cases, burn injury is a manifestation of child abuse. Nonaccidental burns are also seen in some cultures where therapeutic burns are practiced as a means of treating febrile convulsions and epilepsy, based on the belief that heat will terminate the convulsion. Bilateral symmetrical burn of the feet from the immersion of both feet in hot water is a characteristic pattern in such therapeutic burns.

Pathophysiology

The depth of a burn injury depends on the temperature and duration of exposure to the heat source as well as the patient's age. For example, the immersion time needed to induce a burn injury following exposure to water heated to 54°C is 30 seconds in an adult, 10 seconds in a child, and less than 5 seconds in an infant.

The initial local effect of a burn injury is divided into three histological zones (Figure 33.1). An intermediate zone of stasis surrounds a central zone of tissue coagulation composed of irreversibly injured tissue, and both are surrounded by the zone of hyperaemia. Increased vascular permeability in the zone of hyperaemia/inflammation causes transudation of fluid into the interstitial space, leading to oedema. The extravasation continues for 24–48 hours. In extensive burns, this may lead to hypovolaemia and shock, if untreated.

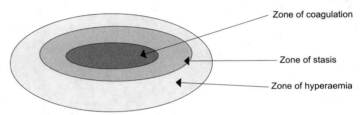

Figure 33.1: The histological effect of burn injury at the site of injury.

Appropriate cooling, fluid resuscitation, and maintenance of tissue perfusion may reverse the changes in the zone of stasis, allowing it to revert to normal. If not properly managed, continued tissue injury in this region may lead to an increase in the clinically apparent area of necrosis of the zone of coagulation.

Oedema

Increased capillary permeability in injured tissue, protein leakage, and the resultant hypoproteinaemia lead to increased osmotic pressure in burnt tissue, hence the oedema. In general, oedema is maximal at 24–48 hours, resolving in 3 to 4 days. However, in children with large burn wounds, the inflammatory response and tissue oedema may be significantly prolonged.

Hypermetabolism

The basal metabolic rate may increase up to 200 times, leading to a hypermetabolic phase associated with increased levels of catecholamines and catabolic hormones. Hypermetabolism slows down with treatment and resolves upon wound closure. The hypermetabolic response leads to increases in oxygen consumption, basal metabolic rate, urinary oxygen excretion, lipolysis, protein catabolism, and decreased synthesis, along with weight loss, that are directly proportional to the size of the burn. Early enteral feeding may attenuate the hypermetabolic response.

Many ongoing studies are focused on modulation of catecholamines in order to decrease oxygen demand, cardiac rate, and energy expenditure. Some of the promising agents include beta adrenergic blockers, insulin, and the anabolic steroid oxandrolone.

Classification of Burns

Burn injuries are classified into first- (superficial thickness), second- (partial thickness), and third-degree (full thickness) burns (Table 33.1). Second-degree burns are further subclassified into superficial and deep second-degree burns.

Table 33.1: Classification of burn injuries.

	First degree	Second degree		Third degree
	Superficial	Superficial	Deep	Full thickness
Cause	Very short flash, ultraviolet exposure	Short flash, spill scald	Flame, scald	Flame, immersion scald, chemical contact, electric current
Injured tissue	Epidermis only	Entire epidermis and part of dermis; dermal appendages intact	Entire epidermis and part of dermis; very few dermal appendages intact	Epidermis and dermis destroyed; no dermal appendages
Clinical appearance	Skin erythematous	Blisters, bullae, oedema	Blisters, bullae, oedema, pseudo-eschar	Leathery, charred skin with thrombosis of vessels
Pain	Pain gone in 48–72 hours	Painful	Painful	No pain
Healing time	1 week	2–3 weeks	More than 3 weeks	Requires grafting to heal
Results of healing	No scarring	Minimal or no scarring; dyspigmentation may occur	Large scar, hypertrophic may develop into keloids and contractures	Chronic wound, incapable of healing without intervention; contractures result

Eschar

An eschar is the necrotic tissue resulting from a burn. It separates slowly from underlying viable tissue and can serve as the substrate for invading microorganisms. Left untreated, it becomes colonised and eventually infected. Infection attracts white blood cells, which digest the interface and cause separation of the eschar from the underlying viable tissue. Circumferential eschars around limbs may impair blood circulation, and if unrelieved may cause distal ischaemia. Immediate relief is obtained by performing an escharotomy by placing vertical incisions through the eschar along the sides of the limb. Chest and abdominal eschars restrict respiration and may also require escharotomies along the sides of the chest wall. There should be no hesitation in early escharotomy if physiologic compromise is suspected.

Blisters

Burn blister management is controversial. Small blisters may be left alone to serve as biological dressings. Larger blisters require debridement to prevent an impairment of function and release the fluid that is rich in potentially deleterious proinflammatory substances.

Initial Resuscitation and Management

As with any trauma, the principles of Advanced Trauma Life Support (ATLS®) must be implemented to ensure that all life-threatening injuries are prioritised and managed. The ABCDE of ATLS must be followed:

Airway: Early intubation should be considered in patients with extensive burns requiring intensive care unit (ICU), those with extensive facial burns, and those with inhalation injuries. Progressive airway oedema is common in these situations.

Breathing: Deep chest and abdominal burns, especially when circumferential, severely impair chest wall breathing and ventilation. Escharotomies should be performed urgently when indicated. Associated chest and abdominal injuries may also impair chest wall excursion.

Circulation: Large-bore intravenous (IV) access should be placed through nonburned tissues. Venous cutdowns are frequently necessary for IV access for initial resuscitation. As an alternative route, intraosseous (IO) access may be used in the paediatric population. The doctor providing burn care must be conversant with the relevant techniques and anatomy. Isotonic salt solutions, most commonly lactated Ringers solution, should be used for resuscitation and maintenance.

Depth of Burn and **D**isability: Assessment of the depth of the burn is discussed under "Secondary Survey" in this chapter. A thorough neurological examination sets a baseline, especially in the setting of an associated head injury. Mental status changes or a history of loss of consciousness in the setting of a flame burn is most likely due to carbon monoxide poisoning. Administration of 100% oxygen, or hyperbaric oxygen where available, may be life saving.

Extent of Injury(s) and controlled **E**xposure of body: The full extent of the burn should be determined and the child examined for additional injuries. The child should be kept warm at all times.

An "F" should be added to ABCDE for paediatric patients:

For children:

• Children have larger heads and smaller limbs in terms of body surface area (BSA) compared to adults.

• Hypothermia is more common due to larger evaporation because the total BSA (TBSA)-to-height ratio in children is higher.

• Children have smaller glycogen stores, so hypoglycaemia is a risk.

• Adequate tetanus prophylaxis must be ensured.

• For any unusual injury patterns, consider child abuse.

Inhalational Injuries

The possibility of inhalational injury should be considered early during burn resuscitation because such patients may require early intubation. Inhalation injury results from exposure of the respiratory tract to superheated steam or air, toxic gases, chemicals, and particulate matter of smoke. Clinical diagnosis is difficult, but inhalational injury should be suspected when the child had been trapped in a closed space and in burns involving the head and neck. Characteristic symptoms indicating severe upper airway injury include hoarseness, change in voice, complaints of throat pain, and odynophagia. The child may cough up carbonaceous sputum and may demonstrate tachypnoea, wheezing, crepitations, rhonchi, and use of accessory respiratory muscles. When available, early diagnostic bronchoscopy will identify most victims.

The presence of inhalational injury is the major predictor of morbidity and mortality after burn injury. The pathogenesis can be differentiated into direct pulmonary and upper airway inhalation injury, and secondary (indirect) pulmonary injury due to activation of the systemic inflammatory response. In addition, secondary delayed pulmonary injury can be caused by sepsis and pneumonia. Ventilator-associated lung injury may be an important contributing iatrogenic factor.

Fluid Resuscitation

Advancements in fluid resuscitation of critically burned patients have made a major impact on patients' survival and have led to a general decrease in complication rates. Burn injury leads to a combination of hypovolaemic and distributive shock by means of generalised microvascular injury and interstitial third-space fluid accumulation.

Fluid resuscitation formulas are based on the child's weight and percentage of the TBSA burned. The goal is to replace ongoing fluid losses during the early postburn period. For burns larger than 15% TBSA, significant fluid losses occur and must be replaced aggressively. The most widely used fluid regimen is probably the Parkland formula or one of its several adaptations. Numerous resuscitation formulae are in use as guides to the initial resuscitation in hypovolaemic shock following thermal injury. Most use various combinations of crystalloid and colloid solutions, but they differ widely in the ratio of crystalloid to colloid as well as the rate of administration. Most formulae give approximately 0.52 mmol of sodium/kg body weight per % TBSA burn. Although no single fluid replacement formula is perfect, physicians should aim for a urine output of 1.0–2.0 ml/kg body weight per hour. This is proof of adequate resuscitation and perfusion.

With the Parkland formula, the child is given 2–4 ml/kg per % TBSA burn over the first 24 hours, with half administered in the first 8 hours and the second half in the next 16 hours. Different physiologic demands in children of various ages and the size of the burn require even more modification of the guideline formula. For children with burns of more than 15% TBSA and weight less than 20 kg, an additional maintenance fluid containing glucose should be administered.

For burns of less than 10% TBSA, oral fluids or maintenance (IV) fluid are usually sufficient. Children with burns between 10% and 15% TBSA generally respond appropriately to 1.5 times the normal calculated maintenance fluid. Maintenance glucose infusion should be given to children younger than 2 years of age, as they may easily become hypoglycemic due to limited glycogen stores.

Frequent measurements of vital signs, hourly urine output, and observation of general mental and physical response are best used to judge the adequacy of resuscitation. If available, monitoring of the central venous pressure is also a helpful guide to the adequacy of intravascular volume.

Children require more fluid for burn shock resuscitation than do adults with similar burns. The presence of inhalation injury increases the fluid requirements for resuscitation from burn shock after thermal injury. Continuous colloid replacement may be required to maintain colloid oncotic pressure in very large burns and in the paediatric burn patient. Serum albumin levels should be maintained above 2.0 g/dl.

Failure of Burn Shock Resuscitation

In some patients, failure of burn shock resuscitation still occurs despite administration of massive volumes of fluid. Such patients are characterised by extreme age, extensive tissue trauma, major electrical injury, major inhalation injury, a delay in initiating adequate fluid resuscitation, or underlying disease that limits metabolic and cardiovascular reserve. In such patients, refractory burn shock and resuscitation failure remain major causes of early mortality. Additional data implicate a myocardial depressant factor as a contributor to early burn shock, despite adequate volume resuscitation.

The Parkland formula, discussed in the last subsection, is well known and is used as an example in this chapter. Crystalloids are preferred with this formula, as they are also cheaper than other fluids, but some centres use colloids or even hypertonic saline. Because of the increased capillary leak, colloids may potentially worsen postburn oedema.

In electrical injuries (high-voltage, including lightning strikes), the goal for urine output should be 2.0 ml/kg per hour, and alkalinisation

of the urine may be necessary (add bicarbonate to the IV fluid). When available, electrocardiogram (ECG) monitoring and measurement of cardiac muscle enzymes and urine myoglobin levels are useful indicators of muscle damage. Urine output is the single most useful index of adequate intravascular replacement. In this regard, systemic blood pressure (BP) and central venous pressure (CVP) are unreliable. However, an overaggressive protocol may lead to complications, such as compartment syndromes and pulmonary oedema. Serial serum potassium and sodium levels are needed to monitor electrolyte changes.

Secondary Survey

Following initial resuscitation, a detailed history and head-to-toe examination should be conducted. The possibility of associated nonburn injuries or a precipitating event (e.g., epilepsy) should always be considered.

History

In addition to the history obtained during the primary survey, more detailed information is needed to determine:

- the cause of the burn injury (hot liquid, hot object, chemical, open flame, etc.);
- the time since injury;
- the duration and location of contact/exposure (a closed-space flame burn suggests a coexistent inhalation injury);
- any preexisting medical conditions, such as epilepsy, diabetes, mental handicap, and so forth;
- other coexisting injuries; and
- a vaccination history.

Physical Examination

Assessment of the burn wound should include the age, height, and weight of the patient; the depth of the burn wound; the extent (total body service area) of the burn; and the anatomical location of the injury.

Age, height, and weight

The age, height, weight, and calculated TBSA are needed to determine the appropriate doses of fluid and medications.

Depth of burn

The depth of the burn may be determined by clinical wound inspection and the pinprick test (see Table 33.1). The depth of the burn is the primary determinant of the patient's long-term appearance and function. It is critical to differentiate between superficial and deep second-degree burns. Whereas superficial second-degree burns heal within 2–3 weeks, deep second-degree burns require early tangential excision and skin grafting to permit relatively uncomplicated healing and a return to normal life.

Extent of burn

The extent of the burn surface involved is determined by careful observation, and should be graphically represented to aid in diagnosis, treatment, prognosis, and epidemiologic surveillance. It is calculated as a percent of total body surface area (% TBSA) using any of the following:

- Wallace's "rule of nines" (Table 33.2), which allows rapid estimation;
- Lund and Browder normogram for a more precise estimation (this table is described in several references);
- the "rule of tens", which is more appropriate for estimation of paediatric burns; or
- the patient's palm (~ 1% of their body surface area), which is useful for children with smaller burns.

Anatomical location

The location of burns has an important bearing on specific treatment, reconstruction, and rehabilitation. The hands, feet, face, eyelids, perine-

Table 33.2: Wallace's "rule of nines" for estimating % TBSA involved in burns.

Anatomic area	% TBSA
Head and neck	9
Anterior trunk	18
Posterior trunk	18
Right upper extremity	9
Left upper extremity	9
Right lower extremity	18
Left lower extremity	18
Perineum & external genitalia	1

um, genitalia, and joints are considered primary areas. They must be given appropriate care to optimise wound healing and prevent cosmetic and functional problems.

Investigation

Burn patients presenting acutely should be resuscitated as described above. The initial therapy aims at restoring normal physiologic parameters and the prevention of life-threatening complications. It is guided by the weight of the patient and the % TBSA injured.

Initial blood samples should be drawn for blood grouping and cross-match, total blood count, electrolytes, glucose, and urea nitrogen. Arterial blood gases and pH are obtained whenever inhalation injury is suspected.

Radiological investigations are generally not necessary except where inhalation injury is suspected or in the multiple trauma patient. Where possible, an initial baseline chest radiograph is useful for later comparisons.

Hospital Care

An assessment of the severity of the burn (Table 33.3) should be established early, as it gives a useful guide of the prognosis and the amount of resources that will be required to care for the child. The following steps should be initiated once the child has been resuscitated

Table 33.3: Classification of burn severity.

	Minor burns	Moderately severe burns	Major burns
BSA	<5%	5–15%	>15%
Special areas involved	No	No	Yes
Full thickness burns	None	None	Present
Comorbidities present (medical or trauma)	None	None or present	Present
Electrical or chemical injury	None	None	Present
Management	Outpatient	Hospital	Hospital

1. Clean the burns with normal saline and dress with saline gauzes, or cover with gauze dressing.

2. Adequate anaelgesia must be administered.

3. Administer tetanus prophylaxis.

4. Prophylactic antibiotics, oral or intravenous, are not indicated. Their use, prophylactically, is indicated only in the following three scenarios:

- early administration of antistreptococcal drugs in a high-risk patient to prevent burn wound cellulitis;

- perioperative administration of antibiotics; and

- administration of broad-spectrum antibiotics pending return of culture information in febrile or hypotensive patients.

Ideally, children with severe burns should be managed in a burn centre

or a hospital with an ICU. Guidelines include:

- children with burns >10% BSA require IV resuscitation;

- children with burns >30% BSA require central line placement;

- resuscitate crystalloids initially, with possible subsequent inclusion of colloids; and

- kaliuresis is common, and K+ losses must be supplemented; however, this should be done with care because the damaged tissue may release large amounts of potassium.

Nutrition

During days 2 and 3 following thermal injury, treatment is directed toward fluid resuscitation and maintenance of haemodynamic stability and electrolyte balance. Starting on postburn days 3 to 5, metabolic expenditure in the thermally injured patient begins to increase and is paralleled by an accompanying increase in nutritional demands. This increased metabolic drive is directed toward support of the healing burn wound by both local and systemic hormonal mechanisms. Due to the catabolic effect of catecholamines and increased energy expenditure, a high-calorie and high-protein diet or nutritional supplementation should be initiated as soon as possible after injury.

The goals of nutritional support are to maintain and improve organ function, prevent malnutrition, and improve overall outcomes. Nutritional support is not without potential complications, which may include sepsis, glucose, and osmolar intolerance, and the mechanical hazards of the administration techniques.

A number of different formulae that may be used to calculate caloric needs for burn patients exist. The Curreri formula is one example:

$$\text{Calories/day} = (\text{wt in kg}) (25) + (40) (\% \text{ BSA})$$

This formula probably overestimates caloric needs, and needs periodic recalculation as healing occurs.

Hypermetabolism is a characteristic physiological response to major injury, and there is a direct relationship between the magnitude and duration of the hypermetabolic response and the severity of the sustained trauma. The hypermetabolic response to burn injury is not temperature dependent, and has been postulated to be mediated through the hypothalamic temperature centre. The reset hypothalamus triggers an increased metabolic rate by elevating the plasma levels of three hormones: catecholamines, glucagon, and cortisol. Because the skin plays a large part in thermoregulation, extensive damage due to burns impairs the body's thermoregulatory capacity.

There is also a marked catabolic response that accompanies severe burns; it is associated with weight loss; poor wound healing; and negative nitrogen, potassium, sulfur, and phosphorus balance. It is also associated with increased levels of glucagon and catecholamines in plasma as well as depressed levels of insulin.

The increased metabolic expenditure persists for several weeks until the burn wound either spontaneously heals or is closed by skin grafting. However, even wound closure does not immediately return metabolic expenditure to normal, and thus increased nutritional support must continue even after closure of the wound surface.

Adequate nutritional support is best monitored by daily measurement of body weight. Postburn weight loss of up to 10% is well tolerated, provided the patient was not nutritionally compromised before the burn. Weight loss exceeding 10% of the preburn weight is associated with increased morbidity. A progressive physical therapy programme enhances the deposition of protein into lean muscle mass, allowing the performance of kinetic work required for the maintenance of normal function.

Enteral feedings are recommended over parenteral feedings in burn patients because they are more physiological and less costly, and they help to preserve gut structure and function, thereby reducing translocation of bacteria and/or toxins. As a result, the incidence of sepsis is lower in enterally fed burn patients. Due to the high incidence of gastric ileus in burn patients, nasoduodenal or nasojejunal tubes may be used for administration of feedings.

Despite the benefits, enteral feeding still carries significant risks, with the potential for disastrous complications if not well managed, including:

- mechanical complications (aspiration pneumonia, sinusitis, nasoa- lar, oesophageal and gastric mucosal irritation and erosion, tube lumen obstruction);
- gastrointestinal (GI) complications, such as diarrhaea and faecal impaction; and
- metabolic complications (dehydration, hyperglycaemia, hyper- or hyponatremia, hyper- or hypophosphataemia, hypercapnia, hyper- or hypokalaemia).

Pain Management

Burn injuries cause significant pain. Untreated, the pain exacerbates the hypermetabolism. This pain can be constant, therefore requir- ing continuous analgesia, including the use of narcotics and sedative agents. It is vital to provide adequate pain relief, especially during dressing changes, when ketamine may be useful. If narcotics are used for pain alleviation, the physicians must remember that tolerance may develop if therapy is prolonged. Sedation and analgesia should not be administered until hypoxia and hypovolaemia have been excluded and/or treated because they both produce anxiety and disorientation in the patient. When given, they must be kept at an absolute minimum to avoid cardiopulmonary depression and to allow evaluation of the sensorium, an important indicator of adequate resuscitation. Analgesics should be given intravenously because intramuscular absorption is erratic and unpredictable. Discontinuation of opiates should be antici- pated and tapered as wounds heal.

Burn Wound Management

The goals of local wound management are the prevention of viable tissue desiccation and control of bacterial loads by use of topical anti- microbial agents and/or biological dressings.

Second-degree wounds usually present as vesicular lesions that should be punctured and the nonviable skin removed to allow for the application of topical chemotherapeautic agents to the underlying viable dermis.

Topical Antibiotics

Several topical antimicrobial agents are available, as shown in Table 33.4. Modern antibacterial topical therapy for burn injuries was advo- cated by Moyer and co-workers in the early 1960s. They used aqueous silver nitrate 0.5% solution.

Silver nitrate is effective against most gram-positive organisms and most strains of *Pseudomonas,* although it has limited effectiveness against other gram-negative bacteria, such as *Klebsiella* and *Enterobacter.* Silver nitrate (0.5%) soaks are also effective in preventing microbial penetration of the eschar when treatment is begun immediately after the burn. Because silver nitrate does not readily penetrate the eschar, however, it has limited ability to control the proliferation of microorganisms already colonising the eschar. Soaks of 0.5% silver nitrate are generally reserved for use in patients allergic to sulfonamides.

Sulfamylon® was introduced in the mid-1960s, and is effective against a wide spectrum of gram-positive and gram-negative organisms, as well as anaerobes. Sulfamylon is an 11.1% suspension of mafenide acetate in a hydrophilic base. The solubility and the high activity of mafenide against gram-negative organisms, particularly *Pseudomonas aeruginosa*, make Sulfamylon burn cream particularly effective in limiting the proliferation of bacteria that have penetrated the eschar and

Table 33.4: Properties of topical antimicrobial agents.

Topical antimicrobial	Fibroblast toxicity	Bacteriocidal	Bacteriostatic
Sodium hydrochloride	✗	0.025%	
Povidone Iodine	✓	0.5%	
	✓	1.0%	
Hydrogen peroxide	0.3%	✗	
	3.0%	✓	
Acetic acid	0.25%	✗	
Silver nitrate	✓		10.0%
	✗		5.0%
	✓		1.0%
Silver sulfadiazine	✗ (with aloe vera/ nystatin)		1.0%

preventing the development of invasive burn wound infection. However, by inhibition of the carbonic anhydrase enzyme, it may induce acid-base derangements. It is also associated with pain on application, as well as occasional hypersensitivity reactions (5–7% of patients).

Silver sulfadiazine as 1% suspension in a hydrophilic base (Silvadene®) has essentially the same spectrum of activity as mafenide acetate, but fewer side effects. It is widely used in Africa as well as in the Western countries.

Betadine is a water-soluble antiseptic, effective against a wide range of gram-positive and gram-negative organisms, as well as some fungi.

Clinical bacteriologic monitoring of the burn wound is imperative in order to diagnose incipient burn wound sepsis and effect immediate treatment.

Traditionally, topical antimicrobial agents have been applied to a burn wound débrided of devitalised skin in a form of ointment, cream, or solution. A secondary dressing should be applied to the burn wound over the antimicrobial agent. These include: gauze, xeroform (3% bismuth tribromophenate in a petrolatum-blend on fine gauze), aquaphor gauze, foam dressings, and polyurethane dressings. These types of dressings are quite painful and, particularly in children, associated with significant anxiety. Recent developments of new silver- based antimicrobial delivery systems have eliminated the disadvantages of daily dressing change. Examples of available products include, among many: Acticoat®, Aquacel Ag®, Mepilex Ag®, and Glucan Silver Matrix®. These products consist of silver-containing pads or hydrocolloid fibre sheets that provide a sustained delivery mechanism for silver and in addition function to absorb excessive exudate from a wound. Applied to the débrided wound surface, these products could be left in place for several days.

Tangential Excision

The current accepted practice involves early excision (3–7 days post- burn)—tangential excision of deep second- and third-degree wounds until viable tissue is reached, as evidenced by capillary bleeding. Tangential eschar excision and skin grafting 3–5 days after the burn injury offers several advantages over full-thickness (fascial) excision, such as removal of only necrotic tissue, salvage of injured tissue that otherwise would have progressed to necrosis, preservation of biological properties of the dermis, and prevention of contractures. The primary closure is achieved by immediate grafting with autograft, and temporary closure is performed with heterograft or homograft, or synthetic barrier dressings. Although technically easy to perform, this procedure requires experience in determining the level of adequate excision. The advantag- es are a shortened hospital stay and potentially improved function when the wounds extend across joints. Tangential excision offers nothing if the burn wound is large and full-thickness. The major disadvantage is performing a major operation, with potential for a lot of blood loss, on a very sick patient, as well as the fact that it does not appear to materially change the pattern of the causes of death in those who die after 3 days of hospitalisation. Due to a lack of resources, in many hospitals in Africa, the eschar is often allowed to separate on its own, leading to an increased risk of infections and prolonged convalescence.

Wound Closure

Biologic dressing and biosynthetic products

Following spontaneous eschar separation or, preferably, after surgical removal by tangential or fascial excision, extensive wounds can be permanently covered with autograft or temporarily covered using a variety of techniques and dressings.

Biologic dressings, such as porcine xenograft or cadaveric allograft, are most commonly used. These provide early temporary wound closure, and therefore contribute to the prevention and control of infection, the preservation of healthy granulation tissue, and the maintenance of joint function. They decrease evaporative water loss and limit heat loss secondary to evaporation; they cover exposed sensory nerves, and thus decrease pain associated with the open wound; and they protect neurovascular tissue and tendons that would otherwise be exposed. The major drawbacks are their variable quality and, depending on donor age and harvesting technique, both have to be removed and both carry potential risk for viral infection. Amniotic membranes have also been used. Tissue engineering and advancements in biotechnology have provided several novel modalities to address those issues. Varieties of products are available, including skin, dermal, and epithelial substitutes.

Biosynthetic products used for temporary wound closure include Apigraf® (allogeneic bilayered skin equivalent, which consists of human keratinocytes and human fibroblasts in a lattice of bovine type I collagen); Biobrane® (nylon mesh coated with porcine collagen type I peptides and bonded to silicone rubber membrane); and TransCyte® (human neonatal fibroblasts seeded on coated nylon of Biobrane). The latter tissue substitute contains multiple growth factors and secreted matrix molecules, and is not only effective in treatment as a temporary closure of excised wound, it is also easy to handle and to remove with reduced bleeding as compared to allograft. Its drawback, however, is a significant cost of production.

Dermal substitutes include: Integra® (bilaminate membrane, which consists of bovine collagen–based dermal analogue covered with silastic sheeting); AlloDerm® (an acellular dermal substitute from cryopreserved human cadaver skin that is deprived of cells of the epidermis and dermis, leaving dermal matrix and basement membrane); and Matriderm® (a bovine noncross-linked collagen/elastin matrix).

Definitive burn wound closure is the ultimate objective of all burn wound care. However, priorities of coverage are dictated by functional and cosmetic considerations. The hands, feet, face (especially the eyelids), neck, and joints should in general be covered prior to nonfunctional surfaces.

Cultured epithelium

The technique of cultured epithelium involves the tissue culture growth of epidermal cells obtained from the prospective recipient, who will require grafting. Often, patients with extensive thermal injury have a disparity between available donor sites and the areas requiring coverage. Additionally, due to the paucity of donor sites, multiple graft harvests from the uninjured areas may be necessary, yielding tissue of progressively inferior quality. Cultured autologous keratinocytes have been used successfully to cover patients with massive skin defects secondary to burn injury.

Use of this technique in major burns may be the only way to prevent major burn complications and the consequent contractures, but it is not without its downsides. Disadvantages include the immensely high cost of the graft as well as its interference with the physical therapy programme (after grafting, the patient has to be immobilised for 7–10 days), easy traumatisation and blistering, breakdown, and lack of long-term durability because of the abnormal histologic architecture.

Complications

Complications after a burn injury may be examined from different perspectives. A thorough knowledge of the potential complications on initial evaluation and admission of the child allows the physician to prevent those complications. Acutely, the most feared complication is death. Others are complications related to the burn injury itself and subsequent organ failure, including death.

Burn complications may be classified as infective and noninfective.

Infective Complications

Infection is the most common and most serious complication of a major burn injury. Sepsis accounts for 50–60% of deaths in burn patients today despite improvements in antimicrobial therapies. Infections include bronchopneumonia, pyelonephritis, thrombophlebitis, and invasive wound infection.

Microbial colonisation of the open burn wounds, primarily from an endogenous source, is usually established by the end of the first week.

After a burn injury, in the absence of topical chemotherapy, the superficial areas of the burn wound contain up to 10^7 organisms per gram of burn tissue within 48 hours following the injury.

Routine administration of prophylactic antibiotics is associated with an increased incidence of yeast colonisation of the gastrointestinal tract and the rapid emergence of resistant gram-negative organisms in the burn wound, although antibiotics do not decrease the incidence of early gram-positive cellulitis. Indeed, even a brief 5- to 7- day course of prophylactic penicillin hastens the emergence of resistant gram-negative organisms. The potential harm caused by widespread use of prophylactic antibiotics has been known since the 1970s, but this practice is still rampart in many African hospitals.

Antimicrobial therapy is directed by bacterial surveillance through routine tri-weekly sputum, urine, and wound cultures, and antibiotics should be given only to treat specific infections. For example, gram-positive cellulitis caused by beta-haemolytic streptococci should be treated with penicillin. It is noteworthy that bacterial counts of <10^3 organisms/gm are not usually invasive and allow skin graft survival rates of >90%, without the use of antibiotics.

Methods of diagnosis of burn wound infection include clinical examination, quantitative cultures of a burn wound biopsy, and burn wound histology.

Generic clinical signs of burn wound infection include any of the following:

• spreading peri-wound erythema;

• oedema and/or discoloration of unburned skin at wound margin (usually due to *Pseudomonas* infections);

• rapid eschar separation (bacterial wound sepsis, may be fungal in some environments);

• punctuate haemorrhagic subeschar lesions;

• conversion of partial-thickness burns to full-thickness wounds;

• black or brown patches of wound discoloration;

• green pigment (pyocyanin) visible in subcutaneous fat (*Pseudomonas* infection);

• ecthyma gangrenosa—violaceous or black, erythematous nodular lesions in unburned skin (typically progress to focal necrosis);

• burn wound cellulitis;

• invasive burn wound infection; and

• burn wound impetigo.

Burn wound sepsis can be difficult to distinguish from the usual hyperdynamic, hyperthermic, hypermetabolic postburn state. Blood cultures are commonly negative, and fever spikes are frequently not proportional to the degree of infection.

Clinical diagnosis of sepsis is made by meeting at least three of the following criteria:

• burn wound infection (>10^5 organisms/gm tissue with histologic or clinical evidence of invasion);

• thrombocytopaenia (<50,000 or falling rapidly);

• leukocytosis or leukopaenia (>20,000 or <3,000);

• unexplained hypoxia, acidosis, or hyper- or hypoglycaemia;

• prolonged paralytic ileus;

• hyper/hypothermia (>39°C or <36.5°C);

• positive blood cultures;

• documented catheter or pulmonary infection;

• altered mental status; and

• progressive renal failure or pulmonary dysfunction.

Noninfective Complications

Noninfective complications may include any of the following:

• contractures—positioning and physiotherapy are preventive manoeuvres;

• hypertrophic scars and keloids—early wound closure and appropriate scar management are important in the functional and cosmetic outcomes;

• smoke inhalation syndrome;

• sterile multiorgan failure;

• anaemia;

• malnutrition;

• Curling's ulcers—H_2 blockers or proton pump inhibitors are effective in protecting against gastric ulceration and bleeding; and

• thrombo-embolic complications—estimated to affect between 0.4% and 7% of burn patients.

Additionally, long-term complications of burn scars include skin dyspigmentation, hypertrophic scars, keloid, and chronic nonhealing or unstable scars that may degenerate into squamous cell carcinomas (Marjolin's ulcers). Cutaneous horns may also develop from burn scars. Alopecia and burn syndactylys, digit or limb amputations, corneal perforations, and blindness are other possible postburn complications.

Prognosis and Outcomes

Prompt and appropriate treatment of burn injuries, including resuscitation and appropriate wound care, have led to a reduction in morbidity and mortality. Poor outcomes are the result of inadequate early management. Inadequate fluid resuscitation may lead to renal failure and needless death. Inappropriate triaging of patients leads to a waste of resources as well as the deaths of otherwise salvageable patients. Poor surgical wound management leads to wound infection, delay in wound closure, prolongation of the inflammatory/hypermetabolic phase, and significant malnutrition, especially in the child.

Delayed wound closure, with wound healing by secondary intention, leads to unsightly scars, dyspigmentation, keloids, and contractures. Resultant low self-esteem coupled with limited mobility may lead to

children being ostracised from society. Unable to attend school or other social activities, children may be unable to develop to their potential, unable to fit into society, and unable to pursue their dreams. Such children are at risk of posttraumatic stress disorder (PTSD) and other psychological disorders; psychological assessment and treatment are important components of rehabilitation from major burn injury.

Prevention

An old adage holds that "prevention is better than cure". Nowhere else is this proverb more applicable than in trauma, and more specifically in burn injuries. The majority of burn injuries occur among the poor urban populations living under deplorable conditions. Poor infrastructure, including overcrowding, poorly planned housing, and no water access points, lead to rapid spread of fires in these shanty communities. Provision of appropriate housing and decent living conditions are important steps in reducing the scourge of burns to children

Education and government action will likely be needed to abolish child labor practices that place children at greater risk of burn injuries (e.g., underage children who handle fires or hot liquids while cooking). Fire drills in schools should be implemented to help avoid deaths among schoolage children, particularly in boarding schools. Finally, first aid should be taught, which will minimise the burn injuries when they do occur.

Ethical Issues

The management of paediatric burn injuries in the African environment, especially in rural areas, may be complicated by traditional beliefs and practices. Many traditional therapies, such as raw egg mixtures, flour, and liquid paraffin, among other practices, remain harmful and delay appropriate care. Consistent education is urgently needed to both prevent these injuries and improve their outcomes, should they occur.

Child abuse by guardians must also be considered where unusual burn injury patterns or suspicious histories are presented, and appropriate safety measures must be undertaken.

Evidence-Based Research

Table 33.5 presents a comparative study of the use of a biosynthetic skin replacement versus cryopreserved cadaver skin to temporarily cover excised burn skin.

Table 33.5: Evidence-based research.

Title	A multicentre clinical trial of a biosynthetic skin replacement, Dermagraft-TC (DG-TC), compared with cryopreserved human cadaver skin for temporary coverage of excised burn wounds
Authors	Purdue GF, Hunt JL, Still JM Jr, et al.
Institution	Department of Surgery, University of Texas, Southwestern Medical Center, Dallas, Texas, USA
Reference	9063788 (PubMed ID)
Problem	Coverage of excised burn skin.
Intervention	Biosynthetic skin replacement.
Comparison/ control (quality of evidence)	Randomised controlled trial, comparative study.
Outcome/effect	DG-TC was equivalent or superior to allograft with regard to autograft take at post-autograft day 14. DG-TC was also easier to remove, had no epidermal slough, and resulted in less bleeding than did allograft, while maintaining an adequate wound bed. Overall satisfaction was better with DG-TC.
Historical significance/ comments	Improvement in burn care, surgical technique of covering wounds and its quality.

Key Summary Points

1. When a child is burned, his or her life is in danger.

2. Burn injuries are preventable.

3. Early and appropriate management of burn injuries significantly reduces associated morbidity and mortality.

4. Tetanus prophylaxis *must* be administered to burn victims. Prophylactic antibiotics are *not* indicated, and should *not* be used.

5. Antibiotics in burn care should be used only in preoperative prophylaxis and in cases of established infection.

6. Making a list of all the potential complications each week—both acute and long term—and taking action to prevent them would improve the outcome. Early splinting of limbs, early tangential excision and skin grafting, and physical therapy should all be instituted promptly.

Suggested Reading

Albertyn R, Bickler SW, Rode H. Paediatric burn injuries in Sub Saharan Africa—an overview. Burns 2006; 32:605–612.

American Burn Association. Hospital and prehospital resources for optimal care of patients with burn injury: guidelines for development and operation of burn centres. J Burn Care Rehabil 1990; 11:98–104.

American College of Surgeons. Resources for Optimal Care of the Injured Patients. American College of Surgeons, 1993, P 64.

Bishop JF. Burn wound and surgical management. Crit Care Nurs Clin N Am 2004; 16:145–177.

Burd A, Yuen C. A global study of hospitalized paediatric burn patients. Burns 2005; 31:432–438.

Cancio LC, Chavez S, Alvrado-Ortega M, Barillo DJ, Walker SC, McManus AT, Goodwin CW. Predicting increased fluid requirements during the resuscitation of thermally injured patients. J Trauma 2004; 56:404–414.

Cone JB., What's new in general surgery: burns and metabolism. J Am Coll Surg 2005; 200:607–615.

Demling RH. Fluid resuscitation. In: Boswick JA Jr, ed. The Art and Science of Burn Care. Aspen, 1987, Pp 189–202.

Duffy BJ., McLaughlin PM., Eichelberger RM. Assessment, triage, and early management of burns in children. Clin Pediatr Emerg Med 2006; 7:2.

Forjuoh SN, Keyl PM, Diener-West M, Smith GS, Guyer B. Prevalence and age-specific incidence of burns in Ghanaian children. J Trop Pediatr 1995; 41:273–277.

Gali BM, Madziga AG, Naaya HU. Epidemiology of childhood burns in Maiduguri north-eastern Nigeria. Niger J Med 2004; 13:144–147.

Ipaktchi K, Arbabi S. Advances in burn critical care. Crit Care Med 2006; 34(9 Suppl):S239–S244.

Kalyai GD. Burn injuries in Zaria: a one year retrospective study. East Afr Med J 1997; 71:317–321.

Moyer CA, Brentano L, Gravens DL, Margraf HW, Monafo WW Jr. Treatment of large human burns with 0.5% silver nitrate solution. Archives of Surgery 1965; 90:812–867.

Munster AM, Smith-Meek M, Shalom A. Acellular allograft dermal matrix: immediate or delayed epidermal coverage? Burns 2001; 27:150–153.

Nthumba PM. Giant cutaneous horn in an African woman: a case report. J Med Case Rep 2007; 1:170. Available at: http://www.jmedicalcasereports.com/content/1/1/170.

Nthumba PM, Oliech JS. Outcome of moderate and severe thermal injuries at Kenyatta National Hospital. Thesis, Master of Medicine in Surgery, University of Nairobi, February 2002.

Onuba O, Udoibok E. The problem and prevention of burns in developing countries. Burns 1987; 3:382–385.

Peck MD, Weber J, McManus A, et al. Surveillance of burn wound infections: a proposal for definitions. J Burn Care Rehabil 1998; 19:386–389.

Pham C, Greenwood J, Cleland H, Woodruff P, Maddern G. Bioengineered skin substitutes for the management of burns: a systematic review. Burns 2007; 33:946–957.

Pizano LR, Davies J, Corallo JP, Cantwell PG. Critical care and monitoring of the pediatric burn patient J Craniofac Surg 2008; 19:929–932.

Purdue GF, Hunt JL, Still JM Jr, et al. A multicenter clinical trial of a biosynthetic skin replacement, Dermagraft-TC, compared with cryopreserved human cadaver skin for temporary coverage of excised burn wounds. J Burn Care Rehabil 1997; 18(1 Pt 1):52–57.

Rennekampff HO, Pfau M, Schaller HE. Acellular allograft dermal matrix: immediate or delayed epidermal coverage? Burns 2002; 28:100–101.

Sheridan RL, Remensnyder JP, Schnitzer JJ, Schulz JT, Ryan CM, Tompkins RG. Current expectations for survival in pediatric burns. Arch Pediatr Adolesc Med 2000; 154:245–249.

Sowemimo GO. Burn care in Africa: reducing the misery index: the 1993 Everett Idris Evans Memorial Lecture. J Burn Care Rehabil 1993; 14:589–594.

Tenenhaus M, Rennekampff HO. Burn surgery. Clin Plast Surg 2007; 34:697–715.

CHAPTER 34
INJURIES FROM CHILD ABUSE

AB (Sebastian) Van As
Dorothy V. Rocourt
Benedict C. Nwomeh

Introduction

Child abuse and neglect can be broadly defined as the maltreatment of children by parents, guardians, or other caretakers. The main responsibilities of all health care workers (HCWs) are the detection, treatment, and reporting of child abuse. Contrary to common belief, child abuse is not a new phenomenon. Many reports indicate that child abuse has been around since early times and is present in all cultures. The child is weak, vulnerable, and an easy target for abuse. The smaller the child, the greater the danger of abuse and the higher the risk for fatal outcome.

Children in low-income countries are particularly vulnerable to death from abuse. Africa has the highest rates of homicide for children younger than 5 years of age, at 17.9 per 100,000 for boys and 12.7 per 100,000 for girls—more than six times the incidence in Western countries.[1] The magnitude of the problem is obscured by differing legal and cultural definitions of abuse and poor reporting and recording of cases.

Definition of Child Abuse

In Africa, child-rearing practices often vary from those in Western countries; therefore, caution is needed in determining what constitutes abuse or neglect. For example, some cultures accept male as well as female circumcision, but others might consider it as clear child abuse. A useful approach is one that defines child abuse as *abuse to an extent that is not acceptable in a particular culture*. However, this can easily lead to problems. According to the World Health Organization (WHO), "child abuse or maltreatment constitutes all forms of physical and/or emotional ill-treatment, sexual abuse, neglect or negligent treatment or commercial or other exploitation, resulting in actual or potential harm to the child's health, survival, development or dignity in the context of a relationship of responsibility, trust or power".[2]

Health Care Workers' Roles in Child Abuse

The roles of health care workers are to:

• recognise child abuse;

• accurately document the extent of the clinical findings (physical or psychological);

• provide appropriate treatment of the injuries sustained; and

• report the case to the appropriate authorities.

Treatment might vary from analgesics to extensive surgical procedures and placement in institutions. Besides medical treatment for the child, support for the patient and family should be provided. The majority of parents have normal human feelings (i.e., they are not mentally ill), so they might be loaded with guilt. To take an adequate history can be very complicated, as the parents or caregivers are often in an excited and anxious state.

It might be very difficult to establish whether the injury was accidental or nonaccidental. However, the role of the physician is to provide accurate diagnosis and not to play detective. The diagnosis might be very difficult, but the following circumstances should raise the suspicion of child abuse:

• unexplained injuries;

• discrepant histories;

• delay in seeking medical care;

• alleged self-inflicted injury;

• alleged third-party–inflicted injury;

• repeated injuries;

• sexualised behaviour; or

• sexually transmitted disease (STD).

Types of Child Abuse

There are several types of child abuse, as outlined here.

1. *Physical abuse* or nonaccidental injury denotes injuries inflicted by the caretaker.

2. *Child sexual abuse* is the use of a child for sexual gratification. Note that this is a broader term than child rape. Besides sexual intercourse it also includes:

• touching, fondling, or other inappropriate contact with the child's genitals or breasts;

• masturbation of a child by an adult or vice versa and masturbation of an adult in the presence of a child;

• body contact with adult genitals;

• exhibitionism; and

• pornography, including photography and erotic talk.

Of note, most of these abuse acts will leave no physical signs on the victim.

1. *Failure to thrive* due to nutritional deprivation most commonly occurs within the first 2 years of life. Approximately 50% of all failure to thrive in this age category is due to maternal neglect.

2. *Intentional drugging* or poisoning takes place when parents give the child a prescribed drug that is harmful and not intended for children.

3. *Medical care neglect* occurs when a child suffers from a (chronic) disease and the condition worsens due to parental neglect of the condition. Children are completely dependent on their parents for medical care.

4. *Safety neglect* is present when there is a gross lack of supervision, especially in younger children.

5. *Emotional abuse* may occur when the child is repeatedly blamed for incidents or rejected by parents and/or caregivers. Severe verbal abuse and berating are common. This is a difficult condition to prove.

6. *Organised abuse* is a form of organised crime, and often involves multiple victims and perpetrators. The so-called paedophilic and pornographic rings are the major contributors to this group, but there is also cult-based abuse, in which the abuse has spiritual or social objectives.

Physical Abuse

Child abuse is a common cause of childhood death, second only to sudden infant death syndrome (SIDS) in the age group under 6 months. The average age of the abused child is 7 years old; the average age of fatality is 3 years. Socioeconomic problems often play a role. Although culture or socioeconomic status may be associated with child abuse, many studies indicate that abuse occurs among all income categories and all cultures.[3] The smaller the child, the bigger the risk. Younger children are at greatest risk because they are more demanding, defenseless, and nonverbal. One-third of physical abuse takes place under the age of 6 months, another third at 6 months to 3 years of age, and the remaining third above the age of 3 years. At particular risk are male children, those born prematurely, and stepchildren.

Modes of physical abuse can be designated as nonaccidental or accidental. Nonaccidental injuries are events resulting from deliberate actions by individuals against themselves or another victim that intentionally threatens, attempts, or actually inflicts physical harm. Accidental injuries result from unforeseen events that cause an external trauma to the body, without the intent to cause harm.

The exact circumstances surrounding an assault are not always clear, but in some cases, the child is used as a shield for an adult under attack. This so-called *shielding phenomenon* encompasses a large spectrum, from the scenario where the child is injured as an innocent bystander to one in which an adult positions the child in self-defence against an attacker.[4] Some injuries, such as knife attacks, are particularly suggestive of shielding because it is not likely that anyone would deliberately assault a child with such a weapon.

Causes of Child Abuse and Predisposing Factors

There is often an assumption that parents of abused children are severely psychotic or criminal, but research indicates that more than 90% of the parents have no psychological problems or criminal nature. Instead, they tend to be lonely, unhappy, and angry adults under tremendous stress. Additional stressful factors include a breakdown of family structure, poverty, financial need, unemployment, being a single parent, and substance abuse. There is also a very strong correlation with child abuse of the parents: more than 90% of abusing parents may have been abused during their own childhoods.

Diagnosing Child Abuse

There are many ways to establish a diagnosis of nonaccidental injury in children. The first occurs when the child readily cites a particular adult as the assailant. The complaint should always be taken very seriously, and every case must be thoroughly investigated. Unexplained injury should prompt a consideration of child abuse, particularly when parents are reluctant to explain the nature of the accident. For instance, parents might claim that they "just found the child like that", or "the child might have fallen down", or "someone else might have hit the child". The majority of the parents know to the minute where and when the child was hurt. A discrepant history is also suggestive of child abuse.

The suspicion of child abuse increases when the history provided does not explain the severity of the physical injuries. For instance, a child who fell from a bed and yet is covered with bruises is unlikely to have suffered such injuries from the stated mechanism. Another is a parental claim that the child "bruises so easily". This history is usually misleading, especially when no new bruises appear during hospitalisation. Claims of self-infliction in children should be treated with suspicion—for example, a report that a small baby had "rolled over her arm and fractured it". Similarly, shifting the blame for the injury to a third party may be an indication of child abuse.

Delayed presentation is a common feature of abuse injuries. In normal situations, it is uncommon for parents to bring their child to the hospital more than 24 hours after an injury. After child abuse, however,

a delay is common. Finally, repetitive injuries in any child may be indicative of child abuse.

Typical Findings of Physical Abuse

A constellation of physical findings characterises the injuries seen in abused children. Some of these are listed in Table 34.1 and explained in more detail below.

Table 34.1: Typical presentations of physical abuse.

- **Head injuries**
  - Fractures,
  - Intracranial injuries
- **Truncal injuries**
  - Fractured ribs
  - Spinal cord injuries
  - Internal organ injuries
- **Extremity injuries**
  - Fractures of long bones
  - Single fracture with multiple bruises
  - Multiple fractures in different stages, possibly with no bruise or soft tissue injury
  - Metaphyseal or epiphyseal injuries, often multiple
- **Superficial injuries**
  - Cuts and bruises
  - Burns and scalds
  - Signs of hypothermia and frostbite
- **Suffocation**
- **Poisoning**

Skin

Lesions can occur everywhere. Bruises on the buttocks and lower back are often related to punishment; bruises on the cheek are usually secondary to being slapped. Other typical findings in child abuse are grip marks, pinch marks, and circumferential bruises. Defining the age of the injuries is difficult. Most skin lesions have an initially red colour, followed by a reddish-purple period within 24 hours, which then gradually progresses to a predominantly purple lesion over the next week. Discoloration to yellow/green/brown is due to degradation of haemoglobin and occurs over a period of 1–3 weeks.

Burns

Approximately 10% of physical abuse involves burns. Typical lesions found in child abuse are cigarette burns and so-called stocking/glove injuries in toddlers from hot water immersion.

Head Injuries

The incidence of abusive head injury ranges from 17 per 100,000 to 40 per 100,000, with the largest group of head injuries seen in infants 0 to 3 months of age.[5] Approximately one-third of abusive head injuries are not recognised at the time of initial visit to a health care provider. Although nonaccidental head trauma in children younger than 3 years of age is difficult to diagnose, one should maintain a high index of suspicion. The spectrum of head injury can range from skull fractures to lethal intracranial bleeding and brain atrophy (Figure 34.1).

Subdural haematomas may also be the result of shaking. The rapid acceleration and deceleration of the shaking head appears to tear bridging veins, with resulting bleeding and subdural haematomas, often bilaterally. Another common finding is diffuse cerebral oedema with loss of normal grey-white matter differentiation (Figure 34.2). Retinal haemorrhages are nearly always present in these cases (Figure 34.3).[6]

Skeletal Injuries

Fractures in small children are rare. In all patients under the age of 3 years, the occurrence of a fracture without an adequate history should prompt the suspicion of child abuse. Approximately one-quarter of cases of physical abuse involve skeletal injury. Two-thirds of fractures involve the long bones, and the fractures can be spiral or transverse. Certain fractures are almost pathognomonic for child abuse, such as a chip fracture (corner or bucket handle fracture) of the long bones (Figure 34.4). This injury occurs due to avulsion of the corner of the metaphysis from the periosteum during wrenching injuries to the long bones. Approximately 10 days after the injury, calcification of the subperiosteal bleeding will give rise to the classical double cortex line.

In all children with suspected child abuse, a skeletal survey should be obtained. The skeletal survey comprises a combination of x-rays of the chest, skull, and extremities only in the anteroposterior (AP) direction. Repeated abuse may manifest as old rib fractures with callous formation in different phases of healing (Figure 34.5). A radionuclear bone scan is a more sensitive method to pick up old injuries, but is unreliable under the age of 1 year.

Differential Diagnosis

Child abuse is common in Africa; however, a number of other conditions may be mistaken for abuse (and vice versa), including the following:

- *Birth trauma:* should be evident from the birth history.

- *Congenital syphilis:* chronic periosteal reaction combined with metaphyseal widening and positive blood tests.

- *Osteogenesis imperfecta:* multiple fractures, blue sclerae, osteopaenia.

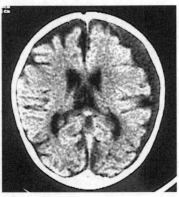

Figure 34.1: Severe brain atrophy in an infant due to physical abuse.

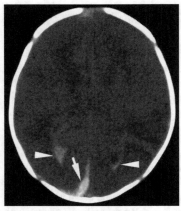

Source: Courtesy of Brian Coley MD, Nationwide Children's Hospital, Columbus, Ohio, USA.

Figure 34.2: Noncontrast CT scan of the brain. There is diffuse cerebral oedema with loss of normal grey-white matter differentiation and abnormal hypodensity in the posterior parietal lobes, indicating early infarction. There is bilateral intraventricular haemorrhage (arrowheads) and a parafalcine acute subdural haematoma (arrow).

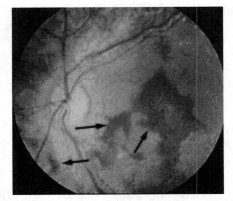

Source: Pressel DM. Evaluation of physical abuse in children. The American Family Physician. (http://www.aafp.org/afp/20000515/3057.html). Reproduced with permission.

Figure 34.3: Retinal haemorrhages (arrows) in a patient with shaken-baby syndrome

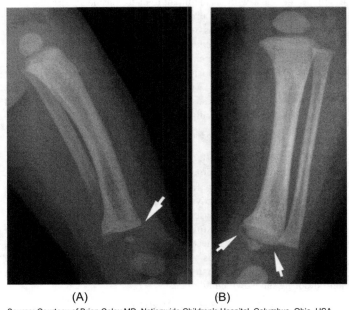

(A)   (B)

Source: Courtesy of Brian Coley MD, Nationwide Children's Hospital, Columbus, Ohio, USA.

Figure 34.4: Classic metaphyseal lesion. (A) Lateral radiograph of the left tibia shows a distal metaphyseal corner fracture (arrow). (B) Frontal radiograph of the same left tibia shows that with a different obliquity the metaphyseal fracture appears as a crescentic fragment (arrows), the "bucket-handle" fracture.

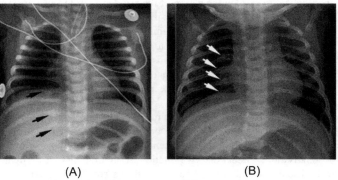

(A)   (B)

Source: Courtesy of Brian Coley MD, Nationwide Children's Hospital, Columbus, Ohio, USA.

Figure 34.5: Rib fractures from physical abuse. (A) Frontal chest radiograph shows healing fractures of the right posterior 8th, 10th, and 11th ribs (arrows). (B) Frontal chest radiograph shows healing fractures of the right posterior 5th, 6th, 7th, and 8th ribs (arrows).

- *Rickets:* renal disease, bowed long bones, blood abnormalities.
- *Scurvy:* poor wound healing, bleeding gums, petechiae.
- *Bleeding disorders:* haemophilia, meningococcaemia.
- *Skin diseases:* impetigo, chicken pox, scaled skin syndrome (may mimic burns).

Of course, genuine accidental trauma may also present—the history, pattern of injury, and interaction with the parents should help to indicate that this is the case.

Initial Management of Injuries

The initial stabilisation of the physically assaulted child uses an ABC approach, as with any injured child:[7]

- primary survey with resuscitation;
- secondary survey with emergency treatment; and
- transfer to definitive care.

Treatment of the child is the priority at this stage; care should be taken to minimise the interference with any forensic evidence on the child's clothes or skin.

Primary Survey

The primary survey consists of ABCDE:

- Airway with cervical spine control
- Breathing with ventilatory support
- Circulation with haemorrhage control
- Disability with prevention of secondary insult
- Exposure

Useful adjuncts at this stage include chest and pelvic radiographs, initial blood tests (including a cross-match sample), an oro- or nasogastric tube, and a urinary catheter.

Secondary Survey

The initial priority is resuscitation and treatment of immediate life-threatening problems, followed by the secondary survey, in which the child undergoes a thorough head-to-toe examination. Physically abused children often have evidence of older injuries at the time of their presentation to the health services, and the evaluating physician should document these accurately. Treatment of specific injuries is discussed in detail in corresponding chapters in this book.

Transfer

The final stage of emergency management is transfer to definitive care. This involves appropriate packaging for transfer—either within the hospital or to another unit—and handover to the receiving staff. Accurate handover is essential in cases of suspected or proven physical abuse, and the presence of accurate contemporaneous notes greatly facilitates continuity of care.

Sexual Assault

Sexual abuse is common in all societies. The overall rate of sexual abuse in children under the age of 18 years is 14% for females, and 7% for males.[8] Any child presenting with perineal injuries or infection should be suspected of being a victim of child abuse. In girls, sexual abuse can be chronic (without signs of fresh injuries, but absent hymen) or acute (often with fresh physical injuries). Small children often present with a bruised perineum. In the majority of cases, the perpetrator is known to the child and is probably a family member.[9]

A child very rarely presents with the history of sexual abuse and therefore the clinician should be alert to the following symptoms and signs of abuse:

- recurrent abdominal pain;
- difficulty walking or sitting;
- painful micturition and recurrent urinary tract infections;
- faecal soiling or retention;
- discharge from penis or vagina;
- abnormal dilatation of vagina/anus;
- genital laceration/bruising;
- vaginal bleeding; and
- signs of sexually transmitted infections.

Guidelines for Examination after Abuse

Examination of a sexually abused child should never be taken lightly; if not performed under ideal circumstances, it may seriously contribute to secondary trauma of the child. Examination should always be performed by a qualified doctor, following a specified protocol:

- A designated private area is needed.
- A third person (mother or nurse) should be present.
- The procedure should be explained to the caregiver as well as to the child.
- A full general examination is necessary; noting weight, height, and nutritional state.
- The genital examination should be performed only once.
- Small children can be examined on the mother's lap with the child's back to the mother and the mother holding the legs.
- Older children can be examined in the supine lithotomy position.
- The lateral decubitus position should be used to examine the anus.
- The stage of sexual development should be noted (using the Tanner scale).

All children with evidence of perineal trauma should be examined under anaesthesia to determine the exact nature of the injury and the need for surgical repair.

Due to the large discrepancy between sexual organs, penetration rarely occurs in sexually abused children. However, forced penetration in small children can cause a mutilating injury. Absence of penetration does not rule out abuse. In a local study, one-third of the paediatric sexual assault victims had no physical injuries.[10]

Bruises and first- and second-degree tears can usually be repaired primarily. However, when there is violation and laceration of the anal sphincter or the rectovaginal septum, a diverting colostomy and washout are needed. When all signs of infection have subsided (usually between 6 weeks and 3 months), the definitive repair can be performed.

The recommended routine investigations for all cases of sexual abuse are the following:

- Full blood count (FBC) and platelets, international normalisation ratio (INR) and partial thromboplastin time (PTT) to exclude a bleeding disorder.
- Vaginal or penile swab where a discharge is present—send for microscopy, culture, and sensitivities (MC&S).
- Blood for Venereal Disease Research Laboratory (VDRL).
- Human immunodeficiency virus (HIV) serology. Post exposure prophylaxis (PEP) is continued only for those who test negative.
- Photographic documentation for legal purposes. Digital photographs have to be printed, dated, and signed immediately to be useful as evidence in court.

The child should be checked for syphilis (the VDRL test) and HIV/acquired immune deficiency syndrome (AIDS). If available, antiretroviral therapy should be instituted. Do not routinely start children on antibiotics, but wait for the results of laboratory tests. Social workers should be involved from the onset, and the child protection unit (police) contacted.

Reporting Cases of Suspected Child Abuse and Court Testimony

There are several pitfalls in dealing with a case of suspected child abuse, some of which are listed below:

• relying on the history provided by the caretakers or parents regarding the mechanism of injury;

• not undressing and examining the whole child;

• not being able to mask emotional display while examining the injured child;

• insufficient experience in examining children, requiring the child to be re-examined;

• blaming the caretakers and/or parents instead of supporting them; and/or

• omission of prophylactic antiretroviral therapy after sexual assault.

To be accused of child abuse is an extremely painful experience for anyone. Some parents will react in an aggressive way once medical staff probes the possibility of child abuse. Parents and other caretakers regularly threaten with legal action. However, the law in South Africa and several other countries protects those who report suspected child abuse in good faith, and no court cases can be pursued against people who report. Even though the investigator must be firm to conduct a thorough investigation, due recognition must be given to the possibility that the accused may be innocent.

In order to be as thorough as possible regarding the medical report, an affidavit should be written within 24 hours of severe abuse cases that might be litigated by court. This will help the doctors tremendously at a later stage. Cases often do not get to court for many years. If the abuse was not well documented or data are missing, the perpetrator nearly always evades justice.

All child sexual abuse cases ought to be investigated by the police. However, in our experience, only 30% of perpetrators end up in court, and only about 7% face prosecution. It is important to realise that child sexual abuse cases cannot be withdrawn (in adult sexual abuse cases, however, the victim can change her or his mind).

Conclusion

Child abuse contributes greatly to the burden of disease among children in Africa, who have the unenviable distinction of having the highest unintentional injury death rates in the world. There is a need in Africa to focus on creating and maintaining awareness about the magnitude, risk factors, and preventability of child injuries among policy makers, donors, practitioners, and parents.[11] In the special case of sexual violence toward children, it is time for African governments to publicly acknowledge the problem, establish systems of reporting, and ensure a system that protects those who report offences and swiftly dispenses justice to offenders.[12]

Evidence-Based Research

Table 34.2 presents a USA-based study that addresses the problem of health care workers missing child abuse cases.

Table 34.2: Evidence-based research.

Title	Child abuse fatalities: are we missing opportunities for intervention?
Authors	King WK, Kiesel EL, Simon HK
Institution	Department of Pediatrics and Emergency Medicine, Emory University, Atlanta, Georgia, USA
Reference	Pediatric Emergency Care 2007; 22:211–214
Problem	Missed pediatric child abuse cases at initial visit with health care provider.
Intervention	Early recognition of child abuse by emergency department health care providers.
Methods	Retrospective review of medical examiners records.
Outcome/ effect	Forty-four cases of abuse were identified, of which 37 (84%) were younger than 4 years of age. Of the 37 cases, blunt head trauma was the leading cause of death (57%), followed by blunt torso injury (13%), gunshot injury (11%), fire (8%), drowning (8%), and poisoning (3%).
Historical significance/ comments	Nonaccidental injury or child abuse is a leading cause of morbidity and mortality in the paediatric population. Fatalities tend to occur in younger children, with blunt trauma being the leading cause of death. The authors conclude that although child abuse is difficult to diagnose, most cases present to a health care provider prior to their fatal event. They suggest a number of measures to capture at-risk children and reduce the incidence of a fatal subsequent event. These include parental questionnaires, biochemical markers, ongoing education to health care providers, and tracking health care utilisation and patterns of injury.

Key Summary Points

1. Child abuse or nonaccidental injury is a leading cause of morbidity and mortality in children.

2. Abuse patients are managed as trauma patients, with a primary and secondary assessment being performed.

3. Management of the abused patient is multidisciplinary.

4. Health care providers need to be continuously educated to identify the child at risk for nonaccidental injury.

5. Children younger than 3 years of age are at highest risk for nonaccidental injury.

6. Head injury is the leading cause of mortality in child abuse, with children 0–3 months of age having the highest risk.

7. Child abuse should be suspected in all cases of unexplained injuries, discrepancy in history, delay in seeking medical care, repeated injuries, presence of sexually transmitted diseases, and sexualised behavior.

References

1. Krug EG, Dahlberg LL, Mercy JA, Zwi A, Lozano R. World Report on Violence and Health. World Health Organization, 2002.

2. Report of the Consultation on Child Abuse Prevention, 29–31 March 1999. World Health Organization, 1999 (document WHO/HSC/PVI/99.1).

3. van As S, Naidoo S, eds. Paediatric Trauma and Child Abuse. Oxford University Press, 2006, ISBN 9780195762594.

4. Fieggen AG, Wiemann M, Brown C, van As AB, Swingler GH, Peter JC. Inhuman shields—children caught in the crossfire of domestic violence. South Afr Med J 2004; 94(4):293–296.

5. Tingberg B, Falk AC, Flodmark O, Ygge BM. Evaluation of documentation in potential abusive head injury of infants in a paediatric emergency department. Acta Paediatr 2009; 98(5):777–781.

6. Pressel DM. Evaluation of physical abuse in children. The American Family Physician. Available at: http://www.aafp.org/afp/20000515/3057.html (accessed 18 January 2010).

7. Advanced Life Support Group. Advanced Paediatric Life Support: The Practical Approach. BMJ Books, 2005.

8. Peden M, Oyegbite K, Ozanne-Smith J, et al., eds. World Report on Child Injury Prevention. WHO and UNICEF, 2008. Available at: http://www.who.int/violence_injury _prevention/child/en/ (accessed 25 February 2009).

9. Barker J, Hodes D. The Child in Mind. A Child Protection Handbook. Routledge, 2004. ISBN 0-415-32175-1.

10. AB van As, M Whithers, AJW Millar, H Rode. Child rape—patterns of injury, management and outcome. South Afr Med J 2001; 91(12):1035–1038.

11. Peden M, Hyder AA. Time to keep African kids safer. South Afr Med J 2009; 99(1):36–37.

12. Jewkes R. Preventing sexual violence: a rights-based approach. The Lancet 2002; 360:1092–1093.

CHAPTER 35
BIRTH INJURIES

Auwal M. Abubakar
Johanna R. Askegard-Giesmann
Brian D. Kenney

Introduction

The majority of birth injuries are minor and often unreported. Occasionally, though, birth injuries may be so severe as to be fatal or leave the child with a permanent disability. They may occur because of inappropriate or deficient medical skills or attention, but they also can occur despite skilled and competent obstetrical care. Birth injuries are mostly iatrogenic, and the legal implications of these should be noted. Most of these injuries can be managed nonoperatively, but prompt identification of those that will need surgical intervention is essential.

Demographics

The incidence of significant birth injuries in the United Sates is 6–8 per 1,000 live births, accounting for less than 2% of perinatal mortality.[1] In Africa, statistics on birth injuries are lacking. However, a survey of rural Egyptian birth attendants in different regions revealed an overall prevalence of birth injuries at 7%, and up to 17% in the Aswan region.[2] Autopsy studies on stillbirths from Accra, Ghana, also estimate the incidence of perinatal deaths due to birth trauma as 5.4%.[3]

Aetiology

The risk factors for birth injuries are as follows:[4–6]

1. primigravida;

2. maternal age younger than 16 or older than 35 years;

3. high neonatal birth weight;

4. maternal parity >6;

5. prolonged or precipitate delivery;

6. cephalopelvic disproportion;

7. foetal presentation (face, breech);

8. type of delivery (forceps, vacuum);

9. prematurity;

10. postmaturity;

11. organomegaly and mass lesions in the abdomen; and

12. coagulopathy.

Injuries are sustained as a result of mechanical impact on the foetus during birth due to pressure in the birth canal or to traction and pressure produced by manipulations during delivery. The risk of injury to infants during breech delivery is about twice that with vertex delivery. Birth injuries can also occur, however, in spontaneous, full-term, apparently uncomplicated deliveries.

Clinical Presentation and Management

Fractures

Most fractures following birth trauma heal spontaneously. Nonunion is almost unknown. The most common bones involved are the clavicle, femur, humerus, and skull. Calcification of these fractures is evident by the second week of life. The absence of such calcifications suggests child abuse rather than birth injury, especially if the bones involved are those other than the ones commonly affected in birth injuries. Dislocations following birth trauma are generally rare.

Clavicle

The clavicle is the most common fracture in the newborn, following from difficulty with delivery caused by shoulder dystocia.[7] Many times, the fracture is noticed only when callous formation begins. It is usually a green stick fracture and occasionally is associated with brachial plexus injury. Fracture of the clavicle requires no treatment.

Long bones

Fracture involving the long bones is not common. The femur may be involved during a difficult breech delivery when traction is applied to extract the foetus;[8] usually the midshaft is involved. This fracture is treated by skin traction or splinting with a spica cast. Fracture of the humerus is encountered during a difficult delivery of the shoulder in a vertex presentation. Humeral fractures may be associated with Erb's or radial nerve palsy. These fractures are treated by restricting the baby's movements by bandaging the arm to the chest for a period of 1 to 3 weeks.

Skull

Linear fracture, especially of the parietal bone, is the most common injury seen; it needs no treatment. Depressed skull fractures may require elevation, depending on severity. Closed elevation of a so-called "ping-pong" fracture can be achieved by the use of the vacuum extractor. Open elevation will be required if there is increased intracranial pressure, neurological deficit, or when bony fragments are projecting into cerebral tissue.

Cephalhaematoma

Cephalhaematoma is a subperiosteal haemorrhage, which is limited to one cranial bone by surrounding cranial sutures (Figure 35.1). It appears on the second day of life; this is an important feature distinguishing it from caput succedaneum. There may be a linear fracture of the underlying bone. Most cephalhaematomas are resorbed within 2 weeks to 3 months of age. A massive cephalhaematoma may require blood transfusion. Aspiration or incision of the swelling is contraindicated. Calcification of the haematoma may require surgical excision.

Neurological Injuries

Brachial plexus

The most common neurological injury is brachial plexus injury. Infants with brachial plexus injuries are typically large, with a difficult labour and frequent shoulder dystocia or breech presentation. The predominance of the right plexus injury is related to the common left occipito-anterior presentation that leaves the right shoulder against the pubic arch. Erb-Duchenne paralysis results if the upper roots (C5, C6) are involved. The arm appears adducted and internally rotated, and the forearm is pronated. The Moro reflex on the ipsilateral side is also absent. The hand muscles, however, are intact and without sensory deficit. The phrenic nerve is involved in 5% of cases, and should always be ruled out.

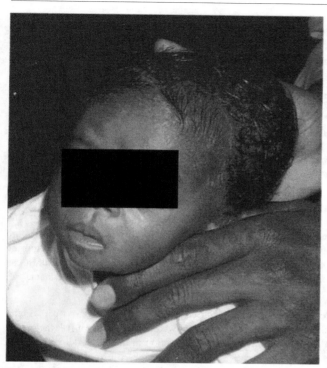
Figure 35.1: The rare occipital cephalhaematoma in an infant.

In the Déjerine-Klumpke palsy, the lower part of the brachial plexus (C8, T1) is involved, causing wrist drop with associated paralysis of the hand. Horner's syndrome is frequently associated with this injury. This has a worse prognosis than Erb-Duchenne paralysis.

Patients are followed up closely with both active and passive exercises. Most patients make a complete recovery on this conservative management. Persistence of deficit for 3 months is an indication for surgical intervention, but this is rare.

Neurolysis, end-to-end anastomosis, and nerve grafting are some of the surgical procedures employed. Primary surgery for brachial plexus lesions with modern microsurgical techniques is an emerging surgical option, with the prospect of improving functional recovery in carefully selected patients who would otherwise be faced with lifelong impairment and secondary skeletal deformities. Grafting and extraplexal neurotisation are the procedures most commonly involved. Donor nerves include the intercostal nerves, phrenic nerve, spinal accessory nerve, and contralateral C7 root.[9–10]

Facial nerve
Facial nerve injury may follow forceps delivery for face presentation or may arise from pressure from the birth canal during labour. Facial nerve injury is of the lower motor neurone lesion in most cases; it usually recovers with nonoperative treatment. In facial nerve paralysis, care of the exposed cornea is important. This is done by instillation of methylcellulose into the conjunctival sac.[11]

Phrenic nerve
The phrenic nerve is rarely involved; this nerve affects diaphragmatic function. It needs to be differentiated from congenital diaphragmatic hernia or eventration of the diaphragm. Chest infections are a serious complication of this injury. Spontaneous recovery is expected in 1–3 months. After 3 months without recovery, operative intervention is indicated. Imbrication or prosthetic replacement of the diaphragm is usually carried out.[12]

Spinal cord
Spinal cord injury is one of the most devastating injuries because in the very severe cases, the babies may be stillborn or die in the immedi-ate postnatal period. The infants who survive with spinal injury may have permanent neurological abnormalities due to the damage to the spinal cord or the vertebral arteries.[13] The mechanism of injury to the spinal cord involves application of strong traction when the spine is hyperextended or when the direction of pull is lateral. It may also occur with a forceful longitudinal pull when the head is firmly engaged. The most common part of the spinal cord involved is the upper cervical C4 with cephalic presentation. Affectation of vertebra above C4 is usually fatal due to compromised respiration because the vital centres in the upper cervical cord and brain stem may be involved.[12] In addition, lower cervical cord injuries (C5–C7) may occur with breech deliveries. Neurological signs may be produced by haemorrhage or oedema. Plain radiography is not very helpful because cord transection can occur without vertebral fractures. Ultrasonography (US) and magnetic resonance imaging (MRI) are best to characterise the site and extent of injuries and are usually confirmatory.

The mainstay of treatment is supportive, with physiotherapy, urology, orthopaedics, and psychology involved. This supportive treatment may mean endotracheal intubation for artificial respiration in the upper cervical injury group. Therefore, great emphasis is placed on prevention.

Intracranial trauma
This trauma is usually intracranial haemorrhage and can be subdural, subarachnoid, or intracerebral. Intracranial trauma usually follows vacuum extraction of the foetus.[11]

Subdural haemorrhage
Acute subdural haemorrhage is a recognised cause of increased head circumference and anaemia soon after birth.[14] The haemorrhage is from dural sinuses or the major cerebral veins. The clinical features are those of a focal neurological deficit, hemiparesis, unequal pupils, or deviation of the eyes. Other symptoms include bulging anterior fontanelle, pallor, vomiting, irritability, and seizures. The diagnosis is suggested by a subdural tap. Computed tomography (CT) scan and MRI are required to confirm the diagnosis. The treatment is by repeated tap of the subdural space by using a size 20G needle.

Subarachnoid haemorrhage
Subarachnoid haemorrhage results from damage to the veins traversing the subarachnoid space. It is the most common form of intracranial haemorrhage related to the trauma of birth. Subarachnoid haemorrhage is suspected on lumbar puncture with frank blood or a tinge of blood. There is no treatment required, as it resolves spontaneously.

Intracerebral haemorrhage
Intracerebral haemorrhage is the least common intracranial trauma. The clinical presentation is that of increased intracranial pressure. Serial US, CT, and MRI are needed to monitor the regression.

Solid Abdominal Visceral Injuries
Solid abdominal visceral injuries are the most serious complications of birth trauma, but, fortunately, they are comparatively rare.[15] The liver is the most common organ involved, followed by the adrenal gland, spleen, and kidney, in that order. The presenting symptoms are severe shock and abdominal distention. These patients may appear normal for the first 3 days, however; therefore, a high index of suspicion is required to make an early diagnosis. Refusal of feeds, listlessness, and rapid respiration in the presence of a rapidly developing anaemia should alert the physician to the possibility of internal bleeding. The presence of scrotal haematoma is an indication of haemoperitoneum usually in a patient with persistence of the processus vaginalis. Abdominal paracentesis will confirm haemoperitoneum. Abdominal ultrasound will confirm the injury and is also used in monitoring patients where nonoperative treatment is used. Coagulopathy and hypoxia are contributing factors to injuries.

In bilateral injuries involving the adrenal gland, acute adrenal insufficiency characterised by pyrexia, convulsions, coma, hypoglycaemia, and hyponatraemia are additional forms of presentation. In fact, in the more severe cases of bilateral adrenal haemorrhage, the diagnosis is usually made at postmortem examination. Patients should be resuscitated from shock and steroid replacement, and electrolytes should be administered in cases with adrenal involvement. Coagulopathy should be corrected.

Liver

One mechanism of injury to the liver is thoracic compression pushing the liver down and applying a pull on the hepatic ligaments, leading to a tear of these ligaments at their site of attachment.[16] Another is direct pressure on the liver during the passage of the foetus through the maternal pelvis, leading to subcapsular haemorrhage.[16] In breech delivery, blood is compressed from the lower parts of the body and venous return is retarded by the compression on the chest by the uterus, leading to marked congestion of the solid abdominal organs. Therefore, if pressure is applied on the trunk instead of the pelvis during delivery, any of these organs may be injured. This is the most common form of hepatic injury encountered—even more so in the premature baby whose liver is more exposed.

The nonoperative approach to correction of liver injury should be considered, as described in Chapter 29 on abdominal injuries. In severe cases, particularly in haemodynamically unstable infants, surgical exploration treatment should be undertaken. Topical haemostatic agents such as fibrin glue are more effective than direct suturing or electrocoagulation of the involved liver surface.[17] In Africa, where these agents may not be available, however, the use of the omentum, which acts as a plug when sutured in place, is advocated.

Adrenal gland

The right adrenal gland is most commonly involved in birth injuries. The vertebra exposes it to mechanical compression. The presence of a neuroblastoma is a risk factor that must always be ruled out in adrenal trauma.[18] Plain abdominal x-ray will show a rim of calcification only in adrenal haemorrhage, as different from the diffuse calcification seen in the diagnosis of the tumour. Biopsy of the adrenal gland should always be taken at laparotomy in suspicious cases.

Nonoperative treatment suffices in most cases of adrenal injuries. Haemorrhage into the perinephric fascia arrests spontaneously. Unilateral adrenalectomy is tolerated, even though steroid replacement may be necessary.

Spleen

Injury to the spleen secondary to birth trauma is rare. The mechanism of injury and clinical presentation are similar to those for the liver. The injury can occur alone but is frequently associated with liver injury. Preservation of the spleen is a high priority to avoid the problem of overwhelming postsplenectomy infection.[19] However, spleen-sparing surgeries are very difficult in the newborn, and splenectomy is frequently carried out.

Kidney

The kidney is rarely involved in birth injuries. Tissue preservation, just as for the spleen, is paramount. Intravenous urography is indicated to assess the extent of renal injuries. CT scan is the modality of choice in more accurate assessment of these injuries.

Genitourinary Injuries

Foetal manipulations in breech delivery have been associated with scrotal and testicular injuries in boys. In one particular report, an iatrogenic injury caused castration in a newborn.[20]

In girls, severe perineal tears have been described following both breech delivery and caesarian section (Figure 35.2). These injuries require prompt surgical intervention by way of a multilayered closure to achieve a good outcome.[21] A significant delay was associated with a fatal outcome from overwhelming sepsis.[22]

Rare (Unusual) Injuries

Injuries to the pharynx, trachea, bronchi, or oesophagus have been

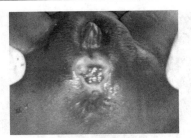

Figure 35.2: A severe form of perineal injury from repeated vaginal examination from the referral hospital. The child was delivered by a caesarian section due to delayed second stage and breech presentation.

described following the use of suction or endotracheal tubes.[1] Dislocation of the triangular cartilage of the nasal septum has been described.[23] Evisceration of the bowel through a wide tear of the umbilical cord during delivery may occur. This may result in bowel injury, requiring resection and anastomosis. If this occurs immediately after birth, it can be confused with gastroschisis by the inexperienced birth attendant.[24]

Prevention

In developed countries, improvements in obstetrics care, particularly antenatal ultrasonography, have allowed identification of risk factors for birth trauma and have led to modification in modes of delivery.[25] Also, more liberal use of caesarian section, decreased use of difficult forceps delivery, and centralisation of high-risk services have reduced the incidence of birth trauma. In developing countries, however, many deliveries still take place outside the orthodox centres. This practice is attended by a higher incidence of birth injuries and increased perinatal mortality.[2,3,26]

Health education and training of traditional birth attendants and reduction of delivery fees in hospitals in Africa will reduce the perinatal morbidity and mortality associated with birth injuries.

Evidence-Based Research

Table 35.1 presents a case control study of the incidence of birth trauma using a five-year review.[27]

Table 35.1: Evidence-based research.

Title	Birth trauma. A five-year review of incidence and associated perinatal factors
Authors	Perlow JH, Wigton T, Hart J, Strassner HT, Nageotte MP, Wolk BM
Institution	Department of Obstetrics and Gynecology, Christ Hospital and Medical Center, Oak Lawn, Illinois, USA
Reference	J Reprod Med 1996; 41(10):754–760
Problem	Birth injury.
Intervention	Case-control study.
Comparison/ control (quality of evidence)	Compares cases with injury to control births without injury to examine the incidence of clavicular fracture, facial nerve injury, and brachial plexus injury at birth to identify possible risk factors.
Outcome/ effect	The injuries are associated with prolonged gestation, epidural anaesthesia, prolonged second stage of labor, oxytocin use, forceps delivery, shoulder dystocia, macrosomia, low Apgar scores, and a previous maternal obstetric history of macrosomia when compared to controls. Other significantly associated variables include the presence of meconium in labor and neonatal hyperbilirubinaemia. Despite the presence of multiple perinatal factors that are individually associated statistically with the injured groups, multiple logistic regression analysis predicted 44.2% of clavicle fractures, none of the facial nerve injuries, and only 19% of the brachial plexus injuries.
Historical Significance/ comments	Most reports of birth injuries are case studies; this study, however, tries to examine for risk factors.

Key Summary Points

1. The majority of birth injuries are minor.

2. Breech delivery is a major risk factor for birth injuries.

3. Fractures from birth injury heal spontaneously; nonunion is almost nonexistent. The clavicle is the most common bone fractured.

4. Brachial plexus injuries are the most common form of neurological injury. The majority (75%) will recover on conservative management.

5. Spinal injuries are rare, but severe, with a fatal outcome or survival with a permanent disability.

6. Solid abdominal visceral injuries, although rare, have the most serious complications of birth trauma.

7. The liver is the most common organ involved. A high index of suspicion is necessary for the diagnosis of these injuries.

8. The presence of a tumour should be ruled out, especially when the adrenal gland is involved.

9. In girls, severe perineal tears have been described; these require prompt surgical intervention to avoid a fatal outcome.

10. Antenatal ultrasonography should be employed to identify risk factors for birth trauma and modify modes of delivery.

11. In Africa, health education, training of traditional birth attendants, and reduction of delivery fees should encourage more women to have supervised antenatal care and delivery, and hence reduce the risk of birth injuries.

References

1. Schullinger JN. Birth trauma. Pediatr Clin North Am 1993; 40:1351–1358.

2. Damstedt GL, Hussein MH, Winch PJ, et al. Practices of rural Egyptian birth attendants during the antenatal, intrapartum and early neonatal period. J Health Popul Nutr 2008; 26:36–45.

3. Wiredu EK, Tettey Y. Autopsy studies on still births in Korle Bu Teaching Hospital: causes of death in 93 still births. West Afr J Med 1998; 17:148–152.

4. Soni AL, Mir WA, Kishan J, Faquih AM, Elzouki AY. Brachial plexus injuries in babies born in hospital: an appraisal of risk factors in a developing country. Ann Trop Paediatr 1985; 5:69–71.

5. Vane DW. Child abuse and birth injuries. In Grosfeld JI, O'Neill JA Jr, Coran AG, Fonkalsrud EW, Caldamone AA, eds. Paediatric Surgery, 6th ed. Mosby Elsevier, 2006, Pp 400–407.

6. Presller JL. Classification of major newborn birth injuries. J Perinat Neonat Nurs 2008; 22:60–67.

7. Oppenheim WL, Davis A, Growdon WA, et al. Clavicle fractures in the newborn. Clin Orthop 1990; 250:176–180.

8. Morris S, Cassidy N, Stephens M, McCormack D, McManus F. Birth-associated femoral fractures: Incidence and outcome. J Pediatr Orthop 2002; 22:27–30.

9. Marcus JR, Clarke HM. Management of obstetrical brachial plexus palsy: evaluation, prognosis, and primary surgical treatment. Clin Plast Surg 2003; 30:289–306.

10. Boome RS, Kaye JC. Obstetrics traction injuries to the brachial plexus: natural history, indications for surgical repair and results. J Bone Joint Surg (Br) 1988; 70-B:571–576.

11. Madan A, Hamrick SEG, Ferriero DM. Central nervous system injury and neuroprotection. In: Taeush HW, Ballard RA, Gleason CA, eds. Avery's Diseases of the Newborn, 8th ed. Elsevier Saunders, 2005, Pp 965–992.

12. Langer JC, Filler RM, Coles M, Edmonds JF. Plication of the diaphragm for infants and young children with phrenic nerve palsy. J Pediatr Surg 1988; 23:749–751.

13. De Souza SW, Davies JA. Spinal cord damage in a newborn infant. Arch Dis Child 1974; 49:70–71.

14. Whitby EH, Griffiths PD, Rutter S, et al. Frequency and natural history of subdural haemorrhages in babies and relation to obstetric factors. Lancet 2003; 362:846–851.

15. Eraklis AJ. Abdominal injury related to the trauma of birth. Pediatrics 1967; 39:421–424.

16. Tank ES, Davis R. Holt J, et al. Mechanisms of trauma during breech delivery. Am J Obstet Gynecol 1971; 38:761–767.

17. French CE, Waldstein G. Subcapsular haemorrhage of the liver in the newborn. Pediatrics 1982; 69:204–208.

18. Murthy TVM, Irving IM, Lister J. Massive adrenal haemorrhage in neonatal neuroblastoma. J Pediatr Surg 1978; 13:31–34.

19. Matsuyama S, Suzuki N, Nagamachi Y. Rupture of the spleen in the newborn: treatment without splenectomy. J Pediatr Surg 1976; 11:115–116.

20. Samuel G. Castration at birth. Br Med J 1988; 297:1313–1314.

21. Patel HI, Moriarty KP, Brisson PA, Feins NR. Genitourinary Injuries in the newborn. J Pediatr Surg 2001; 36:235–239.

22. Bhat BV, Jagdish S, Pandey KK, Chatterjee H. Intrauterine perineal tear: a rare birth injury. J Pediatr Surg 1992; 27:1614–1615.

23. Soboczyski A, Skuratowicz A, Grzegorowski M. Nasal septum deviation in newborns. Acta Otolaryngol Belg 1992; 46:263–265.

24. Abubakar AM. Birth injuries. In: Ameh EA, Nwomeh BC, eds. Paediatric Trauma in Africa: A Practical Guide. Spectrum Books Limited, 2005, Pp 157–165.

25. Mazza F, Kitchens J, Akin M, et al. The road to zero preventable birth injuries. Jt Comm J Qual Patient Saf 2008; 34:201–205.

26. Etuk SJ, Itam H, Asuquo EE. Role of the spiritual churches in antenatal clinic default in Calabar, Nigeria. East Afr Med J 1999; 76:639–643.

27. Perlow JH, Wigton T, Hart J, Strassner HT, Nageotte MP, Wolk BM. Birth trauma. A five year review of incidence and associated perinatal factors. J Reprod Med 1996; 41(10):754–760.

Head and Neck

CHAPTER 36
NECK: CYSTS, SINUSES, AND FISTULAS

James O. Adeniran
Kokila Lakhoo

Introduction

Lumps in the neck are a common problem in children. Some of the lumps may not be obvious at birth but slowly get bigger and become worrying to the parents. Most of the lumps are asymptomatic, but some can cause respiratory or swallowing difficulties.[1,2] Some lumps become infected and require urgent medical attention. Most sinuses are usually not noticed at birth, but as the child grows, there is persistent discharge from the ostia. Many of these lumps and sinuses are remnants of structures that form the face and neck. Some sinuses are due to chronic infections.

Lumps that appear around the necks of children may be due to various conditions, as listed in Table 36.1. This chapter focuses on cysts, sinuses, and fistulas of the neck, which are remnants of branchial apparatus, and remnants of the thyroid gland. Sinuses due to tuberculosis, human immunodeficiency virus (HIV), and fungi also are discussed. Lymphadenopathy is discussed in Chapter 37, sternomastoid tumours in Chapter 38, thyroid masses in Chapter 40, and lymphangiomas in Chapter 44.

Branchial Arches, Clefts, and Pouches

Embryology and Pathology

Branchial arches appear as four pairs of ridges on the lateral side of the face of the 5-week old embryo (Figures 36.1 and 36.2). The arches bulge into the side walls of the foregut and meet each other in its floor, displacing the heart caudally to establish the neck region of the embryo.[3] The ridges are separated by four pairs of external, ectodermal grooves (branchial clefts) matched internally by four pharyngeal, endodermal pouches. The arches form the skeleton, musculature, and blood vessels of the jaws, palate, larynx, and pharynx, as well as the muscles of the face. As the dorsal ends of each arch approach the hindbrain, these structures are invaded by nerve fibres from the branchial efferent column. The ventral ends of the arches also converge on the pericardium to connect capillaries from the truncus arteriosus.[3] Each arch has mesenchyme, which develops into bone, cartilage, blood vessels, and muscles innervated by the nerve of that arch.

First Branchial Arch

Embryology

The first, or mandibular, arch appears on the 22nd gestational day, and by the 6th week fuses in the midline to form the mesenchymal primordium that develops into the anterior two-thirds of the tongue. The core of the arch chondrifies to form Meckel's cartilage, which develops into the malleus and incus bones. The muscles of mastication develop from the first arch mesoderm, all innervated by the motor root of the trigeminal. The first branchial cleft forms the external acoustic meatus.

The first pharyngeal pouch is recognised after the formation of the head fold about the 20th day of embryonic life. The first pair of grooves and pouches persists to form the auditory canal and eustachian tube, which is separated by the tympanic membrane. The first pouch and membrane persist as the pharyngotympanic tube, middle ear cavity, and tympanic membrane.

Table 36.1: Common causes of lumps in the necks of children

Location	Cause
Lateral side of neck	Lymph nodes due to scalp or throat infections, tuberculosis, or lymphomas Cystic hygromas Sternomastoid tumour Teratomas Thyroid masses Branchial cyst—first, second, third, fourth
Midline of neck	Thyroglossal cysts Dermoids Haemangiomas Ectopic thyroid tissue

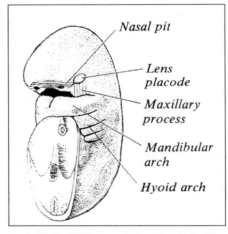

Source: FitzGerald MJT. Human Embryology: A Regional Approach. Harper & Row Publishers, 1978. Used by permission.

Figure 36.1: Five-week embryo showing the position of branchial arches.

Differentiation of the first branchial arch is shown below:

- *Skin:* skin of lower part of face
- *Bones:* malleus, incus, mandible, maxilla
- *Muscles:* muscles of mastication, floor of the mouth, tensor palati, tensor tympani, anterior belly digastric and mylohyoid
- *Nerve:* mandibular branch of trigeminal nerve
- *Artery:* maxillary
- *Membrane:* mucous membrane of nasopharynx

Remnants

Abnormal development of the first branchial arch results in cleft lip and palate, pinna deformities, and malformed malleus and incus, which may produce congenital deafness.[3–5]

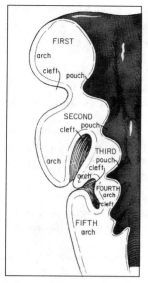

Figure 36.2: Coronal view of 5-week embryo showing branchial arches.

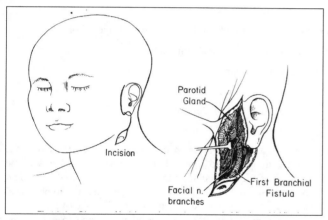

Figure 36.3: Surgical management of first branchial arch fistula.

Clinical presentation

True anomalies of the first branchial cleft are uncommon.[5] Skin tabs, pre-auricular cysts, and sinus tracts around the ear are not of branchial cleft origin but occur from abnormal infolding and entrapment of epithelium during the merger of the six hillocks of His that form the external pinna.[4,6]

When they occur, first branchial cleft cysts present as a swelling in front of or behind the pinna. External openings of the fistula lie below the mandible and above the hyoid bone. The tract may pass superficial or deep to the main branches of the facial nerve and through the substance of the parotid gland with the internal opening into the external auditory canal, which forms the source of recurrent infection (Figure 36.3).

Management

If operation is deemed necessary, a curved incision is made to elevate the pinna and expose the parotid gland. The facial nerve and its trunks are identified and preserved. The tract is then dissected superiorly and then medially to the external auditory canal (see Figure 36.3).

Histologically, the tracts are lined by stratified squamous epithelium with skin appendages. Muscle fibres and cartilages may be seen in the deeper layers.

Second Branchial Arch

Embryology

The first two branchial (or hyoid) arches and clefts, and second pharyngeal pouches appear in the 22-day old embryo. The second arch extends down the neck (as the platysma) to overlap the second, third, and fourth branchial clefts, forming a potential space—the cervical sinus of His. The core of the hyoid arches forms a U-shaped cartilage, which forms the upper part of the hyoid bone. The dorsal end forms the stapes and the styloid process of the temporal bone.

Differentiation of the second branchial arch is shown below:

- *Skin:* lateral and anterior part of neck
- *Bones:* stapes, styloid process, upper part of body and lesser cornu of hyoid
- *Muscles:* posterior belly of digastric, muscles of facial expression, stapedius, stylohyoid, platysma
- *Nerve:* facial nerve
- *Artery:* stapedial (remnant of dorsal part of second aortic arch)
- *Membrane:* membrane of oropharynx

The muscular element of the hyoid arch spreads like a fan to form the muscles of facial expression, innervated by the facial nerve (Figure 36.4). Lymphocytes invade the lateral end of the second pharyngeal pouch to form the palatine tonsils

Remnants

Complete fistulas, external sinuses, and cysts may occur as remnants of the second branchial arch. Although congenital, the tiny openings may not be obvious at birth. Attention is usually drawn to the problem by persistent mucoid drainage and/or recurrent infection. Sinuses present in the first decade of life, and cysts usually in the second decade. The cysts and external openings of the second branchial cleft lie along the anterior border of the sternomastoid muscle at the junction of the upper two-thirds and the lower one-third (Figures 36.4 and 36.5). The tract ascends along the carotid sheath to the level of the hyoid bone, then turns medially between the branches of the carotid artery, behind the posterior belly of the digastric and stylohyoid muscles, and in front of the hypoglossal nerve to end in the tonsilla fossa (see Figure 36.1). Sinuses with external openings at the same site pursue the same course before terminating blindly after variable distances. Secretions in branchial cysts may take a while to accumulate because they are clinically visible or palpable. The cysts may not, therefore, be clinically evident until late in childhood or early adolescence. Bacteria from the oral cavity may contaminate the cysts, leading to an abscess in 25% of cases.[7] The cysts may be bilateral in 10% of the cases.

The cysts contain turbid fluid and therefore do not transilluminate like cystic hygromas. Lymph node enlargement from tuberculosis, tonsillitis, and lymphomas may present with neck masses to form differential diagnosis.

Investigation

A sinogram may be done to outline the course of the fistula, but it is not a substitute for careful dissection at operation. Fine needle aspiration (FNA) cytology or excision may be needed to confirm the diagnosis, and this must be done aseptically to prevent introducing infection.

Management

Sclerotherapy has not been developed as a method of management; therefore, operative excision is the treatment of choice. Unless the whole tract is dissected, recurrences may occur, with the possibility of neoplastic degeneration in adult life.[8,9]

Operations to remove the cyst, sinus, and fistula are all approached the same way, with the patient under general anaesthesia with endotracheal intubation.

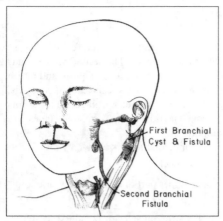

Source: Welch KJ, Randolph JG, Ravitch MM, O'Neill JA Jr, Rowe MI. Pediatric Surgery. Year Book Medical Publishers, 1986. Used by permission.
Figure 36.4: Courses of first, second, and third branchial fistulas.

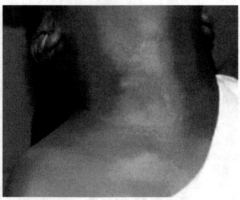

Figure 36.5: Second branchial cyst in a 4-year-old girl (the cyst had discharged and healed 4 or 5 times).

For the procedures outlined below, a sandbag is placed under the shoulders to extend the neck, and a head-ring is applied to steady the head, similar to the standard draping for a thyroid operation. The head is then turned to the contralateral side as convenient.

Brachial cysts

1. In branchial cysts, a transverse incision is made 3–4 cm long over the mass.

2. The skin and platysma are incised and deepened to the edge of the mass.

3. Blunt and sharp dissections are done to identify the tract. It is important to maintain a bloodless field, using mostly diathermy, throughout the dissection and to keep close to the tract. Keeping close to the tract will not only make the tract easily visible, but will prevent inadvertently injuring surrounding structures. It is not necessary to identify all the surrounding structures. If the dissection is very close to the tract, the likelihood of injuring other structures is slim.

Sinus

Preparation and draping for surgery is as above.

1. An elliptical incision is made around the opening.

2. The incision is deepened through the skin and platysma and the tract is identified.

3. The operation then proceeds the same way as for removal of a branchial cyst.

Fistula

In many cysts and sinuses, the tracts end blindly at various distances but must be pursued as a fistula. Again, preparation and draping for surgery is as above.

1. The fistula is traced along the carotid sheath through the bifurcation of the carotid artery, then medially to the tonsilla fossa.

2. The anaesthetist may assist by inserting a gloved finger into the patient's mouth to push the tongue down.

3. Another skin incision may be necessary, as a step-ladder incision, if the original skin incision is too far down in the neck.

Patients with bilateral fistulas can have both sides operated at the same sitting.

Histologically, the cysts are lined by squamous epithelium, surrounded by muscle fibres and lymphoid tissue, but in 10% of patients, respiratory columnar epithelium may also be present.[4,10]

Third Branchial Arch

Embryology

The three pharyngeal arches and four pharyngeal pouches develop by the 27th day of embryonic life. The pouches are tube-like extensions of the pharynx.[11]

The third arch mesenchyme forms the posterior one-third of the tongue. Its cartilage ossifies to form the lower part of the hyoid bone. Its only muscle, the stylopharyngeus, is supplied by the glossopharyngeal nerve from the nucleus ambiguous.[3] The thymus and inferior parathyroid glands develop from the third pharyngeal pouch.

Differentiation of the third branchial arch is shown below:

• *Skin:* lateral part of neck

• *Bone:* lower part of body and greater horn of hyoid bone

• *Muscle:* superior pharyngeal constrictor

• *Nerve:* glossopharyngeal

• *Artery:* common carotid

• *Membrane:* lower part of pharynx

Remnants

Rarely, some cysts may arise from the left side of the neck in close relation to the thyroid gland. The external openings are usually at the anterior border of the clavicular head of the sternomastoid. The tract runs behind the internal carotid artery, the vagus, and the hypoglossal and superior laryngeal nerves, and then turns medially above the spinal accessory nerve and penetrates the thyroid membrane to end in the pyriform sinus.

Management

Incision and drainage may be necessary when the cysts are infected. The tract may need excision if there is recurrent infection.

Histologically, thyroid, thymic, and lymphoid tissue and Hassall corpuscles have been seen, which may suggest their origin from lower pharyngeal pouches.[4]

Fourth to Sixth Branchial Arches

The fourth and sixth arches mingle as they produce the cartilages and ligaments of the larynx, the levator palate, and the intrinsic muscles of the larynx and pharynx, all supplied by the vagus nerve.[3] Part of thymus and the superior parathyroid glands develop from the fourth pharyngeal pouch.

Contributions of the fourth branchial arch are shown below:

• *Skin:* none

• *Cartilage:* thyroid and arytenoids

• *Muscles:* inferior pharyngeal constrictor, cricothyroid, intrinsic laryngeal

• *Nerve:* superior laryngeal branch of vagus

• *Artery:* arch of aorta on left side, first part of subclavian artery on right side

• *Membrane:* hypopharynx

Contributions of the sixth branchial arch are shown below:

- *Skin:* none

- *Cartilage:* cricoid, arytenoids, rings of trachea and bronchi

- *Muscles:* intrinsic muscles of larynx (except cricothyroid, stylopharyngeus, tensor palate)

- *Nerve:* recurrent laryngeal branch of vagus

- *Artery:* pulmonary artery on right side, ductus arteriosus on left side

- *Membrane:* hypopharynx

Remnants

Anomalies of the fourth branchial pouch very rarely may produce a cyst or a fistula very low in the neck behind the sternomastoid muscle. On the right side, the tract goes behind the subclavian artery; on the left side, it goes under the arch of the aorta. It opens into the cervical oesophagus.

Midline Cervical Clefts

Midline cervical clefts (Figure 36.6) are due to imperfect midline fusion of the paired branchial arch tissue about the fourth week of embryonic development. These present as raw, weeping areas in the midline of the lower neck. They may have irregular skin tabs or shallow sinuses. Management is usually conservative. If excision is deemed necessary, a Z-plasty may be done to prevent ugly scars or contractures.

Dermoid Cysts

Dermoid (inclusion) cysts (Figure 36.7) are caused by entrapment of epithelium of branchial arch origin at the time of embryologic midline fusion. Most of the cysts are in the midline, are firm in consistency, and may be attached to overlying skin (Figure 36.7). They do not move with swallowing or protrusion of the tongue. They usually do not have any deep-seated tracts and are easily excised surgically through a transverse collar-stud incision.

Teratomas

Teratomas are tumours composed of multiple tissues foreign to the anatomical locus.[1,2,12] These tissues cannot have resulted from metaplasia. They develop adjacent to normal anatomical structures or organs and are generally attached by limited vascular pedicles. The most common sites for teratomas are the gonads and the sacrococcygeal areas.[2] These sites embryologically allow deviation of early germinal issue to disorganised complex teratomas. Teratomas are also common in the neck region (Figure 36.8). Most teratomas are benign. They produce secondary symptoms due to their pressure effects on adjacent organs.

Investigation

Teratomas may be soft to firm in consistency because they may contain cystic areas. They may be confused with cystic hygromas. Neck ultrasound and/or aspiration, under aseptic conditions, may be necessary to confirm the diagnosis.

Management

Complete excision of the teratoma should be the desired goal. Incomplete excision may lead to recurrence of the mass, recurrent infection, draining sinuses, or the possibility of malignant change.[1,13]

Thyroglossal Cysts

Thyroglossal cysts are the most common midline masses in children, accounting for 70% of all congenital cervical lesions.[14] They can occur at any age, and one-third become obvious in adult life.

Embryology

The thyroid gland develops as a diverticulum from the foramen caecum of the tongue, descending in front of the trachea in company with the thymus and the inferior parathyroid glands. It reaches its final position by the 7th week of embryonic life.[14–16] The hyoid bone develops at about the same time, from the second and third arches, and fuses anteriorly so that the thyroglossal duct may pass anterior to, through, or posterior to the body of the hyoid bone.[3,14] The duct usually spontaneously obliterates, but remnants may be found anywhere from the base of the tongue to the pyramidal lobe of the thyroid gland (Figure 36.9), although 80% are juxtaposed to the hyoid bone.[15]

Clinical Presentation

Most thyroglossal cysts are clinically evident before the child is 10 years old. Males and females are affected equally. The cysts present as round masses in the midline of the neck that move up and down with swallowing and with protrusion of the tongue because of their connection to the hyoid bone. They are soft to firm in consistency, mobile, and nontender unless infected.

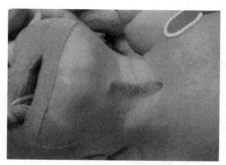

Figure 36.6: Midline cervical cleft.

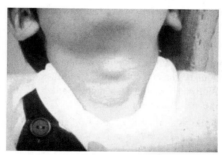

Figure 36.7: Dermoid cyst.

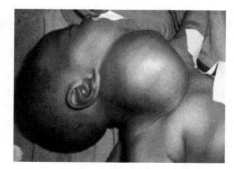

Figure 36.8: Teratoma.

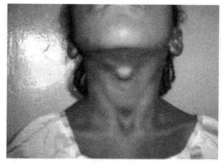

Figure 36.9: Thyroglossal cyst.

Differential Diagnosis

Midline dermoids, which occur commonly in the submental triangle, are the commonest differential diagnosis.[16] Ectopic midline thyroid, enlarged pyramidal lobe of thyroid gland, and thyroid adenomas may also present as midline masses.

Investigations

Neck ultrasonography and thyroid iodine scintigraphy may be needed to confirm the diagnosis and rule out ectopic thyroid tissue.

Complications

Thyroglossal fistula may result from infection of the thyroglossal cyst or after drainage of a thyroglossal abscess. The fistula is usually in the midline. Sinograms are unnecessary for diagnosis, and sclerotherapy as a means of treatment has not been described.

Surgical Management

Both thyroglossal cysts and fistulas are surgically approached by the Sistrunk operation described by Walter Sistrunk in 1920.[17] The aim of the operation is to completely excise the duct with the middle part of the body of the hyoid bone and a cuff of the tongue muscles because side branches of the duct may occur within the muscles of the tongue.[16] Complete excision of the duct is essential to prevent recurrence or malignant degeneration.[18]

For the procedures outlined below, the patient is given general anaesthesia with endotracheal intubation. In the supine position, a sandbag is placed under the patient's shoulders to extend the neck, and a head ring is used to steady the head. The neck, lower jaw, and upper part of the chest are cleaned and draped.

Thyroglossal cyst

1. A transverse skin incision is made at the midpoint of the mass. The incision is deepened through platysma and subcutaneous tissues to reach the edge of the cyst. With strict haemostasis using diathermy, the tract is easily identified on the upper part of the cyst.

2. Thereafter the procedure follows as for a thyroglossal fistula.

Thyroglossal fistula

1. An elliptical skin incision is made around the ostium. This skin incision is deepened through platysma until the tract is identified.

2. Keeping very close to the tract, the tract is dissected between the sternohyoid muscles until the hyoid bone is identified.

3. The body of the hyoid bone is cleared from the sternohyoid muscle inferiorly and the mylohyoid and geniohyoid muscles superiorly with diathermy.

4. An artery forceps is used to separate the body of the hyoid bone from the thyrohyoid membrane inferiorly.

5. The middle portion of the hyoid bone is then excised either with a strong straight scissors or with small bone cutters.

6. The hyoid bone is then held with towel clips and lifted to expose the proximal part of the tract. This is now dissected to the floor of the mouth. The anaesthetist may be asked to depress the tongue with a gloved finger to assist the surgeon to locate the foramen caecum but this manouvre is usually not necessary.[16]

7. At the foramen caecum, a small rectangular piece of hyoglossus and genioglossus are excised with the tract.

8. Strict haemostasis is maintained and the wound closed in layers. It is unnecessary to reapproximate the hyoid bone. Drainage is usually unnecessary unless haemostasis is unsatisfactory or there is previous infection. A subcuticular stitch may be used to close the skin.

9. Perioperative antibiotics are justified if previous infection of a cyst has occurred or after operation on thyroglossal fistula.

Histologically, the tract usually contains pseudostratified ciliated columnar respiratory epithelium in 60% of cases and stratified squamous epithelium in the rest.[19] More than 100 carcinomas have been reported from thyroglossal duct remnants. These are either papillary adenocarcinomas or squamous carcinomas.[14,20] Most of these malignancies arise in the substance of the ducts and not from metastasis from the thyroid glands. The tumours are slow-growing and confined to the neck for long periods.[14] Most, including the affected lymph nodes, can be managed surgically with the Sistrunk operation.

Other Rare Neck Masses

Many rare neck masses appear low in the neck and may have connections to masses in the thoracic cavity.

Bronchogenic Cysts

Bronchogenic cysts are attached to the hilum of the lung and may present as low neck masses, where they may compress the trachea, causing stridor.

Lymphangiomas

Lymphagiomas involving the posterior mediastinum may extend to the lower part of the neck, generally to the left of the trachea.

Thymic Cysts and Mediastinal Tumours

Thymic cysts and mediastinal tumours may rarely present with extensions in the lower part of the neck.

Evidence-Based Research

Table 36.2 presents a retrospective study that reviews the types of congenital cysts, their management, and problems associated with management.

Table 36.2: Evidence-based research.

Title	Congenital cysts and fistulas of the neck
Authors	Nicollas R, Guelfucci B, Roman S, Triglia JM
Institution	Service d'ORL Pediatrique, Federation ORL Hospital de la Timone, Marseille, France
Reference	Intl J Pediatr Otorhinolaryng 2000; 55:117–124
Design	Retrospective study
Aim	To review types of congenital cysts seen, the management given, and problems associated with management.
Period	1984–1999.
Exclusion	Preauricular cysts and cystic hygromas.
Result	Of 191 children with congenital cysts and fistulas, 123 were malformations of the midline, 102 were thyroglossal duct cysts, and 21 were dermoid cysts. Of the 68 malformations of the laterocervical region, 37 were cysts and fistulas of second cleft, 20 were cysts of first cleft, 7 were cysts of fourth pouch, and 4 were thymic cysts.
Problems in management	Diagnosis and management of midline masses are usually straightforward. Misdiagnosis of lateral cysts is common and often leads to inadequate treatment and recurrence.

Key Summary Points

1. Branchial arches develop as six-paired structures on the side of the neck of the embryo. Many congenital neck lumps and fistulas are remnants of branchial arches.

2. The first arch forms the skin of the lower part of face, malleus, incus, mandible, maxilla, and muscles of mastication. Remnants of the first branchial arch are uncommon.

3. The second arch forms skin of the lateral and anterior part of neck; the stapes, body, and lesser cornu of the hyoid bone; and muscles of facial expression. Cysts (and fistulas) of the second arch appear at the anterior border of the sternomastoid muscle.

4. The third arch and pouch develop into the posterior one-third of the tongue, the lower part of the hyoid bone, the thymus, and inferior parathyroid glands. External openings of remnants of the third arch are usually at the anterior border of the clavicular head of the sternomastoid.

5. The fourth to the sixth arches mingle as they produce the cartilages and ligaments of the larynx and pharynx (all supplied by the vagus nerve), part of the thymus, and the superior parathyroid glands.

6. The thyroid gland develops from a diverticulum at the floor of the mouth. Remnants of the thyroid may be found from the base of the tongue to the pyramidal lobe of the thyroid

7. Thyroglossal cysts are the most common congenital midline cysts. Thyroglossal cysts move with swallowing and protrusion of the tongue.

8. Thyroglossal fistulas are best removed by the Sistrunk operation.

9. Extrapulmonary tuberculosis, fungi, and HIV can affect neck glands to produce discharging sinuses in the neck.

References

1. Adeniran JO, Abdur-Rahman LO, Bolaji BO. Cervical teratoma in a neonate: case report. Trop J Health Sci 2006; 13:40–41.

2. Kerner B, Flaum E, Mathews H, et al. Cervical teratoma prenatal diagnosis and long term follow-up. Prenat Diagn 1998; 18:51–59.

3. FitzGerald MJT, ed. Human Embryology: A Regional Approach. Harper & Row Publishers, 1978, Pp 137–168 (Head and neck).

4. Soper RT, Pringle KC. Cysts and sinuses of the neck. In Welch KJ, Randolph JG, Ravitch MM, O'Neill JA, Rowe MI, eds. Pediatric Surgery, 4th ed. Year Book Medical Publishers, 1986, Pp 539–552.

5. Hyndman OR, Light G. The branchial apparatus. Arc Surg 1929; 19:410.

6. Streeter GL. Development of the auricle in the human embryo. Contrib Embryol Carnegie Instit 1921; 14 :113–138.

7. Toomey JJ. Cysts and tumors of the pharynx. In: Paparella MM, Shumrick DA. Otolaryngology. WB Saunders, 1973, Chapter 23.

8. Brauer HO. Congenital cysts and tumors of the neck. In: Brauer, RO. Reconstructive Plastic Surgery. WB Saunders, 1977, Philadelphia,

9. Katubig D, Damjanov I. Branchial cleft carcinoma. Arch Otolaryngol 1969; 89:750.

10. Ackerman LV, Rosai J. Surgical Pathology. Mosby, 1974, Chapter 9 (thyroid gland).

11. Norris EH. The parathyroid glands and the lateral thyroid in man: their mophogenesis, histogenesis, topographic anatomy and prenatal growth. Contrib Embryol Carnegie Instit 1937; 26:247–294.

12. Willis RA: The Borderland of Embryology and Pathology. Butterworth, 1962; P 442.

13. Wooley MM: Teratoma. In: Welch KJ, Randolph MM, eds. Pediatric Surgery, 4th ed. Year Book Medical Publishers, 1986, Pp 265–276.

14. Roback SA, Telanda RL. Thyroglossal duct cysts and branchial cleft anomalies. Semin Pediatr Surg 1994; 3:142–146.

15. Ward PH, Strahan RW, Acquerelli M. The many faces of cysts of the thyroglossal tract. Trans Am Acad Ophthalmol Otolaryngol 1970; 74:310.

16. Brereton RJ. Symonds E. Thyroglossal cysts in children. Br J Surg 1978; 65:507–508.

17. Sistrunk WE. The surgical treatment of cysts of the thyroglossal tract. Ann Surg 1920; 71:121–123.

18. Lui AHF, Littler ER. Thyroid carcinoma originating in a thyroglossal cyst: report of a case. Am Surgeon 1970; 36:546–548.

19. Stahl WM Jr, Lyall D. Cervical cysts and fistulae of thyroglossal tract origin. Ann Surg 1954; 139:123.

20. Shepard GH, Rosenfeld L. Carcinoma of thyroglossal duct remnants. Am J Surg 1968; 116:125.

CHAPTER 37
LYMPHADENOPATHY IN AFRICAN CHILDREN

S. W. Moore
N. Tsifularo
Ralf-Bodo Troebs

Introduction

Lymphadenopathy is an extremely common clinical finding in children in Africa as well as the rest of the world. It is common in children due to their large lymphoid mass and rapid lymphocytic response to allergens or infections. It is therefore most prevalent in the first decades of life; the majority of children between the ages of 2 and 12 years will have an enlarged lymph node at one stage or another.

In broad terms, lymphadenopathy represents an enlargement of lymph nodes resulting from:

• *Reactive state* – acute lymphadenitis

• *Hyperplasia* – e.g., human immunodeficiency virus (HIV), autoimmune disease

• *Granulomas* – tuberculosis (TB), mycobacteria other than tuberculosis (MOTT), toxoplasmosis, syphilis

• *Neoplastic* – primary (lymphomas) or secondary (metastases)

Lymphadenopathy is important because it may be the first (and sometimes only) indication of underlying disease. The major cause is infection, which may be acute bacterial or viral or chronic due to a host of causes, the majority of which give rise to granulomas. It is therefore understandable that the incidence of lymphadenopathy is reportedly higher in sick children than in those attending well baby clinics.

The obvious therapeutic and prognostic implications of lymphadenopathy necessitate an accurate and prompt diagnosis. Size, location, consistency, and nonresponse to empiric antibiotic therapy are the major criteria for further investigation. More than half the cervical lymph nodes examined in children in a developing country display very significant and clinically important pathology, thereby justifying active management of all paediatric patients with persisting lymphadenopathy.

One of the main concerns is the association between malignancy and lymphadenopathy, which may be primary or secondary but particularly includes the lymphoma group of conditions. Lymphadenopathy therefore needs to be actively investigated should it not respond to simple initial treatment so as not to overlook these important conditions. It is important to institute early treatment.

Anatomy

Lymph nodes are discrete encapsulated aggregations of lymphoid tissue that are seldom palpable in the normal child. These bean-like ovoid structures are scattered along lymphatic vessels but increase in number where the vessels converge, such as in the neck, axilla, pelvis, mediastinum, and similar situations (Figure 37.1).

Lymph nodes are structurally divided into three zones (the cortex, the paracortex, and the medulla). The architecture of these areas often is important. These sites appear to have separate functions: the cortex is the main site of B-cell activation; the paracortex is the T-cell dependent region; and the medulla, with abundant sinuses lined by macrophages, has a reticulo-endothelial function.

The primary function of the lymph node is to entrap and mount a response against foreign agents as part of the reticulo-endothelial system.

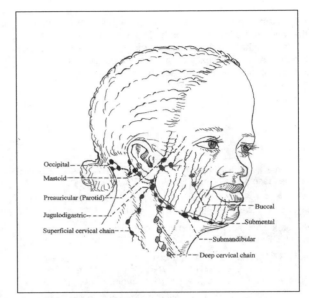

Figure 37.1: Anatomy of lymph nodes.

Demographics

Well-documented geographical differences exist in the epidemiology of lymphadenopathy in childhood. In general, the pathology usually identifies what is common in that particular environment, which has a special significance for Africa, where tuberculosis remains one of the main causes of lymph node enlargement. For example, in one South African series,[1] the incidence of *Mycobacterium tuberculosis* was 28%, similar to the 24.9% reported in children worldwide, but that incidence is higher than in developed countries such as Australia and countries in Europe and North America, where *M. tuberculosis* is less common, and parallels an increase in infections caused by "atypical mycobacteria" (i.e., MOTT). As a result, chronic granulomatous conditions result mainly from MOTT infections and cat scratch disease in those countries.

Aetiology

Chronic lymphadenopathy in children of developing countries has a high incidence of infective causes, including pathogenic bacteria, mycobacteria, and fungi, as well as neoplastic, metabolic, and immunological causes, and other causes of lymph node reaction.

Infective causes may be further classified into acute or chronic.

Acute Suppurative Lymphadenitis

Acute suppurative lymphadenitis is secondary to infections of the upper respiratory tract; ear, nose, and throat (ENT); or scalp. Submandibular lymph nodes are common sites in the 3–6 months age group

Acute lymphadenitis can result from poor dental and mouth hygiene. Involvement of the floor of the mouth is common in developing countries.

Acute lymphadenitis often leads to suppuration and abscess formation (Figure 37.2), and may lead to Ludwig's angina.

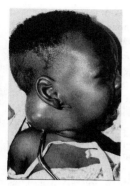

Figure 37.2: Acute suppurative lymphadenitis with abscess.

Chronic Lymphadenitis

Chronic lymphadenitis may be caused by a reactive hyperplasia virus; defined infections, such as toxoplasmosis or infectious mononucleosis; or chronic granulomas, such as mycobacteria (other than TB), cat scratch disease, or possibly TB; or viruses (e.g., Ebstein–Barr, HIV, or cytomegalovirus (CMV)).

Pathology

Lymphadenopathy represents the response to localised or generalised pathology as a result of antigenic stimulation or infiltration by cellular elements. The larger lymphoid mass as well as a brisk lymphogenic response following exposure to new antigens predisposes to lymph node enlargement in children.

Generalised enlargement of lymph nodes is defined as two or more noncontinuous lymph node regions with enlarged nodes (including intraabdominal lymphadenopathy). It most often occurs as a result of systemic disease due to infectious agents, but malignancies, autoimmune disease, and lipid storage diseases, as well as drug reactions and other miscellaneous pathologies, also contribute to the overall picture. It is often accompanied by other generalised symptoms, such as weight loss, night sweats, and ill health, or symptoms typical of the underlying pathological condition.

In contrast, localised lymphadenopathy occurs mainly as a result of diseases or infections in the node or their drainage areas. It can be cervical, axillary, inguinal, or other (e.g., supratrochlear, occipital, etc.).

Reactive Hyperplasia

The majority of enlarged lymph nodes in children occur as a result of infective agents; viral infections show only reactive hyperplasia in the majority (in as many as 48% of patients) without a specific cause being identified. This is not entirely unexpected considering the empiric use of antibiotics, which may mask certain aetiological agents, and the difficulty of identifying causative pathogens, particularly in Africa. This high prevalence of reactive hyperplasia does not exclude the need for careful clinicopathological correlation to improve diagnostic capability, however.

The most probable aetiology guides the diagnosis of lymphadenopathy. Despite the myriad causes, lymph nodes enlarge as a result of proliferation of normal lymphoid elements or infiltration by phagocytic cells or malignant cell deposits. Many are caused by viral infections, which result in small, self-limiting lymph nodes. If a bacterial aetiology is anticipated, an empiric course of antibiotics that cover streptococci and staphylococci is appropriate, with re-evaluation. Abscess formation is treated surgically.

Chronic Granulomas

In our series[1] of 1,877 surgically biopsied lymph nodes, 484 (36.3%) had chronic granulomatous changes. Although *M. tuberculosis* was the causative agent in the majority, in almost 10% the causes of the chronic granulomas were not always clear but included sinus histiocytosis with massive lymphadenopathy (Rosai–Dorfman disease), syphilis, yaws, and toxoplasmosis.

Acute Bacterial Lymphadenitis

Aetiology

Unilateral, large, and tender lymph nodes are commonly due to acute bacterial infection. The most common cause of acute lymphadenitis is a bacterial infection arising in the oropharynx. Submandibular and upper cervical nodes are affected in the majority of cases. Axillary, inguinal, and other locations also may be inflamed. Ultrasonography may detect an abscess not already apparent on physical examination.

Typical organisms are penicillin-resistant *Staphylococcus aureus* and *Streptococcus pyogenes*. Group B streptoccal adenitis may occur in the infant with unilateral submandibular swelling, erythema, tenderness, fever, and irritability. In the older child with dental caries or periodontal disease, anaerobic germs (e.g., *Bacteroides* sp., *Peptococcus* sp., *Peptostreptococcu*) play a role. Following animal (dog) bites or animal scratches, *Pasteurella multocida* may cause acute lymphadenitis.

Without treatment, the lymph node usually enlarges and becomes fluctuant. Thinning over the overlying skin and spontaneous perforation may occur. Laboratory findings include an elevation of white blood cell and neutrophil count.

Treatment

Initial treatment of acute lymphadenitis consists of administration of a beta-lactamase–resistant antibiotic for 2 weeks, at least 5 days beyond resolution of acute signs and symptoms. In older children with dental or periodontal infection, the antibiotic therapy should include an anti-anaerobic antibiotic, such as penicillin V or clindamycin.

If the child appears toxic (high fever, cellulites, respiratory problems) or is quite young, hospitalisation and intravenous (IV) administration of antibiotics are often necessary. In these cases, blood cultures should be obtained. However, the incidence of bacteremia associated with pediatric acute adenitis seems to be low.

Fluctuance of the lesion is a clear indication for surgical evacuation. Needle aspiration and drainage of the purulent material can be both diagnostic and therapeutic. It is particularly attractive when treating in cosmetically important areas. However, repeated aspirations may be necessary, and judicious antibiotic therapy is required.

The aspirated material should be cultured for aerobic and anaerobic germs as well as for mycobacteria. In addition, it is helpful to examine the material by Gram and Ziehl–Neelsen acid-fast stain. In the immunocompromised child, fungal infections have to be taken into account.

An alternative to node aspiration is open drainage under general anaesthesia, which is safe and highly successful. The node can be incised and packed loosely with a Penrose drain or a gauze strip. An attempt should be made to open and drain all loculations. The drain can usually be removed after a period of several days.

Complications

Major and life-threatening complications reported in children with suppurative cervical lymphadenitis are fasciitis, carotid artery aneurysm, and rupture, thrombosis of the jugular vein, generalised septic embolisation, mediastinal abscess, and purulent pericarditis.

Mycobacterial-Related Lymphadenitis

Tuberculosis and Lymphadenopathy

Although the incidence of TB has stabilised or declined in most world regions, it is increasing in Africa, Southeast Asia, and the eastern Mediterranean countries, being fuelled by the HIV pandemic with which it is closely associated. Tuberculous lymphadenitis and malignant nodal spread remain the most frequently encountered reasons for lymph node enlargement. Tuberculosis (TB) is the most frequent form of extrapulmonary tuberculosis and is identified in at least 28% of most series of cervical lymphadenopathy. Given the historical difficulties in diagnosis, the actual figure for Africa is probably somewhat higher.

Cervical lymphadenopathy has been reported to occur in 4–9% of children with pulmonary tuberculosis, with 57% occurring between the ages of 1 and 3 years. Clinical suspicion of cervical TB is high in children with a previous history of TB or close contact with a TB patient from an endemic region. The significance increases in the presence of a markedly positive tuberculin skin test (i.e., Mantoux test). The finding of nontender, painless, unilateral cervical lymph nodes on physical examination further strengthens this suspicion. Objective diagnosis is then fairly difficult and relies on cervical lymph node sampling.

Particular difficulties exist in making a clinical diagnosis in children with HIV disease, who may have atypical presentations. When clinically indicated, screening for pulmonary and laryngeal disease depends heavily on lymph node sampling. Fine needle aspiration (FNA) with culture or polymerase chain reaction (PCR)–based identification are rapidly overtaking the more conventional methods of diagnosis, with the more traditional method of excisional biopsy being reserved for selected cases.

Nontuberculous Mycobacterial Infections

BCG lymphadenitis
A special situation exists in lymphadenopathy related to the Danish strain of bacille Calmette-Guérin (BCG; Figure 37.3), which is estimated to occur at the rate of 36 per 1,000 vaccinations. This may be partly strain specific, and the association of the current Danish-strain BCG and regional lymphadenitis has been recognised especially in HIV-positive children. Similarly, disseminated BCG disease occurs almost exclusively in immunocompromised children and has an extremely high mortality. In HIV-positive children with suspected BCG-regional axillary lymphadenitis, the diagnosis should be confirmed by means of FNA, pus swab, or gastric washout. The investigative protocol in these patients should include a chest radiograph to exclude disseminated mycobacterial disease. If a positive BCG mycobacterium is cultured from the lymph nodes, initial treatment should be by means of tuberculostatics, and surgery should be avoided and reserved for complicated patients and cases where diagnostic doubt exists.

In BCG adenitis, if the lymph nodes are <3 cm in size, the diagnostic FNA should be followed by a "wait and see" policy, which avoids the use of ineffective tuberculostatics, with the inherent problem of acquired drug resistance, as well as affording a lower incidence of surgically related complications. In nodes >3 cm in size with a negative FNA culture, other concerns of underlying disease need to be taken into account in evaluating surgical intervention. This is especially so if the patient is not responding to conventional therapy.

Mycobacteria other than tuberculosis
Mycobacteria other than tuberculosis can be a cause of chronic localised cervicofacial lymphadenitis. Due to MOTT's perceived resistance to

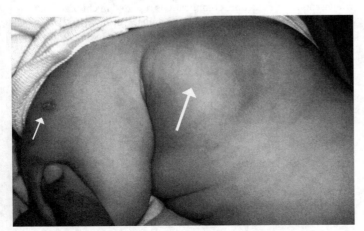

Figure 37.3: BCG ulcer (small arrow) and axillary lymphadenopathy (large arrow) in a neonate.

antituberculous therapy, surgical excision has become the treatment of choice for nontuberculous mycobacterial lymphadenopathy. Surgical management encompasses total excision or curettage of the affected lymph node(s) and remains the treatment of choice due to the high cure rate with a single procedure. For lesions in proximity to the facial nerve or with extensive skin necrosis, curettage can be performed as an alternative to total excision as the initial procedure. This is usually part of a staged process followed by subsequent excision and wound closure.

Immunocompetent patients with nontuberculous cervical lymphadenitis do, however, appear to show some response to medical therapy alone. A recent study[2] of 92 immunocompetent children with nontuberculous mycobacterial lymphadenopathy (90% *M. avium* complex or *M. hemophilum*) showed a natural history of violaceous skin changes with discharge of pus for 3–8 weeks. The infection then seemed to settle, with 71% achieving total resolution within 6 months and resolution of the remaining 29% within 9–12 months. This raises the question of a possible conservative approach to nontuberculous mycobacterial infestations of the cervicocranial region.

Cervical lymphadenopathy caused by nontuberculous mycobacteria can thus be managed by a variety of therapeutic options in immunoincompetent children, with infection resolution being the eventual outcome regardless of management option selected. The best management option in this group appears to be an individualised approach with excisional biopsy as the recommended option; its feasibility is determined by the length of history, the danger of facial nerve injury (due to position), and the presence of hypertrophic scarring.

In immunocompromised (e.g., HIV-affected) children, the management option may change depending on the CD4 count. The potential for systemic disease in these patients remains (see the preceding section on bacille Calmette-Guérin lymphadenitis).

Other Causes of Chronic Granulomas in Lymph Nodes

Rosai-Dorfman disease
Rosai-Dorfman disease, or sinus histiocytosis with massive lymphadenopathy (SHML), is an uncommon but well-defined cause of chronic lymphadenopathy in childhood. It is a histiocytic proliferative disease. Patients may present with a low-grade fever and cervical lymphadenopathy. It is a benign self-limiting disorder. Histological features include numerous large histiocytes with prominent emperipolesis (a halo observed around the cell), fine vacuoles in the cytoplasm, and lymphocytes and plasma cells in the background.

Diagnosis has successfully been made with a FNA biopsy in a number of reports demonstrating the characteristic SHML features, namely, large histiocytes with abundant pale, eosinophilic cytoplasm containing well-preserved lymphocytes and occasional plasma cells and granulocytes. Additional immunostaining may demonstrate typical positive S-100 protein and alpha-1-antichymotrypsin staining, but no reaction when stained for lysozyme.

Cat scratch disease
Cat scratch disease is caused by infection by the *Bartonella henselae* organism. Cat scratch disease occurs in many countries (including some developing ones), but may be difficult to diagnose in children. It is a self-limiting zoonotic condition that may occur at any age, but it is most common among children and adolescents. It usually involves enlargement of only a single node regionally, which is usually the cervical or axillary and very rarely inguinal lymph nodes. It is diagnosed on careful history taking and specific serological test and histopathological examination.

Castleman disease
Castleman disease (angiofollicular lymph node hyperplasia) has been reported in Africa both in the cervicofacial area and intraabdominally. Although presentation as an asymptomatic neck mass is not uncommon, it most frequently presents with mediastinal lymphadenopathy.

Other lymph node groups (e.g., cervical, intraabdominal) may occasionally be involved. Castleman disease is not always a benign disorder in children,[3] and associated systemic manifestations may or may not be present. There are two clinical types, localised and multicentric, as well as three histological variants (hyaline-vascular, plasma cell, and mixed type). Of these, the plasma cell and mixed type appear to be more aggressive than the hyaline-vascular type.

Although the aetiology of Castleman disease is uncertain, multicentric Castleman disease (a lymphoproliferative disorder) and Kaposi sarcoma have both been reported to have an increased occurrence in patients with HIV infection. This is as a result of the ability of the human herpes virus (HHV) 8 to persist in B-lymphoid cells and endothelial cells, and the current HIV epidemic has raised a new awareness of this association.

Surgical excision is the treatment of choice for Castleman disease, but it is not always possible to obtain a complete clearance.

Malignancy and Lymphadenopathy

Problems still exist in excluding malignancy in lymphadenopathy in childhood, which results in difficult clinical management decisions. All efforts should be taken to achieve a definitive diagnosis. Repeated sampling of deeper nodes may be indicated if difficulties persist, and results may be further improved by sampling multiple lymph nodes and taking cultures.

The differential diagnosis of cervical lymphadenopathy includes malignant tumours. The overall risk of malignancy is approximately 12% (1 in every 8 lymph nodes biopsied) in chronic cervical lymphadenopathy. The similar incidence of reactive lymphadenopathy and chronic granulomatous infections (of different kinds) in most series suggests a similar incidence of lymph node malignancy in both developed and developing countries.

In our own series,[1] lymphomas were prominent in 70% of patients. These may be divided into Hodgkin's disease, non-Hodgkin's lymphomas, and Burkitt lymphoma in children. Each of the above groups represented approximately one-third of the total cases.

Age

The mean age of patients with a malignancy was 8.5 years in our own series (Figure 37.4),[1] but some age differences are evident. Burkitt lymphoma, for instance, usually presents almost exclusively in younger children (mean age of 5 years), whereas Hodgkin's and other lymphomas occur predominantly in the older age group. Nonlymphoma-related malignancies in the head and neck region have been reported to occur more frequently at the age of 5 years of less. In our series of 1,877 specimens, these included neuroblastomas (13) and rhabdomyosarcomas (4), as well as local spread from thyroid tumours (3) and nasopharyngeal carcinoma (5). There were also a number of cervical metastases from advanced tumours at distant sites (e.g., Wilm's tumours, hepatocellular carcinomas, sarcomas, malignant melanomas, teratomas, and ovarian tumours).

Burkitt lymphoma

A special situation occurs with Burkitt lymphoma, a childhood cancer common in sub-Saharan Africa. Burkitt lymphoma has an extremely rapid growth and a 24-hour doubling time. It has a relationship to the Epstein-Barr virus (EBV, an important cause of a variety of viral conditions as well as malignancy) and malaria, but its association with HIV is not clear as yet. The HIV pandemic as well as the increase of malaria in Africa have resulted in an increase of Burkitt lymphoma in HIV-endemic areas, particularly in HIV-infected children. Recent studies[4] suggest that EBV and malaria, and possibly HIV, act jointly in the pathogenesis of Burkitt lymphoma. Malaria prevention may thus potentially decrease the risk of Burkitt lymphoma. As the diagnosis and introduction of chemotherapy is urgent, there is an acute need for improved rapid diagnostic methods as well as early, appropriate oncologic management. In addition, less toxic drug combinations need to be utilised for HIV-infected patients.

Age for lymph nodes

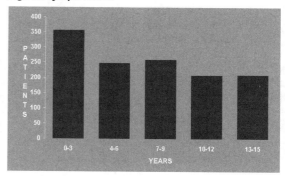

Age for neoplastic nodes

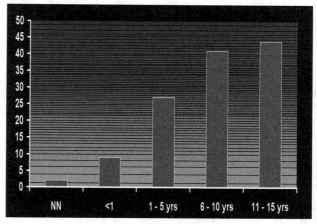

Figure 37.4: Age range of 1,877 patients with biopsy of enlarged lymph nodes. Note the increased incidence of neoplastic nodes with increasing age (right) when compared to the overall decrease in general (left).

Oncology patients

Oncology patients warrant special consideration as far as tuberculosis is concerned, and active TB should be excluded before commencing chemotherapy in patients at risk. Further identification of latent TB in oncology patients from endemic areas and the early introduction of prophylactic anti-TB treatment during the early stage of chemotherapy might be indicated in these patients. The importance of follow-up of patients with nonspecific reactive nodes is illustrated by the fact that 15 cases (3%) in our series[1] were subsequently diagnosed with lymphoma, and patients identified as having an "atypical hyperplasia" should therefore undergo repeat biopsy.

Rarer Causes of Lymphadenopathy

Other less obvious causes of lymphadenopathy (e.g., CMV, toxoplasmosis, cat scratch disease) can be identified only with special tests.

Lymphadenopathy and viruses

Many childhood viral diseases (e.g., measles, rubella, infected chicken pox) are associated with lymphadenopathy but are not the primary presenting feature. CMV, EBV, and HHV, especially types 6, 7, and 8) have been associated with lymphadenopathy.

Cytomegalovirus and lymphadenopathy

Most CMV infections are subclinical, including those acquired congenitally. The course of CMV mononucleosis infection is generally mild, lasting 2 to 3 weeks. The later stages may have lymphadenopathy as a feature, but that is usually atypical.

It is generally accepted that immunosuppressed or immunocompromised patients (especially those with HIV and bone marrow transplant patients) may experience more severe human CMV (HCMV) infection and disease. Control of HCMV infection and prevention of associated diseases in immunocompetent hosts are ensured mainly by CD8+ T cells.

Epstein-Barr virus

The Epstein-Barr virus causes the acute form of infectious mono-nucleosis, presenting with fatigue, malaise, fever, sore throat, hepato-splenomegaly, and a generalised lymphadenopathy. After the primary infection, EBV (similar to other herpes viruses) gives rise to lifelong latent infection. Because the virus is harboured in the oropharyngeal cells and B lymphocytes in the blood, it is therefore not surprising that both epithelial (e.g., nasopharyngeal Ca) and B lymphocyte activation (Burkitt lymphoma) occur. EBV is associated with up to 98% of cases of endemic Burkitt lymphoma.

Failure to control the EBV infection in immunocompromised patients may have severe consequences. The decrease in T-cell populations allows EBV to escape immune surveillance. It may be associated with conditions such as X-linked lymphoproliferative syndrome and the T/NK-cell lymphoproliferative disorders (LPDs) of children and young adults. These are also sometimes termed severe chronic active EBV (CAEBV) infections, which have an aggressive clinical course.

Kikuchi-Fujimoto disease

The cause of Kikuchi-Fujimoto disease (histiocytic necrotising lymph-adenitis) is unknown, although viruses such as herpes and EBV have been associated with this condition. This disease appears to represent a common pattern of response to a variety of aetiological factors rather than a single clinicopathological entity.

This relatively newly described condition has sparked recent interest. Although appearing to be largely confined to the Far East, where it was described in young women in Southeast Asia, it has also been described in the Americas and other parts of the world. There are no reports of this condition in Africa as yet, although it is being reported from other developing countries. Reasons for this may be specific to geography or the overwhelming prevalence of tuberculosis in Africa.

Tropical diseases and lymphadenopathy

- Lymphadenopathy is a feature of acquired toxoplasmosis *(Toxoplasma gondii)*, mainly occurring in cervical nodes. The congenital form of the disease does not show lymphadenopathy as much as hepatosplenomegaly.

- The regional lymphadenopathy that occurs with rickettsial infections such as tick bite fever is often generalised, but if localised, it may indicate the site of the bite and assist in diagnosis. Widespread trematode infections (e.g., schistsomiasis) may also produce gener-alised lymphadenopathy.

- Dengue fever is transmitted by the Stegomyia family mosquitoes and not infrequently presents with lymphadenopathy in addition to the myalgia, gastrointestinal upset, and rash usually associated with this condition.

- Lymphadenopathy may also be present in association with trypano-somiasis and West African sleeping sickness.

- Kala azar is associated with lymphadenopathy in certain areas of northern Africa, the Middle East, and South America. It needs to be differentiated from tuberculosis and malignancies such as leukae-mia and lymphoma.

- Lymphadenopathy may also occur with certain zoonotic infections such as toxocariasis (visceral larva migrans).

- *Wuchereria bancrofti* infection affects the lymphatic system, is dis-tributed throughout tropical and subtropical areas of Africa as well as many other parts of the world, and causes filariasis. Lymphatic filariasis can be disabling in the long term, but the problem relates more to lymphangitis than lymphadenopathy per se. Acute infec-tions are characterised by fever, lymphangitis, headaches, and myal-gia, mostly in the second decade of life with chronic manifestations occurring later (>30 years).

Clinical Presentation

History

Clinical evaluation of a child with enlarged lymph nodes includes careful history and examination. The following questions should be answered:

- When did it arise?

- Is there any association with infections?

- How fast is it growing?

- Is there any other lymphadenopathy?

- Are there any systemic symptoms (e.g., night sweats, loss of weight, bone pain)?

Physical Examination

Note the following features:

- position (supraclavicular/posterior triangle neck, etc.);

- size (significant if >1 cm);

- consistency (hard/matted/immobile); and

- presence of other lymphadenopathy/visceromegaly.

Clinical Evaluation

Age of Patient

Age plays a role because lymph nodes are usually not palpable in neo-nates, making neonatal lymphadenopathy suspicious. In our large series of 1,877 biopsied lymph nodes,[1] the mean age was 7 years (for TB, it was 5.8 years, and for neoplastic disease, 8.5 years). A comparison of the ages of all the lymph nodes sampled compared with those with malignancy shows a rather striking difference in those children older than 5 years of age, when malignancy appears to increase in prevalence.

Size of Significant Lymph Nodes

The size of lymph nodes should be recorded in the initial evaluation and prior to commencing treatment. Although the majority of studies avoid giving specific measurements for significant lymph nodes, nodes greater than 1 cm were considered abnormal in the cervical region (normal being <3 mm). Lymph nodes in the axilla are not considered to be enlarged unless their diameter exceeds 1 cm for axillary nodes and 1.5 cm for inguinal nodes.

Pathological lymph nodes are abnormal in size and site for the particular age of the child but also include those with an irregular or hard surface as well as lymph nodes that persist for more than 4 to 6 weeks despite adequate antibiotic treatment.

Position of Enlarged Lymph Nodes

The main peripheral groups of nodes involved in pathology are the cer-vical (46%), axillary (23%), inguinal (13%), and submandibular (8%) groups of nodes, as well as deeper areas such as the mediastinum and intraabdominal lymph nodes. The most important area is in the neck, where cervical lymphadenopathy is the most common initial presenta-tion site of the majority of head and neck malignancies and a number of other pathologies (e.g., lymphoma).

A special risk situation exists with mediastinal nodes that may not be clinically obvious but may have exerted pressure on the trachea, thus compromising the airway. A chest x-ray (CXR) on which the mediastinum is broadened in the absence of a thymic shadow is suggestive of mediastinal lymphadenopathy. The outline of the trachea and respiratory tree can be traced on CXR, but if suspect, a computed tomography (CT) scan should be performed prior to any anaesthetic procedures being performed (Figure 37.5).

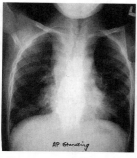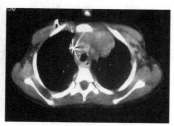

Figure 37.5: Chest x-ray (left) and CT scan (right) showing mediastinal node effect on airway.

Localised Lymphadenopathy

Cervical Lymphadenopathy

Cervical lymphadenopathy is a common clinical problem in children; two-thirds of affected patients are older than 5 years of age. Cervical lymphadenopathy is extremely common in developing populations and could therefore be expected to include a higher percentage of patients with acute infection, tuberculosis, neoplasia, and related diseases.

Lymphadenopathy in the posterior triangle of the neck is viewed with suspicion because lymphoma often presents there (Figure 37.6). In addition, the presence of an enlarged post auricular node in children older than 2 years of age is likely to be clinically significant. Lymphadenopathy in the supraclavicular region is highly significant, as up to 60% are caused by malignant tumours.

The clinicopathological spectrum of lymphadenopathy is not always predictable on clinical grounds, and cervical lymph nodes are often asymptomatic. The differential diagnosis largely encompasses reactive hyperplasia, specific infective agents, or malignancy. The obvious therapeutic and prognostic implications necessitate an accurate and prompt diagnosis. Nonresponse to empiric antibiotic therapy is a major criterion for further investigation. Surgical intervention provides material to establish an early diagnosis and is thus a vital part of management.

Although chronic lymphadenopathy in children of developing countries has a high incidence of infective causes, including mycobacteria; it has an approximate 11% risk of malignancy. More than half the cervical lymph nodes examined in children in a developing country displayed very significant and clinically important pathology, thereby justifying active management of all paediatric patients with persistent cervical lymphadenopathy.

The largest safely accessible node is selected for biopsy. Correct handling of a lymph node biopsy is essential. Nodes are divided in half, with half going fresh to histopathology for imprints and histology. The remaining half is further subdivided in two, with one section being sent for tissue culture and the remaining section for TB culture.

The causes of lymphadenopathy may vary from upper respiratory viral infections (e.g., adenovirus, rhinovirus, enterovirus) to the more common childhood diseases (e.g., measles, mumps, rubella, herpes) and other specific viral infections (e.g., cytomegalovirus, EBV, and HIV/AIDS (acquired immune deficiency syndrome) within endemic regions). A number of noninfective causes should also be considered in addition to the viral diseases, such as sarcoidosis, Kawasaki disease, and cat scratch disease in addition to the mycobacterial group of organisms. Axillary lymphadenopathy is mostly associated with malignancy (e.g., Hodgkin's) and cervical lymphadenopathy mostly associated with TB (although a significant number are malignant).

Lymphadenopathy is not an uncommon feature of viral and rickettsial infections and may be a part of infectious diseases such as rubella, infectious mononucleosis, and certain tropical diseases (e.g., dengue fever). In infectious mononucleosis, the lymphadenopathy is mostly cervical and epitrochlear.

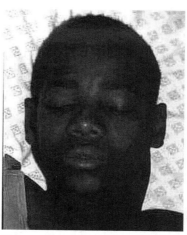

Figure 37.6: Cervical lymphadenopathy as a result of Hodgkin's lymphoma in a 10-year-old boy.

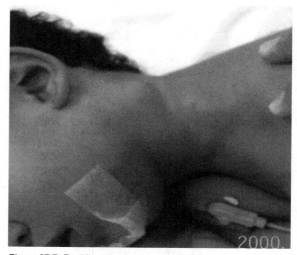

Figure 37.7: Rapidly enlarging lymph nodes in a 4-year-old boy with lymphoma.

Rapidly enlarging lymphadenopathy suggests malignant disease (Figure 37.7). The highest incidence of malignancy occurs in the supraclavicular lymph nodes.

Axillary and Inguinal Nodes

Enlarged lymph nodes of the axilla and groin are unusual presenting sites for lymphomas, which are the most common forms of malignancy seen involving lymph nodes. Hodgkin's lymphoma may present with enlarged axillary nodes.

The presence of lymphadenopathy in atypical anatomic regions, persistence despite appropriate treatment, absence of previous pyogenic infection, geographical prevalence, history of cat scratch, and a positive TB history are all significant clues for suspecting the diagnosis of lymphoma.

Early tissue sampling may be indicated if the postauricular, epitrochlear, mediastinal, and abdominal lymph nodes are involved in the presence of generalised symptoms of unexplained fever and weight loss. The presence of large mediastinal and hilar nodes may lead to anaesthetic hazards and must be evaluated prior to a surgical procedure (e.g., biopsy) being undertaken.

Special Investigations

Depending on the clinical presentation, the initial visit may require little or no special investigations if an empiric trial of antibiotics for proven or suspected infection is anticipated. In a subsequent visit, basic special investigations, such as a white cell count, Mantoux test, and a chest x-ray become the initial screening tools. Further investigation depends on the clinical findings, response to antibiotic therapy, and Mantoux and CXR results. Tuberculosis should be excluded by the Mantoux skin test and chest x-ray in addition to gastric washings and cultures.

The majority of cases of lymphadenopathy are related to infection, so it is logical to rule out acute infection as a possible cause. Many clinicians would thus advocate the use of empiric antibiotics in the initial stages in the absence of other worrying signs. A 7–10 day trial of antibiotics is therefore advocated.

Biopsy and Sampling

Fine needle aspiration biopsy (FNAB) and sampling are indicated by any of the following conditions of the lymph nodes:

• no response to antibiotic therapy in 4–6 weeks (>2 cm);

• rapid increase in size;

• hard, matted lymph nodes in the posterior triangle or the supraclavicular region of the neck; and

• difficulty in diagnosis.

Malignancy in lymph nodes may be difficult to assess, particularly in the early stages when they appear as small blue round cells. There is a real risk of malignancy. Specialised tests such as immunostaining and flow cytometry remain useful adjuncts where available.

Fine Needle Aspiration

Although excision biopsy remains the gold standard in diagnosis, FNA has changed the practice in adult surgery in the modern era and may provide material to establish an early diagnosis in children.

Technically, FNA makes several passes with a 22-gauge needle from a variety of angles, using suction in the syringe once the capsule of the gland is entered on each occasion before the needle is withdrawn. A small amount of saline may be aspirated, and the obtained cells are expressed onto a glass slide and fixed in the same way as for a Papanicolau test (Pap smear). It is then submitted to the laboratory for analysis.

FNA is a means of a rapid and definitive diagnosis of tuberculosis in the majority of cases of suspected tuberculous lymphadenitis. Expert care should therefore be expressed in interpreting negative FNA results to exclude a false sense of security. It must be stressed, however, that the interpretation of a FNA in a child is a highly specialized area of expertise, and in most cases cannot be completely sufficient to make the diagnosis of lymphoma. Its major value is probably in establishing metastatic spread from a known tumour and providing material for culture.

The definitive diagnosis is then based on cytomorphology and identification of the organism. FNA is, however, difficult to perform without sedation in the younger child and should be regarded as a diagnostic triage tool, being accurate only as far as its positive findings are concerned. It yields a smaller sample and gives no information on lymph node architecture so it must lead to a more difficult diagnosis in the absence of flow cytometry.

In a recent study,[5] cultures for the TB organism were positive in 79/175 patients (45%) of those subjected to FNA. In these, 61 (77%) were identified as *Mycobacterium tuberculosis* with *M. bovis* (bacille Calmette-Guérin) being identified in the remainder. Where Burkitt lymphoma is a possibility, flow cytometry techniques identify the abundance of B lymphocytes in the specimen.

Surgical Lymph Node Biopsy

Lymph node biopsy remains an important and valuable surgical diagnostic tool in the evaluation of lymphadenopathy with very minimal risk to the patient (Figure 37.8). It allows the assessment of gland architecture in addition to the cytological features, thereby allowing for early diagnosis. It should be the endpoint of all cases of lymphadenopathy where a diagnosis is not readily forthcoming.

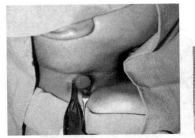
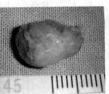

Figure 37.8: Surgical biopsy of cervical lymph node (lymphoma).

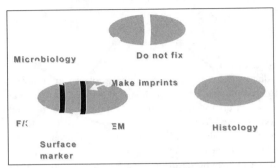

Figure 37.9: Schematic outline for handling lymph node biopsy specimens.

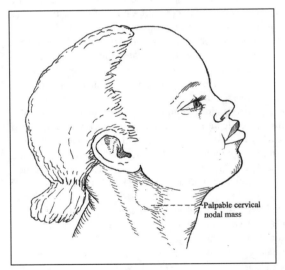

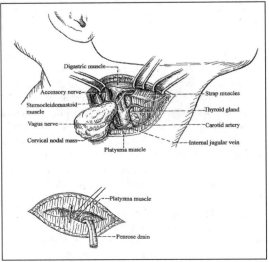

Figure 37.10: Surgical technique to excise lymph nodes.

The node sampled should be a representative node, preferably from a deep site. The node should be divided into specimens for histology and specimens for tissue culture (and TB culture). The specimen for histology should be further divided into a formalin fixed section and a section sent fresh for imprinting. Figure 37.9 outlines the handling of biopsy specimens.

The surgical technique for lymph node excision is shown in Figure 37.10.

Immunocompromised Patient
Lymphadenopathy may be a much more serious problem in the immunocompromised patient.

Up to 18% of HIV-affected patients in Africa have lymphadenopathy on presentation. A generalised lymphadenopathy (particularly cervical and axillary nodes) has been reported as the most common presentation of children with symptomatic HIV in Zimbabwe, but concomitant tuberculosis needs to be excluded. The histological picture of HIV-affected lymphadenopathy is usually nonspecific with the immunologic reaction to HIV being the most prominent feature. The picture is further complicated by the clinical and multiple HIV virus subtypes in sub-Saharan Africa and Nigeria.

Key Summary Points

1. Lymphadenopathy is an extremely common clinical finding in the children of Africa as well as the rest of the world.

2. It is most prevalent in the first decades of life and the majority of children between the ages of 2 and 12 will have an enlarged lymph node at one stage or another.

3. A significant lymph node is >2cm.

4. Lymphadenopathy may be the first (and sometimes only) indication of underlying disease.

5. Active management is justified of paediatric patients with persisting lymphadenopathy.

6. Atypical anatomic regions, persistence despite appropriate treatment, absence of previous pyogenic infection, geographical prevalence, history of cat scratch, a positive TB history, are all important in assessment.

7. The aetiology is mostly infective. This may be acute bacterial, viral or chronic inflammation due to many different infective agents.

8. Granulomas suggest chronic infective causes such as mycobacteria (e.g., M. tuberculosis and other mycobacteria] organisms.

9. A special situation exists in lymphadenopathy related to the Danish strain of bacille Calmette-Guérin, (BCG) particularly in immunocompromised children.

10. Up to 18% of HIV affected patients in Africa have lymphadenopathy on presentation.

11. Malignancy in enlarged lymph nodes occurs in 12% and 2/3 are lymphomas.

12. Fine needle Aspiration biopsy (FNAB) is a useful triage for the rapid and definitive diagnosis of tuberculosis but may miss malignancy.

13. Early tissue sampling indicated with generalized symptoms of unexplained fever and weight loss.and lymphadenopathy (especially mediastinal and abdominal lymph nodes).

14. Where malignancy is suspected biopsy of an entire representative lymph node is required and submitted for appropriate culture and histology.

References

1. Moore SW, Schneider JW, Schaaf HS. Diagnostic aspects of cervical lymphadenopathy in children in the developing world: a study of 1,877 surgical specimens. Pediatr Surg Int 2003; 19:240–244.

2. Zeharia A, Eidlitz-Markus T, Haimi-Cohen Y, Samra Z, Kaufman L, Amir J. Management of nontuberculous mycobacteria-induced cervical lymphadenitis with observation alone. Pediatr Infect Dis J 2008; 27:920–922.

3. Foucar E, Rosai J, Dorfman R. Sinus histiocytosis with massive lymphadenopathy (Rosai-Dorfman disease): review of the entity. Semin Diagn Pathol 1990; 7:19–73.

4. Mutalima N, Molyneux E, Jaffe H, Kamiza S, Borgstein E, Mkandawire N, et al. Associations between Burkitt lymphoma among children in Malawi and infection with HIV, EBV and malaria: results from a case-control study. PLoS ONE 2008; 3(6):e2505.

5. Wright CA, van der BM, Geiger D, Noordzij JG, Burgess SM, Marais BJ. Diagnosing mycobacterial lymphadenitis in children using fine needle aspiration biopsy: cytomorphology, ZN staining and autofluorescence—making more of less. Diagn Cytopathol 2008; 36:245–251.

CHAPTER 38
STERNOMASTOID TUMOUR OF INFANCY AND CONGENITAL MUSCULAR TORTICOLLIS

Lukman O. Abdur-Rahman
Brian H. Cameron

Introduction

Sternomastoid tumour (SMT) of infancy is usually associated with congenital muscular torticollis (CMT); these will be discussed together in this chapter. The term "tumour" is a misnomer because it is a congenital fibrotic process; it also is referred to as congenital fibromatosis coli. The terms "torticollis" and "wryneck" actually describe the tilting and rotation of the head and neck that results from the contracture of the sternocleidomastoid muscle. The torticollis, when untreated, results in plagiocephaly, hemifacial hypoplasia, and body distortion. The key to preventing deformity is early diagnosis and passive stretching exercises (PSEs) of the affected muscle, with only 5% of cases needing surgical intervention in a large prospective series.[1]

Demography

The prevalence of SMT and CMT in Africa is unknown.[2] At the University of Ilorin Teaching Hospital in Nigeria over a period of 10 years (1999–2008), only 15 cases presented at the outpatient clinic and only one had surgical intervention at 10 months of age because of severe torticollis. CMT is reported to occur in 0.3–2% of all births, with a slight male preponderance. The right side is affected in 60% of the cases, and 2–8% are bilateral.[3]

Aetiology

The sternocleidomastoid muscle is enveloped by the deep cervical fascia as it attaches to the clavicle, manubrium, and mastoid process. The aetiology of SMT is unknown, but the current theory is that it results from abnormal intrauterine positioning, leading to intramuscular compartment syndrome and ischaemic muscle injury with subsequent fibrosis and contracture of the sternomastoid muscle.[4] Muscle biopsy shows replacement of muscle bundles with a mass of maturing fibrous tissue—evidence that the pathology may begin prenatally.[3]

Contracture of the sternomastoid muscle on one side causes the head and neck to tilt (flex) to the ipsilateral side and the face to turn toward the contralateral side (Figure 38.1).

If untreated, the sternomastoid tumour naturally resolves completely in 50–70% of the cases by 6 months of age, with muscle shortening persisting in 5–7% after 1 year.[1,5] Hence, late presentations are usually accompanied by fibrotic and shortened sternocleidomastoid muscle from a missed or unrecognised sternomastoid tumour.

Clinical Presentation

History

Infants present with either a lump in the neck, or with a head tilt that is not correctable by repositioning. SMT is usually absent at birth and presents between 3 weeks to 3 months of age. There is a high incidence of breech presentation or assisted delivery. It is important to reassure the parents that the obstetric difficulty is thought to be the result rather than cause of the shortened sternomastoid muscle.[4]

Many parents present their children after 3 months of age in the African setting because they presume the abnormal position to be due

to poor neck control in infants before this age (Figure 38.2). Some of the cases are first noticed by grandmothers while doing the traditional body massage for the babies.

Physical Examination

A sternomastoid tumour is defined by the presence of a palpable, hard, spindle-shaped, painless, 1–3 cm diameter swelling within the substance of the sternocleidomastoid muscle, usually located in the lower and middle third of the muscle. The mass may be confused with a lymph node or neoplasm, which is far less likely at this age.

Children presenting with CMT should have the entire length of the sternomastoid muscle palpated to determine whether the swelling or area

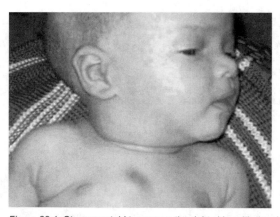

Figure 38.1: Sternomastoid tumour on the right side, with the child's head turned away from the affected side.

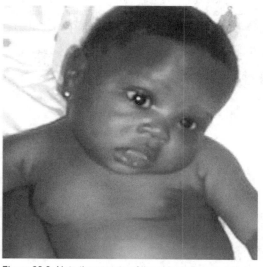

Figure 38.2: Note the posture of the older baby with left sternomastoid tumour.

of fibrosis is present and in what proportion. More than 50% of children with CMT will have SMT at the time of presentation.[1] The anterior border of the sternomastoid muscle may reveal a tight band of muscle, especially in older children. Bilateral sternomastoid tumour with torticollis creates difficulty in confirming the diagnosis from examination.

Infants with a head tilt will prefer to look away from the affected muscle. The most important part of the physical exam is to determine the presence and severity of limitation of passive neck rotation. Gentle neck rotation with the baby supine and head held over the side of the examining table should normally allow the chin to reach to or past the shoulder, 90–110 degrees from the neutral position (Figures 38.3 and 38.4). With CMT, there is limited rotation towards the affected side, which can be graded as mild (>80 degrees), moderate (45–80 degrees), or severe (<45 degrees) (Figure 38.5).[6]

The head should be examined from the back and top of the baby to document any plagiocephaly, a flattening of the contralateral occiput that results from persistent lying on one side; this is sometimes accompanied by contralateral flattening of the forehead (Figure 38.6).

Mild facial asymmetry may be noted, even at an early presentation; this asymmetry worsens when the torticollis is severe and untreated. The degree of hemifacial hypoplasia can be determined by the angle between the plane of the eyes and the plane of the mouth (Figure 38.7).

Older children with long-standing torticollis may have secondary compensation resulting in musculoskeletal deformities, including elevation of the ipsilateral shoulder to maintain a horizontal plane of vision, twisting of the neck and back to maintain a straight line of sight, and wasting of the neck muscles from disuse atrophy (Figure 38.8).There may be accompanying muscle spasm with cervical and thoracic scoliosis.

Developmental dysplasia of the hip (DDH) is seen in 5–8% of children with CMT, so this should be screened for on the initial physical examination. Clues on inspection are asymmetric thigh folds and apparent leg length discrepancy; the Ortolani and Barlow tests for hip stability should be done. The American Academy of Pediatrics recommends an ultrasound at 6 weeks of age or radiographs of the hips at 4 months of age in children at higher risk, which includes girls having breech presentations.[7] No specific mention is made of torticollis as a risk factor, but DDH may occur in at least 4% of infants with torticollis,[5] so it may be prudent to screen children with hip ultrasound if it is available. Metatarsal adductus and calcaneovalgus may also be associated with abnormal intrauterine positioning.

Differential Diagnoses
The clinical features of SMT when associated with CMT are pathognomonic and should not be confused with other lateral neck masses, such as cystic hygroma, branchial cyst, or hemangioma. Enlarged cervical nodes are rare in infancy, as are neoplasms.

Congenital torticollis may present without an SMT, but most will still have some palpable thickening and shortening of the muscle. If there is a head tilt without any limitation of rotation of the neck, then causes of postural torticollis should be considered. These would include congenital hemivertebra, Klippel-Feil syndrome (atlanto-axial fusion), strabismus, and Sandifer syndrome caused by chronic gastro-oesophageal reflux (see Table 38.1). Familial and hereditary sternomastoid muscle aplasia have also been reported.[8,9]

Investigations
Clinical examination confirms the diagnosis of sternomastoid tumour and torticollis in most cases, and no investigations are routinely required. However, imaging studies can occasionally be used to exclude other conditions when the clinical findings are equivocal or atypical.

Plain cervical radiographs are of limited use in nontraumatic infant torticollis due to their low true-positive yield; more false-positives were identified in one retrospective review.[10] In only 1 of 502 cases was there a craniocervical anomaly, and the study concluded that physical examination could safely eliminate the need for routine radiography in infant torticollis.

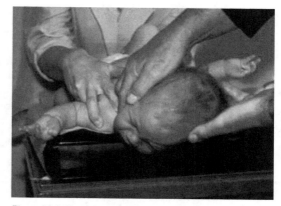

Figure 38.3: Normal rotation of the neck to the left past the shoulder.

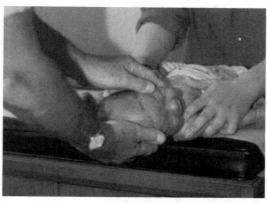

Figure 38.4: Limitation of passive neck rotation towards the right (affected) side.

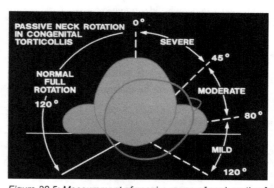

Figure 38.5: Measurement of passive range of neck motion from the midline.

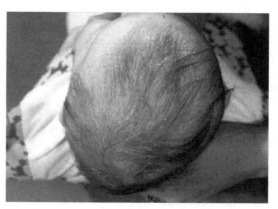

Figure 38.6: Right occipital flattening (plagiocephaly) with left sternomastoid shortening.

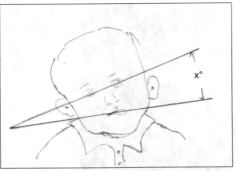

Figure 38.7: Degree of hemifacial hypoplasia measured by the angle between the plane of the eyes and mouth (x°).

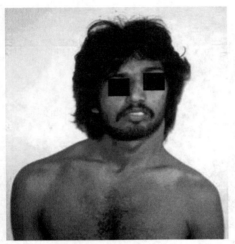

Figure 38.8: Long-standing right sternomastoid shortening causing facial asymmetry with secondary neck, shoulder, and back deformities.

Table 38.1: Differential diagnoses of torticollis.

Congenital
1. Sternomastoid tumour
2. Muscular torticollis
3. Congenital vertebral anomalies (cervical hemivertebral)
4. Klippel-Feil syndrome (atlanto-axial fusion)

Trauma
1. Rotary subluxation of atlantoaxial or atlanto-occipital joints (post ear, nose, throat (ENT) surgery, such as tonsillectomy; retropharygeal abscess drainage)
2. Cervical spine fracture
3. Clavicular fracture

Inflammatory
1. Grisel syndrome
2. Diskitis
3. Vertebral osteomyelitis
4. Juvenile rheumatoid arthritis
5. Cervical disc calcification
6. Retropharyngeal abscess
7. Cervical lymphadenitis
8. Acute lymphoblastic leukaemia

Neurologic
1. Posterior fossa tumour
2. Syringomyelia
3. Arnold-Chiari malformation
4. Paroxysmal torticollis of infancy
5. Cerebral palsy
6. Strabismus

Others
1. Sandifer syndrome in chronic gastro-oesophageal reflux
2. Thymitis
3. Thyroiditis
4. Postural; familial

Ultrasonography has been used to classify, monitor progress, and predict outcome of congenital muscular torticollis (Table 38.2).[11] However, it is not used routinely in most centres, and treatment decisions should be based on clinical findings. Fine needle aspiration (FNA) cytology and open muscle biopsy are not necessary and may be misleading because the histology may look similar to a fibrous neoplasm. These procedures should be reserved for atypical cases or when the muscle tumour does not resolve as expected (Figure 38.9).

Management

Most cases of SMT and CMT are managed nonoperatively. Babies are encouraged to actively look towards the affected side. In the University of Ilorin Teaching Hospital, mothers are encouraged to be turning the face of the child in the ipsilateral direction while "backing" their babies in the traditional way (Figure 38.10). This position also helps in keeping the hip flexed and abducted, preventing or reducing the chance of a hip dislocation; this could serve as treatment for associated hip dysplasia. This management replaces the Pavlik harness in the African setting. For kangaroo bag (frontal child carrier bags) users, this affords the mother the opportunity to do the massage of the neck and manual stretching even when in transit.

Minor cases will resolve spontaneously with or without treatment, but there is evidence that early PSEs are effective in almost all cases when initiated prior to 3 months of age.[5,6,12,13]

Passive Stretching Exercises

The PSE technique is as follows:[6] With the baby supine and head suspended over the side of the examining table, one adult holds the baby's shoulders while the other rotates the neck to the same side as the affected muscle. Gentle but firm pressure and some flexion are applied at the limit of rotation to maximally stretch the muscle for 10–15 seconds (Figure 38.11). This procedure is repeated 10 times, twice daily.

The keys to success are to explain the diagnosis and prognosis to the parents, demonstrate the PSE, watch them do the PSE in the clinic, and then follow-up in the clinic at 2 and 6 weeks to ensure progress. Parents are motivated by telling them that PSE prevents the need for surgery in most cases. Reassure the parents that babies get used to the exercises and do not remember the discomfort when they are older. With proper instruction, PSE will not harm the child. The sternomastoid scar will occasionally "snap", which may lead to some temporary swelling, but this often results in an improved range of motion.[14]

The PSE should be consistent and continuous until the muscle tumour and contracture resolve, generally within 6–8 months.[12] PSE treatment is successful in more than 90% of cases when commenced within the first 3 months of life.[1,6,13] Emery[15] followed 101 children who started treatment at a mean age of 4 months and found that the average PSE treatment duration was 4.7 months, with all but one child achieving a full passive range of motion.

A child older than 6–8 months of age is less cooperative with the PSE, and surgery is more likely to be necessary because the contracture is tighter and more fibrotic.

A physiotherapist can be engaged to do the initial demonstration and follow-up of progress, especially when mothers are afraid to do the stretching or there is no response to this treatment as expected. Physiotherapy would need to be done at least three times a week to be effective;[5] a professional physiotherapist service is an additional cost that many families would want to avoid and may lead to hospital default. To prevent this, the confidence of the parents is gained by providing adequate information and instruction on the pathology and the treatment options.

A neck brace has been used in older children as an adjunct to PSE or after surgical treatment.[16] If used, the neck brace should be carefully fitted and not worn at night.

Plagiocephaly can be prevented or treated by positioning the head to avoid persistent lying on the same side of the occiput. Measures tried

Table 38.2: Ultrasound prediction of outcome of congenital muscular torticollis.

Type I, 15%	Fibrotic mass	Spontaneous resolution
Type II, 77%	Diffuse fibrosis mixing with normal muscle	Spontaneous resolution
Type III, 5%	Without normal muscle in the involved muscle	Surgical intervention
Type IV, 3%	Fibrotic cord in the involved muscle	Surgical intervention (odds ratio = 31.54, p = .0196)

Source: Adapted from Hsu TC et al. Correlation of clinical and ultrasonographic features of congenital muscular torticollis. Arch Phys Med Rehabil 1999; 80:637–641.

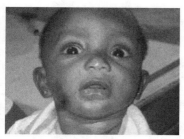

Figure 38.9: Residual left sternomastoid swelling in a five-month-old infant at 8 weeks of physiotherapy. The tumour progressively reduced over 4 months.

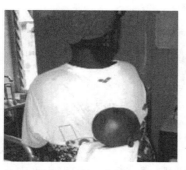

Figure 38.10: A woman backing an infant with the head turned to the ipsilateral side of the sternomastoid tumour.

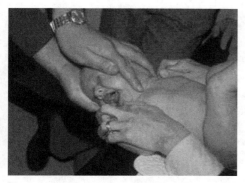

Figure 38.11: The baby's mother does PSE assisted by a friend, while the surgeon watches.

have included placing toys and desirable objects on the ipsilateral side of the lesion so that the child turns towards it. The child could also be put to sleep with the head facing the ipsilateral side. Helmet treatment has been described in some children with severe plagiocephaly,[17] but it is usually impractical.

Operative Treatment

Surgical treatment is required in only about 5% of patients seen early, but is necessary in half of those presenting after 6 months of age.[6] The indications for surgery are:

1. late diagnosis, after 12 months of age; and

2. failure after at least 6 months of PSE with a significant head tilt, persistent deficit of passive neck rotation, and a tight band in the sternomastoid muscle, often with hemifacial hypoplasia.

There is evidence that surgical release of the sternomastoid contracture between 12 and 18 months of age maximises spontaneous correction of plagiocephaly. Surgical correction also results in adequate mobility and acceptable cosmetics in more than 90% of cases, with some benefit even in older children.[18] Other authors recommend delaying operative treatment until after 5 years of age, when the patient can comply with postoperative bracing and physiotherapy.[19]

Operative Procedure—Open Technique

1. The patient is placed under general anaesthesia with endotracheal intubation or the use of a laryngeal mask airway. Anaesthetic intubation difficulty may arise from abnormal tilt in the trachea, so a prior cervical x-ray will guide the anaesthetist. Where available, fibreoptic guided endotracheal intubation is the best.

2. The patient is positioned supine with the shoulder raised and neck rotated to the contralateral side.

3. A 3–4cm transverse skin incision is made 1 cm above the sternal and clavicular origin of the sternomastoid muscle.

4. The platysma is carefully divided along the line of incision to avoid injury to the external jugular vein and accessory nerve.

5. The two heads of the sternomastoid muscle are dissected free from the anterior and posterior layers of the investing fascia and are subsequently divided using diathermy to prevent bleeding; some advocate excision of a 1-cm segment of the muscle.[18]

6. Tight deep cervical fascia should be released, testing lateral and rotational movement carefully under anaesthetic.

7. In severe cases of contracture, division of the upper end of the sternomastoid may be necessary.

8. The platysma is then sutured with 4-0 interrupted absorbable suture, and the skin is closed with 5-0 absorbable suture. There is no need for a drain provided haemostasis is well secured.

Postoperatively, physiotherapy is resumed after wound healing to maintain a full range of motion; some authors recommend using a neck brace for several months.[18]

Alternative surgical approaches that have been described are a sternomastoid lengthening technique using a Z-plasty,[20] and endoscopic tenotomy of the sternomastoid contracture.[21]

Postoperative Complications

1. A hematoma usually will resolve, but sometimes requires aspiration or drainage.

2. Residual contracture from incomplete division of both heads of sternomastoid or cervical fascia over the posterior triangle of the neck would need a reoperation.

3. Recurrent CMT is rare.

The cosmetic appearance may be disfiguring, especially in the older child with severe contracture. This is usually due to anomalous reattachment of the clavicular head of sternomastoid or loss of the sternomastoid column of the neck.

Prognosis and Outcome

The prognosis for sternomastoid tumour is generally excellent if treated early. The child is able to achieve full range of head movement, and the swelling resolves within 6 months. The majority of those who have surgery also do well.

Follow-up should continue until the sternomastoid muscle resolves and feels normal, and full neck rotation is achieved. Older children should be monitored for development of scoliosis.

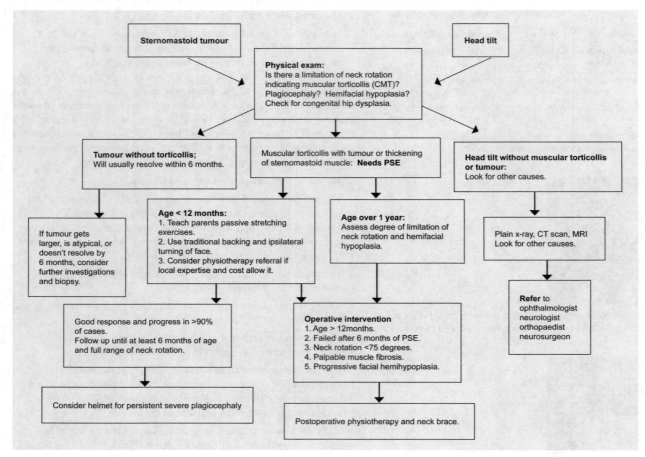

Figure 38.12: Flow chart.

Prevention

There is no primary prevention because the aetiology of sternomastoid tumour is unknown. Secondary and tertiary prevention strategies will identify early cases of CMT in children with SMT or breech presentation, initiate early PSE to prevent further deformity, and avoid the need for surgery. The contracture and torticollis resulting from the sternomastoid tumour should be prevented by early identification, adequate physiotherapy, and good follow-up.

Ethical Issues

Full involvement and education of the parents in the PSE programme requires time and compassionate commitment on the part of the surgeon. Giving information that the mass and head tilt will resolve spontaneously in many of the children may make mothers default from regular visits due to the constraint of cost, distance to the hospital, and long waits in the outpatient clinic. Referral to a costly supervised stretching programme by the physiotherapist should be avoided if it will discourage the parents and lead them to default further outpatient visits. The accessibility and affordability of care make follow-up challenging in the African setting.

Summary

The flow chart presented in Figure 38.12 summarises the recommendations of this chapter.

Evidence-Based Research

Many prospective studies have been conducted to predict the outcome of congenital muscular torticollis, but none were randomised. The study in Table 38.3, however, involves a standardised programme of manual stretching.

Table 38.3: Evidence-based research.

Title	Clinical determinants of the outcome of manual stretching in the treatment of congenital muscular torticollis in infants. A prospective study of 821 cases
Authors	Cheng JCY, Wong MWN, Tang SP, Chen TMK, Shum SLF, Wong EMC
Institution	The Chinese University of Hong Kong and the Prince of Wales Hospital, Hong Kong, China
Reference	J Bone Joint Surg Am 2001; 83:679–687
Problem	The natural history of congenital muscular torticollis and the outcome of different treatment modalities have been poorly investigated, and the results of treatment have varied considerably.
Intervention	Standardised program of manual stretching.
Comparison/ control (quality of evidence)	The study involved three groups: 1. Palpable sternomastoid tumour group 2. Muscular torticollis group (thickening and tightness of the sternocleidomastoid muscle) 3. Postural torticollis group (torticollis but no tightness or tumour). Level 2 evidence.
Outcome/ effect	Controlled manual stretching is safe and effective in the treatment of congenital muscular torticollis when a patient is seen before the age of 1 year. The most important factors that predict the outcome of manual stretching are the clinical group, the initial deficit in rotation of the neck, and the age of the patient at presentation. Surgical treatment is indicated when a patient has undergone at least 6 months of controlled manual stretching and has residual head tilt, deficits of passive rotation, lateral bending of the neck of >15°, a tight muscular band or tumour, and a poor outcome according to a special assessment chart.
Historical significance/ comments	A sternomastoid tumour was involved in 55% of the patients in the study. Eight percent of the sternomastoid tumour group needed surgical intervention, compared to 3% and 0% in the muscular and postural torticollis groups, respectively. The worse the neck rotator deficit, the higher the need for surgical intervention.

Key Summary Points

1. Sternomastoid tumour is usually associated with congenital muscular torticollis.

2. All children with sternomastoid tumour should be thoroughly examined for associated conditions, such as torticollis, facial and cranial asymmetry, and hip dysplasia.

3. The degree of limitation of rotation of the neck towards the affected side should be assessed. Congenital muscular torticollis is a clinical diagnosis that does not require other investigations.

4. Differentials should be considered and investigated in the absence of sternomastoid mass or nonresolving torticollis with nonoperative treatment.

5. With early diagnosis and treatment, more than 90% of the cases resolve with an adequately supervised passive stretching exercise programme.

6. Surgery is indicated in late presentation (>1 year), persistent limitation of neck rotation with head tilt, and progressive facial asymmetry.

7. Follow-up should continue until the tumour resolves and neck rotation normalises.

References

1. Cheng JC, Wong MW, Tang SP, Chen TMK, Shum SLF, Wong EMC. Clinical determinants of the outcome of manual stretching in the treatment of congenital muscular torticollis in infants. A prospective study of 821 cases. J Bone Joint Surg Am 2001; 83:679–687.

2. Nwako FA. Torticollis. In: Nwako FA, ed. A Textbook of Pediatric Surgery in the Tropics. MacMillan Press Limited, 1980, Pp 277–278.

3. Beasley S. Torticollis. In: Grosfeld JL, O'Neill JA Jr, Fonkalsrud EW, Coran AG. Pediatric Surgery, 6th ed. Mosby, 2006, Pp 875–881.

4. Davids JR, Wenger DR, Mubarak SJ. Congenital muscular torticollis: Sequela of intrauterine or perinatal compartment syndrome. J Pediatr Orthop 1993; 13:141.

5. Cheng JC, Tang SP, Chen TM, Wong MWN, Wong EMC. The clinical presentation and outcome of treatment of congenital muscular torticollis in infants—a study of 1086 cases. J Pediatr Surg 2000; 35:1091–1096.

6. Cameron BH, Langer JC, Cameron GS. Success of nonoperative treatment for congenital muscular torticollis is dependent on early therapy. Pediatr Surg Intl 1994; 9:391–393.

7. Goldberg MJ. Early detection of developmental hip dysplasia: synopsis of the AAP Clinical Practice Guideline. Pediatr Rev 2001; 22:131–134.

8. Adams SB Jr, Flynn JM, Hosalkar HS. Torticollis in an infant caused by hereditary muscle aplasia. Am J Orthop 2003; 32:556–558.

9. Hosalkar HS, Gill IS, Guyar P, Shaw BA. Familial torticollis with polydactyly: manifestation in three generations. Am J Orthop 2001; 30:656–658.

10. Snyder EM, Coley BD. Limited value of plain radiographs in infant torticollis. Pediatr 2006; 118:e1779–e1784.

11. Hsu TC, Wang CL, Wang MK, Hsu KH, Tang FT, Chen HT. Correlation of clinical and ultrasonographic features of congenital muscular torticollis. Arch Phys Med Rehabil 1999; 80:637–641.

12. Celayir AC. Congenital muscular torticollis: early and intensive treatment is critical. A prospective study. Pediatr Int 2000; 42:504–507.

13. Demirbilek S, Atayurt HF. Congenital muscular torticollis and strenomastoid tumour. Result of non operative treatment. J Pediatr Surg 1999; 34:549–551.

14. Cheng JC, Chen TM, Tang SP, Shum SL, Wong MW, Metreweli C. Snapping during manual stretching in congenital muscular torticollis. Clin Orthop 2001; 384:237.

15. Emery C. The determinants of treatment duration for congenital muscular torticollis. Phys Ther 1994; 74(10):921–929.

16. Symmetric Designs: The TOT Collar for Torticollis Treatment. Available at: www.symmetric-designs.com/tot-collar-.html (accessed 30 July 2009).

17. Losee JE, Mason AC, Dudas J, Hua LB, Mooney MP. Nonsynostotic occipital plagiocephaly: factors impacting onset, treatment, and outcomes. Plast Reconstr Surg 2007; 119(6):1866–1873.

18. ChengJC, Tang SP: Outcome of surgical treatment of congenital muscular torticollis. Clin Orthop 1999; 362:190.

19. Azizkhan RG, DeColl JM. Head and neck lesions. In: Ziegler MM, Azizkhan RG, Weber TR, eds. Operative Pediatric Surgery. McGraw-Hill Professional, 2003, Pp 221–240.

20. Shim JS, Jang HP. Operative treatment of congenital torticollis. J Bone Joint Surg Br 2008; 90(7):934–939.

21. Sasaki S, Yamamoto Y, Sugihara T, Kawashima K, Nohira K. Endoscopic tenotomy of the sternocleidomastoid muscle: new method for surgical correction of muscular torticollis. Plast Reconstr Surg 2000; 105:1764–1767.

CHAPTER 39
SALIVARY GLAND DISEASES IN CHILDREN AND ADOLESCENTS

Sunday Olusegun Ajike

Kokila Lakhoo

Introduction

Salivary glands are found in and around the oral cavity, and they are divided into major and minor salivary glands. The major salivary glands are the parotid, submandibular, and sublingual glands; the minor salivary glands are located in the lips, buccal mucosa, palate, and throat. Generally, salivary gland diseases are not common in the paediatric population. The classification of salivary gland diseases is very complex because it encompasses different entities; however, precise classification and terminology are necessary for accurate diagnosis and management. As in adults, diseases of the salivary glands may be nonneoplastic or neoplastic (tumours) (Table 39.1). The pattern of incidence in the paediatric population differs greatly from that in the adult group. Most salivary gland lesions in children are either inflammatory or vascular in origin. Of the developmental salivary gland diseases, haemangiomas are the most common. In the African paediatric population, mumps is the most common in the inflammatory/infection group, but in the developed world, only sporadic cases of mumps are now reported, and rhabdomyosarcomas are the most common nonodontogenic mesenchymal tumours in children.

Neoplastic changes in the paediatric population are very rare compared to the inflammatory groups. In the population as a whole, salivary gland neoplasms constitute 2.8% of all head and neck tumours, but in children it accounts for about 10% of all childhood neoplasms and between 3% and 22% of epithelial salivary gland neoplasms. The majority (88.5%) of salivary gland tumours are benign; the remaining 11.5% being malignant. In children, the most common benign epithelial tumour is pleomorphic adenoma, and the most common malignant tumour is mucoepidermoid carcinoma.

Salivary gland tumours in children have the same clinical and biologic behavior as those in the adult. The majority (76.7%) occur in the major glands, with the remainder in the minor glands, a ratio of 3.3:1. The ratio of occurrence of parotid to submandibular to sublingual tumours in the major salivary glands is 30:6:1. Globally, these tumours occur predominantly in girls and at any childhood age. A detailed clinical history with imaging features narrows the differential diagnosis while providing useful information for management and prognosis. Incisional biopsy must be avoided due to the possibility of tumour spillage and facial nerve damage.

The treatment of salivary gland diseases is categorised into medical and surgical, depending on the nature of the disease condition. The neoplastic lesions usually require surgical intervention, with or without radiation and chemotherapy, whereas the nonneoplastic/inflammatory diseases are managed symptomatically and conservatively. A protracted conservative medical management is strongly advised, however, before surgical ablation is considered in children.

Investigations

Salivary gland enlargement is a diagnostic challenge to the attending surgeon because the glands could be involved in a wide spectrum of diseases.

Table 39.1: Classification of salivary gland diseases in children.

Nonneoplastic tumours
Congenital/developmental
Agenesis/aplasia, hypogenesis/hypoplasia
Aberrant/ectopic salivary gland
Haemangioma
Lympangioma
Inflammatory and infection.
Acute sialadentis
Mumps, cytomegalovirus, Coxasackie A or B or parainfluenza virus)
Human immunodeficiency virus (HIV)-associated salivary glands
Recurrent parotitis in children (RPC)
Autoimmune
Sjogren's syndrome
Cysts
Ranula mucocele (mucous retention cyst)
Salivary gland dysfunction
Xerostomia
Sialorrhea/ptyalism
Neoplastic tumours
Benign
Pleomorphic adenoma
Warthin's tumour
Malignant
Mucoepidermoid carcinoma
Acinic cell carcinoma
Adenoid cystic carcinoma
Mesenchymal tumours
Neural tissue
Neurofibroma
Muscular tissue
Rhabdomyosarcoma

Investigative modalities in the diagnosis of salivary gland disorders in children are listed below. In an African setting, however, the cost of computed tomography (CT) and magnetic resonance imaging (MRI) systems usually limits investigations to ultrasonography and fine needle aspiration (FNA) cytology.

1. Ultrasonography (US) is useful in assessing the size of the gland and the vascularity of the lesion. It differentiates between a focal and diffuse disease, cystic and solid lesions, and is a useful adjunct for the assessment of adjacent vascular structures. US also guides FNA. The normal gland is hyperechogenic, whereas the diseased gland varies in hypogenicity.

2. A CT scan defines the nature and exact extent of the disease. It is useful in the diagnosis of acute inflammatory glands, abscess, and solid tumours. This is the imaging modality of choice in salivary gland diseases in children.

3. MRI defines the extent of the lesion similar to the CT scan. It is superior to CT, though, in that MRI also demonstrates the facial nerve within the parotid gland.

4. FMA cytology is a useful diagnostic tool. It can be used to establish whether a lesion is inflammatory benign or malignant. When used in children, however, there may be a need for sedation due to lack of cooperation. FNA cytology accurately diagnoses whether a lesion is benign or malignant in about 84–97% of the cases.

5. Sialography is very useful in the evaluation of autoimmune and chronic inflammatory diseases. The appearance is described as "cherry-blossom" or "branchless fruit laden tree" or '"snow storm".

6. Sialochemistry is useful in inflammatory and nonneoplastic diseases of the salivary glands. In inflammatory diseases, the IgA, IgG, IgM, albumin, transferring, lysozyme, Na, and protein are raised, and the phosphate level is decreased.

7. Sialometry is the determination of salivary flow rate. It is useful in the detection of salivary gland hypofunction.

8. Chest x-rays are used to detect any lung metastasis.

9. Radiographs of the jaws are used for the localisation of ectopic salivary gland tissues.

Congenital and Developmental Diseases

Aplasia (Agenesis) and Hypoplasia
Aplasia is the absence of any or a group of salivary glands; they could be unilaterally or bilaterally absent. Hypoplasia of the gland is reduced glandular tissue associated with hypofunction. Aplasia and hypoplasia are very rare, and only case reports have been documented.

Aplasia is of unknown aetiology; it may be isolated or occur in association with other developmental defects, such as hemifacial micostomia and the mandibulo-facial dysostosis (Treacher Collins syndrome), Down syndrome, and ectodermal dysplasia.

Aplasia presents with the development of xerostomia and its effects; however, other causes of xerostomia should be excluded. The effects of aplasia (agenesis) include dryness of the mouth, difficulty in mastication and swallowing of solid foods, an unusual pattern of dental caries, erosion of teeth, the presence of plaque, periodontal disease, soft tissue infection, chelitis, atrophic mucositis, and the absence of the salivary ducts. CT and MRI indicate the absence of the glands and replacement with fatty tissues; a salivary flow rate lower than 50% of its normal value is diagnostic.

Treatment is usually conservative; artificial saliva is used for frequent lubrication of the oral cavity. Comprehensive dental preventive and restorative therapy is strongly advocated.

Aberrant/Ectopic Salivary Gland
In aberrant/ectopic glandular anomaly, there is the presence of the salivary gland tissue in an abnormal location. This condition is rare in children, probably due to the difficulty in localising the lesion with a periapical radiograph in children and because it is usually asymptomatic. Locations include the tonsils, rectum, and the mandible. Inclusion of the gland in the angle of the mandible is seen frequently and referred to as Stafne's idiopathic bone cyst. Radiographically, this anomaly presents as a round or oval radiolucency between the mandibular canal and the inferior border of the mandible. The usual treatment is exploration of the cavity, whereas others believe it should just be kept under observation.

Haemangiomas
Haemangiomas are congenital malformations of the vascular system. They are the most common benign salivary gland lesion in children and the commonest benign tumour of children and adolescents. They have a female predilection. The majority are capillary in nature, occurring during the first year of life. Haemangiomas are usually soft masses noted shortly after birth, mainly in the parotid region, and rarely in the sublingual gland (Figure 39.1). They grow rapidly during the first year, with slow spontaneous complete regression at adolescence. They could be unilateral or bilateral.

At ultrasound, haemangiomas are hypoechoic relative to the gland, with a variable abnormal flow at Doppler US; contrast-enhanced CT reveals hypervascular mass with variable intensity of enhancement with an occasional demonstration of phleboliths. FNA cytology demonstrates elongated spindle cells arranged in coils and arcades.

Histopathologic analysis shows areas composed of an unencapsulated mass of closely packed, thin-walled capillaries with plump endothelial cells. Immunochemistry reveals vascular spaces lined by CD34 and factor VIII-positive flattened endotheliail cells.

Most capillary haemangiomas regress spontaneously, so surgical treatment should be delayed. Treatment options include injection of sclerosants, such as injection of boiling water normal saline, steroid, alfa 2a or 2b interferone (3 million units/m² per day, occlusion of feeder vessels, ligation of feeder vessels, surgical and laser ablation, or a combination of these modalities. Surgery is indicated in rapidly growing haemorrhagic tumours or following failure of the tumour to regress after achieving fibrosis postsclerotherapy.

Complications of haemangiomas include infection, ulceration, and occlusion of the larynx.

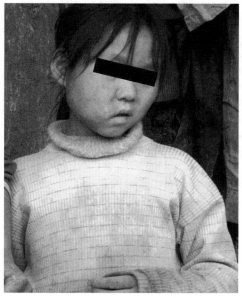

Figure 39.1: Haemangioma involving the parotid gland in a 13-year-old girl.

Lymphangiomas

Lymphangiomas are congenital malformations of the lymphatic system usually involving the parotid gland. They are the second most common nonneoplastic salivary gland tumours in children, occurring from birth to about 12 years of age, with a majority at 4 years of age and younger. About 65% are present at birth and 90% are detected during the second year, with a peak during the first decade. Lymphangiomas occur more in girls than boys. They present as a soft, asymptomatic swelling with facial asymmetry (Figure 39.2). Unlike haemangiomas, lymphangiomas rarely undergo spontaneous regression due to the extent of involvement and multispatial character of the lesion. Lymphangiomas are classified on the basis of the size of cystic spaces as simplex, cavernous, and venolymphatic.

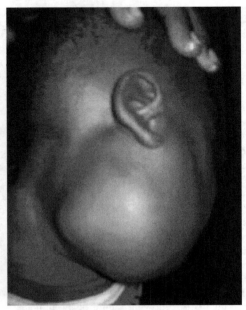

Figure 39.2: Lymphangioma of the parotid gland.

Ultrasonography typically reveals thin-walled septations with occasional solid areas, CT shows a multispatial mass with heterogeneous septation and cystic areas often containing fluid levels; however, solid portions of the lesion may show enhancement. MRI demonstrates heterogeneous multiple cystic areas. Contrast-enhanced imaging may show enhancement of the solid portions of the lesion.

Treatment options for lymphangioma include intralesional injection of sclerosing agents; OK432 (picibalin), bleomycin, or surgical excision. Complications include infection and haemorrhage.

Parotid Swelling

Several nonspecific conditions are characterised by unilateral or bilateral enlargement of the parotid gland. Differential diagnosis of bilateral parotid swellings in a child may have the following aetiologies:

• viral (mumps, HIV-associated salivary disease);

• immunological (Sjogren's syndrome); and

• nutritional (obesity, hypervitaminosis A, beri-beri, hypoproteinaemia).

In addition, of unknown aetiology are hypertrophy of the masseter muscle and juvenile recurrent parotitis (JRP, also known as recurrent parotitis in children, or RPC).

Viral

Mumps

Mumps (epidemic parotitis) is now rare in the developed world due to the availability of the measles-mumps-rubella (MMR) vaccines, except for sporadic outbreaks that occur in adolescents and adults. However, in the developing world, it is the most common cause of parotitis in children, primarily affecting children younger than 15 years of age. Mumps frequently occurs as an epidemic between ages 5 to 15 years. It is usually contagious, with an attack conferring a lifelong immunity.

The aetiology of mumps is due to the paramyxovirus group with an incubation period of about 21 days. A similar clinical picture may present in Coxasackie A or B or parainfluenza virus. It is characterised by mild fever, malaise, and pain and sudden distention of the involved gland, usually the parotid gland. Initially, it involves one side, but within 3 to 5 days both glands become involved. The involved gland feels tensed and tender with congested punctum.

Mumps is a self-limiting disease. The treatment is primarily symptomatic: analgesic for pain, antibiotic to prevent secondary infection, and rehydration with adequate bed rest. Its postpuberty complications are orchitis and oophoritis in the male and female, respectively. Prevention is by the administration of the MMR vaccine.

HIV-associated salivary gland lesions

HIV-associated salivary gland lesions have become common in the African setting following the HIV/AIDS pandemic. The pandemic is a leading cause of immunodeficiency in infants and children. Lesions commonly involve the parotid glands; however, parotid involvement in the paediatric group is associated with a better prognosis. Typical lesions are of the benign lympyhoepithelial types and cystic. Other presentations are with xerostomia and sialorrhea. On ultrasonography, 70% show multiple hypoechoic or anechoic areas, with the remaining 30% being anechoic. CT and MRI demonstrate bilateral parotid enlargement with intraglandular cystic and solid masses. No surgical intervention is needed, as resolution of swellings occurs following the administration of antiretroviral drugs.

Immunological: Sjogren's Syndrome

Sjogren's syndrome is an autoimmune disease characterised by mononuclear infiltration and destruction of the salivary and lacrimal glands. Two types are recognised: primary Sjogren's is a sialolacrimal disease without associated autoimmune disease, and secondary Sjogren's is a sialolacrimal disease with an autoimmune disease, usually rheumatoid arthritis.

Clinical features include those due to xerostomia with dryness of the eye and keratatis. Diagnosis is based on determination of the parotid rate lower than 1–2 ml/min; ultrasonography studies showing a snowstorm, cobblestone appearance; labial gland biopsy; detectable rheumatoid factor; antinuclear and antisalivary duct; and antithyroid antibodies. Histologically, it is characterised by infiltration, replacement, and destruction of the salivary and lacrimal glands by lymphocytes and plasma cells.

Treatment for Sjogren's syndrome is symptomatic, as for xerostomia: treat connective tissue diseases and keratoconjuctivitis with artificial saliva and ophthalmic lubricants.

Unknown Aetiology

Recurrent parotitis in children

RPC is a nonobstructive, nonsuppurative inflammatory disease of the parotid salivary gland of unknown aetiology in children, although congenital autoimmune duct defects are implicated. It is the second most common salivary gland disease in children after mumps. Clinically, it is characterised by a sudden onset of intermittent unilateral or bilateral parotid swellings over a period of years. The child is usually not ill, although there may be a mild rise in temperature; leucocytic count differentiates it from mumps. This lesion should also be differentiated from Sjogren's syndrome and HIV-associated salivary gland diseases. It predominates in male children between 3 months and 16 years of age with remission at puberty. There is usually a widening of the Stenson's duct with mucopurulent discharge.

Diagnosis is usually from parental history and a report of recurrent unilateral or bilateral parotid gland infections. Sialographic studies show a pattern of sialectasis similar to Sjogren's syndrome strictures, dilations, and kinks. Salivary chemistry is usually altered as it also is in adult patients: increased amounts of sodium, and protein, IgA, IgG, IgM, albumin, transferrin, and myeloperoxidase.

Treatment is conservative by lavage, ductal dilatation and hydrocortisone (100 mg) injection via sialoendoscopy, glandular massage salivary stimulation with sugarless sour candy, and antibiotics augmentin (25 mg/kg) or clindamycin (150 mg, 8-hourly, for 7 days). In an African setting, glandular massage of the parotid with antibiotics may be very helpful.

Masseteric hypertrophy

This is an asymptomatic bilateral enlargement of the masseter muscles as a result of hypertrophy. It is associated with bruxism and clenching of the teeth. Treatment usually involves debulking the masseter.

Cysts

Ranula

A ranula is a cyst-like soft swelling in the mouth. It presents as a translucent bluish colour under the tongue (Figure 39.3). The appearance is that of a frog's belly. Its aetiology is as a result of mucous extravasation of the sublingual gland following trauma, and obstruction or infection of the gland ducts, resulting in leakage and escape of secretion into the surrounding tissue. Simple ranula occurs when the extravasation is into the oral aspect of the mylohyoid muscle, whereas involvement of the hernited sublingual gland through the mylohyoid muscle results in a plunging ranula manifesting extraorally in the neck (Figure 39.4). Simple ranulas are noted more commonly in females, and plunging ranulas noted more frequently in males. CT scan demonstrates a cystic mass in the suprahyoid anterior neck.

Marsupialisation of the simple intraoral ranula involves deroofing of the cyst, suturing of its wall to the surrounding mucosa with packing of lumen. Plunging ranula is excised with the involved sublingual gland. Recurrence usually necessitates excision of the involved sublingual gland (see Figure 39.4).

Mucoceles

A mucocele (mucous extravasation cyst) develops mostly in children and young adults and mainly from the minor salivary glands following trauma and leakage of saliva into the surrounding submucosal tissue. The most common sites are the lower lip and inner aspect of the cheek, which are areas susceptible to trauma during oral function. A mucocele has no epithelial lining; rather, it is contained within a wall of fibrous and inflammatory tissue. It typically presents as a slow-growing and superficial soft wall fluctuant fluid containing mass of diameter 1.0–2.0 cm.

The overlying mucosa is usually of a translucent bluish color. A mucocele causes little or no discomfort. Marsupialisation of the cyst with overlying mucosa leads to recurrence of this pseudocyst. Occasionally, it ruptures spontaneously and forms again because of the accumulation of secretions beneath the healed surface. Excision of the cyst with the overlying mucosa lining is the treatment of choice.

Salivary Gland Dysfunctions

Xerostomia

Xerostomia is dryness of the mouth. The major cause in children is dehydration. Other causes are the use of antihistamine-containing drugs or decongestants; autoimmune diseases such as Sjogren's syndrome, sarcoidosis, and HIV; agenesis/aplasia or salivary gland hypofunction; and ectodermal dysplasia.

Symptoms of xerostomia include dryness of the oral cavity, burning sensation, soreness of the lips, difficulty with speech, difficulty with mastication and swallowing of solid foods, and altered taste sensations.

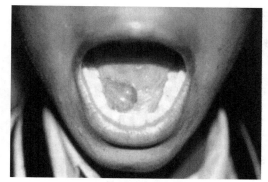

Figure 39.3: Simple ranula in a 6-year-old boy.

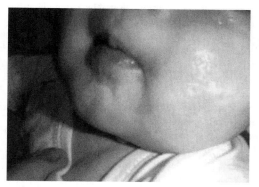

Figure 39.4: Plunging ranula.

Signs of xerostomia are dryness of the oral mucosa, mucositis, angular chelitis, dental plaques, dental smooth surface caries and demineralisation of the enamel, inflamed gingivae with periodontal diseases, and candidiasis. Diagnosis is based on history, clinical examination, sialometry (salivary flow is decreased), sialography, scintigraphy, sialochemistry (sodium and chloride lactofarrin levels), gland biopsy, and whole saliva immunotesting for antinuclear antibodies.

Treatment is conservative. The use of stimulants, sugarless candies and gums, artificial saliva; increased fluid intake; oral lubricants; and nonirritating toothpastes is recommended. Oral rehabilitation may be required to correct rehydration in some cases. Comprehensive dental management is strongly advocated.

Sialorrhea

Sialorrhea (ptyalism) is a persistent increase in salivary flow rate. It differs from drooling. In children, the most common cause is teething. Other causes are childhood epilepsy, HIV parotid enlargement, mental retardation, cerebral palsy, and herpes infection. In children, it requires the constant change of clothing and the use of bibs.

Treatment for sialorrhea is usually conservative, involving the use of anticholinergic agents (atropine) and antidepressants. However, surgical management such as parotid duct rerouting (Wilkie procedure), submandibular duct rerouting, tympanic neurectomy, or excision of the glands may be carried out when conservative management fails.

Neoplastic Epithelial Tumours

The parotid gland is the most common site of tumours (85.1%), followed by the submandibular (11.7%) and the sublingual (3.2%). In the minor salivary gland, the most common site is the palate. Overall, salivary gland tumours occur more in girls than in boys.

The majority of salivary gland neoplasms in children are benign. The pleomorphic adenoma is the most common benign neoplasm, and the most common malignant tumour is mucoepidermoid carcinoma. About 11.5–35% of salivary gland tumours in children are malignant, and 60–90% of these are mucoepidermoid carcinomas; adenoid cystic and acinic cell carcinomas follow in frequency, each occurring at approximately 5–10%. The mainstay of treatment of salivary gland tumours is surgery.

Pleomorphic Adenoma

Pleomorphic adenoma (mixed tumour) is the most common childhood salivary gland tumour, occurring mostly in the parotid gland. Typical features are as a hard or firm or fluctuant, painless, slow-growing, freely mobile, bossellated mass. Facial nerve paralysis in association with pleomorphic adenoma never occurs, even in large grotesque swellings seen in Africans (Figure 39.5). The most common intraoral site is the palate, followed by the buccal mucosa and the lip (Figure 39.6).

In the minor salivary glands, the features include bossellated ulcerated swelling, causing ill-fitting dentures and difficulty in speech, which may occasionally erode the palatine bone. Ulceration is usually as result of trauma or following topical application of herbal medication. No childhood age is exempt, with a median of 15 years from some studies, occurring predominantly in females.

At ultrasound, the pleomorphic adenoma varies from hypoechoicity to isoechoicity relative to the rest of the gland, with occasional hyperechogenic foci due to some calcifications within the mass. CT and MRI demonstrate varying findings depending on the tumour size. Small lesions are homogenous with well-defined margins, whereas larger lesions are more heterogeneous with less well defined margins. FNA cytology confirms the benignity of this tumour.

Microscopically, the pleomorphic adenoma tumour is composed of varying proportions of glandular-like epithelium and connective tissue stroma. Epithelial cells may show nests, solid sheets, or ductal structures with varying stroma, which may be myxoid, chondroid, fibroid, or osteoid with some areas of squamous metaplasia and foci of keratin.

Treatment is parotidectomy (superficial or total) with facial nerve sparing. In the submandibular gland; treatment is submandibulectomy. In the minor salivary glands, wide local excision with a circumscribed incision of 3–5 mm of apparent normal tissue is made around the tumour. There is a high recurrence, usually due to enucleation of the tumour.

Parotidectomy procedure

1. The external auditory canal is blocked with a pledget of cotton wool to prevent blood from entering into the ear canal.

2. A lazy S incision starts anterior to the ear helix, extends posteriorly over the mastoid bone, and curves anteriorly parallel to the angle of the mandible or running along the submandibular incision line up to about 3 cm.

3. A skin incision is raised, exposing the superficial parotid fascia, and is retracted and sutured down (Figure 39.7).

4. The mastoid, the anterior border of the sternocleidomastoid muscle, and the posterior belly of the digastrics muscles are identified. Finger pressure is applied medial to feel for the styloid process.

5. The posterior belly of the digastrics muscle is retracted, exposing the facial nerve as it exits from the stylomastoid foramen (see Figure 39.7).

6. The nerve is followed into the parotid gland, where it divides into its five terminal branches under the superficial lobe.

7. For superficial parotidectomy, the gland is dissected off the nerve. For total parotidectomy, the superficial lobe is removed and the deep lobe is excised after elevating the nerve.

8. The surgical site is irrigated and a suction drain is inserted.

9. The wound is closed in layers and a compression dressing is applied (Figure 39.8).

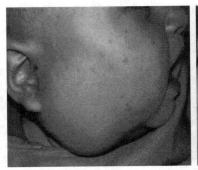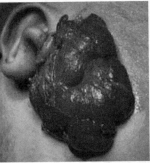

Figure 39.5: Pleomorphic adenoma of the parotid gland

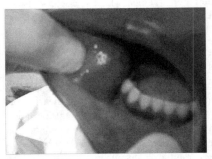

Figure 39.6: Pleomorphic adenoma of the buccal mucosa.

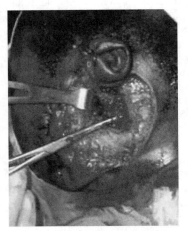

Figure 39.7: Skin incision exposed and sutured down. The posterior belly of digastrics and facial nerve are identified with forceps.

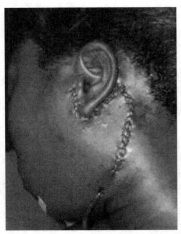

Figure 39.8: Wound closure with an in situ drain.

Complications of parotidectomy

An immediate complication of parotidectomy is bleeding. Delayed complications include haematoma, infection, transient facial nerve paralysis, facial nerve paralysis, Frey's syndrome, salivary fistula, and recurrence.

Warthin's Tumour

The second most common benign salivary gland neoplasm in children is Warthin's tumour (papillary cystadenoma lymphomatosum, or adenolymphoma). This occurs mainly in the parotid gland. It is a slow-growing, painless swelling, usually unilateral with multiple masses in the gland. Developmentally, there is incorporation of the lymphatic element, salivary gland tissue, and the paraparotid lymph nodes.

CT and MRI demonstrate a well-circumscribed, homogenous cystic or solid lesion in the parotid gland.

Grossly, the tumour appears as multiple cysts of varying diameters containing viscous fluid with solid areas of lymphoid follicles. Microscopically, the tumour comprises tall eosinophilic columnar cells with papillary projections into cystic spaces in a background of lymphoid stroma.

Treatment is surgical excision (parotidectomy) of the tumour with preservation of the facial nerve.

Carcinomas

Acinic Cell Carcinoma

Acinic cell carcinoma (also known as acinic cell adenocarcinoma or acinous cell carcinoma) is a malignant epithelial neoplasm of salivary glands demonstrating serous acinar cell differentiation. It is second in occurrence to mucoepidermoid carcinoma in the paediatric population. It is of varying malignancy, accounting for 6–37% of the total malignancies in children. It is more common in girls than boys, and 4% of the patients are younger than 20 years of age.

The majority occur in the parotid gland. It typically presents as a painless, slow-growing, enlarging solitary mass in the parotid, occasionally multinodular and fixed to the skin and underlying tissues. It is occasionally painful, with associated facial nerve paralysis.

The treatment modality is parotidectomy (superficial or deep) with preservation of the facial nerve. Nodal and distance metastasis with recurrence may occur.

Mucoepidermoid Carcinoma

Most studies agree that mucoepidermoid carcinoma (mixed epidermoid and mucus-secreting carcinoma) is the most common salivary gland malignancy in children. The majority are in the major salivary glands, with about 45% in the parotid. The most frequent intraoral sites are the palate and the buccal mucosa. It has a female predilection, and occurs in the 5- to 15-year-old age group, peaking between 12 and 14 years of age.

The clinical features depend on the grade of the tumour. They are classified as low, intermediate, or high grade. In children, the majority are of the low-grade variety with a very good prognosis. The low-grade presentation may simulate a benign tumour. Otherwise, it typically presents as a rapidly growing swelling with perineural and soft tissue invasion. High-grade tumours are usually found in children younger than 5 years of age.

Diagnosis is based on clinical, radiological, and pathological findings. The low-grade type shows smooth "benign appearing" margins at US, CT, and MRI, containing cystic low attenuation and

occasional calcified foci at CT. The high-grade type is more solid and homogenous at both CT and MRI.

The cut surface may contain cystic or solid areas, or both. Cystic areas contain viscous or mucoid materials. Microscopically, this tumour contains two types of cells—mucous and epidermoid cells; the proportion determines the grade of the tumour. The low-grade tumour is characterised by prominent cystic structures and mature cellular elements; the intermediate-grade tumour has fewer and smaller cystic structures and occasional solid islands of epidermoid cells; and the high-grade tumour is a hypercellular solid tumour with cellular atypia and high mitotic figures.

The treatment of mucoepidermoid carcinoma is surgery, depending on the grade, location, and tumour extent. Wide local excision is adequate for low-grade tumours. Block composite excision with radical neck dissection is appropriate for the intermediate- and high-grade varieties. This may involve excision of the gland and facial nerve; petrosectomy; mastoidectomy; or resection of the ramus of the mandible, zygomatic arch, and the overlying skin, with subsequent nerve grafting and facial reconstruction. In the palate, palatoalveolectomy, maxillectomy with or without radiotherapy, and chemotherapy are used postoperatively. Radiation should be used with caution in children due to the long-term effects. Tumour grading and subtype have a tremendous predictive effect on the prognosis.

Rhabdomyosarcoma

Rhabdomyosarcoma is the most common childhood soft tissue sarcoma, usually of the embryonic subtype. About 40% of all rhabdomyosarcomas arise in the head and neck region, and the parotid and the adjacent structures are usually involved by direct invasion. It is common between 1 and 13 years of age, with most patients dying a few months after initial diagnosis. Prognosis is usually poor because of late presentation (Figure 39.9).

CT demonstrates heterogeneous attenuation of the tumour, and MRI shows a poorly defined, heterogeneous mass. The treatment is wide surgical excision of the tumour and adjacent structures with reconstruction of the lost tissues. For advanced inoperable tumours, as is commonly seen in the African population, palliative chemotherapy is recommended.

Neurofibroma

Neurofibroma is a benign nerve sheath tumour that may arise from the facial nerve within the parotid gland. It is rarely in the submandibular gland. It may be solitary with gross facial disfigurement (Figure 39.10) or have multiple lesions, as seen in von Recklinghausen's disease. Clinically, it feels like a bag of worms. CT demonstrates it as well-demarcated, homogenous, and isoattenuated relative to muscle. It shows moderate enhancement following injection of contrast media. Occasionally, it may push the larynx or the trachea, causing respiratory difficulty (Figure 39.11). MRI may show low to intermediate signal intensity.

Histologically, neurofibroma consists of loose collagen fibre with long, thin processes of nerve fibre and darkly stained elongated nuclei. The treatment is surgical excision. Recurrence occurs because of inadequate excision.

Evidence-Based Research

Table 39.2 presents a study of surgical procedures on tumours of the salivary glands in children and adolescents.

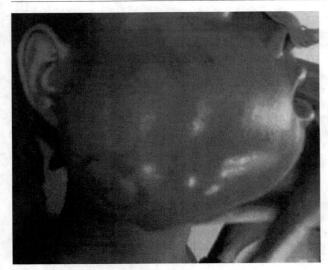

Figure 39.9: Rhabomyosarcoma in a 15-year-old girl.

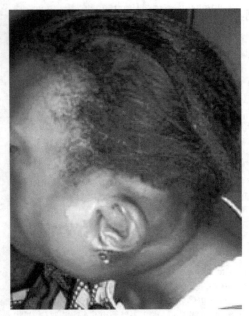

Figure 39.10: Neurofibroma involving the parotid gland in a 16-year-old girl.

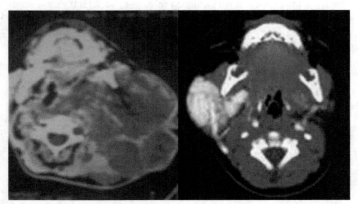

Figure 39.11: CT scan of neurofibroma pushing the airway in a 16-year-old girl.

Table 39.2: Evidence-based research.

Title	Tumours of the salivary glands in children and adolescents
Authors	Ellis M, Schaffranietz F, Arglebe C, Lawskawi R
Institution	Department of Otorhinolaryngology, Head and Neck Surgery, Universitats-HNO-Klinic, Germany
Reference	Int J Oral Maxillofac Surg 2006; 64:1048–1058
Problem	To examine the outcome and side effects of therapy and recurrence of 52 salivary gland tumours in juveniles and adolescents.
Intervention	Surgical procedures.
Outcome/ effect	Forty benign and 12 malignant tumours underwent various surgical procedures. For the benign tumours, 20 cases (50%) were parotidectomies; 2 (5%) of these with facial nerve graft, 14 (35%) had lateral parotidectomies, 2 (5%) had subtotal parotidectomies, 3 (7.5%) had submandibulectomies, and 1 (2.5%) had enucleation. For the malignant tumours, 11 (91.75%) had total or radical parotidectomies; 4 (33.3%) had total parotidectomies with excision of facial nerve and facial nerve grafting with the greater auricular nerve; 5 (41.7%) had radical parotidectomy with facial nerve and adjacent structures (ascending ramus, temporomandibular joint, zygomatic bone, and mastoid); 2 (22.2%) had parotidectomies with neck dissection; and 1 (11.1%) had superficial parotidectomy.
Historical significance/ comments	This report of 52 cases of salivary gland tumours demonstrates the various types of salivary gland tumours in the parotid region, provides a useful practice guide, and attests to the rarity of these tumours in the paediatric population. Irrespective of the type of tumour, surgery is the preferred mode of treatment. However, the postoperative complications of the parotidectomy procedure should be noted. The authors recommend a multidisciplinary approach involving the paediatrician, the surgeon, the radiotherapist, and the oncologist. The findings of this report have important implications for the African setting in that primary surgery is most effective and the surgeons and paediatricians are readily available, whereas the radiotherapists and oncologists are not. Furthermore, in the African setting, microscopic surgery for nerve grafting is still elusive.

Key Summary Points

1. Salivary gland tumours in children are rare.

2. Most salivary gland lesions in children are either inflammatory or vascular in origin.

3. Classification of salivary gland diseases is complex but important for management planning.

4. Major glands are more readily affected.

5. In Africa, investigation may be limited to ultrasound and fine needle aspiration.

6. Most lesions are self-limiting or require medical management.

7. Surgical management is reserved for tumours and nonresolving lesions.

8. Facial nerve damage is the major morbidity in salivary gland surgery and should be avoided.

Suggested Reading

Abiose BO, Oyediji O, Ogunniyi J. Salivary gland tumours in Ibadan, Nigeria. A study of 295 cases. Afr J Med Sci 1990; 19(3):195–199.

Adebayo ETO, Ajike SO, Adekeye EO. Tumours and tumour-like lesions of the oral and perioral structures of Nigerian children. Int J Oral Maxillofac Surg 2001; 30:250–253.

Ajike SO, Adebayo AT, Adekeye EO. Minor salivary gland tumours in Kaduna, Nigeria. Nig J Surg Res 2003; 5(3-4):100–105.

Al-Khateeb T, Al Hadi Hamasha A, Almasari NM. Oral and maxillofacial tumours in Northern Jordanian children and adolescents: a retrospective analysis over 10 years. Int J Oral Maxillofac Surg 2003; 32:78–83.

Al-Salam AH. Lymphangioma in infancy and childhood. Saudi Med J 2004; 25(4):466–469.

Bentz BG, Hughes CA, Ludemann JP, Maddalazzo J. Masses of salivary gland region in children. Arch Otolaryngol Head Neck 2000; 126:135–139.

Bradly P, McCliand L, Mehta D. Paediatric salivary epithelial neoplasms. Otolaryngol 2007; 67:137–145.

Callender DL, Frankenthaler RA, Luna MA, Lee SS, Goepfert H. Salivary gland neoplasms in children. Act Otolarngol Head Neck Surg 1992; 118:472–476.

Ethunandan M, Ethunandan A, Macpherson D, Conroy B, Pratt C. Parotid neoplasm in children: experience of diagnosis and management in a district general hospital. Int J Oral Maxillofac Surg 2003; 32:373–377.

Greene AK, Rogers GF, Mulliken JB. Management of parotid haemangiomas in 100 children. Plast Reconstr Surg 2004; 113(1):53–60.

Jaber MA. Intraoral minor salivary gland tumours: a review of 75 cases in a Libyan population. Int J Oral Maxillofac Surg 2006: 35:150–154.

Kolude B, Iawoyin JO, Akang EEU. Salivary gland neoplasms: a 21 year review of cases seen at the University College Hospital, Ibadan. Afr J Med Sci 2001; 30:95–98.

Malata CM, Camilleri IG, McLean NR, et al. Malignant tumours of the parotid gland: a 12-year review. Br J Plastic Surg 1997; 50:600–608.

Malik, NA. Diseases of the salivary glands. In: Malik NA. Textbook of Oral and Maxillofacial Surgery, 1st ed. Jaypee Brothers Medical Publishers (P) Ltd., 2002, Pp 479–503.

Otoh EC, Mandong BM, Danfillo IS, Jalo PH. Salivary gland tumours: a 16 year review at Jos University Teaching Hospital, Jos, Nigeria. Nig J Clinic Biomed Res 2006; 1(1):53–58.

Owotade FJ, Fatusi OA, Adebiyi KE, Ajike SO, Ukpong MO. Clinical experience with parotid gland enlargement in HIV infection: a report of five cases in Nigeria. J Contemp Dent Pract 2005; 6(1)136–145.

Shikhan AH, Johns ME. Tumours of the major salivary glands in children. Head Neck Surg 1988; 10(4): 257–263.

Yu GY; Li ZL; MA DQ; Zhang Y. Diagnosis and treatment of epithelial salivary gland tumours in children and adolescents. Brit J Oral Maxillofac Surg 2002; 20(5):389–392.

Zhao YF, Jio Y, Chen XM, Zhang WF. Clinical review of 580 ranulas. Oral Surg Oral Med Oral Pathol Oral Radiol Endod 2004; 98(3):281–287.

CHAPTER 40
THYROID AND PARATHYROID GLANDS

Abdulrasheed A. Nasir

Emmanuel A. Ameh

Ashley Ridout

Demographics

Diseases of the thyroid gland were demonstrated to occur in 3.7% of 4,819 school-aged children at initial examination in the United States; in a followup examination 20 years later, the prevalence had increased to 10.5%.[1] About half of these are diffuse gland hypertrophy or simple goiter. Thyroiditis was the second most common abnormality, followed by thyroid nodules and functional disorders. Malignant neoplasms are exceedingly rare, with only two papillary thyroid carcinomas found in a population of nearly 5,000 children followed up for three years. Data on thyroid diseases in African children are scanty. One series reported four cases of thyroid tumours in children over a ten-year period in Enugu, Nigeria.[2] Three of these were adenomas and the remaining one was a papillary carcinoma. All of the patients were girls younger than 10 years of age. Data from the United States, based on the National Cancer Registry, reported the annual incidence of thyroid tumours as 0.54 per 100,000 individuals.[3]

Evaluation of Thyroid Diseases

Assessment of Thyroid Function

It is often necessary to determine whether a patient has a hyperactive, normal, or hypoactive thyroid function. A detailed history and careful clinical examination will reveal the diagnosis.

Measurement of Thyroid Hormones in the Serum

Thyroid functional status can be established by estimating the serum thyroid hormones and thyroid-stimulating hormone (TSH, or thyrotropin), which are the most important diagnostic tests. Levels of free T_4 and free T_3 in serum provide a better assessment of the thyroid status than total T_4 and T_3. The levels of T_4 and T_3 are decreased in hypothyroidism, and they are increased in hyperthyroidism. Free T_4 and TSH are the most common useful tests in paediatric thyroid disorders, but test results must be interpreted in conjunction with the child's overall clinical condition. T_3 levels usually need to be measured only when a patient is suspected of having hyperthyroidism but has normal T_4 levels, particularly in cases of toxic nodule, multinodular goiter, or recurrent Graves' disease.[4] Graves' disease is discussed later in this chapter.

Thyrotropin is nearly always decreased in the hyperthyroid state and elevated in hypothyroidism and is an extremely sensitive measure of hypothyroid state. The plasma free T_4 level is a measure of biologically active thyroid hormone, unaffected by protein binding. When total plasma T_3 and T_4 are measured, it is necessary to consider the level of unbound biologically active hormone.

Serum Thyroid Antibodies

The autoantibody status is important in determining thyroid autoimmune diseases. Serum thyroid antibodies are frequently elevated in autoimmune thyroid disorders. Approximately 80% of patients with Hashimoto's disease have elevated antimicrosomal autoantibodies,[5] and most patients with Graves' disease have detectable thyroid-stimulating immunoglobulins. The presence of these antibodies is helpful in the diagnosis of autoimmune thyroid disorders.

Test of Hypothalamic Pituitary Axis

The test for thyrotropin-releasing hormones (TRH) is given intravenously. The basal level of serum TSH is raised in a normal individual at 20 minutes and returned to normal in 120 minutes. In hypothyroidism, the already elevated TSH shows a much higher rise, but there is no response in hyperthyroidism. This is known as the TRH stimulation test.

Imaging

Several imaging modalities are available to assist in evaluating the thyroid gland, among them ultrasonography (US), computed tomography (CT), magnetic resonance imaging (MRI), and scintigraphy.

Ultrasonography

Ultrasound imaging is very useful in the evaluation of thyroid disease and can determine whether a neck mass actually arises from the thyroid and whether multiple nodules are present. It allows differentiation of solid and cystic lesions. It is useful in detection of thyroid nodules and measurement of their volume. Goiter volume can be assessed precisely with US and is a useful guide in the assessment of goiter shrinkage response under medical treatment. Although this modality can be used in a clinical setting, it may not be appropriate for mass surveys.

Computed tomography and magnetic resonance imaging

A CT scan is useful in the study of the architecture of the thyroid gland and its relation to the surrounding organs. It can be useful in assessing retrosternal extension of the thyroid. Pituitary or hypothalamic tumours can be seen, as can metastatic lesions of thyroid carcinoma, which are usually solitary. MRI provides a good soft tissue resolution and helps in further ascertaining the architecture of the thyroid gland.

Scintigraphy

Scintigraphy tests are based on the avidity or otherwise of the thyroid to absorb or release the isotope of iodine or technetium and the distribution of the isotope within the gland. Isotopic scanning provides information on the size, shape, position, function, and possible nature of thyroid swelling. The uptake by the thyroid of a low dose of either radioiodine ^{123}I or ^{131}I and technetium-99m pertechnetate will demonstrate the distribution of activity in the whole thyroid gland. The test is of value in a toxic patient with a nodule or nodularity of the thyroid. Localisation of overactivity in the gland will differentiate between a toxic nodule with suppression of the remainder of the gland and toxic multinodularity goiter with several areas of increased uptake with important implications for therapy.[6] Scintigraphy may also be useful in detecting ectopic thyroid tissue or metastatic thyroid carcinoma.

Fine Needle Aspiration Biopsy and Cytology

Thyroid tissue is obtained percutaneously with a 22–25-gauge needle attached to a 20-ml syringe fixed in a syringe holder. Fine needle aspiration (FNA) is useful in diagnosing papillary, medullary, and anaplastic carcinomas. There is small risk of false negative results. It is difficult to differentiate between simple and malignant follicular tumours by FNA cytology.

Nonneoplastic Diseases of the Thyroid Gland

Congenital Anomalies

Lingual thyroid

Lingual thyroid occurs when the thyroid gland fails to descend to its normal cervical location. Approximately 1 in 600,000 live births present in childhood or adolescence with lingual thyroid.[7] In cases of undescended thyroid, 90% were found within the tongue and 10% in the anterior neck above the hyoid bone.[8] The posterior part of the tongue around the foramen caecum is the most common site of lingual thyroid. It is most common in females. Symptoms usually consist of dysphagia and dyspnea. Diagnosis is confirmed by radioactive iodine scintigraphy. Of patients with lingual thyroids, 75% have no functional thyroid tissue.[9] Therefore, testing for location of thyroid tissue in addition to gland function is necessary.

Treatment consists of complete excision of the lingual thyroid followed by lifelong thyroid hormone therapy. Autotransplantation of the excised lingual gland or pedicle transfer—retaining a vascular pedicle and moving part of the thyroid into the neck—has been successful in several cases.[8,10]

Goiters

An enlarged thyroid gland due to any cause is called a goiter. Goiters are classified as diffusely enlarged or nodular and either toxic or euthyroid. A diffuse thyroid enlargement is the most common form of goiter in small children. Physiologically, diffuse thyroid enlargement may be related to autoimmune diseases, or can be an inflammatory or compensatory response. In a study of 152 school children with goiters, most patients (83%) had adolescent colloid goiter.[11] Goiters may be endemic or sporadic.

Endemic goiters

Endemic goiters exist when more than 10% of any community has goiters,[12] usually in high rocky mountain regions of the world. Endemic goiter has been described in nearly all African countries. Endemic goiter is mainly caused by insufficient iodine intake in the diet. The iodine content of the water supply and the soil in granite mountain regions are very low. Other causes of endemic goiter are goitrogens in food and excessive calcium salts in the water supply. Cassava, which is a common foodstuff in most African communities, contains cyanogenic glycosides, which yields thiocyanate as a metabolic by-product. Thiocyanate inhibits iodine uptake by the thyroid.[12]

The physiologic changes to iodine deficiency are usually accompanied by an increase in the size of the thyroid gland. Generalised epithelial hyperplasia occurs, with cellular hypertrophy and reduction in follicular spaces. In chronic iodine deficiency, the follicles become inactive and distended with colloid accumulation. These changes persist into adulthood, and focal nodular hyperplasia may develop, leading to nodular formation. Some of these nodules retain the ability to secrete thyroxin and form functioning thyroid nodules. Others do not retain this ability, become inactive and form cold nodules. Necrosis and scarring result in fibrous setae, which contribute to the formation of multinodular goiters (Figure 40.1). Some multinodular goiters eventually become toxic. One study reports an increasing risk of toxicity developing in nodular goiters in children and adults in Africa, and 10.7% of adult nodular goiters may develop infective thyroiditis (thyroid abscess), although whether this infective complication occurs in children is not clear.[13,14]

Sporadic goiters

Sporadic goiters occur in areas where goiters are not endemic. Sporadic goiters affect relatively few people and are usually pathological. The persistence of goiters in some areas with adequate iodine prophylaxis and the unequal geographic distribution of goiters in iodine-deficient areas suggest the existence of other goitrogenic factors. Cyanoglucosides are naturally occurring goitrogens found in several

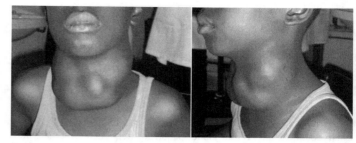

Figure 40.1: A ten-year-old boy with endemic multinodular goiter.

staple foods in the tropics, namely, cassava, maize, bamboo shoots, and sweet potatoes. The brassica family of vegetables is a well-known example producing thioglycosides. Flavonoides from millet, a staple food in Sudan, are also known to have antithyroid activity.

Congenital goiter

The majority of neonatal goiters result from maternal ingestion of goitrogens. In the newborn infant, the most commonly implicated drugs are iodides and thiourea derivatives used for treatment of maternal thyrotoxicosis. Congenital goiter has also been described in a newborn with Prader-Willi syndrome.[15] Most goiters in the newborn are of the hyperplastic type and disappear a few weeks after birth.[16]

Ultrasonography provides a useful noninvasive investigation in assessing the size of the goiter as well as the response to therapy. Rarely, goiters may be large enough to produce severe respiratory distress by tracheal compression. These patients may require division of the isthmus or subtotal thyroidectomy to relieve tracheal compression.

Physiologic goiter

In physiological states such as puberty, menstruation, and pregnancy or lactation, the body's requirement for thyroid hormones is increased due to the increased metabolic activity. If this requirement is not met, TSH secretion is increased to stimulate the thyroid. The thyroid gland undergoes physiological hyperplasia and may therefore enlarge. The thyroid gland is enlarged evenly, and feels comparatively soft. This occurs at puberty and is almost exclusively confined to females. Involution takes place when the hormones are increased in a sufficient amount or the need for an increased amount is over, usually by the twenty-first year.[6,12]

Colloid goiter

Colloid goiter is diffuse hyperplasia of the thyroid gland due to iodine deficiency. It is commonly seen in endemic areas but may also occur sporadically. In endemic areas, children may be affected, but girls from puberty to 20 years of age are most commonly involved.[12] The gland is enlarged, smooth-surfaced, may be firm in areas and soft in others, and has some degree of elasticity. All goiters of puberty that do not subside completely must be considered colloid goiters. The gland may occasionally be big enough to cause tracheal compression. The degree of lateral lobe enlargement determines the extent of displacement or narrowing of the trachea. Spontaneous regression is common, although, on occasion, minimal amounts of thyroxine preparation may be necessary.

Classification of goiter in general is according to the size of the thyroid gland on physical examination and the grading system recommended by the World Health Organization (WHO) in 1960 and modified in 1994:[17]

• Grade 0: No palpable or visible goiter

• Grade 1: Mass consistent with enlarged thyroid that is palpable but not visible when the neck is in the neutral position; it also moves upwards in the neck as the subject swallows.

• Grade 2: Swelling visible in a neutral position of the neck and consistent with an enlarged thyroid when the neck is palpated.

Prevention

The supply of adequate iodine in the diet and the elimination of goitrogens are the means used to prevent endemic goiter. Global iodisation of salt has been successfully introduced with remarkable results worldwide.

Thyroiditis

Hashimoto's disease

Hashimoto's disease (chronic lymphocytic thyroiditis) is an uncommon entity in young patients. This is a common cause of diffuse enlargement of the thyroid gland, occurring frequently in female adolescents. This condition is part of the spectrum of autoimmune thyroid disorders. It is thought that CD_4 T cells are activated against thyroid antigens and recruit cytotoxic CD_8 T cells, which kill thyroid cells, to cause hypothyroidism. In this autoimmune self-destructive state of lymphadenoid goiter, the gland is firm and uniformly enlarged, usually pebbly and granular in nature. Children are initially euthyroid and slowly progress to become hypothyroid. About 10% of children are hyperthyroid (hashitoxicosis).[18] Ninety-five percent of patients with chronic lymphocytic thyroiditis have elevated antithyroid microsomal antibodies or antithyroid peroxidase antibodies. The plasma level of thyroid hormones is normal or low, and TSH levels are elevated in 70% of patients.[18] This condition may also be associated with Down syndrome, Turner syndrome, Noonan syndrome, juvenile diabetes, treated Hodgkin's disease, and phenytoin therapy.[19]

Thyroid imaging may not be necessary if clinical and laboratory findings are strongly suggestive of the diagnosis.

An ultrasound finding is not specific, showing diffuse thyroid hypoechogenicity.

A radionuclide scan usually shows patchy uptake of the tracer and may mimic the findings in Graves' disease or multinodular goiter.

Fine needle aspiration may be needed to confirm the diagnosis.[18] Histology usually reveals the characteristic Askanazy cells.[2]

Treatment

Thyroiditis resolves spontaneously in about one-third of adolescent patients, with the gland becoming normal and the antibodies disappearing. Exogenous thyroid hormone should be given in the hypothyroid patient, but it is not effective in reducing the size of the gland in euthyroid children.[18]

Subacute Thyroiditis

Subacute (de Quervain's) thyroiditis is a viral inflammation of the thyroid gland. It is unusual in children. The thyroid is swollen, painful, and tender. Mild thyroitoxicosis results from injury to the thyroid follicles, with release of thyroid hormone into circulation. Serum T_3 and T_4 levels are elevated and TSH is decreased. Findings of reduced radioactive iodine uptake due to thyroid follicle dysfunction differentiate it from Graves' disease. Histologically, granulomas and epitheliod cells may be seen.[18]

The treatment of subacute thyroiditis is symptomatic, consisting of nonsteroidal anti-inflammatory agents or steroids. The condition typically lasts 2 to 9 months, and complete recovery is expected.

Acute Suppurative Thyroiditis

Acute suppurative thyroiditis is a bacterial infection of the thyroid glands. The gland is acutely inflamed, and the patient is septic. Patients are usually euthyroid. The patient may have a preexisting multinodular goiter.[14] Staphylococci or mixed aerobic and anerobic flora are common causative agents, and a pharyngeal sinus tract may predispose the patient to infection.

Management consists of intravenous antibiotics. Drainage of the abscess may be needed. The thyroid gland may recover completely.

Hyperthyroidism: Graves' Disease

Primary hyperthyroidism (thyrotoxicosis) is a disease associated with an elevation in the circulating long-acting thyroid stimulating (LATS) hormones. Graves' disease, or diffuse toxic goiter, is the most common cause of hyperthyroidism in childhood. The condition is an autoimmune disease caused by the presence of immunoglobulin (Igs) of the IgG class directed against components of the thyroid plasma membrane, possibly including the TSH receptor. These autoantibodies stimulate the thyroid follicles to increase iodide uptake and cyclic adenosine monophosphate production, leading to thyroid growth and inducing the production and secretion of increased thyroid hormones.

TSH receptor antibodies are present in more than 95% of patients with active Graves' disease. The inciting event eliciting the antibody response against TSH is unknown. Reports have suggested the possibility of bacterial infection eliciting antibodies that react with the TSH receptor.[20]

Graves' disease is seen in girls more than boys, with a ratio of 5:1. The incidence steadily increases throughout childhood, peaking in the adolescent years.[18] Thyrotoxicosis is uncommon in African children; a relative incidence of a case or two per year is recorded.[2] A study in conjunction with the British Paediatric Surveillance Unit (BPSU) that analysed data collected between September 2004 and September 2005 from the UK and Ireland reported 110 cases of acquired congenital childhood thyrotoxicosis. This incidence (0.9 cases per 100,000 individuals younger than 15 years of age) is lower than has previously been reported in European studies. Data from Hong Kong report an even higher incidence of thyrotoxicosis: 6.5 cases per 100,000 per year between 1994 and 1998. Ninety-six percent of the cases were due to autoimmune thyrotoxicosis, and the incidence increased with age for both males and females. The incidence in females was significantly higher than in males in the 10–14 year age group.[21]

Congenital Graves' disease, resulting from transplacental passage of maternal antibodies, occurs in about 1% of babies born to women with active Graves' disease. The onset may be delayed until 2 to 3 weeks after birth.[18] In most children, the onset of Graves' disease develops over several months. The clinical manifestations of Graves' disease include goiter (virtually 100%), thyrotoxicosis, and exophthalmus (Figure 40.2). The systemic manifestations of thyrotoxicosis can be classified as initial and later presentations:

• *Early:* Nervousness, emotional lability, decline in school performance.

• *Late:* Weight loss, sweating, palpitations, heat intolerance, staring gaze, increase in appetite, diarrhoea, and general malaise.

Amenorrhea and a swelling above the ankles called pretibial myxoedema may sometimes be present. Above all, thyrotoxicosis must

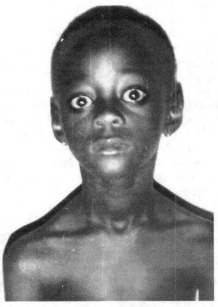

Figure 40.2: Thyrotoxicosis in an 8-year-old girl.

be considered in any child with an unexplained growth spurt, sympathy (e.g., muscle weakness, paraesthesia) or behavioural problems. The gland is uniformly enlarged, smooth, firm, and nontender. It may be so vascular that a bruit is audible over it.

Laboratory evaluation generally reveals elevated free T_4 and decreased TSH levels. In 10–20% of patients, only the T_3 level is elevated, a condition referred to as T_3 toxicosis. The diagnosis of Graves' disease is established by the presence of TSH-receptor antibodies.

Management

The treatment of Graves' disease is palliative, with the goal to allow natural resolution of the underlying autoimmune process. The natural course of untreated Graves' disease is unpredictable.[18] The treatment is designed to reduce the production and secretion of the thyroid hormone. This could be specific or nonspecific. Specific measures include the use of antithyroid drugs (carbimazole, neomercazole, potassium perchlorate). Nonspecific measures include rest and sedation.

Initial therapy is with methimazole or propylthiouracil, which reduces thyroid hormone production by inhibiting follicle cell organification of iodide and the coupling of iodotyrosines. Propylthiouracil also inhibits peripheral conversion of T_4 to T_3, and may be the drug of choice if rapid alleviation of thyrotoxicosis is desired. Both agents may possess some immunosuppressive activity. Methimazole is preferred in most cases due to its increased potency, longer half-life, and associated improved compliance. The initial dose in adolescents is 30 mg once daily, adjusted for younger patients. The dosage is reduced to 10 mg when the patient becomes euthyroid with normal T_3 and T_4.

The thyroid gland decreases in size in about half of the patients. Thyroid enlargement with therapy signals either an intensification of the disease or hypothyroidism with overtreatment.[18]

In general, the disease remission rate is approximately 25% after 2 years of treatment, with a further 25% remission every 2 years.[22] The resolution rate is decreased if TSH-receptor antibodies persist during and after treatment.

Surgery

Surgery is usually contraindicated in children due to the high postoperative incidence of hypothyroidism (35%), recurrence, tetany (17%), and of permanent hypoparathyroidism (10%).[12]

Indications for surgery in children with Grave's disease include:

• idiosyncratic reaction to antithyroid drugs;

• progressive enlargement of the gland, even in a euthyroid state;

• contraindication to radioactive iodine;

• recurrent hyperthyroidism;

• patients who refuse radioiodine;

• failed medical therapy; and

• large thyroid gland compressing the airway.

Surgery in the form of either subtotal thyroidectomy or total thyroidectomy in the suitably prepared patient may be performed. Preoperative antithyroid medication should be administered to decrease T_3 and T_4 levels to the normal range. Beta-blocking agents such as propranolol may be used to ameliorate the adrenergic symptoms of hyperthyroidism.

In addition, Lugol's iodine solution, 5 to 10 drops per day, should be administered for 4 to 7 days before thyroidectomy to reduce the vascularity of the gland.

The incidence of hypothyroidism after subtotal thyroidectomy is 12–54%, and the hypothyroidism may be subclinical in up to 45% of children.[23] The rate of recurrent hyperthyroidism is approximately 13%. The relapse rate may increase with time after surgery. Near total thyroidectomy is advocated by some authors.[2]

Hypothyroidism

Hypothyroidism is a clinical state in which there is reduced thyroid hormonal activity. This is rarely due to thyroid hypofunction secondary to reduced TSH stimulation resulting from hypopituitarism. Hypothyroidism may result from a defect anywhere in the hypothalamic-pituitary-thyroid axis (Table 40.1).

Table 40.1: Causes of hypothyroidism.

Type of hypothyroidism	Cause
Iatrogenic	Following subtotal thyroidectomy
	Hypophysectomy
	Radio-iodine treatment for thyroitoxicosis
	Excessive ingestion of para-aminosalicylic (PAS) acids, phenylbutazone, or antithyroid drugs
Iodine deficiency	Area of endemic goiters
Autoimmune thyroiditis	Secondary to thyroid antibodies
Dyshormonogenesis	Deficiency or absence of enzymes needed for thyroid hormone synthesis
Congenital	Absence of thyroid gland (very rare) or ectopic thyroid gland
	Antenatal goitrogens
	Pituitary-hypothalamic disease

Congenital hypothyroidism

Ninety percent of paediatric hypothyroidism is congenital, detected by neonatal screening programmes, and results from dysgenesis of the thyroid gland. Screening programmes have dramatically altered detection and management of congenital hypothyroidism. In the United Kingdom, all newborns are screened for congenital hypothyroidism as part of a national screening programme, which also includes tests to exclude phenylketonuria and cystic fibrosis. The worldwide incidence of congenital hypothyroidism is reported as 1 in 4,000 infants. However, the true incidence is lower in African Americans and higher in Hispanic and Native American populations.[19] Two-thirds of these babies have a rudimentary gland, and complete absence of thyroid tissue is noted in the rest of the patients. The rudimentary gland may be ectopic.[18]

The severe form of hypothyroidism in children is cretinism, which is also congenital, and the child may be born with or without a goiter. The child is usually underdeveloped both physically and mentally. There may be associated deafness, mutism, and neuromotor disorders (e.g., spastic paraplegia, dysarthria).[12]

Evaluation

Infants with congenital hypothyroidism are often normal size at birth, which is a reflection of the fact that thyroid hormones do not appear to be necessary for foetal growth. Physical features are not apparent in the first week of life. Prolonged neonatal jaundice is usually the first symptom, followed by feeding problems, lethargy, constipation, and poor tone. Examination often reveals coarse facies; a large protruding tongue; large open fontanelles; a hoarse cry; coarse, dry, and mottled skin; umbilical hernia; and delayed growth. In severe cases, these features appear within 4 to 8 weeks of birth.[24]

Serum T_4, T_3, and resin uptake are decreased, whereas TSH is elevated. Assessment of skeletal age (by x-ray of the knee) may show bone maturation of less than 36 weeks gestation, suggesting intrauterine hypothyroidism.

Treatment

Treatment is by lifetime thyroid hormone replacement. Synthetic (laevo-) thyroxin is used at a dosage of 10 mg/kg per day, starting with 25 mg per day and increasing to 100 mg per day.

The aim of treatment is to maintain the serum T_4 level in the high to normal range (10–14 µg/dl). Treatment is monitored with the reversal of clinical signs, linear growth, and TSH levels.[24]

The prognosis is good for linear growth and skeletal maturity. Intellectual progress depends on the age at which treatment is started, and usually poor after 3 months of age.[24]

Acquired hypothyroidism

Acquired, or juvenile, hypothyroidism is commonly caused by autoimmune destruction of the thyroid gland secondary to chronic lymphocytic thyroiditis (Hashimoto's disease). Other rarer causes are goitrogens (e.g., iodide cough syrups, antithyroid drugs), ectopic thyroid dysgenesis, infiltration of the thyroid gland in storage disorders, and secondary involvement from pituitary disorders with TSH deficiency or hypothalamic lesions and TRH deficiency. Onset is usually insidious. There is slowing of linear growth; there may be changes in personality, cold intolerance, diminished appetite, lethargy, and constipation. Girls may have breast development, hypertrophy of labia minora, galactorrhae, and cystic ovarian enlargement; boys may have testicular enlargement without a corresponding development of pubic hair.

Evaluation

Low serum T_4, decreased T_3 resin uptake, and elevated TSH are diagnostic. Skeletal maturation is markedly delayed. There is occasional association with a slipped femoral epiphysis. Assays of circulating thyroid antibodies imply an autoimmune basis for the disease. Low or normal TSH may suggest hypopituitary or a hypothalamic lesion. A TRH stimulation test may be useful in this situation.

Treatment

Thyroid hormone replacement with L thyroxin, 3-5 µg/kg as a single daily oral dose, is given for life. Adequacy of treatment is monitored with measurement of serum T_4, reversal of clinical symptoms, and increased linear growth.

Prognosis is good for catch-up growth and skeletal maturation. Catch-up is not expected if hypothyroidism develops around the time of puberty, when skeletal maturation is nearly complete. Intellect is usually not impaired.[24]

Hypothyroidism is rarely treated surgically.

Neoplastic Diseases of the Thyroid Gland

Thyroid Nodules

A solitary nodule of the thyroid is an uncommon lesion in children.[2,18] This lower incidence may be because fewer children have been exposed to irradiation. It may represent an area of functional hyperplasia (adenoma), which can be associated with secondary hyperthyroidism. Other possible causes of thyroid nodules include:

• adenoma;

• thyroglossal duct remnant;

• cystic hygroma;

• germ cell tumour; and

• infected thyroid cyst.

Thyroid nodules are twice as common in girls than in boys. Most patients present with an asymptomatic anterior neck mass. A thyroid nodule may be a slowly growing, potentially curable, papillary carcinoma.[2] This is frequently clinically indistinguishable from benign lesions, although the former demonstrates a reduced uptake of iodine [131]I.

Thyroid imaging studies are unreliable in distinguishing benign from malignant nodules, but ultrasound may reveal multiple nodules. One report has documented an 18% malignant rate by FNA of thyroid nodules in children.[25]

Surgical resection of a thyroid nodule should be performed if it is malignant, of indeterminate cytology, is a benign nodule that is increasing in size, or is an aspirated thyroid cyst that recurred.[18] Thyroid

nodules in prepubertal children have a higher risk of malignancy. The natural history of benign lesions in younger children is unknown, and the safety of nonoperative treatment has not been documented. In children younger than 13 years of age, it is currently recommended that all thyroid nodules be removed.[18]

Thyroid Carcinoma

Thyroid carcinoma represents about 3% of all paediatric malignancy in United States.[18] The peak incidence is between the ages of 10 and 18 years, with a female preponderance of 2:1. Thyroid carcinoma is the second most common cancer in females aged 15–19 years in the United States.[19] The incidence of childhood thyroid malignancy was reported to be decreasing in most parts of the world due to the reduced use of radiation to treat benign diseases. Individuals who have been exposed to radiotherapy to the neck have a significantly increased chance of development of thyroid dysfunction. The incidence has been reported as being up to 64%, increasing with time of irradiation, radiation dose, and age at time of irradiation.[19]

The incidence of thyroid carcinoma in children is low in the African community,[2] with four cases over 10 years reported in Enugu, Nigeria. Three were adenoma, and the remaining one was papillary carcinoma. All the patients were girls younger than 10 years of age.[2] In one report, there was only one case of follicular carcinoma, in a 10-year-old girl seen over a 10-year period in Ilorin.[26]

In Nigeria, about 90% of thyroid carcinomas in children are of the well-differentiated type: 70% papillary and 20% follicular. The undifferentiated type, such as medullary carcinoma, is rare.[2] Data from the United States, collected retrospectively for the period from 1973 to 2004, reported 1,753 cases of thyroid carcinoma occurring under the age of 20 years. The condition was more common in females than males, and mean survival was 30.5 years. Sixty percent of the tumours were papillary, 23% were the follicular variant of papillary, 10% were follicular, and 5% were medullary. Tumours of the medullary subtype are often associated with the familial syndrome of multiple endocrine neoplasia type 2 (MEN2). Worse predictors of outcome were male sex, nonpapillary tumour subtypes, the presence of distant metastases, and nonsurgical treatment.[3]

Follicular carcinoma has been described in a neonatal dyshormogenetic hyperplastic goiter. Total thyroidectomy is necessary in this instance.

Lateral aberrant thyroid tissues, previously thought to be ectopic thyroid glands, are now known to represent thyroid carcinoma secondary to the cervical lymph nodes.[2]

Thyroid carcinoma is usually first seen clinically as a thyroid mass, sometimes with an enlarged cervical lymph node. The most common presentation in childhood is indolent, palpable lymph glands in the lateral side of the neck. Solitary or multiple nodules in the thyroid glands are usually secondary. The cancer is usually more advanced at presentation in children when compared to adults, and regional lymph node metastases are present in 75% of children when the disease is first detected.[27]

Evaluation

Pathologic diagnosis can be made by either FNA or frozen-section biopsy at operation. Most surgeons, however, recommend surgical resection of all thyroid lesions due to concern over false negative interpretation of FNA.[18]

The functional status of the mass is determined by preoperative scintiscan. A preoperative chest radiograph is necessary because of the high incidence of pulmonary metastases in children.

Burkitt lymphoma of the thyroid gland has also been reported in the tropics.[2]

Treatment

Surgical excision is the treatment of choice with or without lymph node dissection.

Lobectomy with isthmus resection may be sufficient for tumours clearly isolated to one lobe. Because thyroid cancer has been documented to be bilateral in as many as 66% of cases, with about 80% of these exhibiting multifocality, most paediatric surgeons recommend either a total or near total thyroidectomy for a differentiated thyroid cancer.

Lymph node dissection is recommended if regional nodes are suggestive of metastasis.

The parathyroid gland can be preserved by identifying and autotransplanting one or two of the glands into the sternocleidomastoid muscle or into the nondominant forearm. The recurrent laryngeal nerve should also be identified and protected.

It is generally recommended that exogenous thyroid hormones be used to treat all endocrine thyroid cancer, to suppress TSH-mediated stimulation of the gland.

Radioiodine ablative therapy is successful in eradicating residual tumours. It is more effective, however, after removal of the entire gland because less functioning endocrine tissue takes up the radionuclide.

Overall survival rate in nonmedulary thyroid carcinoma is 98%.[28] A higher recurrence rate is seen in children who did not receive postoperative radio iodine [131]I.

Medullary Thyroid Carcinoma

Medullary thyroid carcinoma (MTC) accounts for approximately 5% of thyroid neoplasms in children. It arises from the parafollicular C cells. MTC may occur sporadically or in association with multiple endocrine neoplasia IIA or IIB or the familial MTC syndrome. The neoplasm is particularly virulent in patients with MEN IIB, and may occur in infancy.

The clinical diagnosis of MTC is usually made only after metastatic spread to the adjacent cervical lymph node or to distant sites.

It is recommended that early detection of MTC with RET (REarranged during Transfection) proto-oncogen mutation may improve survival.

Total thyroidectomy is the recommended surgical management of MTC in children. Lymph nodes in the central compartment of the neck, medial to the carotid sheaths and between the hyoid bone and the sternum, should be removed. Surgery is recommended at approximately 5 years of age, especially in children with MEN IIA, before the cancer spreads beyond the thyroid gland.[29] Due to the high virulence of MTC in children with MEN IIB, prophylactic thyroidectomy is recommended at approximately 1 year of age.

Parathyroid Glands: Hyperparathyroidism

Hyperparathyroidism is associated with an increased secretion of parathormone (PTH). This can be primary, secondary, or tertiary.

Primary Hyperparathyroidism

Primary hyperparathyroidism is an unstimulated and inappropriately high parathormone secretion.[6] In childhood, it usually results from a solitary hyperfunctioning adenoma in about 70–90% of patients,[12] and more rarely (10–20%) diffuse hyperplasia of all the four glands.[12] The hyperparathyroidism resulting from hyperfunctioning of all four glands is a feature of MEN-I. Primary hyperparathyroidism of infancy is a rare, often fatal, condition that usually develops within the first 3 months of life. Signs include hypotonicity, respiratory distress, failure to thrive, lethargy, and polyuria. The serum PTH is elevated. There is usually diffuse parathyroid gland hyperplasia. A familial component of the disease is found in about half of the patients. Early recognition and treatment are essential to allow normal growth and development of the baby.[18]

The management of primary hyperparathyroidism in children is surgical. All four parathyroid glands should be identified and biopsies performed. An enlarged and adenomatous gland should be removed. If the other glands are normal, they should be marked with nonabsorbable sutures and left in place.

Secondary Hyperparathyroidism

Increased PTH is secondary or compensatory to conditions that cause low plasma calcium level. Secondary hyperparathyroidism occurs in children with renal insufficiency, malabsorption, or Ricketts. Affected patients typically respond to medical treatment designed to decrease intestinal phosphorus absorption, but, in rare cases, severe renal osteodystrophy develops, manifested by skeletal fracture and metastatic calcifications. Very severe cases can be candidates for total parathyroidectomy with autotransplantation.

Tertiary Hyperparathyroidism

Tertiary hyperparathyroidism occurs when persistent hyperfunction of the parathyroid glands occurs, even after the inciting stimulus has been removed. This is often seen in patients with chronic renal failure and secondary hyperparathyroidism who undergo renal transplantation. It is commonly due to hyperplasia of all four glands, and children with this condition are candidates for total parathyroidectomy with autotransplantation.[18]

Evidence-Based Research

Table 40.2 presents a study that compares the female-to-male prevalence of thyroid disease. Table 40.3 presents a study to evaluate the effect of clinical and treatment factors on thyroid carcinoma control, complications, and recurrence.

Table 40.2: Evidence-based research.

Title	Thyroid diseases in a school population with thyromegaly
Authors	Jaksic J, Dumic M, Filipovic B, Ille J, Cvijetic M, Gjuric G
Institution	Department of Pediatrics, University School of Medicine, Zagreb, Croatia; Department of Pediatrics, Medical Centre, Sibenik, Croatia
Reference	Arch Dis Childhood 1994; 70:103–106
Problem	Goiter is common in childhood and adolescence despite the widespread practice of iodising table salt, which has eliminated the dietary lack of iodine, This study concerns the prevalence and nature of diffuse and nodular goiters found during a survey of 5,462 schoolchildren in Sibenik, Croatia, a seaside region where iodised (0-01% potassium iodide) table salt is regularly available.
Comparison/control (quality of evidence)	The study compared the prevalence of thyroid disease in boys and girls.
Outcome/effect	Thyroid enlargement was found in 152 children (2.8%). The most common disorder was simple goiter, which was established in 126 (2.3%) of these—12 (0.45%) boys and 114 (4.07%) girls. Juvenile autoimmune thyroiditis was found in 19 of the children (prevalence, 0.35%), with a female-to-male sex ratio of 8:1.
Historical significance/comments	This survey of large series of children shows that it is necessary to conduct a thorough examination of the thyroid, even in apparently healthy children in regions where regular iodine intake is established.

Table 40.3: Evidence-based research.

Title	Childhood and adolescent thyroid carcinoma
Authors	Grigsby PW, Gal-or A, Michalski JM, Doherty GM
Institution	Department of Radiation Oncology, Washington University Medical Center, St. Louis, Missouri, USA; Department of Surgery, Washington University Medical Center, St. Louis, Missouri, USA
Reference	Cancer 2002; 95:724–729
Problem	Reports on the specific factors that predict the risk of developing recurrent disease in children are scanty. This study was performed to evaluate the influence of clinical and treatment factors on local tumour control, control of distant metastasis survival, and complications in children and adolescents with thyroid carcinoma.
Outcome/ effect	The study involved 56 children, ages 4–20 years; there were 43 females and 13 males. The overall survival rate was 98% with a follow-up of 0.6–30.7 years (median follow-up, 11.0 years). The 10-year progression-free survival rate was 61%. Nineteen patients (34%) experienced a recurrence of their thyroid carcinoma. The time to first recurrence of disease ranged from 8 months to 14.8 years (mean, 5.3 years). None of those with disease confined to the thyroid developed recurrent disease. The recurrence rate was 50% (17 of 34) in patients with lymph node metastasis and 29% (2 of 7) in patients with lung metastasis ($P = 0.02$).Thyroid capsule invasion ($P = 0.02$), soft tissue invasion ($P = 0.03$), positive margins ($P = 0.006$), and tumour location at diagnosis (thyroid only versus thyroid and lymph nodes versus thyroid, lymph nodes, and lung metastasis, $P = 0.02$) were significant for developing recurrent disease. Patients younger than 15 years of age at diagnosis were more likely to have more extensive tumours at diagnosis than patients who were 15 years of age and older (thyroid only versus thyroid and lymph nodes versus thyroid, lymph nodes, and lung metastasis, $P = 0.02$).
Historical significance/ comments	Carcinoma of the thyroid in children and adolescents has little risk of mortality but a high risk of recurrence. Younger patients present with a more advanced stage of disease and are more likely to have disease recurrence. Total thyroidectomy and lymph node dissection, followed by postoperative ^{131}I therapy, thyroid hormone replacement (suppressive) administration, and diligent surveillance are warranted

Key Summary Points

1. Simple goiter occurs with a wide range of prevalence (1–6%) in different populations of children and adolescents.

2. A diffuse thyroid enlargement is the most common form of goiter in small children.

3. Graves' disease is relatively uncommon in children.

4. Thorough examination of the thyroid, even in apparently healthy children in regions of regular iodine intake, is necessary to detect thyroid disorder.

5. Although thyroid nodules are unusual in childhood and adolescence, they demand careful consideration because of the likelihood that they may represent malignancy.

6. Juvenile autoimmune thyroiditis is one of the most frequent thyroid diseases in childhood.

7. Thyroid hormone treatment is used in established cases of goiter before cystic degeneration sets in to decrease the size of the goiter or arrest its further growth.

8. Endemic goiter can be reversed with iodide and/or thyroxin in the early stages. Response is generally poor or negligible after the formation of nodules and onset of cystic degeneration.

9. Carcinoma of the thyroid in children and adolescents has little risk of mortality but a high risk of recurrence.

References

1. Rallison ML, Dobyns BM, Meikle AW, et al. Natural history of thyroid abnormalities: prevalence, incidence, and regression of thyroid disease in adolescents and young adults. Am J Med 1991; 91:363–370.

2. Nwako FA. Surgical lesions of the neck. In: Nwako FA (ed). A Textbook of Pediatric Surgery in the Tropics. Macmillan, 1980, Pp 128–137.

3. Hogan A, Zhuge Y, Perez E, et al. Pediatric thyroid carcinoma: incidence and outcomes in 1753 patients. J Surg Res 2009; 156:167–172.

4. Thompson NM, Geiger JM. Thyroid/parathyroid. In: O'Neil JA, Rowe MI, Grofeld JI, Fonkalsrud ER, Coran AG, eds. Pediatric Surgery. Mosby, 1998, Pp 743–755.

5. Bogner U, Hegedüs L, Hansen JM, Finke R, Schleusener H. Thyroid cytotoxic antibodies in atrophic and goitrous autoimmune thyroiditis, Eur J Endocrinol 1995; 132:69–74.

6. Krukowski ZH. The thyroid gland and thyroglossal tract. In: Russell RCG, Williams NS, Bulstrode CJK, eds. Bailey and Love's Short Practice of Surgery. Arnold, 2000, Pp 707–733.

7. Gills D, Brnjac L, Perlman K, Sochett EB, Daneman D. Frequency and characteristics of lingual thyroid not detected by screening. J Pediatr Endocrinol Metab 1998; 11:229–233.

8. Wertz ML. Management of undescended lingual and subhyoid thyroid glands. Larygoscope 1974; 84:507–521.

9. Dilley DC, Sieger MA, Budnick S. Diagnosis and treating common oral pathologies. Pediatr Clin N Am 1991; 5:1227–1264.

10. Steinwald OP, Muehrcke RC, Econmous SG. Surgical correction of complete lingual ectopia of the thyroid gland. Surg Clin N Am 1970; 50:1177–1186.

11. Jaksic J, Dumic M, Filipovic B, Ille J, Cvijetic M, Gjuric G. Thyroid diseases in a school population with thyromegaly. Arch Dis Child 1994; 70:103–106.

12. da Rocha-Afondu JT. The thyroid and parathyroid glands. In: Badoe EA, Archampong EQ, da Rocha-Afondu JT, eds. Principles and Practice of Surgery Including Pathology in the Tropics. Ghana Publishing Corporation, 2000, Pp 315–338.

13. Ameh EA, Nmadu PT. Thyrotoxicosis in Zaria, Nigeria: an update. East Afr Med J 1997; 74:433–434.

14. Ameh EA, Sabo SY, Nmadu PT. The risk of infective thyroiditis in nodular goiters. East Afr Med J 1998; 75:425–427.

15. Insoft RM, Hurvitz J, Estrella E, Krishnamoorthy KS. Prader-Willi syndrome associated with fetal goiter: a case report. Am J Perinatol 1999; 16:29–31.

16. Mahomed A. Miscellaneous conditions of the neck and oral cavity. In: Prem Puri (ed). Newborn Surgery. Arnold, 2003, Pp 227–235.

17. Egbuta J, Onyezili F, Vanormelingen K. Impact evaluation of efforts to eliminate iodine deficiency disorders in Nigeria. Public Health Nutr 2003; 6:169–173.

18. Skinner MA, Safford SD. Endocrine disorders and tumors. In: Ashcraft KW, Holcomb GW, Murphuy JP, eds. Pediatric Surgery. Elsevier, 2005, Pp 1088–1104.

19. Babcock D. Thyroid disease in the pediatric patient: emphasizing imaging with sonography. Pediatr Radiol 2006; 36:299–308.

20. Tomer Y, Davies TF. Infection, thyroid disease and autoimmunity. Endocr Rev 1993; 14:107–120.

21. Williamson S, Greene S. Incidence of thyrotoxicosis in childhood: a national population based study in the UK and Ireland. Clin Endocrinol (Oxf) 2010; 72:358–363.

22. Lippe BM, Landaw EM, Kaplan SA. Hyperthyroidism in children treated with long-term medical therapy. Twenty-five percent remission every two years. J Clin Endocrinol Metab 1987; 64:1241–1245.

23. Waldhausen JHT. Controversies related to the medical and surgical management of hyperthyroidism in children. Sem Pediatr Surg 1997; 6:121–127.

24. Azubuke JC. Endocrine and metabolic disorders. In: Azubuke JC, Nkanginieme KEO, eds. Pediatrics and Child Health in a Tropical Region. African Educational Services, 1999, Pp 456–473.

25. Raab SS, Siherman JB, Elsheikh TM, et al. Pediatric nodules: disease demographic and clinical management by fine needle aspiration biopsy. Pediatrics 1995; 95:46–49.

26. Adeniran JO, Adekanye AO. Follicular carcinoma in a 10-year-old girl: case report. Trop J Health Sci 2002; 9:23–24.

27. Hames JA, Thompson NW, McLead MK, et al. Differentiated thyroid carcinoma in children and adolescents. World J Surg 1992; 16:547–554.

28. Grigsby PW, Gal-or A, Michalski JM, Doherty GM. Childhood and adolescence thyroid carcinoma. Cancer 2002; 95:724–729.

29. Szinnai G, Meier C, Kaomminoth P, Zumsteg UW. Review of multiple endocrine neoplasm type 2A in children: therapeutic results of early thyroidectomy and prognostic value of codon analysis. Pediatrics 2003; 111:E132–E139.

THORAX

CHAPTER 41
LARYNGOSCOPY, BRONCHOSCOPY, AND OESOPHAGOSCOPY

V. T. Joseph
Michael Laschat
Catharine Mngongo

Introduction

Endoscopic visualisation of the airway and digestive tract has made huge progress in the past decade due to the technological advances in light and image transmission. The early designs followed Nitze's method of providing illumination with an incandescent bulb. These have now been completely replaced with fibre-optic light systems and Hopkins rod lens telescopes. A further development has been the introduction of flexible fibre-optic endoscopes with high-definition videocameras providing real-time, high-quality images. At the same time, manufacturers have miniaturised endoscopic instruments so that a wide range of these are now available for use in infants and children.

Laryngoscopy

Examination of the larynx is carried out for both diagnostic and therapeutic indications.

Diagnostic

Diagnostic indications for laryngoscopy include:

- stridor, either congenital or acquired;
- subglottic stenosis;
- cysts or masses causing airway obstruction;
- vocal cord palsy; and
- foreign bodies.

Therapeutic

Therapeutic indications for laryngoscopy include:

- subglottic stenosis;
- aspiration/injection of mucous cysts, cystic hygromas;
- papillomas;
- lingual thyroid; and
- webs.

Instruments/Equipment

Laryngoscopy can be performed by using rigid or flexible instruments, each of which has certain specific advantages.

Rigid laryngoscopy

A rigid laryngoscopy may be done by using the indirect or direct method.

Indirect laryngoscopy

Indirect laryngoscopy is performed by using specially designed laryngeal mirrors in combination with a headlight. This enables the larynx and the nasopharynx to be visualised. This method is frequently used in adults, but in children it is often difficult to carry out this procedure.

Direct laryngscopy

Direct laryngoscopy is performed with handheld curved- or straight-blade instruments or by using the suspension laryngoscope, which leaves both hands free to manipulate instruments. The curved Macintosh blade and the straight Miller blade laryngoscopes are routinely used by

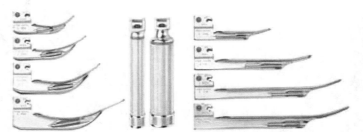

Figure 41.1: Curved blade (Macintosh) and straight blade (Miller) laryngoscopes with locking handles.

anaesthetists to intubate patients (Figure 41.1).

Technique

Direct laryngoscopy

Curved-blade laryngoscope

The patient is placed supine with the neck slightly flexed and extension at the atlanto-occipital joint. The neck should not be extended fully, as this displaces the larynx anteriorly and moves it away from the line of vision. The curved blade is passed along the right side of the tongue, displacing it to the left. The tip of the blade is inserted into the vallecula, and the laryngoscope is lifted upward and forward so that the epiglottis is carried up and away from the laryngeal inlet to expose the vocal cords.

Straight-blade laryngoscope

The tip of the blade is passed under the epiglottis and is used to lift it up to expose the cords. This method is particularly useful in babies and young infants.

Note that direct laryngoscopy with the handheld laryngoscope is useful in providing rapid visualisation of the larynx, but because the surgeon has to hold the laryngoscope by hand, it is difficult to carry out therapeutic manoeuvers.

Suspension laryngoscope

Direct laryngoscopy performed by using the suspension laryngoscope (Figure 41.2) is frequently carried out by ear, nose, and throat (ENT) surgeons. The equipment consists of a short tubular laryngoscope that is locked to a supporting arm that rests on a base plate lying against the anterior chest wall. This arrangement leaves the surgeon's hands free to use instruments and even to position an operating microscope for precise surgery.

The surgical procedures that can be done with the suspension laryngoscope include aspiration/marsupialisation of cysts, excision of nodules, laser vaporisation of papillomas, and injection of bleomycin in cystic hygromas with laryngeal involvement.

Flexible laryngoscopy

The instruments used for flexible laryngoscopy include the ultrathin bronchoscope, the standard flexible bronchoscope, and the specially designed flexible nasopharyngoscope (Figure 14.3). The ultrathin bronchoscope has no suction or instrument channel and is mostly used by anaesthetists for intubation in difficult head and neck cases. The standard bronchoscope has an instrument/suction channel and can be used for therapeutic indications, although the rigid instrument is greatly superior in this respect. Both the standard flexible bronchoscope and the nasopharyngoscope are used to evaluate laryngomalacia and vocal cord paralysis.

The image can be viewed directly through the eyepiece of the scope; in more advanced systems, it is displayed on a high-resolution monitor. The newer nasolaryngoscopes have the camera chip at the tip and can provide extremely high quality images. The ultrafine scopes have an outer diameter of 2.2 mm but do not incorporate a suction/irrigation channel. The instruments with a working channel are larger, with an outer diameter of 4.9 mm, and can be used to remove foreign bodies and to perform biopsies.

Complications

Diagnostic laryngoscopy is generally a very safe procedure. The patient needs to be carefully monitored throughout the endoscopy to ensure that the airway and ventilation are not compromised. Facilities for intubation should always be at hand, and in cases where a difficult airway is anticipated (see Figure 41.4), tracheostomy instruments must be kept in the operating theatre next to the patient. The surgical team must be prepared to carry out a tracheostomy if the anaesthetist fails to intubate the patient.

Therapeutic interventions are potentially at risk of compromising the airway, due to either oedema or collapse of the larynx/trachea following removal of large neck masses. The complications that may occur include laryngeal oedema, haemorrhage, and perforation. The surgeon must decide whether the patient should be left intubated with postoperative intensive care support until the airway is stable.

Bronchoscopy

Paediatric bronchoscopy is indicated for a wide variety of diseases. It allows an assessment of the anatomy and function of the complete upper airway from the nasal passage, pharynx, and larynx to the segment bronchi. Diagnostic procedures such as bronchoalveolar lavage, as well as interventional procedures such as extraction of foreign bodies, can be performed with special instruments.

Diagnostic Bronchoscopy

Stridor is a clinical sign for obstruction of the upper airway. Inspiratory stridor usually indicates an obstruction of the extrathoracic part of the airway. Expiratory stridor indicates an obstruction of the intrathoracic part of the airway.

In most cases, congenital inspiratory stridor is caused by laryngomalacia. It should be investigated endoscopically when it is progressive or causes apnoea, feeding difficulties and growth retardation, or when symptoms point to a diagnosis other than laryngomalacia. In these cases, one may find bilateral vocal cord paralysis, subglottic hemangioma, or laryngeal cysts. Proper diagnosis of congenital inspiratory stridor can be done only with the child breathing spontaneously.

Acquired inspiratory stridor may originate from subglottic scar tissue, ductal cysts, or laryngeal papillomas. Expiratory stridor may be caused by asthma but also may be due to inhaled foreign bodies and tracheomalacia as a result of tracheobronchial or vascular malformations.

Recurrent aspiration with bronchopneumonias can be caused by broncho-oesophageal fistulas or laryngeal clefts. H-type broncho-oesophageal fistula takes an oblique course from the cephalad opening on the posterior wall of the upper trachea to a more caudal position on the anterior wall of the oesophagus. Diagnosis can be very difficult due to the small diameter of some fistulas, but usually can be achieved with combined bronchoscopy and oesophagoscopy. The tracheal aspect of the fistula usually appears as a small prominence in the midline of the posterior membranous wall of the cervical trachea. A fine catheter can be passed through a ventilation bronchoscope into the tracheal opening

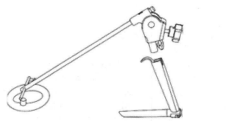
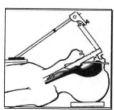

Figure 41.2: Rigid suspension laryngoscope for surgical procedures in the upper airway

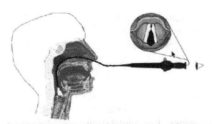
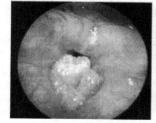
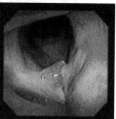

Figure 41.3: Flexible fibre-optic nasopharyngoscope (left) showing normal view (centre) and laryngeal papilloma (right).

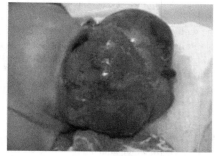

Figure 41.4: Massive tumour (teratoma) occupying whole oral cavity. Intubation could be done only by using a flexible fibre-optic scope to guide placement of the endotracheal tube.

of the fistula into the oesophagus. Diagnosis is then affirmed by oesophagoscopy, demonstrating the catheter entering the oesophagus. Surgical identification is facilitated with a catheter or a wire in the fistula during the operative repair.

Laryngeal clefts are easy to overlook because redundant mucosa fills the cleft. Careful inspection of the interarytenoid and posterior glottis region with a Hopkins rod telescope is mandatory.

Interventional Bronchoscopy

Foreign body inhalation

Symptoms of foreign body inhalation vary. There can be complete obstruction with hypoxia, bradycardia, and cardiac arrest, but if the object is small and passes beyond the main bronchi, the child may quickly become asymptomatic and be presented only when symptoms of distal obstruction occur.

The majority of inhaled foreign bodies are radiolucent. A chest x-ray may show unilateral hyperinflation of the affected side as well as collapse and consolidation distal to the obstruction, but it may also be without pathologic findings.

Indication for bronchoscopy is a positive history and clinical signs of aspiration.

Usually a rigid technique is used for the removal of foreign bodies. With the patient deeply anaesthetised, a rigid ventilation bronchoscope is introduced under direct view into the trachea. The foreign body is extracted with special grasping forceps. In most cases, the foreign body is too large to be removed through the bronchoscope, so the object, forceps, and the bronchoscope have to be removed together as a single unit.

Great danger ensues when the foreign body is lost in the trachea or in the subglottic space obstructing the airway. If the object cannot be removed quickly, it should be pushed down into a main stem bronchus to allow oxygenation. Then a second attempt at removal can be made. After removal of the foreign body, the presence of a second foreign body should be excluded.

Airway stenosis

An important indication for interventional bronchoscopy is treatment of airway stenoses. Laser therapy of subglottic haemangiomas is favoured by some, whereas others use application of intralesional steroids followed by intubation. Subglottic granulation tissue and viral papillomas can be treated with the intralesional injection of drugs (corticosteroids and chemotherapeutic agents). Subglottic cysts, which can develop after intubation, can be resected with a laser or with special forceps. These interventions require the availability of an intensive care unit because many children need to remain intubated due to secondary swelling of the subglottic area.

Technique

In many parts of the world, the use of flexible endoscopes for diagnostic purposes is regarded as a standard, but in many other locations, the availability and cost of flexible bronchoscopes limit the use of these expensive and fragile instruments. Adequate assessment of the supraglottis, subglottis, and the trachea is possible in most cases, however, by using a telescopic rod alone with the patient breathing spontaneously with 100% oxygen and a volatile agent, usually halothane or sevoflurane. Rigid endoscopy is ideal for therapeutic interventions such as foreign body extraction or laser surgery. The main disadvantage of the rigid technique is that it can be used only under anaesthesia, whereas flexible bronchoscopes can be used under sedation and local anaesthesia.

Rigid bronchoscopes

Rigid ventilation bronchoscopes consist of a light metal tube. A port at the distal end allows the attachment of an anaesthetic T-piece for ventilation. Light is transmitted over a prism at the distal end of the tube. The ventilation scope can be used with spontaneous or controlled breathing. The scope can be used with the Hopkins rod telescope for diagnostic procedures (Figure 41.5). With the telescope in place, ventilation and examination are possible under excellent visual conditions. However, the telescope narrows the lumen of the bronchoscope, increasing airflow resistance and making breathing difficult. This is particular a problem with the smallest bronchoscopes. For therapeutic procedures the ventilation bronchoscope is used with special equipment, such as grasping forceps, for extraction of foreign bodies.

The Hopkins rod telescope is an endoscopic telescope in which the air-containing spaces between the conventional series of lenses are replaced with glass rods with polished ends separated by small air lenses. This system transmits more light, yields greater magnification, and provides greater depth and breadth of field than conventional lens systems. The instrument is inserted under direct laryngoscopy with a standard laryngoscope through the mouth under general anaesthesia, with the patient lying in a supine position. The smallest available telescope has a diameter of less than 2 mm. With this instrument, diagnostic bronchoscopy is possible even in very small newborns. In this case the Hopkins rod telescope alone can be inserted either

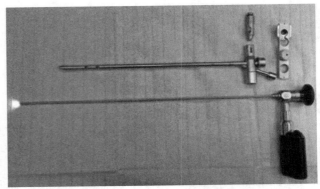

Figure 41.5: Storz ventilation bronchoscope with Hopkins rod telescope. A battery-powered light source is connected to the telescope.

by using an apnoeic technique or alternatively with the newborn breathing spontaneously.

Flexible bronchoscopes

The flexible fiberscope consists of a flexible tube that contains a fibreoptic system that transmits an image from the tip of the instrument to an eyepiece (Figures 41.6 and 41.7). Another technical advance is the video scope. In these instruments, a video chip positioned at the tip of the bronchoscope replaces the glass fibre bundle. This design avoids the inherent susceptibility of a fibre bundle to damage. Digital processing of the image is also possible. Using Bowden cables connected to a lever at the handpiece, the tip of the instrument can be oriented, allowing the practitioner to navigate the instrument into individual lobe or segment bronchi. Small fibre-optic endoscopes down to 2.2 mm in external diameter are available, but these very small instruments lack a channel for suctioning and instrumentation. The fiberscope can be inserted through the nose or the mouth under local anaesthesia with or without sedation. Very young children often need deep sedation or anaesthesia. Otherwise, only suboptimal information can be obtained due to movement, coughing, and obstructed view.

Complications

Complications include hypoxia, hypoventilation, and hypercapnia for many reasons, including obstruction of the airway or deep sedation.

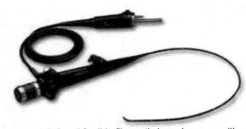

Figure 41.6: Small flexible fibreoptic bronchoscope with suction/irrigation and biopsy channel.

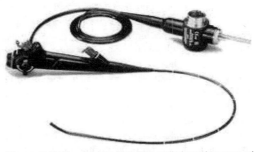

Figure 41.7: Standard flexible fibre-optic bronchoscope with full deflection, suction/irrigation channel, and biopsy channel for instruments.

Trauma to lips, teeth, epiglottis, and larynx with subsequent airway oedema, especially subglottic oedema, are complications associated mainly with rigid bronchoscopes. If stridor is present in recovery, nebulised epinephrine should be administered. Intravenous administered dexamethasone also produces relief of stridor but takes 1 to 2 hours to act.

Damage to the tracheobronchial tree with pneumothorax or pneumomediastinum is rare. Pneumothorax or pneumomediastinum can also be the consequence of air trapping, as passive expiration cannot overcome the resistance in the airway obstructed by the instrument. Air trapping can also lead to diminished venous return and reduced cardiac output.

Local anaesthetic overdose may cause serious bradycardia and even death.

Infections are a problem, especially in flexible bronchoscopy. A major problem is proper disinfection of the suction channel and valves. Leak detection should be performed regularly because bacteria may penetrate into fissures around the optic fibres and cables.

Haemorrhage from granulations or haemangiomas is usually a minor problem and settles spontaneously.

Oesophagoscopy

In the earliest endoscopic procedures to visualise the oesophagus, only rigid instruments were available. These instruments are similar to rigid bronchoscopes except they lack side holes at the distal end and the ventilation channel is not required (Figure 41.8). The fibre-optic light is connected to a light prism, giving proximal illumination, or to a light rod, which is inserted through the lumen of the scope and locks into place to provide distal illumination.

The great advance in endoscopy came with the introduction of fibre-optic technology, which resulted in the development of flexible endoscopes for examination and therapeutic procedures in both the upper and lower gastrointestinal tracts.

Examination of the oesophagus is carried out for both diagnostic and therapeutic indications.

Diagnostic

Diagnostic indications for oesophagoscopy include:

• gastro-oesophageal reflux;

• dysphagia;

• corrosive ingestion;

• upper gastro-intestinal bleeding;

• trauma; and

• strictures.

Therapeutic

Therapeutic indications for oesophagoscopy include:

• balloon dilatation of strictures;

• percutaneous endoscopic gastrostomy (PEG) insertion;

• foreign body removal; and

• injection sclerotherapy.

Technique

Rigid endoscopes

Rigid endoscopes are most useful for removal of foreign bodies because instruments can easily be inserted through the lumen for retrieval. The procedure is done under general anaesthesia with endotracheal intubation. It is important that the endotracheal tube be slightly smaller than what would normally be used and the balloon be deflated; otherwise, it may be difficult to pass the scope down the oesophagus.

Entry into the oesophagus is guided by the use of a laryngoscope with the neck in the flexed position. Once the scope has entered the

oesophagus, the neck is extended by placing a roll under the shoulders. This brings the axis of the scope into a straight line with the oesophagus and it is advanced under direct vision to the cardia. It is sometimes helpful to use a 0-degree telescope to view the distal lumen as the scope is advanced. In this case, the videocamera can be attached to the eyepiece to provide an image on the monitor (Figure 41.9).

Flexible endoscopes

Currently, most of the diagnostic and therapeutic procedures are performed with flexible endoscopes. Although it is possible to insert the flexible scope in an awake patient under sedation, most children will require general anaesthesia for this procedure. The patient is generally placed in the lateral position lying on the left side, although some surgeons prefer the supine position. The tip of the scope is angulated into a curve to follow the back of the tongue. On insertion, the phar-

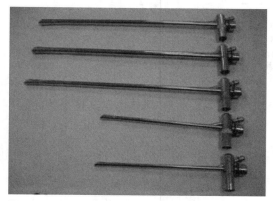

Figure 41.8: Rigid oesophagoscopes for infants to older children.

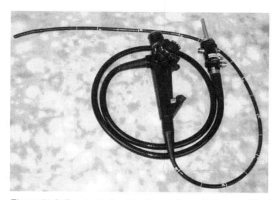

Figure 41.9: Paediatric flexible fibre-optic gastroscope with videocamera head. The image is viewed on a high-resolution monitor.

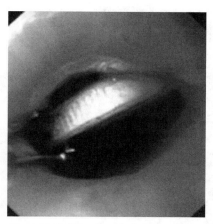

Figure 41.10: Extraction of a lodged coin from the oesophagus with a grasp forceps inserted through the instrument channel of a flexible gastroscope

ynx is seen. Secretions are sucked out and the scope is guided behind the endotracheal tube to the cricopharyngeal inlet, where it enters the oesophagus. Further passage of the scope is assisted by gently insufflating air to distend the lumen and by aspirating any secretions along the way. The scope is passed all the way down into the stomach; Then, on withdrawal, a careful note is made of any pathology that has been noted previously. Any procedures that need to be carried out are then done with the scope positioned at the appropriate site. Many devices, such as forceps, needles, and electrosurgical knives, among others, available for therapeutic and diagnostic purposes can be inserted through an instrument channel (Figure 41.10).

Dilatation of strictures (Figures 41.11 and 41.12) can be done either with the direct endoscopic view or with radiological screening. For this purpose, contrast is used to fill the balloon, and the procedure is observed on the x-ray screen.

Complications

Complications are rare and include minor haemorrhage, injury to the larynx and hypopharynx and infections. Perforation can occur especially following deep biopsy, forceful dilation of strictures, or during removal of foreign bodies.

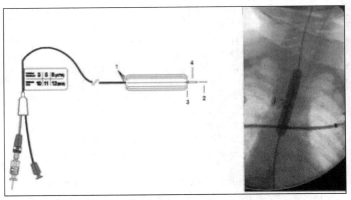

Figure 41.11: Oesophageal balloon (left) for dilatation of stricture (right) – accurate placement of the balloon and monitoring of the pressure used are essential.

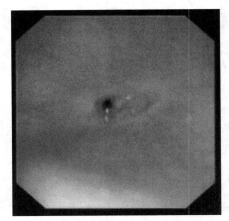

Figure 41.12: Direct endoscopic view to a stricture after repair of oesophageal atresia with a flexible fibre-optic gastroscope. The diameter of this stricture is about 3 mm.

Key Summary Points

1. Rigid bronchoscopes and oesophagoscopes are used for foreign body removal and biopsy. For all other cases, use flexible fibre-optic instruments.

2. The appropriate size of scope must be used in keeping with the age and physical size of the patient.

3. Use video systems whenever possible because the image is magnified and much clearer. Also, the anaesthetist and other team members can see what is being done.

4. Before starting the procedure, always assemble the equipment and make sure that every component is working exactly as intended.

5. It is always helpful to use a laryngoscope to guide passage of the bronchoscope or oesophagoscope. The anaesthetist will be able to do this to display to the surgeon the exact anatomical structures at the upper end of the aerodigestive tract.

6. An emergency tracheostomy set must be ready in the operating theatre in case of airway problems or difficult intubation.

7. During the procedure, careful monitoring of the patient is mandatory. If any problems are noted, the endoscopy must be suspended. If necessary, the instruments must be removed and the anaesthetist allowed to re-establish satisfactory ventilation.

Suggested Reading

Edwards MJ, Greenland KB, Allen P, Cumpston P. The correct laryngoscope blade for the job. Anaesthesia 2009; 64:95.

Holm-Knudsen RJ, Rasmussen LS. Paediatric airway management: basic aspects. Acta Anaesthesiol Scand 2009; 53:1–9.

Lobe TE. Pediatric gastrointestinal endoscopy. In: Scott-Conner CEH, ed. The SAGES Manual: Fundamentals of Laparoscopy, Thoracoscopy, and GI Endoscopy, 2nd ed. Birkhauser, 2005, Pp 747–751.

Mathur NN, Pradhan T. Rigid pediatric bronchoscopy for bronchial foreign bodies with and without Hopkins telescope. Indian Pediatrics 2003; 40:761–765.

Nicolai T. Pediatric bronchoscopy. Pediatr Pulmonol 2001; 31:150–164.

Shinhar SY, Strabbing RJ, Madgy DN. Esophagoscopy for removal of foreign bodies in the pediatric population. Int J Pediatr Otorhinolaryngol 2003; 67: 977–979.

CHAPTER 42
PAEDIATRIC UPPER AIRWAY OBSTRUCTION

Andrew P. Freeland
John Kimario

Introduction

Upper airway obstruction in children is a serious and a potentially life-threatening problem. As such, the most important aspect is to establish the level of obstruction to instigate appropriate treatment without worrying too much about the diagnosis in the first instance.

Listening to the breathing is vital.

Stertor is a pharyngeal noise that sounds like a rough, bubbly snore and is usually inspiratory. Swellings in the pharynx, such as tonsillitis, glandular fever, burns, diphtheria, and space-occupying lesions (e.g., lymphoma) will often have stertor. Obstruction at this level can be bypassed with intubation or tracheostomy.

Stridor can be inspiratory, bifid (two way), or expiratory:

- *Inspiratory stridor* is usually caused by problems at the vocal cord level and above. It can be relieved by intubation or tracheostomy.

- *Bifid stridor* may involve the larynx but comes largely from the trachea, which is not distensible, hence the two-way nature of the noise. It may be relieved by intubation or tracheostomy providing the lesion is not at the distal end of the trachea.

- *Expiratory stridor* is termed *bronchospasm*, and comes from the bronchus. It is due to an inhaled bronchial foreign body and cannot be relieved by tracheostomy or intubation.

Neonates are obligate nose breathers and congenital bilateral choanal atresia (see below) is therefore an acute airway problem that needs immediate recognition and management.

The volume of the noise of breathing is not important, but the breathing characteristics (quality) are important. In addition, a rising pulse and respiratory rate with increasing recession of intercostal muscles and indrawing of the neck are signs that the obstruction is worsening. Cyanosis is a very late sign and one of impending doom.

The minimal requirements for successful management of upper airway obstruction are:

- oxygen;

- hydrocortisone and/or dexamethasone;

- nebulised adrenaline (epinephrine);

- antibiotics: chloramphenicol, ampicillin, and/or cefuroxime; and

- facilities and an ability to perform endotracheal intubation and tracheostomy.

Classification

For convenience it is easier to think along the lines of congenital and acquired airway obstructions. The congenital group normally presents at birth. The acquired group can be divided into acute and chronic. The acute group is further divided into *infective or noninfective* upper airway obstruction.

Congenital Upper Airway Obstruction

Choanal Atresia

Choanal atresia is due to failure of the buccopharyngeal membrane to canalise in embryonic life. This may leave a membranous or bony atresia or occasionally just a stenosis. It is often seen with the CHARGE association. (CHARGE is an acronym for coloboma, heart defects, choanal atresia, developmental retardation, genitorenal defects, and ear abnormalities.) It may be unilateral or bilateral. If the atresia is unilateral, there is usually no need for any acute treatment and feeding and a good airway is possible by suction of mucus from the patent nasal airway. If bilateral, the oral airway is kept in place and oral tube-feeding may be necessary until surgery can be carried out in the first few days of life, provided the child is fit enough and features of the CHARGE association have been excluded.

Diagnosis

Since babies are obligate nose breathers bilateral atresia presents acutely at birth. If the standard midwife practice is followed and nasal catheters are routinely passed the obstruction is easily diagnosed.

Management

The first aid management is to introduce an oral airway. If computed tomography (CT) scanning is available, the nose is cleared of mucus by suction prior to the scan to allow the radiologist a clear view to determine whether it is a stenosis or a bony or membranous atresia. If there is no CTscanner, then a plain x-ray, instilling a drop of radio-opaque dye into the previously cleaned out nose with the child supine will give an indication as to whether there is a stenosis or atresia present.

Surgery

There are many ways of dealing with the problem of upper airway obstruction, but the most sophisticated is via endoscopic nasal surgery by using minute endonasal drills, but these are not always available. The technique described here, however, is reliable and safe with the equipment readily available.

Under general anaesthesia (GA) and with the child intubated, the mucosa of the nose is vasoconstricted with 0.5% ephedrine nose drops. The child is placed supine, and a tonsil gag is used to open the mouth. Curved urethral bougies are gently passed through the nose, using a small size first with the curved tip pointing to the nasal surface of the hard palate. Even if there is a bony stenosis, it is penetrated easily and the tip of the bougie appears in the oral cavity from behind the soft palate. Gradually, larger bougies are introduced to dilate the atresia. Finally, it is necessary to splint the stenosis open with cut-down endotracheal tubes, which will need regular suctioning and should stay in place for about a month.

Results

Sadly, all techniques often need revision, and this one is no exception. The revision rate is about 33%. By the time the child reaches about 3 months of age, oral breathing is established and the acute problem is over.

Unilateral cases need have no surgery until the child is 5 or 6 years of age, and then only if unitateral nasal discharge is a problem.

Laryngomalacia

Laryngomalacia is the most common cause of neonatal obstruction. The pathology is vague, but it is assumed that the laryngeal and often the tracheal cartilages are immature, resulting in lack of stiffness and support for the larynx on inspiration.

Clinical features

Usually, there are no signs of obstruction until the baby is a few days old and becomes more active. Classically, there is an inspiratory stridor only when the baby is agitated or crying. The stridor is more obvious when the child is supine, and it improves when the child is prone. The voice is normal. Feeding can be difficult, however.

Natural history

The vast majority of cases settle down within 6 months and no audible stridor is presnt at 18 months of age. Failure to thrive is the main reason to interfere.

Diagnosis

The classic history is usually enough for diagnosis, but if in doubt, microlaryngoscopy under GA with spontaneous breathing is necessary.

The findings are of an omega-shaped epiglottis that is pulled backwards as the aryepiglottic folds are pulled forward on inspiration. This results in a supraglottic obstruction. The rest of the larynx and upper trachea are inspected to rule out coexisting lesions.

Management

If the failure to thrive is mild, a wait-and-see policy can be tried. In more severe cases, aryepiglottopexy, which is an easy procedure whereby the aryepiglottic folds are snipped with sharp micro scissors or divided with a laser, is a successful blood-free operation, usually with immediate results.

Tracheostomy should be avoided because often there is coexistent tracheomalacia, and extubation becomes very difficult.

Vocal Cord Palsy

Bilateral abductor vocal cord palsy is very rare, but is sometimes associated with hydrocephalus, causing prolapse at the foramen magnum affecting the vagus nerves. Acute inspiratory stridor and a weak cry are present. Laryngoscopy will confirm the diagnosis and tracheostomy is necessary.

Unilateral palsy is usually on the left side and due to inadvertent damage during ligation of a congenital patent ductus arteriosis. A weak cry and usually mild stridor are present, and if the recurrent laryngeal nerve has been traumatised rather than divided, it may recover in about 6 weeks.

Congenital Subglottic Stenosis

Congenital subglottic stenosis is far less common than acquired stenosis, which is often due to prolonged intubation in neonatal life. There will often be a bifid stridor because the lesion is a congenital narrowing of the only complete ring of the trachea, namely, the cricoid cartilage. The cry is normal, but due to respiratory distress, urgent intubation is necessary when the expected diameter tube for the weight of the child is determined to be too wide and a narrower tube is necessary, and often that is also too tight.

Mild stenosis will often grow with the child, and no action is necessary in early life.

More severe stenosis requires treatment. An anterior cricoid split is sometimes effective whereby a vertical incision is made through the anterior arch of the cricoid and a larger endotracheal tube inserted as a dilator for a period of time. Failing this, a tracheostomy will be necessary and reconstruction of the trachea carried out at about the age of 2 years.

Laryngeal Web

A total laryngeal web is incompatible with life and is due to lack of canalisation of the developing larynx. Additional minor webs usually occur between the anterior ends of the vocal cords. The presenting features are inspiratory stridor and a very weak voice. The web is often thin and can be split surgically.

Posterior Laryngeal Cleft Larynx

Posterior laryngeal cleft larynx is rare and difficult to diagnose and may range from a small defect in the interarytenoid muscles to a complete division of the posterior arch of the cricoid. The symptoms are very similar to a tracheo-oesophageal fistula, and complex repair surgery is necessary to stop aspiration.

Haemangioma

Inspiratory or bifid stridor in a child with a cutaneous haemangioma should always raise suspicion of a laryngeal haemangioma. Diagnosis is made via laryngoscopy; symptoms are often absent at birth but become more severe as the lesion grows naturally. The commonest site is the subglottis. Usually there is no more enlargement and at about 6–12 months, natural regression takes place and often no treatrment is necessary. If the airway is becoming compromised, a tracheostomy while waiting for natural regression is the safest option.

External Compression

Rare lesions, such as cystic hygroma (see Chapter 41), may compress the pharynx, larynx, or trachea.

Acquired Upper Airway Obstruction

The acquired causes can be divided into *acute* or *chronic*. The acute causes can be further subdivided into *infective* or *noninfective*. The infective causes will be *pyrexial*, and the noninfective will be *apyrexial*. A simple thermometer (not placed in the mouth) will distinguish between these two groups.

Acute Acquired Airway Obstruction

Acute noninfective upper airway obstruction

Foreign bodies, burns, and angioneurotic oedema need to be considered.

- *Foreign bodies* (FB) in any body cavity are common in children, but an inhaled FB constitutes an emergency. There is usually a history of ingestion or inhalation, and the child will be apyrexial. The level at which the FB is trapped now needs to be determined.

  Gagging will be the main symptom of a pharyngeal FB, such as a fish bone stuck in the tonsil. This may be seen and removed with forceps.

  Inspiratory stridor suggests the FB is at the laryngeal level, and urgent removal by thumping the child on the back with the child in the prone and head-down position or carrying out the Heimlich manoeuvre is mandatory.

  The technique most useful for infants is as follows (see Figure 42.1):
  1. Lay child prone with head down over the knee.
  2. Give five pats on the child's back with the heel of the hand.
  3. Check the child's mouth for a foreign body that can be removed.
  4. Repeat.

  The Heimlich manoeuvre for older children, to be used if the technique shown in Figure 42.1 isn't successful, is as follows (see Figure 42.2):
  1. Stand behind the child.
  2. Make a fist with one hand and place it just below the child's lower sternum.
  3. Place your other hand over the fist.
  4. Pull into and upwards to the child's upper abdomen five times.
  5. Check the child's mouth for a foreign body that can be removed.
  6. Repeat as necessary.

  If either of these techniques is not successful and a skilled laryngologist is not available, then emergency cricothyrotomy or tracheostomy will be necessary to bypass the obstruction. A FB lodged in the upper oesophagus may give very similar symptoms.

  Expiratory stridor preceded by bouts of coughing suggests

a bronchial FB, usually in the right main bronchus in older children, but in either bronchus in infants. Vegetable FBs (such as peanuts) are more dangerous than inert objects because vegetables contain oil that can cause a local pneumonitis and they tend to crumble. Antibiotics are probably wise while waiting for treatment. The situation is usually not desperate, and assessment and investigation can be carried out.

Clinical examination may show the trachea deviated to either side. If there is a valve effect, then air will go in but little will go out due to bronchospasm, in which case the affected lung will be hyperinflated and the trachea deviated away from the affected side. If there is complete obstruction, then the lung will collapse and the trachea will deviate towards the affected side. Percussion of the chest and a chest x-ray in inhalation and exhalation will confirm the diagnosis.

Treatment is rigid ventilation bronchoscopy by a skilled ear, nose, and throat (ENT) surgeon and removal using appropriate forceps. Physiotherapy prior to bronchoscopy is not advised because the FB might be impacted further, compounding the situation. Postoperative physiotherapy is essential to help the lung expand.

- Burns: Inhalational burns are extremely dangerous. The cause may be chemical—from ingestion of bleaches or other caustic chemicals often stored in inappropriate containers (e.g., soda bottles) or from inhalation of smoke and flame. Airway obstruction may not develop immediately and may be missed while dealing with burns to other parts of the body. If there is airway obstruction, intensive care unit (ICU) admission, large doses of hydrocortisone (4mg/kg body weight, intravensously (IV), 6-hourly), antibiotics, and intubation or tracheostomy are required.

- Angioneurotic oedema is usually caused by ingestion or inhalation of an allergen to which the child is sensitive. Common allergens are nuts, penicillin, and some foods. There may well be other signs of systemic shock that need appropriate management, but airway obstruction from a grossly swollen tongue or larynx is an urgent problem, as is acute asthma. Early recognition of the problem can avoid emergency tracheostomy. Adrenaline (10 mgm/kg body weight, intramuscular (IM)), nebulised adrenaline (5 ml of 1 in 1000 with 100% oxygen), and hydrocortisone (4 mg/kg body weight, IV, over 15 minutes) is the first aid management and usually will avoid intubation or tracheostomy.

Acute infective upper airway obstruction

The following infective causes need to be considered and a diagnosis rapidly made because, especially in the case of the epiglottitis, acute deterioration will lead to asphyxiation and death: laryngotracheobronchitis (common "croup"), epiglottitis, bacterial tracheitis, tonsillitis (rarely), glandular fever, retropharyngeal abscess, and diphtheria.

Certain rules exist for the safe management of upper airway obstruction, the most important being not to frighten the child, which will often make the stridor worse. The child's temperature is taken, preferably with an ear thermometer; if there is no fever, the diagnosis is not one of the infective causes discussed in this section. The mother can give a good relevant history, with the child staying on her knee without any interference such as blood tests or throat examination, especially if the stridor has come on rapidly, suggesting epiglottitis.

Table 42.1: Various symptoms of acute infective causes of upper airway obstruction.

Symptoms	Laryngotracheobronchitis (LTB)	Epiglottitis	Retropharyngeal abscess	Diphtheria	Glandular fever/ tonsillitis
Speed of onset	Days	Hours	Days	Days	Days
Age	18 months	2–5 years	Any	Any	Any
Preceding upper respiratory tract infection (URTI)	Yes	No	Yes	Yes	Yes
Voice	Hoarse	Muffled/"hot potato"	Normal	Normal	Normal
Position	Lying down	Sitting up and leaning forward	Sitting up	Any	Any
Drooling/swallowing	No drooling/can swallow	Copious drooling and unable to swallow	Some	Some	Some
Stridor	Noisy	Quiet	Often none or stertor	Variable	Often nil or stertor
Appearance	Pale lips and struggling	Pale lips and frightened	Toxic	Toxic	Variable
Need for alternative airway	Less than 5%	90%	Surgical drainage usually relieves obstruction	If antibiotics and antitoxins fail	Rareluy

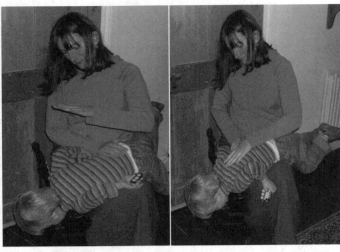

Figure 42.1: Technique for thumping child on the back in a prone position to remove foreign body.

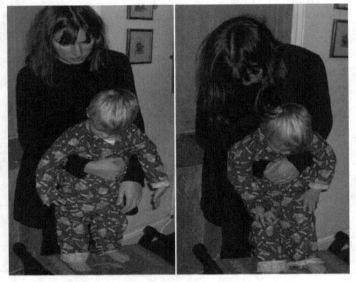

Figure 42.2: Heimlich maneouvre to remove foreign body.

X-rays for the diagnosis of acute epiglottitis are dangerous in that they distress the child and waste valuable time; if a retropharyngeal abscess is suspected, however, a lateral neck film is useful. Cyanosis is a sign of imminent disaster and indicates the child needs an urgent alternative airway. Increasing pulse and respiration rates are also good signs that the child's condition is worsening.

Table 42.1 distinguishes among the various causes of acute infective upper airway obstruction that can be determined from the history and observation of a child. It particularly distinguishes epiglottitis from other causes so that urgent action may be taken with reasonable diagnostic certainty.

Laryngotracheobronchitis

Laryngotracheobronchitis (LTB, or croup) is a viral condition and is the most common infection that causes stridor. Most cases occur at around 18 months of age, and there is always a history of upper respiratory infection in the preceding week. There may be a history of previous attacks. Mild cases present with a barking seal-like cough with a hoarse cry and inspiratory stridor, which is worse if the child gets agitated when an expiratory component can also be heard.

Rarely is there any need for intubation (less than 5%) and the management is to calm the child and reassure the mother. Avoid

injections and nasal airways, as they only upset the child

Observations and management of LTB are as follows:

- A slowing pulse and reduced respiration rate are good signs.

- Humidified air, or oxygen if necessary, is given via a mask held in front of the child's face.

- Oral fluid is given.

- Antibiotics are not necessary except for the more severe cases when oral cephalexin (25 mg/kg body weight, every 6 hours) or chloramphenicol (2.5 mg/kg body weight, every 6 hours) are given.

- Steroids (dexamethasone, 0.6 mg/kg body weight) given orally twice a day as necessary will help.

- Nebulised adrenaline (5 ml of 1 in 1000) given via a face mask is a good way to reduce oedema in the more severe cases. This may need repeating every 2 hours while the condition is monitored with a transcutaneous oxygen probe and careful pulse and respiratory rates are recorded.

- Severe cases will need intubation or, occasionally, tracheostomy.

As children grow, the subglottic lumen increases oedema from LTB has less effect on narrowing the airway, which is why this condition is usually seen only in children under 2 years of age.

Acute Epiglottitis

Epiglottitis is a frightening emergency airway problem to deal with, but if handled correctly will lead to a child rapidly restored to health from a potentially fatal situation. It is an infection caused by *Haemophilus influenza* in a nonimmunised child, usually around the age of 5 years. It is very much rarer than LTB, especially in countries where *H. influenza* vaccine immunisation is routinely given. Rapid diagnosis is essential to ensure urgent life-saving treatment. It is safe to assume all children will require a temporary alternative airway, usually intubation if the skills are present to carry out what is a potentially difficult procedure; otherwise, a tracheostomy is necessary.

The following points should be heeded in the management having suspected the diagnosis based on the information in Table 42.1:

- *Never* examine the throat except in a facility where intubation can be immediately carried out.

- *Never* do anything invasive or attempt to lie the child down. The child is much safer sitting up, leaning forward, drooling, and in the clothes in the child had been wearing.

- *Never* carry out a lateral neck x-ray. The thumb sign seen in most textbooks is not necessary to make the diagnosis, and the performance of moving and positioning a child for a neck x-ray may precipitate a sudden airway crisis.

- *Always* reassure the child and the mother.

- *Always* arrange urgent transfer to an anaesthetic room, having first called an anaesthetist and ENT surgeon to be present so that an alternative airway can be performed.

- *Always* use humidified oxygen given by a face mask held close to the child's face while being transferred to a resuscitation room.

Once the appropriate personnel are present, general anaesthesia is induced while the child is in the sitting position, and the child is laid prone once asleep. The diagnosis is now made with an intubating laryngoscope when a "cherry red" epiglottis is seen. Intubation is carried out at the same time. If this is impossible, a thump on the chest will often produce a bubble of air, indicating where the tube should be aimed. If the swelling is so great that a flexible tube will not pass, the ENT surgeon should be able to pass a rigid bronchoscope through the obstruction. A useful trick is to use a Magill nasal sucker, which has a blunt end and a gentle curve, allowing easy intubation. If either of these rigid instruments has been used, do *not* remove them but continue anaesthesia via the bronchoscope and carry out a tracheostomy onto the rigid bronchoscope.

Once the airway is secure, blood cultures and a throat swab are carried out and IV chloamphenicol (50mg/kg body weight) is given, followed by 25mg/kg every 6 hours.

The next step is to transfer the child to an ICU where the alternative airway can be managed. Rapid response to treatment is usual, and extubation is possible within 24–72 hours.

Retropharyngeal Abscess

Retropharyngeal abscess is a condition most often seen in infants and young children and may mimic epiglottitis in that the symptoms of inspiratory stridor, drooling, and a muffled voice are similar, but there is always a long period of fever and general debility prior to the diagnosis. It is due to the breakdown of a retropharyngeal adenitis into an abscess and is frequently associated with tonsillitis. The child will usually have a stiff, painful neck, which is held to one side because the midline raphe attached to the anterior cervical spine pushes the abscess to one side. The organisms are usually *Streptococcus haemolyticus*, *Staphylococcus aureus*, or anaerobes. This condition is sometimes seen in cases of tuberculosis (TB) where the cervical spine is involved and caseous breakdown occurs.

Due to the long history of preceding URTI symptoms, unlike for epiglottitis, it is permissible to examine the throat where an asymmetric pharyngeal swelling is seen. The next stage is a lateral neck x-ray, which shows a lack of the normal lordosis and a widened space between the spine and the pharyngeal airway. If the organism is anaerobic, a gas bubble may be seen in the soft tissue swelling.

The management involves urgent surgical drainage and culture of the drained pus. If GA and intubation are difficult, then a No 11 blade wrapped in tape (except for its point) can be used to lance the abscess. A large IV cannula could also be tried. IV antibiotics depending on the gram stain of the organism are necessary in large doses. Mediastinitis is the most serious complication, with a mortality rate of 40–50%.

Diphtheria

Diphtheria is seen only where low immunisation levels are present. Infants are often protected by maternal antibodies, and the usual age group for diphtheria is 2–4 year olds.

The disease nearly always affects the pharynx, and a thick white/gray membrane caused by the toxin covers the tonsils and pharyngeal walls and bleeds if it is separated from the underlying structures. The membrane may extend to the larynx, causing stridor. Frequently, large cervical lymph nodes give the appearance of a "bull neck."

Toxaemia, which may vary from mild to severe, is the other main feature of diphtheria apart from the respiratory symptoms. Severe toxaemia may result in cardiovascular collapse and neuropathy and include myocarditis and palatal palsy.

The diagnosis is made by examining the throat and sending a piece of membrane for urgent gram stain. The management is to deal with the toxins and support the airway:

- *Benzylpenicillin* (50 mg/kg body weight, IV, 4-hourly). Once drinking is established and the child is less toxic, a change is made to oral penicillin. Erythromycin is an alternative.

- *Dexamethasone* (0.6 mg/kg, twice daily, IV) if there is stridor or gross neck swelling.

- *Antitoxin* is essential (60,000 units IM/IV). A test dose should be given first to ensure there is no reaction (0.1 ml of 1 in 1000 in saline intradermally).

- Consider *tracheostomy* if airway compromised.

- Oxygen.

- Cardiac monitoring.

- *Bed rest* for 2 weeks.

- *Nasogastric feeding* if there is palatal palsy.

- *Immunisation* of patient and close contacts before discharge.

Glandular Fever

Glandular fever (infectious mononucleosis) is a viral infection due to the Epstein-Barr virus, which may cause airway obstruction due to massive tonsillar enlargement. Stertor rather than stridor is evident, examination of the neck shows large cervical glands, and the tonsils are covered with a white membrane. The other main symptom is extreme tiredness and lethargy. The liver and spleen may be enlarged and a general lymphadenopathy may be present.

Treatment is mainly symptomatic with bed rest, fluids and analgesia. Ampicillin should not be given since a widespread rash may occur.

If the airway obstruction is present large doses of IV steroids will usually relieve the obstruction and intubation or tracheostomy is rarely necessary.

Bacterial Tracheitis

Bacterial tracheitis is a rare but nasty condition in which the tracheal mucosa sloughs off to form thick crusts in the airway that are difficult to remove. Measles is not infrequently complicated by this bacterial infection, often due to *Streptococcus pneumoniae* or *Haemophilus influenza B*.

Children with bacterial tracheitis frequently require intubation and ICU management if only to clear the thick secretions. The child is much more toxic with this bacterial infection than in viral LTB and the absence of swallowing and drooling problems distinguish it from epiglottitis. Bronchial complications are common, and prolonged treatment with antibiotics, humidification, and physiotherapy are necessary once the acute airway management has been completed.

Key Summary Points

1. If epiglottitis is suspected, do not examine the throat except at the time of resuscitation.
2. Hypoxaemia and cynanosis are very late signs.
3. Dexamethasone (0.6 mgm/kg body weight orally) should be given early. (The oral form is as effective as injected if the child is able to swallow.)
4. Nebulised epinephrine (1 ml in 1/1000 in 3 ml of 0.9% saline) should be available.
5. History taking and resuscitation should take place at the same time.
6. Immunisation against *H. influenzae* should be administered.
7. In recurrent croup, suspect subglottic stenosis.
8. Antibiotics chloramphenicol, cefuroxime, and ampicillin should be available.
9. Oxygen must be available.
10. If intubation is considered, make sure personnel are available to carry out tracheostomy in case intubation fails.

Suggested Reading

Gleeson M, ed. Scott-Brown's Otorhinolaryngology, Head and Neck Surgery, 7th ed, Vol. 1. Hodder Arnold, 2008. See, especially:

- Chapter 86, Stridor, David Albert, pages 1114–1126.

- Chapter 87, Acute laryngeal infections, Susanna Leighton, pages 1127–1134.

- Chapter 88, Congenital disorders of the larynx, trachea and bronchi, Martin Bailey, pages 1135–1149.

Lissauer T, Clayden G. Illustrated Textbook of Paediatrics. St. Louis, MO: Mosby Elsevier, 1997.

CHAPTER 43
TRACHEOMALACIA

Vivien M. McNamara
David P. Drake

Introduction

The normal trachea is supported by up to 20 horseshoe-shaped cartilage rings completed by a posterior membranous wall. In tracheomalacia, these cartilages may be abnormally shaped, small, or even absent, with a detrimental effect on the support of the trachea. The anteroposterior (AP) diameter of the tracheal lumen becomes reduced, especially during periods of increased airflow. The dynamic movement of the malacic segment becomes most pronounced during the exertion of feeding, crying, or coughing. Symptoms can range from mild to severe, the latter culminating in complete airway obstruction. Mild cases can be managed conservatively with the expectation of spontaneous recovery, usually within the first two years of life.

Associated medical problems including gastro-oesophageal reflux and pneumonia, require aggressive treatment. More severe cases of tracheomalacia require supportive therapy, diagnostic imaging and endoscopic evaluation, and a few may require early surgical intervention to prevent acute life-threatening airway collapse.

Aetiology

Tracheomalacia may be primary (congenital absence or deformity of tracheal rings; the cause is often unknown) or secondary (in conjunction with another pathology) (see Table 43.1). The latter group includes oesophageal atresia (OA), with or without tracheo-oesophageal fistula (TOF); a vascular ring (e.g., double aortic arch); vascular compression (aberrant innominate artery or pulmonary artery sling); or extrinsic compression from another source (e.g., a mediastinal mass). It may also occur in association with prolonged positive pressure ventilation or following a tracheostomy. It is rarely seen in association with connective tissue disorders (e.g., Larsen's syndrome). Tracheomalacia commonly affects the distal third of the trachea, but can rarely extend into the bronchi. When associated with TOF in infants with OA, the malacic segment is located in the middle third of the trachea. Isolated bronchomalacia is usually associated with major cardiac pathologies and is frequently fatal.

The incidence of tracheomalacia is unknown, but it is the most common cause of expiratory stridor in infants and children. It is most often identified secondary to OA/TOF.[1, 2, 3] In affected infants, the tracheal cartilage rings fail to develop normally, especially at the site of the previously ligated fistula.[4] This has long been thought to occur as a result of extrinsic pressure of the adjacent dilated upper oesophageal pouch, although more recent evidence suggests an early embryological disturbance of tracheal development.[5]

Localised tracheomalacia secondary to extrinsic compression, from either a vascular ring (double aortic arch) or an aberrant aortic arch or pulmonary artery (PA) vessel, form a small but important group of affected infants. A double aortic arch results from persistent left and right dorsal aortic segments, compared to the normal aortic arch in which there is regression of the right dorsal aorta by week 8 postconception. The extent and location of tracheal compression is variable; therefore, so is the degree of malacia. In addition, compression of the oesophagus may present with dysphagia. A double aortic arch will compress both the trachea and oesophagus.

Table 43.1: Causes of tracheomalacia.

Primary	Cause usually unknown.
	Absent or deformed tracheal cartilage rings.
Secondary	Oesophageal atresia with or without tracheo-oesophageal fistula.
	Extrinsic vascular compression: vascular ring (e.g., double aortic arch), aberrant vessel (e.g., anomalous innominate artery or pulmonary artery sling), or (mediastinal mass).
	Prolonged tracheal intubation and ventilation (especially cuffed tubes).
	Tracheostomy.
	Connective tissue disorder (e.g., Larsen's syndrome).

Chronic inflammation of the tracheal cartilages occurs with prolonged intubation or following a tracheostomy. This deleterious effect of mucosal ischaemia caused by the localised pressure of the intratracheal tubing, especially with cuffed tubes, will compound airway compromise and can delay successful decannulation.

Presentation

Signs and symptoms of tracheomalacia vary from mild to severe and life threatening (Table 43.2). Many infants exhibit a simple barking cough but otherwise are not troubled by their mild tracheomalacia. For those with OA/TOF, the term "TOF cough" is frequently used to describe the characteristic sound made. Expiratory stridor indicates increasing airway obstruction. Crying, agitation, and coughing make the degree of malacic collapse more pronounced. Signs of respiratory distress, including tachypnoea and intercostal recession, herald further airway compromise, and the stridor may become biphasic. Increasing severity with infections, including the respiratory syncytial virus (RSV) infection, is to be expected, and recurrent respiratory sepsis is common.

Feeding provides particular challenges, especially in an infant with tracheomalacia following surgery for OA. Distention of the proximal oesophagus, especially with a solid bolus, may cause compression of the posterior trachea and worsen the symptoms. This is further compounded by poor oesophageal motility, anastomotic strictures, and gastro-oesophageal reflux (GOR). Feeding difficulties may lead to poor weight gain.

The most severe tracheomalacia is complicated by hypoxia and cyanosis. With major airway collapse, following a period of significant respiratory distress, complete obstruction may supervene and the infant will lose consciousness. At this stage, the collapsed airway will relax and open again, but with no guarantee that normal ventilation will resume. These events are often referred to as "dying spells" or acute life-threatening events (ALTEs). The resulting hypoxia may be severe and prolonged, leading to bradycardia, cerebral anoxia, asystole, and even death. Immediate resuscitation, often by the parents, is vital and is an indication for prompt surgical referral.

Most infants will demonstrate a gradual improvement of symptoms over the first year or two of life as the tracheal cartilages become more

Table 43.2: Signs and symptoms of tracheomalacia.

Mild	Harsh, barking TOF cough
Exacerbating events	Crying
	Coughing
	Feeding (especially food bolus)
	Acute distress
Moderate	Expiratory stridor
	Wheeze
	Chronic cough
	Recurrent respiratory infections
	Feeding difficulties
	Failure to thrive
	Respiratory distress (tachypnoea, intercostal recession, hypoxia)
Severe	Severe hypoxia
	Biphasic stridor
	Cyanosis
	Reflex apnoea (vagal stimulation)
	"Dying spells" or acute life-threatening events, which may be fatal.

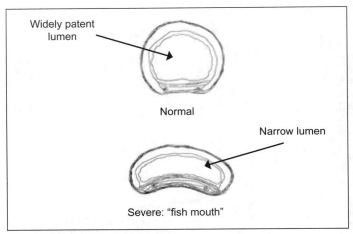

Figure 43.1: Airway in cross section showing varying degrees of tracheomalacia.

Table 43.3: Management of tracheomalacia.

Supportive	Frequent, small oral feeds
	NGT feeding (during times of acute respiratory infections)
	CPAP
	Intubation and positive pressure ventilation
Co-morbid pathology	Antibiotics for acute pneumonia
	Supplemental oxygen (pneumonia, RSV infections)
	Antireflux therapy for GOR
Surgical	Aortopexy
	Tracheostomy
	Correction of vascular rings or extrinsic compression (vascular, mediastinal mass)
	Endobronchial stenting
	Glossopexy
	Antireflux surgery (fundoplication)

rigid and afford better support of the airway. However, it may take many years for a TOF cough to disappear, and for some this clinical sign will persist into adult life.

Assessment

The need for investigation should be guided by the severity of symptoms demonstrated by the child. For infants who have already had surgical correction for OA, a high index of suspicion should alert the clinician to signs of developing tracheomalacia. Close observation and timely investigation are recommended. For older children presenting with significant tracheomalacia, vascular or mediastinal compression should be considered. Other conditions that may cause diagnostic confusion, including a laryngeal cleft, laryngomalacia and H-type TOF (H-TOF), should be excluded or confirmed by laryngobronchoscopy.

A plain chest x-ray is of limited diagnostic value, although it may show a mediastinal mass. A lateral chest x-ray may demonstrate localised narrowing of the trachea. Flow volume loops are able to demonstrate major airway compromise, but the impracticalities of performing them in babies and infants limit their use except in specialist research facilities.

A bronchoscopy performed under general anaesthetic is the initial investigation of choice. This will both establish the diagnosis and assess the degree and location of any airway collapse. It is important to ensure that the child continues to breathe spontaneously and does not receive intravenous muscle relaxation. A rigid bronchoscopy will allow visualisation of the supraglottic, laryngeal, and tracheobronchial tree. Flexible bronchoscopy, ideally via a laryngeal mask, provides superior assessment of any airway collapse. The AP diameter of the airway reduces during expiration, and in severe cases, the anterior and posterior tracheal walls will touch and occlude the airway entirely. The site of collapse is confirmed by a typical "fish mouth" appearance (Figure 43.1).

An upper gastrointestinal (UGI) contrast study with both AP and lateral views of the entire oesophagus is recommended. This can clearly suggest a vascular ring and may demonstrate GOR. A double aortic arch is suggested by both a right and left lateral indentation of the oesophageal outline seen in the AP view and a posterior indentation on the lateral view. This differs from the normal left-sided indentation by the normal aortic arch.

Cross-sectional imaging of the chest with computed tomography (CT) or magnetic resonance imaging (MRI) will identify either abnormal vascular anatomy or a mediastinal mass. These methods are less helpful in identifying tracheomalacia, which is a dynamic process. Vascular anomalies may require further specialist investigations.

Management

The management of tracheomalacia is summarised in Table 43.3. Treatment is initially focused on managing predisposing conditions. In cases of compression from a vascular ring or aberrant vessel, surgical correction may be required. This should be performed by a paediatric cardiothoracic surgeon and is tailored to the underlying vascular anomaly. Most commonly, surgical correction involves division of the smaller arch in cases of a double aortic arch, division of the ligamentum arteriosum when seen with other vascular rings, or reimplanting an aberrant vessel (typically the pulmonary artery in cases of a PA sling). However, tracheomalacia may persist or progress following correction of an underlying pathology, such as a OA/TOF.

Not all children will require intervention, especially when symptoms are mild. Appropriate medical treatment for GOR is started, and, when necessary, antireflux surgery may be undertaken. Respiratory infections require appropriate antibiotic therapy. RSV infections often require hospital admission and even respiratory support in the acute phase. Oral feeding may be problematic during this time, and nasogastric tube (NGT) supplementation may be required.

As the degree of tracheomalacia increases, conservative measures will not suffice. Supplemental oxygen may be required and should be available at home. The parents should receive resuscitation training. Adjustment of oral dietary regimens and periods of NGT feeding may be required. Support of the airway with continuous positive airway

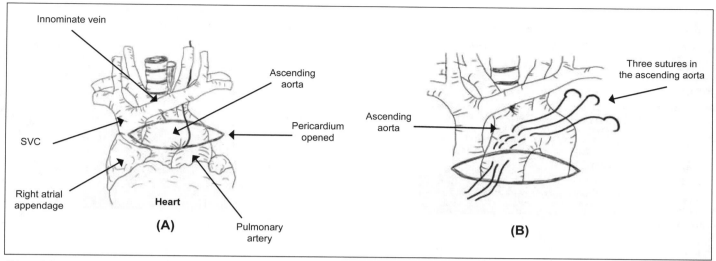

Figure 43.2: (A) Surgical approach to ascending aorta; (B) suture placement.

pressure (CPAP) may provide temporary assistance but is not suitable for long-term therapy.

Aortopexy

For severe tracheomalacia, especially for cases complicated by "dying spells" or ALTEs, and those infants who remain CPAP dependent, aortopexy offers an excellent surgical option.[6,7,8] The crucial step in an aortopexy is to ventrally suspend the ascending aorta, suturing it to the underside of the sternum, thereby creating space anterior to the trachea. Access to the aortic arch is achieved via either a median sternotomy or a left anterior thoracotomy (through the bed of the third rib), with resection of the thymus gland. Three nonabsorbable Prolene™ sutures are placed in the wall of the ascending aorta, each suture taking bites of the vessel from its intrapericardial segment to the innominate artery. These sutures can be passed through the infant sternum or sutured to its deep periosteum. The assistant depresses the sternum as the sutures are tied with minimal tension (Figure 43.2). Complications from surgery include bleeding from major vessel injury and phrenic nerve damage with subsequent ipsilateral diaphragm paralysis. Alternatively, a low cervical skin crease incision with a manubrial split affords excellent access for surgery under direct vision, with improved cosmesis.[9]

The surgical approach to aortopexy now includes thoracoscopy, with repair of the primary OA/TOF having already been undertaken endoscopically.[10] It has also been employed in aortopexy undertaken for vascular compression.[11]

In specialist cardiothoracic units, short segments of tracheomalacia may be resected and a primary anastomosis performed.

Glossopexy may offer an alternative surgical approach. This serves to anchor the tongue forward, although aortopexy may still be required.[13]

Endoluminal Stenting

Endoluminal stenting appears an attractive treatment modality, initially arising from a need to manage malignant airway compromise in the adult population. Technology used in endovascular stenting has further advanced the techniques. Balloon-expandable metallic or silicone-type stents placed at bronchoscopy are available in some specialist units. However, they carry potentially life-threatening complications of bleeding, granulation tissue formation, luminal obstruction, and erosion into adjacent blood vessels. Removal of these stents is also hazardous but they can offer an alternate mode of management in selected cases.[12]

Outcome

Long-term follow-up of children with significant tracheomalacia is mainly derived from studying infants previously treated with oesopha-geal atresia. Aortopexy leads to immediate relief of symptoms in the majority of infants.

Aortopexy may be required in up to 10% of infants following repair of OA/TOF, at a median age of 7 months. Ninety-five percent of these cases have resolution of their symptoms, although almost half require antireflux surgery (fundoplication) for severe reflux.[6] Overall, aortopexy affords good symptomatic improvement in such infants, with indications for surgery being "dying spells", inability to be extubated, expiratory stridor, and recurrent pneumonia.[14] When aortopexy fails, insertion of an airway stent or a tracheostomy may be required.

Evidence-Based Research

Tables 43.4 and 43.5 present case reviews involving management of tracheomalacia by aortoplexy.

Table 43.4: Evidence-based research.

Title	Management of tracheomalacia by aortopexy
Authors	E M Kiely, L Spitz, and R Brereton
Institution	The Hospital for Sick Children, Great Ormond Street, London, UK
Reference	Pediatr Surg Int 1987; 2:13–15
Problem	The problem is symptomatic tracheomalacia in infants with congenital tracheo-oesophageal anomalies. Indications for surgery included respiratory distress, recurrent apnoea, cyanosis or "dying spells", worsening stridor, or repeated hospital admissions for respiratory infections
Intervention	Aortopexy
Comparison/ control (quality of evidence)	Case review (level 4). A review of 210 infants with tracheo-oesophageal anomalies admitted over a six and a half year period. Twenty-five infants underwent an aortopexy, 22 having had repair of an oesophageal atresia and three who had primary tracheomalacia.
Outcome/ effect	Seventeen infants had immediate and dramatic relief of symptoms, and the other five were greatly improved. The operation failed in one patient.
Historical significance/ comments	Aortopexy had previously been described as a surgical option for the treatment of symptomatic vascular compression of the trachea. This was the first description of this surgical procedure for patients with congenital oesophageal anomalies. It demonstrated an excellent outcome from aortopexy for children with significant tracheomalacia, and recommended early surgery.

Table 43.5: Evidence-based research.

Title	Aortopexy for tracheomalacia in oesophageal anomalies
Authors	Corbally MT, Spitz L, Kiely E, Brereton RJ, Drake DP
Institution	The Hospital for Sick Children, Great Ormond Street, London, UK
Reference	Eur J Pediatr Surg 1993; 5:264–266
Problem	The problem is significant symptomatic tracheomalacia in association with repaired congenital oesophageal anomalies. Indications for surgery included recurrent apnoea/cyanosis (31), "near fatal episodes" (16), recurrent respiratory distress and infections (20), and worsening stridor (15).
Intervention	Aortopexy
Comparison/ control (quality of evidence)	Case review (level 4). A review of 48 patients over a ten-year period who underwent an aortopexy for tracheomalacia following repair of an oesophageal anomaly.
Outcome/ effect	Gastro-oesophageal reflux was also noted in 30 cases. Aortopexy cured near fatal episodes in all patients and resulted in improvement of airway obstruction in 95%. Failure in two patients was due to unrecognised bronchomalacia.
Historical significance/ comments	Aortopexy was recommended as the primary procedure of choice for significant tracheomalacia.

Key Summary Points

1. An association exists between oesophageal atresia and/or tracheo-oesophageal fistula (OA/TOF) and tracheomalacia.

2. Expiratory stridor should be investigated by bronchoscopy in a self-ventilating patient.

3. Anterior-posterior collapse of the tracheal lumen indicates severe tracheomalacia, and urgent intervention should be considered.

4. An aortopexy gives excellent results for localised tracheomalacia in association with OA and TOF.

5. Severe gastro-oesophageal reflux may be associated with tracheomalacia and may require a fundoplication.

6. Vascular anomalies associated with tracheomalacia require specialised investigations and management in a paediatric cardiothoracic unit.

References

1. Stringer MD, Oldham KT, Mouriquand DE. Pediatric Surgery and Urology: Long-Term Outcomes, 2nd ed. Cambridge University Press, 2006.

2. Filler RM, et al. Life-threatening anoxic spells caused by tracheal compression. J Pediatr Surg 1976; 11:739–748.

3. Benjamin B, et al. Tracheomalacia in association with T.O.F. Surgery 1976; 79:504–508.

4. Wailoo MP, Emery JL. The trachea in children with T.O.F. Histopathology 1979; 3:329–338.

5. Pole RJ, Qi BQ, Beasley SW. Abnormalities of the tracheal cartilages in the rat fetus with tracheo-oesophageal fistula or tracheal agenesis. Pediatr Surg Int 2001; 17:25–28.

6. Kiely EM, Spitz L, Brereton R. Management of tracheomalacia by aortopexy. Pediatr Surg Int 1987; 2:13–15.

7. Kimura K, et al. Aortosternopexy for tracheomalacia, technical refinement. J Pediatr Surg 1990; 25:769–772.

8. Corbally MT, Spitz L, Kiely E, Brereton RJ, Drake DP. Aortopexy for tracheomalacia in oesophageal anomalies. Eur J Pediatr Surg 1993; 3:264–266.

9. Morabito A, MacKinnon E, Alizai N, Asero L, Bianchi A. The anterior mediastinal approach for management of tracheomalacia. J Pediatr Surg 2000; 35(10):1456–1458.

10. van der Zee DC, Bax KN. Thoracoscopic treatment of esophageal atresia with distal fistula and of tracheomalacia. Semin Pediatr Surg 2007; 16(4):224–230.

11. Kane TD, Nadler EP, Potoka DA. Thoracoscopic aortopexy for vascular compression of the trachea: approach from the right. J Laparoendoscopic Adv Surg Tech A. 2008; 18(2):313–316.

12. Anton-Pacheco J.L. Cabezali D, Tejedor R, et al. The role of airway stenting in pediatric tracheobronchial obstruction. Eur J Cardiothorac Surg 2008; 33(6):1069–1075. Epub 2008 Mar 4.

13. Cozzi F, Morini F, Casati A, et al. Glossopexy as an alternative to aortopexy in infants with repaired esophageal atresia and upper airway obstruction. J Pediatr Surg 2002; 37(2):202–206.

14. Filler RM, Messineo A, Vinograd I. Severe tracheomalacia associated with esophageal atresia: results of surgical treatment. J Pediatr Surg 1992; 27(8):1136–1140; discussion 1140–1141.

CHAPTER 44
CONGENITAL CYSTIC LUNG LESIONS

Kokila Lakhoo
Catherine Mngongo

Introduction

Congenital lesions of the lung are rare with an unknown true rate of incidence. An overall incidence of 1/10,000 to 1/25,000 births (and 2.2% when compared to acquired lesions) has been reported. Presentation varies from life-threatening symptoms at birth to incidental findings at autopsy. Diagnosis is either made in utero or due to complications of the lesion, such as lung abscess, pneumonia, or pneumothorax. At an early stage, there is a good argument for describing these lesions simply as cystic lung malformations because the precise diagnosis may need to await later pathological examination or other postnatal investigations. Embryology and classification of the lesions are attempted. Classic lesions of congenital cystic or pulmonary adenomatous malformation (CCAM or CPAM) of the lung, bronchopulmonary sequestration (BPS), congenital lobar emphysema/overinflation, congenital lung cysts, and other less common anomalies are described. Although described as a number of separate and seemingly distinct entities, these lesions often overlap.

Embryology

In the third week of the embryonic phase, the lung appears as a ventral out-pouching of the endodermal foregut. At the end of the fourth gestational week, the caudal growth of the respiratory diverticulum becomes separated into the dorsal oesophagus and ventral trachea by the formation of the tracheo-oesophageal septum from the tracheo-oesophageal septum (Figure 44.1). The larynx, which develops from the fourth to the sixth branchial arches, maintains communication with the trachea. Pleural cavities are formed on either side of the foregut by caudal migration of the developing lung bud into the coelomic cavity. At the 6th embryonic week the right lung bud divides into three lobes and the left bud into two. Pulmonary vasculature develops in the mesoderm at 7–8 weeks of gestation. Bronchial division, which forms the conductive airways, is complete in mid-trimester, and the terminal airways and alveoli, which are the sites for gaseous exchange, continue to develop until early childhood (i.e., 8 years of age). Gaseous exchange is possible at 7 months gestation.

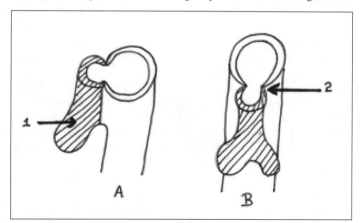

Figure 44.1: Embryology of lung bud: (A) week 3, showing lung bud (1); (B) week 4, showing tracheo-oesophageal septum (2).

Classification

The historic histologic classification by Stocker (type 0 = total lung involvement; type 1 = >2 cm cyst; type 2 = <2 cm cyst; type 3 = <0.5 cm cyst; type 4 = >5 cm cyst) and prenatal ultrasound classification of Adzick (macrocystic = >5 mm; microcystic = <5 mm) have been replaced by a pathological classification recently proposed by Langston (Table 44.1).

Pathogenesis

The pathogenesis of congenital cystic lung lesions is controversial, and many theories have been proposed. The historic vascular traction theory, vascular insufficiency theory, vascular maldevelopment theory, accessory bud theory, and the more recent molecular markers and signalling protein theories have not been confirmed.

Prenatal Diagnosis and Management of Congenital Lung Lesions

Most congenital lung cysts are diagnosed at the 20-week anomaly scan. The diagnostic accuracy is 100% for congenital cysts, but specificity for distinct lesions are variable. Doppler ultrasound may identify an abnormal vessel from the aorta to suspect pulmonary sequestration, but it cannot confirm hybrid (mixed) lesions. Large lesions may cause cardiac compression, resulting in hydrops foetalis and fetal demise. Fetal intervention, fortunately, is indicated in only 10% of prenatally diagnosed lesions that are at risk of developing hydrops foetalis. These are amenable to foetal intervention through thoracentesis, pleuroamniotic shunting, or laser ablation of the feeding artery. Postnatal symptomatic lesions are subject to early surgical treatment; however, the management of postnatal asymptomatic lesions remains controversial. Most centres now propose postnatal computed tomography (CT) scan imaging followed by surgery at 3–6 months of age for asymptomatic lesions due to the risk of infection and malignancy. Small lesions of less than 1 cm on CT scan may be managed conservatively. Proponents of conservative management follow all asymptomatic lesions with serial CT scanning (Figure 44.2).

Congenital Cystic Adenomatous Malformation

Congenital cystic adenomatous malformation (CCAM) is the commonest congenital lung lesion, accounting for 50–70% of these lesions. It is a hamartomatous malformation characterised by the lack of normal alveoli and an excessive proliferation and cystic dilatation of terminal respiratory bronchioles with varying types of epithelial lining. The lesions are mainly cystic and intrapulmonary, usually unilobar with a slight predilection for the lower lobes of the lung. The side of the lung, race, and gender are equally affected. In the absence of prenatal scanning the presentation may be at birth with respiratory distress. Distinction from diaphragmatic hernia may be assisted by the position of the stomach on chest radiograph (Figure 44.3). Multicystic lesions are usually noted on chest radiograph. Presentation outside the neonatal period includes nonresolving pneumonia, lung abscesses, empyema, reactive lung disease, failure to thrive, and malignancy. At this stage,

Table 44.1: Langston's classification of congenital lung malformations.

Bronchopulmonary malformation

- Bronchogenic cyst (noncommunicating broncho-pulmonary foregut malformation)
- Bronchial atresia
  - Isolated
  - With systemic arterial/venous connection (intralobar sequestration)
  - With connection to gastrointestinal tract (intra-lobar sequestration/complex or communicating bronchopulmonary foregut malformation)
  - Systemic arterial connection to normal lung
- **CCAM: large cyst type (Stocker type 1)**
  - Isolated
  - With systemic arterial/venous connection (hybrid lesion/intralobar sequestration)
- **CCAM: small cyst type (Stocker type 2)**
  - Isolated
  - With systemic arterial/venous connection (hybrid lesion/intralobar sequestration)
- **Extralobar sequestration**
  - Without connection to gastrointestinal tract (with/without CAM, small cyst type)
  - With connection to gastrointestinal tract (complex/communicating bronchopulmonary foregut malformation)

Pulmonary hyperplasia and related lesions

- Laryngeal atresia
- Solid or adenomatoid form of CCAM (Stocker type 3)
- Polyalveolar lobe

Congenital lobar overinflation

Other cystic lesions

- Lymphatic/lymphangiomatous cysts
- Enteric cysts
- Mesothelial cysts
- Simple parenchymal cysts
- Low-grade cystic pleuropulmonary blastoma

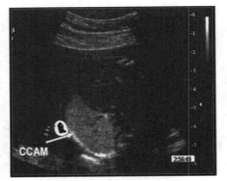

Figure 44.2: Prenatal ultrasound of CCAM.

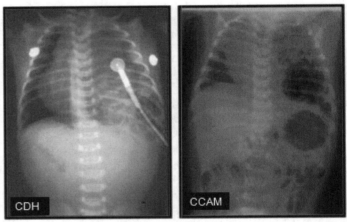

Figure 44.3: Chest radiographs showing congenital diaphragmatic hernia (CDH) and congenital cystic adenomatous malformation of the lung (CCAM).

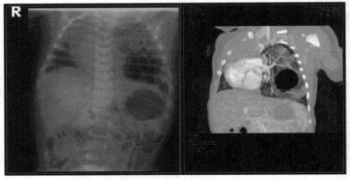

Figure 44.4: CCAM on chest radiograph (left) and CT scan (right).

a distinction should be made from infected pneumatocoele, which resolves with antimicrobial treatment. In difficult cases, a CT scan may help in confirming the diagnosis (Figure 44.4).

Surgical Procedure

The surgical procedure is performed via thoracotomy or more recently thoracoscopically. Lobectomy is preferred to segmentectomy to avoid recurrence of disease infection and development of malignancy in the incomplete resection. At surgery, abnormal vasculature should be looked for in the event of a hybrid lesion. Hybrid lesions are CCAM with intra-lobar pulmonary sequestration (see below). Prenatally diagnosed lesions are discussed above.

Malignant Transformations with CCAM

Bronchioloalveolar carcinoma (BAC) and rhabdomyosarcoma in associ-ation with CCAM have been repeatedly reported in children and adults. Since 1980, more than 25 cases of malignancy have been reported

in children as young as 1 month to 13 years of age. These malignant transformations were noted in primary CCAM lesions and those that were incompletely resected. The long-term malignant potential of in situ CCAMs has been further reported, suggesting postnatal surgical excision by means of lobectomy rather than segmentectomy as well as surgical preference to long-term radiological surveillance. Thus, with the increasing number of reports and case series of malignancy within CCAM, together with the possibility of lung infection, surgical resection in nearly all cases of CCAM is recommended.

Bronchopulmonary Sequestration (BPS)

Bronchopulmonary sequestrations (BPSs) make up 10–30% of congeni-tal cystic lung lesions. These are solid, nonfunctioning congenital lung lesions that have a blood supply originating from the aorta rather than the pulmonary artery and an absence of communication with the bron-chial tree (Figure 44.5). They can be subdivided into *intralobar* BPS or

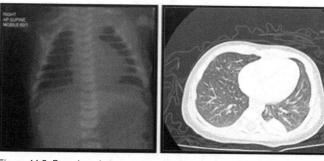

Figure 44.5: Bronchopulmonary sequestration on chest radiograph (left) and CT scan (right).

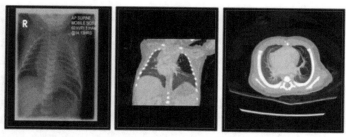

Figure 44.6: Congenital lobar emphysema on chest radiograph (left) and CT scan (right images).

extralobar BPS, with the former enveloped by normal lung parenchyma and the latter are an entirely separate entity with a complete covering of visceral pleura.

Intralobar Sequestration

Intralobar sequestrations usually affect the left lower lobe with an aberrant vessel from the thoracic aorta; however, branches from the abdominal aorta, intercostal vessels and brachiocephalic vessels have been noted. Presentation includes nonresolving pneumonia, lung abscess, and, rarely, haemoptysis. Chest radiography demonstrates a nonaerated atelectatic mass, and a contrast CT should confirm the mass with an aberrant vessel. Management consist of resection via thoracotomy or thoracoscopy.

Extralobar Sequestration

Extralobar sequestration is most commonly found in the left lower chest, with 80–90% above the diaphragm and 10–20% below. The aberrant blood supply is mainly from the thoracic aorta, and 20% arise from the abdominal aorta. Associated anomalies such as diaphragmatic hernia, cardiac defects, arterio-venous malformations, and other anomalies are present in 50% of extralobar sequestration. Presentation is often asymptomatic at birth, but due to arteriovenous shunting may develop congestive cardiac failure in infancy or hydrops prenatally. Chest radiography typically depicts a left posterior mediastinal mass; however, further imaging with contrast CT scan is recommended. A prenatal scan with Doppler ultrasound may identify the aberrant blood supply. Resection via thoracotomy/thoracoscopy in early infancy is recommended.

Congenital Lobar Emphysema

Congenital lobar emphysema (CLE), also known as congenital lobar overinflation (CLO), is characterised by air trapping and overdistention of one or more pulmonary lobes, possibly secondary to a defect in the bronchial cartilage. Less frequent aetiology is extrinsic compression from lymphadenopathy, anomalous vessels, and masses. Antenatal diagnosis of CLE has been reported, and spontaneous regression in the third trimester may occur. The typical postnatal presentation is of respiratory distress, which may necessitate excision of the affected lobe. Asymptomatic patients may be managed expectantly. Diagnosis is confirmed on chest radiograph, and echocardiogram is recommended for the 15–20% associated with congenital heart disease (Figure 44.6).

Bronchogenic Cyst

Bronchogenic cysts contain a lining of respiratory epithelium and have smooth muscle, glandular tissue, and cartilage in the wall and cysts. Bronchogenic cysts may share an embryological origin with that of foregut duplications. Such lesions are found in the mediastinum in up to two-thirds of cases, lying adjacent to the major airways, heart, or oesophagus, with the remainder found within the lung parenchyma. Most cases present postnatally, usually with pulmonary infection, but a proportion are diagnosed incidentally. Surgical excision is curative and can be achieved by segementectomy, lobectomy, or simple cyst removal (peripheral lesions). Malignant transformation has not been reported in relation to these lesions.

Hybrid Lesions

Many lateral series have shown that some cystic lung lesions have features of both CCAM and BPS, suggesting that they share the same developmental ancestry and perhaps represent two ends of a broad spectrum of pathology. Any time a congenital lung lesion is approached surgically, the surgeon should be aware of the possibility of an aberrant arterial supply, even if this is not demonstrated by advanced imaging techniques. The possibility of separate coexisting lesions should also be considered.

Communicating Bronchopulmonary Foregut Malformations

Congenital bronchopulmonary foregut malformations are sequestrations that communicate with the upper digestive tract, usually the oesophagus. Diagnosis is suspected with recurrent chest infection and air-filled mass in the mediastinum. Upper gastrointestinal contrast may confirm the diagnosis.

Surgical Technique

Detailed surgical technique is beyond the scope of this book; however, salient points for a left lower lobectomy are described as follows:

1. The patient is positioned in the right lateral decubitus position, left side up, with the arm extended and placed over the head and a rolled towel under the chest for support.

2. A posteriolateral incision is performed over the fourth or fifth intercostal space marked just lateral and below the nipple.

3. Latissimus muscle is divided along the line of incision with serratus anterior muscle spared if possible.

4. Rib space is identified by elevating the scapula to count the ribs and the space entered by dividing the intercostal muscles on the upper border of the lower rib to avoid the intercostal neurovascular bundle.

5. The pleura are entered without damaging the underlying lung, and access to the chest cavity is obtained by using a rib spreader.

6. The interlobar fissure is exposed and the lingular artery identified before the lower lobe artery is ligated and divided.

7. The lung is retracted anteriorly to expose the pulmonary ligament in the basilar region. The ligament is divided to expose the inferior pulmonary vein, which is again ligated and divided.

8. The bronchial attachment to the lobe is divided and sutured with non absorbable suture using the interrupted suturing technique. Air leaks are checked with saline test and lung inflation.

9. Damage to the adjacent structures such as pericardium, aorta and phrenic nerve is avoided.

10. A chest drain with an underwater seal is placed for drainage, and the wound is closed in layers following rib approximation with absorbable sutures. The drain is removed after 24hours provided no air leak is demonstrated.

Outcome

The outcome for lung surgery is excellent except where previous infection existed. Air leaks, residual disease, infection, and damage to adjacent structures are noted morbidities.

Evidence-Based Research

Title	Management of congenital lung lesions.
Authors	Stanton M, Davenport M
Institution	King's College, London UK
Reference	Early Hum Dev 2006; 82(5):289–295.
Problem	Conservative versus surgical management of prenatally diagnosed lesions
Intervention	Surgery
Comparison/ control (quality of evidence)	Review
Outcome/effect	Surgery recommended to avoid long-term complications.

Key Summary Points

1. Cystic lung lesions are rare.

2. Accepted classification is now descriptive.

3. Symptomatic lesions require surgical intervention.

4. Management of asymptomatic lesions is controversial; however, most institutions recommend operative treatment.

5. A chest radiograph may diagnose most symptomatic lesions. A CT scan, where available, should provide better imaging of the lesion.

6. Lobectomy or cystectomy is the treatment of choice in most conditions.

7. Morbidity is due to air leaks and infection, but overall outcomes are good.

Suggested Reading

Calvert JK, Lakhoo K. Antenatally suspected congenital cystic adenomatoid malformation of the lung: postnatal investigation and timing of surgery. J Pediatr Surg 2007; 42(2):411–444.

Farugia M-K, Raza SA, Gould S, Lakhoo K. Congenital lung lesions: classification and concordance of radiological appearance and surgical pathology. PSI 2008; 24:973–977.

Groenman F, Unger S, Post M. The molecular basis for abnormal human lung development. Biol Neonate 2005; 87(3):164–177.

Laberge JM, Puligandla P. Congenital Malformations of the Lungs and Airways. In: Taussig and Landau, eds. Pediatric Respiratory Medicine, 2nd ed. Elsevier, Amsterdam, 2008, chapter 64.

Laberge JM, Puligandla P, Flageole H. Asymptomatic congenital lung malformations. Semin Pediatr Surg 2005; 14(1):16–33.

Langston C. New concepts in the pathology of congenital lung malformations. Semin Pediatr Surg 2003; 12(1):17–37.

Rahman N, Lakhoo K. JPS A comparison between open and thoracoscopic resection of congenital lung lesions. JPS 2009; 44(2):333–336.

CHAPTER 45
CONGENITAL DIAPHRAGMATIC HERNIA AND DIAPHRAGMATIC EVENTRATION

Merrill McHoney
Kokila Lakhoo

Introduction

Congenital diaphragmatic hernia (CDH) is a group of conditions characterised by developmental defects in the diaphragm. The cause is disordered embryogenesis, resulting in incomplete fusion of elements giving rise to the diaphragm. CDH occurs at distinctive sites. The diagnosis can be made in the antenatal period, and can present in the early postnatal period with respiratory distress. Associated lung, vascular, and cardiac abnormalities lead to a high mortality (almost 50% overall), and prompt neonatal management is the most important influence on outcome. In this regard, surgical correction has become a nonurgent secondary intervention. Chromosomal abnormalities are found in 5–30% of cases (trisomy 18 and 13 are the most common). CDH can present outside the neonatal period in patients with minimal physiological compromise. The mortality is negligible in this naturally selected group.

Demographics

The incidence of CDH is 1 in 2,500 to 1 in 3,500 live births. Left-sided CDH is more common than right-sided, with a ratio of 6:1. Bilateral lesions are reported, but they are invariably fatal. Ninety percent of CDH cases are found in a postero-lateral defect (Bochdaleck hernia), and 9% are found in an anterio-medial defect (Morgagni hernia). The remainder of cases comprise the relatively rarer forms of total absence of the diaphragm, absence of the central portion of the diaphragm, and oesophageal hiatal hernia. There is no gender or race predisposition.

Aetiology/Pathophysiology

The diaphragm arises from four mesodermal elements in the embryo:

1. the pleuro-peritoneal membrane (fold);

2. the septum transversum (developing central tendon);

3. the dorsal mesentery of the oesophagus (crural precursor); and

4. somites of the body wall.

Fusion of these elements between the 5th to 8th week of intrauterine life separates the abdominal cavity from the thoracic cavity. The last element to close is the pleuroperitoneal membrane, the site of the Bochdaleck hernia, the commonest form of CDH. Return of the intestinal organs from the umbilicus around the 10th week of gestation can herniate into the chest if there is defective diaphragmatic development. Bowel loops within the chest compress the developing lung and cause lung hypoplasia (in both lungs, but in particular in the lung on the affected side). Development of type II alveolar cells that produce surfactant is also inhibited, resulting in relative surfactant deficiency.

Abnormal development of the pulmonary vasculature leads to pulmonary hypertension and increased pulmonary vasculature reactivity. Thus, the affected neonate is prone to episodes of hypoxia and hypercapnia, which in turn further increase the pulmonary hypertension and cause persistent foetal circulation. Persistent foetal circulation is a state of reduced pulmonary blood flow and pulmonary hypertension with severe right-to-left shunting through the patent ductus atreiosus

and formanen ovale, which further worsens the hypercapnia and hypoxia. This vicious positive cycle can lead to severe physiological consequences in those most affected, and lung hypoplasia/pulmonary hypertension is the most detrimental pathophysiological process that affects outcome.

Clinical Presentation

History
Antenatal

In countries where routine antenatal ultrasound scanning is performed, approximately 50–85% of CDH are diagnosed on antenatal ultrasound scan. The features present antenatally are:

- polyhydramnios;

- absent stomach bubble or stomach bubble in chest;

- bowel loops in chest;

- mediastinal shift; and

- hydrops.

Foetal magnetic resonance imaging (MRI; see Figure 45.1) is also used in some centres for clarification of the diagnosis, to rule out associated anomalies, for planning, and for prognostic features. This is not widely practiced nor available.

Some features in the antenatal scan are associated with a poorer outcome. These are (1) hydrops, (2) contralateral lung-to-head circumference ratio <1.0, (3) diagnosis before 25 weeks gestation, and (4) associated cardiac abnormality. The role of antenatal contralateral lung-to-head circumference ratio in predicting outcome and indication

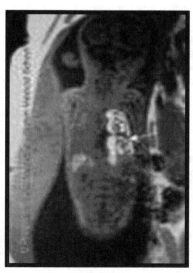

Figure 45.1: Antenatal MRI scan showing a left CDH at a 32-week scan. Bowel loops are seen in the chest, and there is mediastinal shift.

for foetal surgery is being questioned in recent studies, however.[1] Foetal surgery for CDH is being assessed in specialist centres, but as yet, there are no clear indications and benefit from this approach.[2,3]

Postnatal

Postnatally, the infant presents with respiratory distress. The timing of presentation is proportional to the degree of respiratory reserve; the later the presentation, the better the reserve and the baby's outcome. Grunting, tachypnoea, cyanosis, and poor feeding may be present.

Physical examination

A general physical examination may reveal respiratory distress with grunting, use of accessory muscles and cyanosis. The affected hemithorax will have decreased respiratory movement. The trachea and apex beat may be deviated to the contralateral side. Diminished breath sounds with audible bowel sounds may be heard in the affected side. The abdomen is generally scaphoid in those presenting early. If presentation is delayed, however, this sign may not be present.

One particular presentation of CDH is with the constellation of the five malformations making up the pentalogy of Cantrell, a rare defect resulting from a severe mesodermal fusion failure:

1. Diaphragmatic hernia;

2. Lower sternal defect;

3. Pericardial defect;

4. Major cardiac anomaly; and

5. Epigastric exomphalos.

Late and atypical presentations

In the absence of antenatal scanning and the absence of neonatal symptoms, some children may present later in childhood. They may present with poor feeding or vomiting and failure to thrive, poor respiratory reserve to strenuous exercise, or almost incidentally on an x-ray for a suspected chest infection. Subtle respiratory signs may be noted.

Cases are reported of children subject to minimal trauma, with severe respiratory symptoms, who undergo a chest x-ray and a diagnosis of tension pneumothorax is made (mistaking the herniated stomach for air in the pleural space). Needle or tube thoracocentesis of the chest is an avoidable iatrogenic complication if the x-ray is scrutinised carefully and the absence of a diaphragm noted, confirming a diaphragmatic hernia. Most of these cases are found to be a CDH at operation, although a traumatic rupture of the diaphragm is an alternative diagnosis.

Differential diagnosis

The main differential diagnosis and the key features in differentiating them are:

• *Eventration of the diaphragm:* A thin rim of soft tissue shadowing may appear on the chest x-ray, suggesting that some diaphragmatic tissue is present. The diagnosis is best distinguished by using fluoroscopy to demonstrate paradoxical chest movement during respiration, but the distinction is sometimes made only at operation.

• *Congenital pulmonary airway malformations:* Congenital malformations of the airway and lung with cysts in the lower chest can mimic CDH on a plain x-ray of the chest. In these cases, however, the abdominal x-ray demonstrates a normal gas pattern with the nasogastric tube (NGT) in the abdomen, and a good diaphragmatic rim is usually seen. Usually no further imaging is needed to differentiate them, but a computed tomography (CT) scan is helpful in difficult cases.

Investigations

A plain anterior-posterior radiograph of the chest is diagnostic in most cases. The x-ray should be combined with a plain abdominal x-ray with a nasogastric tube in place. Features of the common Bochdaleck hernia on the radiograph are (see Figures 45.2–45.4):

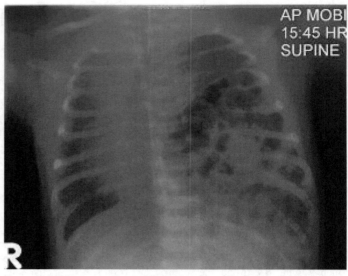

Figure 45.2: Chest x-ray showing a left CDH. Bowel loops are seen in the chest, and there is mediastinal shift. The appearances could be similar to congenital lung cysts, and an abdominal x-ray is needed to confirm the diagnosis.

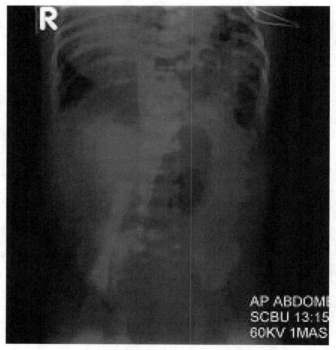

Figure 45.3: Abdominal x-ray of the same patient as in Figure 45.2. Bowel loops are seen in the chest, and there is paucity of gas in the abdomen, confirming herniation. In this patient, the stomach did not herniate; therefore, the NGT is in the abdomen.

• absence of the diaphragm;

• bowel loops seen in the chest, with paucity of loops in the abdomen;

• tip of NGT in the chest (only if stomach is herniated);

• mediastinal shift; or

• with right-sided lesions, a radio-opaque lesion replaces the lung tissue.

With a Morgagni hernia (see Figure 45.5) the features include a radiolucent shadow overlying the heart. A lateral view is helpful in showing this to be in the anterior mediastinum.

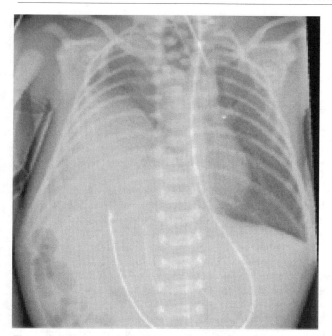

Figure 45.4: Chest and abdominal x-ray of patient showing a right-sided CDH. A soft tissue shadow is seen in the chest and represents the herniated liver. Also note in this patient the presence of a dilated trachea (dilated radiolucent pouch in lower neck/upper chest) as a result of antenatal tracheal occlusion. Remnants of the balloon used is seen as a radio-dense dot in the left side of the chest.

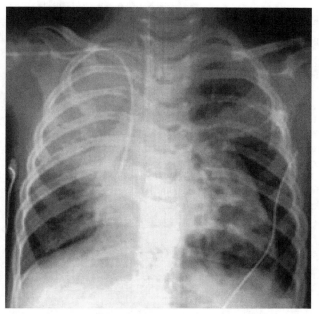

Figure 45.5: Chest X-ray of patient showing a left-sided Morgagni hernia. The bowel loops are seen overlying the cardiac shadow, and loops can be traced from the abdomen just to the left of the midline

Other investigations and their indications are:

• *An echocardiogram* is useful in evaluating cardiac function (shunting, ejection fraction, cardiac output, and changes with inotropic support) and in outlining any cardiac anomalies associated with CDH (atrial and ventricular septal defects).

• *A contrast study* may be indicated in cases of suspected Bochdaleck hernia that do not have a definitive diagnosis on plain radiograph. A contrast enema or meal with follow through may delineate bowel contents in the chest.

• *A renal ultrasound scan* is useful in ruling out any renal abnormalities.

• *Fluoroscopy* of the diaphragm may help differentiate between eventration and CDH in cases that are difficult to distinguish. *Ultrasound* of the diaphragm is less sensitive in picking up paradoxical movement than fluoroscopy, and is sometimes false negative.

Management

The most important management is the resuscitation and stabilisation of the newborn by an experienced neonatologist. If the diagnosis is suspected, avoid bag and mask positive-pressure ventilation (to avoid intestinal distention and possible worsening of respiratory compromise).

The management of CDH is a complex one that involves specialist neonatal ventilatory and cardiovascular support in severe cases.[4,5] The essence of neonatal management can be summarised as follows:

• Prompt endotracheal intubation in the delivery room for respiratory distress.

• Replogle tube or wide-bore nasogastric tube insertion.

• Chest and abdominal x-ray to confirm diagnosis, assess NGT position, and exclude other diagnoses.

• Early measurement of blood gases, repeated at regular intervals to aid management.

• Surfactant administration, used in some centres in selected cases.

• Preductal oxygen saturations maintained at 85–90%.

• Minimal ventilation pressures to reduce barotrauma (iatrogenic injury from ventilation strategies may be significant and should be minimised).

• Volume resuscitation and vasopressors (dopamine and dobutamine) often required to maintain systemic blood pressure (BP) and reduce right-to-left shunting.

• Pulmonary vasodilatation with inhaled nitric oxide and occasionally other vasodilators (e.g., nitroprusside).

• Consideration of high-frequency oscillatory ventilation when conventional ventilation fails or when peak airway pressures remain high (>30 cm H_2O).

• Extracorporeal membrane oxygenation (ECMO), which has not offered consistent beneficial results in most studies. Oxygenation index (FiO_2 × mean airway pressure × 100/PaO_2) can be used to predict the need for ECMO in centres where this is offered. An oxygenation index value of >40 is an indication of severe respiratory failure and the need for ECMO.

• Initially not feeding by mouth (but trophic feeding is not strictly contraindicated in those stabilising with no signs of obstruction). Reliable central venous access is required for administration of drugs or fluids and/or parenteral nutrition.

One method used to predict outcome in the postnatal period is a formula developed at the Red Cross Hospital in South Africa,[6] (respiratory rate × PCO_2 × FiO_2 × mean airway pressure/PaO_2 × 6000), based on the first arterial blood gas obtained on initiation of resuscitation. A value greater than 5 was used as a cutoff between survivors and nonsurvivors, with 16/16 (100%) of patients above this value dying and 17/20 (85%) below this value surviving. Overall, it had a 91% predictive value.

Surgery

Surgery is usually contemplated only in those who stabilise and improve on medical management. Stability is indicated by a decreased ventilatory requirement (transition from high frequency to conventional ventilation being a good sign of improvement), decreased oxygen requirements, return of haemodynamic stability, and weaning off inotropes and pulmonary vasodilators if they were required. In those patients who have little cardiorespiratory compromise, a period of 24 hours (the so-called "honeymoon period" in CDH) to allow any instability to announce itself is prudent. Although there may be no long-term advantage of early versus delayed surgery,[7] a somewhat delayed approach (24 to 48 hours) may allow patients with significant cardiopulmonary disease, who would not survive despite any operative intervention, to be selected. In an otherwise stable patient, however, any long delay can be detrimental.[8]

The infant is taken to the operating theatre, and antibiotics, if not already administered, are given at induction. The operative steps are summarised as follows:

1. A transverse supra-umbilical incision is made.

2. Rarely, for large right-sided lesions with a larger proportion of the liver in the chest, a thoracoabdominal incision is required.

3. The intestines or viscera are inspected and gently and gradually reduced from the chest. Often, on the left, the spleen is particularly difficult to reduce without causing injury, and a finger or retractor introduced into the chest can be use to guide it into the abdomen. Rarely, the defect in the diaphragm needs to be enlarged to facilitate this. In right-sided lesions, reduction of the liver can be associated with altered venous return to the heart due to reconfiguration of the inferior vena cava; this should be anticipated and communicated to the anaesthetist.

4. After reduction of the abdominal contents, the chest is examined for a hernia sac. This is best done by grasping and incising over a lower rib to free a sac if present. The entire sac should be excised. The hypoplastic lung can then usually be seen in the chest.

5. The defect in the diaphragm is inspected, and the decision for primary or reinforced closure is assessed. Mobilisation of the leafs of muscle, in particular on the posterio-lateral aspect, can increase the amount of muscle available.

6. Primary closure is then achieved with interrupted nonabsorbable sutures. With large defects, sutures can be placed individually and tied at the end. Sutures may need to be placed around lower ribs in large defects.

7. If the defect is too large for primary closure, a prosthetic patch of artificial or natural graft material is fashioned in the size and shape of the defect, allowing for a small amount of curvature. The choice of material will depend on local availability, but can include polypropylene, Dacron®, Gore-Tex® (polytetrafluoroethylene), Surgisis®, and Permacol®. The patch is sutured in place with nonabsorbable sutures in a manner similar to that described above; again, the lower ribs may need to be used to anchor the stitches. A chest drain is not mandatory, but is used by some judiciously.

8. If artificial material is not available, a muscular graft (e.g., abdominal wall or a lattissimus dorsi graft) is created to close the defect.

9. Abnormalities of rotation can be associated with CDH, and if a narrow midgut mesentery is present, a Ladd's procedure is performed.

10. Abdominal wall closure can be difficult due to the increased tension caused by return of the intestines into the abdomen. Occasionally, to avoid a tight abdominal wall closure with the consequences of respiratory compromise and abdominal compartment syndrome, the abdomen may need to be closed with a patch.

11. A postoperative chest x-ray is performed to check the position of the diaphragm.

Laparoscopic and thoracoscopic approaches for CDH repair have been described by some centres in select cases. These approaches are suitable for specialised personnel in experienced centres, as they can impose further physiological stresses on the infant.

Postoperative Complications

Bleeding due to trauma to liver or spleen can occur intraoperatively and should be anticipated with cross-matched blood. Trauma to the intestines, leading to perforation and peritonitis, is also possible.

Postoperative pleural effusion is expected in the immediate postoperative period. Persistence of this can impair lung expansion and weaning off the ventilator. This complication is increased if a hernia sac is not identified and left in situ. The sac then will act as a compartment for fluid to accumulate. Intraoperative excision of the hernia sac, if present, is therefore the best prevention. Management usually consists of inactivity to allow the fluid to resorb. In those cases where this is delayed, thus causing respiratory symptoms or delayed recovery, drainage via a chest drain may be required; this is seldom necessary.

Mediastinal shifts can occur in the postoperative period, as pressure and volume changes due to reducing the abdominal contents ensue. The mediastinal shift induced by CDH does not usually shift back to the central position immediately, but does so slowly. The space is initially filled by air (Figure 45.6) and later on by fluid.

Misinterpretation of the postoperative changes can lead to unnecessary insertion of a chest drain. This can cause large changes in volumes and pressures, with consequential changes in lung expansion, resulting in a true pneumothorax (especially in the contralateral lung, which will then require drainage).

An incisional hernia can occur in patients with tight abdominal wall closure and those with patch closure of the abdominal wall. Semielective or elective repair after a period of stabilisation and growth is advisable.

Recurrence is seen in 5–15% of patients.[9,10] The incidence of recurrence is higher in patients in whom a patch repair is needed (up to 50%) and in those in whom the closure is under tension. The incidence of recurrence is reported to be lower in patch repair using biological-based material (e.g., Permacol);[11,12] however, this is not a universal finding.[13] Management of recurrence is surgical, with principles similar to those for primary surgery. With large defects and those with multiple recurrences, the need for muscle-based (e.g., abdominal wall or latissimus dorsi) flaps[14,15] should be considered.

Gastro-oesophageal reflux is seen in 50–90% of patients,[9] and should be treated as in any other patient. Overall, however, the requirement for surgical fundoplication is higher than in normal children.

Poor feeding and growth are also seen in some (sometimes needing gastrostomy placement).

Intestinal obstruction caused by adhesions can occur,[10] and initially is treated conservatively or operatively, depending on clinical status.

Chest wall deformities can occur in the forms of pectus carinatum (approximately 30%) and scoliosis (20%).[9] The incidence is higher in those patients with a large defect requiring a tight closure, or those

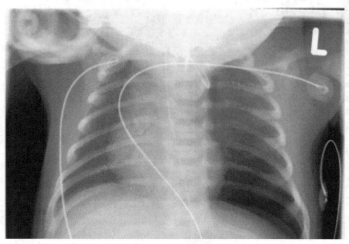

Figure 45.6: Early postoperative chest x-ray in same patient as in Figure 45.2. The lower right chest cavity is filled with air and a small amount of fluid. There is still some mediastinal shift.

requiring a patch repair. Management is usually conservative, as these deformities tend to be mild. Operative intervention is reserved for those with severe deformities.

Chronic lung disease is common in severely affected patients.[9] A mild restrictive pattern of lung function is seen in most patients, but is not necessarily associated with clinical symptoms. Alveolar growth continues up to 8 years of age, and children can outgrow any mild restrictions to exercise tolerance and susceptibility to chest infections. An increased incidence of asthma is seen. Those with severe neonatal lung disease develop chronic lung disease. Continued pulmonary hypertension into infancy and childhood are associated with poor outcome. There is a late mortality, due to chronic lung disease and associated or secondary cardiac dysfunction, which can be as late as 4 years of age.[16]

Neurodevelopmental delay and hearing loss are nonsurgical complications that are consequences of poor oxygenation; they are twice as common in children who receive ECMO support.[9,16]

Prognosis and Outcomes

A summary of the major significant outcome measures and their main determinants (in parentheses) follows.

- death (pulmonary hypertension, associated cardiac anomalies, chromosomal abnormalities, early severe disease);

- neurological impairment and hearing loss (pulmonary hypertension, size of defect, early severe disease);

- chronic lung disease (pulmonary hypertension, size of defect, early severe disease); or

- recurrence (size of defect, need for patch repair).

Thus, the main adverse determinants of outcome seem to be associated chromosomal and cardiac anomalies, severity of the pulmonary hypertension, and size of the defect.

Prevention

There are no known preventive measures for CDH.

Ethical Issues

Two main ethical issues surround the management of CDH. Both are outside the scope of this text, but are discussed here briefly. The first is the indication and benefit of any antenatal intervention in the foetus. Antenatal plugging of the trachea is theoretically advantageous by allowing increased foetal lung growth.[17] The indications for intervention are not clear from the research done to date. It is said that infants with adverse features on antenatal scan could benefit from plugging. Intervention is possibly too late to affect the developmental consequences at this stage, however; this may be borne out in the lack of convincing benefit to date.[2] The resources and personnel necessary to run such a programme (or even research into it) are huge, and the debate on cost versus benefit is likely to continue.

Second, the use of ECMO as "rescue therapy" for infants with severe lung disease remains contentious. In one large trial in the United Kingdom,[16] the benefit of ECMO on survival in CDH could not be established. A meta-analysis of randomised trials also failed to show a long-term benefit (late mortality was similar in ECMO and non-ECMO CDH patients).[18] Furthermore, the morbidity induced in those that do survive (related complications included intracranial infarct or bleed, major bleeding, seizures, and infection) is significantly high[16] and can be costly. Around one-fifth have severe neurodevelopmental problems.[16] The use of ECMO continues, and its advantages need to be continually investigated to resolve this issue.

Eventration of the Diaphragm

Eventration of the diaphragm is defined as an abnormal elevation of an otherwise intact diaphragm due to poor or absent musculature. Although some of the mechanical effects are similar to those of CDH, the incidence of pulmonary hypertension is low and the degree of associated pulmonary hypoplasia is minimal. Thus, the presentation is less dramatic and usually somewhat delayed and the outcome is significantly better.

Demographics

Like CDH, eventration of the diaphragm is more common on the left. Bilateral lesions are rare. There is no gender or race predilection.

Aetiology/Pathophysiology

Eventration of the diaphragm is thought to result from failure of myoblastic transformation of the diaphragm or faulty ingrowth of muscle into the dome during embryogenesis. The involved hemidiaphragm is therefore inactive and demonstrates paradoxical movement with respiration.

Although the elevated diaphragm can lead to lung compression and hypoplasia with associated pulmonary vasculature hypertension, as in CDH, this complication is uncommon or mild in eventration. The incidence of other anomalies is low.

Paralysis of the diaphragm due to phrenic nerve palsy or traumatic/iatrogenic phrenic nerve damage can give a picture similar to eventration. The distinction is sometime difficult in those with a potential cause (birth trauma, cardiac/thoracic surgery). To some extent, the distinction is not important because the treatment, *in the symptomatic child,* is usually the same.

Clinical Presentation

History

Respiratory distress, tachypnoea, and cyanosis may be present in the early neonatal period in severe cases of eventration of the diaphragm. Presentation is more often less dramatic and later than for those with CDH. Due to the limited respiratory reserve, poor feeding or sucking, associated with tiring, is common. Failure to thrive may be the presenting complaint due to poor feeding. Vomiting may be the presenting complaint. Failure to recover from a lower respiratory tract infection or recurrent infections may prompt a chest x-ray that brings the diagnosis to light.

Physical

The physical findings may be minimal. There may be signs of respiratory distress. Decreased air entry may be present in both lungs but more marked on the affected side. The cardiac impulse may be shifted away from the affected side.

Investigations

A plain chest x-ray is suggestive of the diagnosis in most cases. Signs on the radiograph are that the right hemidiaphragm is more than two rib spaces higher than the left (Figure 45.7), or the left is more than one rib space higher than the right (Figure 45.8).

It is sometimes difficult to distinguish the radiological picture of eventration of the diaphragm from that of CDH. Unlike the case with CDH, however, there is usually a suggestion of a thin rim of diaphragm.

Fluoroscopy is diagnostic in most cases. Paradoxical movement of the affected diaphragm is seen during screening. (This sign is lost in patients who are ventilated.)

Ultrasound screening to demonstrate paradoxical movements can also be used to make the diagnosis, but this process is less sensitive than fluoroscopy, mainly due to the inability to see both diaphragms simultaneously.

Management

Patients who are asymptomatic or patients who improve without intervention may be treated conservatively. Conservative treatment for asymptomatic cases suspected to be due to phrenic nerve injury can also be advocated, with hope for recovery if possible. Operative management is the treatment of choice in symptomatic cases.

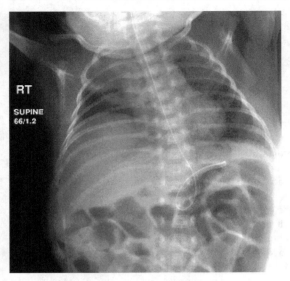

Figure 45.7: Right-sided eventration of the diaphragm.

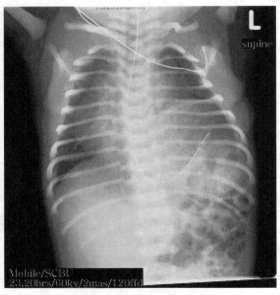

Figure 45.8: Left-sided eventration of the diaphragm.

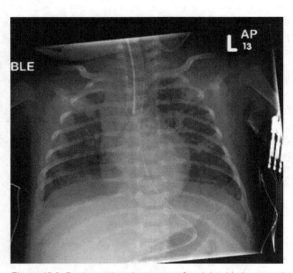

Figure 45.9: Postoperative chest x-ray after right-sided eventration repair for the same patient as in Figure 45.7.

Surgery

For left-sided lesions, the approach can be either abdominal or thoracic. For lesions on the right side, a thoracic approach is preferential. The thoracic approach is through a posterolateral 7th to 9th rib space. The abdominal approach is usually subcostal. Bilateral cases can be approached through a transverse upper abdominal incision. A thoracoscopic approach may be used if skills and resources are available.

The key features of the operation are:

• Confirmation of the diagnosis (versus CDH).

• Plication of the diaphragm by using several rows of pledgeted nonabsorbable sutures to obtain a relatively flat diaphragm.

• Bites of the diaphragm are taken at suitable intervals (~1 cm) in a radial fashion (usually, three or four rows of sutures are needed).

• These sutures can be placed individually without tying, and tied sequentially at the end.

• Identification and avoidance of the branches of the phrenic nerve, if possible.

• A chest drain may be left after a thoracic approach, although this is not mandatory.

A postoperative chest x-ray is suggested to check the position of the diaphragm (Figure 45.9).

Postoperative Complications

There are relatively few postoperative complications with this surgery.[19] Trauma to the intestines and liver during a thoracic approach is avoided by careful placement of sutures into the diaphragm. Postoperative pneumothorax is also uncommon, and usually resolves with chest drainage. Adhesive intestinal obstruction is possible after an abdominal approach. Recurrence is possible, but is much less common than in CDH.

Prognosis and Outcomes

The prognosis is very good in the absence of other anomalies. Respiratory mechanics are improved by plication, with increased tidal volume and vital capacity and improvement of symptoms. In a follow-up study 1 to 5 years postplication, there was no recurrence of symptoms,[19] with only one of nine patients having an elevated diaphragm. In the rest, the diaphragm was flat but immobile.

Prevention

Avoidance of the phrenic nerve during surgery and procedures that put it at risk is preventive in cases due to phrenic nerve injury.

Evidence-Based Research

Table 45.1 presents a meta-analysis that evaluates the use of ECMO in infants with CDH.

Table 45.1: Evidence-based research.

Title	Extracorporeal membrane oxygenation in infants with congenital diaphragmatic hernia: a systematic review of the evidence
Authors	Morini F, Goldman A, Pierro A
Institution	Great Ormond Street Hospital for Children NHS Trust, London, UK
Reference	Eur J Pediatr Surg
Problem	The aim of this study was to evaluate the evidence supporting the use of extracorporeal membrane oxygenation (ECMO) in infants with congenital diaphragmatic hernia (CDH).
Intervention	A meta-analysis of randomised controlled trials (RCTs) comparing ECMO and conventional mechanical ventilation (CMV)
Comparison/ control (quality of evidence)	Meta-analysis
Outcome/ effect	The early mortality was significantly lower with ECMO compared to CMV (RR 0.73 [95 % CI 0.55-0.99]; p < 0.04); however, late mortality was similar in the two groups (RR 0.83 [0.66-1.05]; p = 0.12).
Historical significance/ comments	Nonrandomised studies suggest a reduction in mortality with ECMO. However, differences in the indications for ECMO and improvements in other treatment modalities may contribute to this reduction. The meta-analysis of RCTs indicates a reduction in early mortality with ECMO but no long-term benefit.

Key Summary Points

1. Congenital diaphragmatic hernia is associated with a relatively high mortality related to the associated pulmonary and cardiovascular abnormalities present, and carries some long-term morbidity in most cases. However, self-selected patients who present late have little long-term morbidity.

2. Ventilatory and support mechanisms for patients with congenital diaphragmatic hernia have evolved significantly, but with minimal impact on survival in the severe cases.

3. At present, advanced support for congenital diaphragmatic hernia using ECMO is costly and does not seem to reduce the long-term mortality; it may contribute to more morbidity.

4. The most important factors influencing outcome and long-term morbidity seem to be associated chromosomal and cardiac anomalies, the severity of the pulmonary hypertension, and the size of the defect.

5. Surgery for congenital diaphragmatic hernia is simple in most cases, but can be technically demanding in those with a large defect, requiring knowledge of methods available for secondary closure. Surgery for recurrence can also be demanding, calling for advanced flap procedures.

6. Other surgical procedures for gastro-oesophageal reflux and feeding difficulties or other complications may be required.

7. Unlike congenital diaphragmatic hernia, eventration of the diaphragm is not usually associated with severe morbidity and mortality in most cases. Surgical correction of symptomatic cases is most often rewarded with prompt recovery with little long-term outcome.

References

1. Ba'ath ME, Jesudason EC, Losty PD. How useful is the lung-to-head ratio in predicting outcome in the fetus with congenital diaphragmatic hernia? A systematic review and meta-analysis. Ultrasound Obstet Gynecol 2007; 30(6):897–906.

2. Harrison MR, Keller RL, Hawgood SB, et al. A randomized trial of fetal endoscopic tracheal occlusion for severe fetal congenital diaphragmatic hernia. N Engl J Med 2003; 349(20):1916–1924.

3. Kitano Y. Prenatal intervention for congenital diaphragmatic hernia. Semin Pediatr Surg 2007; 16(2):101–108.

4. Mohseni-Bod H, Bohn D. Pulmonary hypertension in congenital diaphragmatic hernia. Semin Pediatr Surg 2007; 16(2):126–133.

5. Logan JW, Rice HE, Goldberg RN, Cotten CM. Congenital diaphragmatic hernia: a systematic review and summary of best-evidence practice strategies. J Perinatol 2007; 27(9):535–549.

6. Numanoglu A, Morrison C, Rode H. Prediction of outcome in congenital diaphragmatic hernia. Pediatr Surg Int 1998; 13(8):564–568.

7. Moyer V, Moya F, Tibboel R, et al. Late versus early surgical correction for congenital diaphragmatic hernia in newborn infants. Cochrane Database Syst Rev 2002; (3):CD001695.

8. Grant H, Rode H, Cywes S. Potential danger of "trial of life" approach to congenital diaphragmatic hernia. J Pediatr Surg 1994; 29(3):399.

9. Lally KP, Engle W. Postdischarge follow-up of infants with congenital diaphragmatic hernia. Pediatrics 2008; 121(3):627–632.

10. St Peter SD, Valusek PA, Tsao K, et al. Abdominal complications related to type of repair for congenital diaphragmatic hernia. J Surg Res 2007; 140(2):234–236.

11. Mitchell IC, Garcia NM, Barber R, et al. Permacol: a potential biologic patch alternative in congenital diaphragmatic hernia repair. J Pediatr Surg 2008; 43(12):2161–2164.

12. Smith MJ, Paran TS, Quinn F, Corbally MT. The SIS extracellular matrix scaffold-preliminary results of use in congenital diaphragmatic hernia (CDH) repair. Pediatr Surg Int 2004; 20(11-12):859–862.

13. Grethel EJ, Cortes RA, Wagner AJ, et al. Prosthetic patches for congenital diaphragmatic hernia repair: Surgisis vs Gore-Tex. J Pediatr Surg 2006; 41(1):29–33.

14. Barbosa RF, Rodrigues J, Correia-Pinto J, et al. Repair of a large congenital diaphragmatic defect with a reverse latissimus dorsi muscle flap. Microsurgery 2008; 28(2):85–88.

15. Masumoto K, Nagata K, Souzaki R, et al. Effectiveness of diaphragmatic repair using an abdominal muscle flap in patients with recurrent congenital diaphragmatic hernia. J Pediatr Surg 2007; 42(12):2007–2011.

16. Davis PJ, Firmin RK, Manktelow B, et al. Long-term outcome following extracorporeal membrane oxygenation for congenital diaphragmatic hernia: the UK experience. J Pediatr 2004; 144(3):309–315.

17. Jani JC, Nicolaides KH, Gratacos E, Vandecruys H, Deprest JA. Fetal lung-to-head ratio in the prediction of survival in severe left-sided diaphragmatic hernia treated by fetal endoscopic tracheal occlusion (FETO). Am J Obstet Gynecol 2006; 195(6):1646–1650.

18. Morini F, Goldman A, Pierro A. Extracorporeal membrane oxygenation in infants with congenital diaphragmatic hernia: a systematic review of the evidence. Eur J Pediatr Surg 2006; 16(6):385–391.

19. Tiryaki T, Livanelioglu Z, Atayurt H. Eventration of the diaphragm. Asian J Surg 2006; 29(1):8–10.

CHAPTER 46
PLEURAL EFFUSION AND EMPYEMA

Francis A. Uba
Donald E. Meier
Eric S. Borgstein

Introduction

In Africa, as elsewhere, the surgeon is often requested to insert a chest tube for the drainage of pleural fluid. The most common reason for such a request is a postpneumonic infected effusion, or empyema. A chest tube, however, is often an adequate solution to this problem; in some cases, more complicated therapy is required. It is therefore important that the paediatric surgeon appreciates all aspects of pleural space infections (PSIs) in children.

A pleural effusion (PE) is any collection of fluid in the pleural space. Parapneumonic exudative effusions occur in up to 50% of pneumonias. Empyema thoracis (ET) is the accumulation of pus in the pleural space. ET remains a very significant cause of childhood mortality and morbidity in the developing world. Poverty, ignorance, inappropriate antibiotic use, malnutrition, delay in seeking treatment, and lack of supportive care are major impediments to adequate treatment.[1-3]

Empyema is an infected pleural effusion and is usually the result of uncontrolled pulmonary infection or pneumonia. Indiscriminate use of antibiotics and the emergence of antibiotic-resistant organisms have resulted in an increase in the frequency of empyema complicating pneumonia. ET has the reputation of being the worst treated of the common disorders of the chest. Empyema is often recognised after the patient has already received antibiotics, and culture and gram stain may be negative in up to 30% of patients. Reports of anaerobic bacteria isolated from pleural fluid have ranged from 38% to 76%.[4,5] Current treatment of empyema in children is highly variable, due in part to both provider experiences and the variable clinical presentations.

The management of ET in children has evoked considerable controversy.[6,7] The literature provides many options but assists little in establishing the ideal treatment.[6-15] Generally, recommendations have been based on institutional traditions, personal experience, and limited case reviews. Decisions about individual cases are further influenced by varying criteria, such as patient age, clinical status, antibiotic response, stage and duration of the empyema, and the organism cultured.[16]

Demographics

The incidence of empyema thoracis is unknown, although about 50–70% of children admitted with ET have pneumonia.[17] ET affects both sexes equally.

Aetiology/Pathophysiology

A pleural effusion is either an exudate or a transudate, which are distinguished on the basis of protein content. An exudate is characterised by a protein content of >3 g/l. A lactate dehdrogenase (LDH) level of >200 is also diagnostic. Plasma/serum ratios of protein (>0.5) or LDH (>0.6) are more accurate but seldom available. A transudate is usually caused by medical conditions such as congestive heart failure, nephrotic syndrome, and liver cirrhosis; the pleural tap is generally clear and straw-coloured. Exudates are found in postinfective effusions, malignancy, tuberculosis (TB), and other conditions. ET is never a primary condition. A parapneumonic effusion is the most common cause of empyema in childhood.

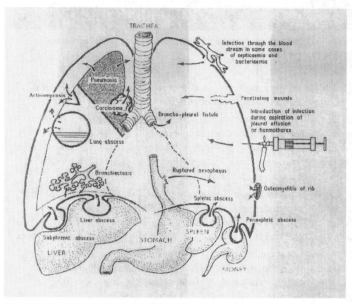

Source: Adeloye A, ed. Companion to Surgery in Africa, 2nd ed. Churchill Livingstone, 1987.

Figure 46.1: Empyema. Sources of infection.

The causes of ET in children include (see Figure 46.1):

1. Pneumonia (usually caused by *Staphylococcus aureus*, *S. pneumoniae*, group A streptococci or *Haemophilus influenza*). There may be anaerobic infections, infections secondary to aspiration, or infections with *Mycoplasma pneumoniae* and viruses.

2. Mycobacterial infections (especially in immunosuppressed patients) and fungal infections.

3. Ruptured lung abscess (usually caused by *S. aureus*).

4. Trauma (e.g., penetrating trauma to the lungs, fracture of ribs, or perforated oesophagus).

5. Amoebiasis (from amoebic abscess).

6. Contiguous infections of the oesophagus, mediastinum, or subdiaphragmatic region.

7. Spread of infections of the retropharyngeal, retroperitoneal, paravertebral, or subphrenic spaces.

8. Malignancy, including Kaposi sarcoma in children with human immunodeficiency virus (HIV) infection.

Host factors that contribute to alterations in pleural permeability, such as noninfectious inflammatory diseases, infection, trauma, or malignancy, may allow accumulation of a thin serous fluid (pleural effusion or parapneumonic effusion) in the pleural space, which may become secondarily infected. As the body attempts to fight off infection, the cavity starts filling up with pleural fluid, pus, and dead pleura cells.

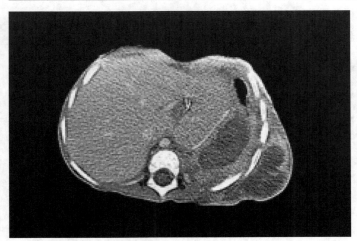

Figure 46.2: Empyema with extension forming subcutaneous abscess and empyema necessitans.

The development of parapneumonic pleural effusions is gradual, and progression to empyema occurs in three phases:

1. *Exudative stage*, or acute phase: This stage is characterised by increased permeability and a small serous fluid collection. At this stage, the pleural cavity fills with an abnormal amount of pleural fluid containing some pus from the infectious condition, contains mostly neutrophils, and is often sterile.

2. *Fibrinopurulent stage:* This second phase is marked by a thickening of the fluid, the accumulation of fibrin—a fibrous, protein-based coagulant—in the cavity, and the formation of fibrin membrane deposition, which forms partitions or loculations within the pleural space.

3. *Organising stage,* or chronic phase: If left untreated, the chronic phase begins, during which a pleural peel is created by the resorption of fluid, forming a thick fibrous material that can entrap the lung parenchyma.

Left untreated, the ET burrows through the parietal pleura, usually into the chest wall, to form a subcutaneous abscess that eventually may rupture through the skin and discharge spontaneously, forming an empyema necessitans[18] (Figure 46.2).

Clinical Features

For both pleural effusion and empyema, the most common preceding factor is pneumonia. The usual presenting symptoms are a general discomfort or uneasiness, with fever, cough, and dyspnoea with nasal flaring.

Depending on the underlying condition, there may also be haemoptysis, chest pain, night sweats, dehydration, and/or weight loss. The inflammation of the pleural space may cause abdominal pain and vomiting. Symptoms may be blunted, and fever may not be present in patients who are immunocompromised.

In more progressive cases, the patient might develop very foul breath or cough up bloody or offensive-looking sputum with a strong fetid odour. There may be a history of TB contact or treatment for other manifestations of Kaposi sarcoma.

Clinically, there is not much to differentiate a pleural effusion and empyema. The usual findings are dullness to percussion, decreased breath sounds, decreased vocal fremitus, and tracheal shift. These signs may vary, however, depending on the causative organism and the duration of the illness.

Auscultation may reveal crackles, decreased breath sounds, and possibly a pleural rub if the process is recognised before a large amount of fluid accumulates. Dullness to percussion and decreased breath sounds are likely findings, but they are difficult to elicit in the younger child, who, because of discomfort, may be less cooperative with the examination.

Failure to improve after pneumonia, the classical physical signs, and radiological evidence of pleural fluid are diagnostic.

Investigations

Imaging

- Plain chest radiography (upright views) should show obliteration of the diaphragmatic margins (costophrenic angles) with pleural fluid collections (Figure 46.3). Because up to 400 ml may be required before these costophrenic angles are obscured in older children and adolescents, further diagnostic imaging may be needed.

- The erect chest x-ray may show an air fluid level (Figure 46.4) if there is lung collapse, an associated pneumothorax, and/or infection with anaerobic bacteria.

- Indistinct diaphragmatic contours merit lateral decubitus views of the chest. This may show layering of fluid. The absence of free layering on the decubitus films does not exclude the possibility of a loculated pleural effusion.

- In moderate effusion, the radiograph may demonstrate displacement of the mediastinum to the contralateral hemithorax, as well as scoliosis.

- Free-flowing pleural effusions suggest less complicated parapneumonic processes, which may not require extensive diagnostic and therapeutic interventions.

- An ultrasound scan is a sensitive test and can also be used to localise loculated effusions and to guide targeted drainage.

- Computed tomography (CT) may identify the presence of consolidated lung or fibrinous septations. In situations of complex fluid collections, chest CT imaging is the study of choice because it can detect and define pleural fluid and image the airways, guide interventional procedures, and discriminate between pleural fluid and chest consolidation.

- Viewing the pleural space by using a thoracoscope to examine its characteristics may also help the diagnosis in complex cases.

Other Investigations

- Thoracocentesis is the standard diagnostic test. Aspirated pus or fluid should always be cultured; in a febrile patient, blood cultures should be done also. Where the cause of the pleural effusion is not clear or if the fluid is bloodstained, cytological investigation should also be done.

- Blood culture is obtained to assist in the identification of the offending organism. In paediatric patients, where sputum production is uncommon, identifying the cause of the pulmonary symptoms early in the course of a pulmonary infection is difficult. However, with parapneumonic effusions, the patient may become bactaeremic as the organism invades the pleural space, and a blood culture may reveal the organism.

- Total serum protein.

- Total white cell blood count.

- Culture and serologic studies of the aspirated pleural fluid, which may reveal bacterial, mycobacterial, and fungal isolates.

- Cell count and differential of aspirated pleural fluid are taken. Although the pleural fluid obtained at thoracentesis is typically purulent, with an elevated white blood count (WBC) count and a predominance of leucocytes, an effusion evaluated early in the infectious process may well be more transudative, with a less cellular WBC and a differential that has fewer leucocytes predominant. Regardless of the cell count and differential, the treatment should be based on clinical course, pending the culture results. Cytokine analyses of pleural fluid have been performed in experi-

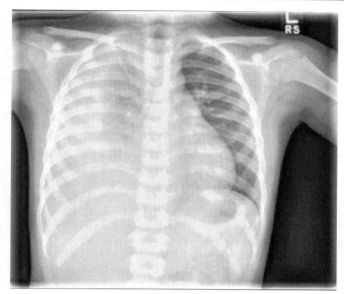

Figure 46.3: Empyema with lung entrapment.

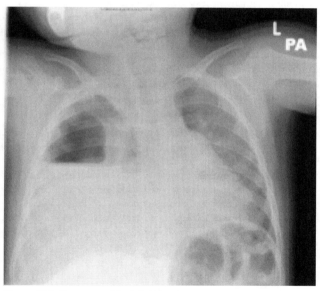

Figure 46.4: Empyema with air fluid levels.

mental settings and may prove to add prognostic value on the degree of inflammation present; these may be beneficial in determining treatment course in the near future.

• Where malignant effusion is suspected, cytological investigation is mandatory. Rarely, a pleural biopsy may be indicated.

• Pleural fluid latex agglutination (or counterimmunoelectrophoresis (CIE) for specific bacteria) may be helpful if the cause of the infection cannot be ascertained from the usual culture results.

Management

There is contention regarding the management of empyema in children. The greatest discrepancies occur between nonsurgical and surgical specialists. The most controversial area in the management of empyema concerns which patients would benefit from pleural drainage and the selection of the appropriate drainage intervention. For uncomplicated free-flowing empyema, surgical intervention is rarely needed; however, surgery is usually indicated for the multiloculated persistent empyema for which initial therapy may have been delayed or failed.

Because many of the infections that cause empyema are indolent, a physician often sees patients after their empyema has already reached the fibrino-purulent or organising stage. These patients often are subjected to multiple surgical procedures and long hospital stays before the empyema is successfully treated.

Thoracentesis, tube thoracostomy, intrapleural thrombolytics (urokinase), thoracoscopic drainage, open drainage, and decortication all have success rates ranging from 10 to 90%.[23,24] The variability in the success rates of these procedures can be attributed, in part, to the stage of the empyema at presentation. In the initial exudative stage, an exudative effusion forms during the first 72 hours; this will usually resolve as the pneumonia clears up following antibiotics therapy.

Antibiotic therapy and drainage of fluid collection are the mainstays of treatment. Broad-spectrum intravenous antibiotic cover should be commenced as soon as pus is aspirated from the chest and before culture results are available. For a simple pleural effusion, aspiration of the pleural space by thoracocentesis is usually adequate but may be repeated as required. A malignant pleural effusion, such as that found in Kaposi sarcoma, should be treated with repeated aspirations and chemotherapy.

The initial treatment of ET is medical. Appropriate antibiotic selection should be based on the gram stain and culture of the pleural fluid; however, because a large number of patients may have already received antibiotics at the time of thoracentesis, an empiric selection of the most appropriate antibiotics is necessary.[19] The choice of antibiotics should be based on the most common pathogens that cause pneumonia within the patient's age range and geographic location. When the organism is identified, the antibiotics may be changed to most specifically cover for the pathogen.

The duration of treatment is determined by the response to therapy; a patient usually receives 10–14 days of intravenous antibiotics and receives treatment until he or she responds appropriately to therapy, with pyrexia reduced and supplemental oxygen no longer required. Continuation of oral antibiotics may be recommended for 1–3 weeks after discharge.

Surgical Management
Treatment of parapneumonic effusions aims to control the infection and effect drainage of the pleural fluid to achieve full re-expansion of the affected lung tissue[1,20]. Optimal treatments include antibiotics alone (for small effusions or empyemas) or in combination with surgical procedures. Numerous surgical options include thoracentesis,[16] tube thoracostomy, fibrinolytics,[7,13] thoracoscopy,[10,21,22] minithoracotomy,[15] open window drainage,[16] or formal thoracotomy and decortication,[14,22] which are described in the following sections.

Thoracentesis and Simple Tube Thoracostomy
Thoracentesis or chest tube placements may be required to effect a cure. In the second, fibrino-purulent stage, antibiotics with properly positioned chest tube drainage usually resolve the empyema thoracis. Failures may be due to an improperly positioned tube, pleural loculations, high fluid viscosity, or early peel on the lung. Failures are managed with open drainage involving rib resection, decortications, intrapleural thrombolytics, or thoracoscopic drainage. Prompt drainage of a free-flowing effusion prevents the development of loculations and a fibrous peel. The tube is removed when the lung re-expands and drainage ceases. If the fluid is not free flowing, further radiologic imaging is undertaken to better define the pleural space disorder.

In addition to the benefit of CT and ultrasonographic imaging to characterise loculated pleural effusions, the radiologist has become significantly involved in the treatment of empyema. The ability of the interventional radiologist to assist in the placement of small-bore catheters, specifically localised to loculated pleural fluid collections, has helped to facilitate drainage. Furthermore, with smaller-diameter tubes, patients have tolerated tube placement better, with less associated morbidity. In addition, radiologists can lyse adhesions directly by using imaging during the tube placement. Finally, interventional radiologists, using fibrinolytics, have further improved the care of complicated empyema by improved management of loculations and amelioration of fibrous peel formation and fibrin deposition. Numerous studies have documented the effectiveness of intrapleural fibrinolytics (e.g., urokinase or tissue plasminogen activator (TPA)) to treat obstructed thoracostomy tubes, increase drainage in multiloculated effusions, and lyse adhesions. Cost may limit its more widespread use.

Open Drainage

Thoracotomy or minithoracotomy (with decortications) to remove the pleural peel and lyse the adhesions (in advanced empyema) if the patient does not respond promptly to treatment is very effective, with a reported 95% success rate for patients with fibrinopurulent empyema.

Customarily, rib resection has been required to manage the organised empyemas. Empyemas that have reached the organised phase are characterised by the presence of thick pleural peel, causing varying degree of pulmonary parenchymal entrapment. Limited thoracoplasty and muscle flap rotation are also needed in some instances to obliterate the pleural space problem.

Video-Assisted Thoracoscopic Surgery

Video-assisted thoracoscopic surgery (VATS) has proven to be an effective and less-invasive replacement for the limited decortication procedure. Thoracoscopic debridement closely imitates open thoracotomy and drainage. Mechanical removal of purulent material and the breakdown of adhesions can be easily accomplished via this route. VATS results in more rapid relief of symptoms, earlier hospital discharge, and significantly less discomfort and morbidity. For the paediatric population of many developed centres, VATS is the preferred method to alternative procedures such as rib resection and open drainage or pleural obliteration.

The Eloesser Procedure

The Eloesser procedure and its modification are important options in the surgical treatment of chronic, complicated ET.

Postoperative Complications

To encourage lung re-expansion, adequate analgesics are administered, and the patient is encouraged to take deep breaths and undergo basic chest physiotherapy including, where possible, blowing up (inflating) balloons.

Specific postoperative complications include:

- *Air leak* (bronchpleural fistula). This may spontaneously or it may require pneumonectomy (lung resection).

- *Persistence and chronicity* (from inadequate drainage due to the premature removal of the drainage tube or failure to establish drainage at the dependent position of the empyema cavity). Management may involve open drainage by rib resection, pneumonectomy (if there is associated lung disease, such as bronchopleural fistula), or obliteration of the pleural space by collapsing the chest wall to meet the lung by performing thoracoplasty.

Prognosis and Outcomes

Mortality-related prognostic factors of empyema thoracis in children include age, causative bacteriological agents such as *Streptococcus milleri*, concomitant disease, and history of operation.[25,26] Morbidity and mortality may be reduced through early diagnosis and therapy.[23,24,27,28]

A significant proportion of children with chronic disease develop a thoracic scoliosis, which is always directed towards the side of the effusion. This is thought to be due to pleuritic pain from the infection/inflammation and discomfort from the chest drainage tube.

Empyema necessitans is another long-term complication of poorly or uncontrolled empyema thoracis. The pus collection bursts and communicates with the exterior, forming a fistula between the pleural cavity and the skin.

The main determinants of outcome of empyema thoracis are early and adequate treatment, access to proper care, nutritional status of the patient, and the causative agent (tuberculous empyema).

Prevention

Early, aggressive, and adequate treatment of pneumonia; good hygiene; and adequate nutrition are imperative to preventing empyema thoracis in children in Africa. Public education and management of patients at risk by medical experts and specialists will play a crucial role in this regard.

Evidence-Based Research

In the literature of the last 10 years, only two reports are available in English from Africa on the treatment of postpneumonic pleural space infection.[29,30] Both reports are of descriptive studies. The mean age at presentation of the patients is 5 years. Fever, cough, and dyspnoea are the standard presentations, together with radiologic evidence of pleural effusion. Pneumococci and staphylococci were the most common organisms isolated. In the Ethiopian study, no patient required thoracotomy and decortication, and in the Nigerian study, only one patient did. Mortality ranged from 7% to 16%.

Key Summary Points

1. Pleural effusion is aspirated and protein content is measured; exudates are cultured, and have cell count, gram staining, and acid-fast staining evaluated.

2. *Streptococcus pneumonia* and *Staphylococcus aureus* are the major pathogens in children; antibiotic treatment should be started before culture results are available.

3. Tuberculous pleurisy needs to be distinguished from TB empyema.

4. Tube thoracostomy (with antibiotics) is the treatment of choice for empyema; and it must be carried out as soon as the diagnosis is made.

5. If an empyema does not resolve promptly with tube drainage, an ultrasound examination should be done and a new drain inserted if necessary.

6. In children, thoracotomy is rarely necessary and is a last resort.

7. The failure of an empyema to resolve is a good indication for VATS.

8. In areas with high HIV prevalence, a bloodstained pleural effusion is usually caused by Kaposi sarcoma.

References

1. Bilgin M, Akcali Y, Oguzkaya, F. Benefits of early aggressive management of empyema thoracis. ANZ J Surg 2006; 76:120–122.

2. Cekirdekci A, Köksel O, Göncü T, et al. Management of parapneumonic empyema in children. Asian Cardiovasc Thorac Ann 2000; 8:137–140.

3. Chan W, Keyser-Gauvin E, Davis GM, Nguyen LT, Laberge J-M. Empyema thoracis in children: a 26-year review of the Montreal Children's Hospital experience. J Pediatr Surg 1997; 32(6):870-872.

4. Varkey B, Rose HD, Kutty CPK, Politis J. Empyema thoracic during a ten year period: analysis of 72 cases and comparison to previous study. Arch Intern Med 1981; 141:1771–1776.

5. Barlett JG, Gorback SL, Thadepalli H, Finegold SM. Bacteriology of empyema. Lancet 1974; 1:338–340.

6. Campbell PW III. New developments in pediatric pneumonia and empyema. Curr Opin Pediatr 1995; 7:278–282,

7. Schropp IQ: Empyema and intrathoracic infection in children. Pedtat Thorac Surg 1993; 3:443-460.

8. Kern JA, Rodgers BM. Thoracoscopy in the management of empyema in children. J Pediatr Surg 1993; 28:1128–1132.

9. Silen ML, Weber TR. Thoracoscopic debridement of loculated empyema thoracis in children. Ann Thorac Surg 1995; 59:1166–1168.

10. Stovroff M, Teague G, Heiss KF, et al. Thoracoscopy in the management of pediatric empyema. J Pediatr Surg 1995; 30:1211–1215.

11. Mangete EDO, Kombo BB, Legg-Jack TE. Thoracic empyema: a study of 56 patients. Arch Dis Child 1993; 69:587–588.

12. Robinson LA, Moulton AL, Fleming WH, et al. Intrapleural fibrinolytic treatment of multiloculated thoracic empyemas. Ann Thorac Surg 1994; 57:802–814.

13. Gustafson RA, Murray GF, Warden HE. Role of lung decortications in symptomatic empyemas in children. Ann Thorac Surg 1990; 49:940–947.

14. Van Way C III, Narrod J, Hopeman A. The role of early limited thoracotomy in the treatment of empyema. J Thorac Cardiovasc Surg 1988; 96:436–439.

15. Vardhan MV, Tewari SC, Prasad BNBM, and Nikumb SK. Empyema thoracis—study of present day clinical and etiological profile and management techniques. Ind J Tub 1998; 45:155.

16. Bono MJ. Recognizing and managing thoracic empyema. Emerg Med 2004; 36(12):37–40.

17. Miller JI. Infections of the pleura. In Shields TW (ed), General Thoracic Surgery, Philadelphia, PA: Lea & Febiger, 1989; pp 633–649.

18. Mandal AK, Thadepalli H, Mandal AK, Chettipally U. Outcome of primary empyema thoracis: therapeutic and microbiologic aspects. Ann Thorac Surg 1998; 66:1782–1786.

19. Rosen H, Nadkarm V, Theroux M: Intrapleural streptokinase as adjunctive treatment for persistent empyema in pediatric patients. Chest 1993; 103:1190–1193.

20. Kern JA. Rodgers BM. Thoracoscopy in the management of empyema in children. J Pediatr Surg 1993; 28:1128–1132.

21. Stovroff M, Teague G, Heiss KF, et al. Thoracoscopy in the management of pediatric empyema. J Pediatr Surg 1995; 30:1211–1215.

22. Miller JI. Empyema thoracis. Ann Thorac Surg 1990; 50:343–344.

23. Mclaughlin JS, Krasna MJ. Parapneumonic empyema. In: Shields TW (ed), General Thoracic Surgery, 4th ed. Philadelphia, PA: Lippincott Williams & Wilkins, 2000; pp 699–708.

24. Lee KS, Im JG, Kim YH. Treatment of thoracic multiloculated empyema with intracavitary urukinase: a prospective study. Radiology 1991; 178:771–775.

25. Waller DA, Rengarajan A. Thoracoscopic decortication: a role for video-assisted surgery in chronic postpneumonic pleuralempyema. Ann Thorac Surg 2001; 71:1813–1816.

26. Lawrence DR, Ohri SK, Moxon RE, Townsend ER, Fountain SW. Thoracoscopic debridement of empyema thoracis. Ann Thorac Surg 1997; 64:1448–1450.

27. Mwandumba HC, Beeching NJ. Pyogenic lung infections: factors for predicting clinical outcome of lung abscess and thoracic empyema. Curr Opin Pulm Med 2000; 6:234–239.

28. Lindstrom ST, Kolbe J. Community acquired parapneumonic thoracic empyema: predictors of outcome. Respirology 1999; 4:173–179.

29. Hailu S. Paediatric thoracic empyema in an Ethiopian referral hospital. E African Med J 2000; 77(11):618–621.

30. Tagbo O, Uchenna O, Anthony H. Childhood parapneumonic pleural effusion in Enugu. Nigerian Postgrad Med J 2005; 12(1):28–32.

Suggested Reading

Baranwal AK, Singh M, Marwaha RK, Kumar L. Empyemathoracis: a 10-year comparative review of hospitalised children from South Asia. Arch Dis Childhood 2003; 88(11):1009–1014.

Eastham KM, Freeman R, Kearns AM, Eltringham G, Clark J, Leeming J, et al. Clinical features, aetiology and outcome of empyema in children in the northeast of England. Thorax 2004; 59(6):522–525.

Schultz KD, Fan LL, Pinsky J, Ochoa L, Smith EO, Kaplan SL, et al. The changing face of pleural empyemas in children: epidemiology and management. Pediatrics 2004; 113(6):1735–1740.

CHAPTER 47
LUNG ABSCESS

Jonathan Karperlowsky

Introduction

A lung abscess is a cavity in the lung parenchyma that contains purulent material resulting from pulmonary infection. This chapter focuses on pyogenic lung abscesses and does not consider other causes of pulmonary cavitations with or without air fluid levels, such as tuberculosis or a complicated hydatid cyst. The role of surgery in lung abscesses is limited, with the vast majority being treated with antimicrobials and percutaneous techniques.

Demographics

Lung abscesses in previously well children are uncommon and are usually the complication of a virulent necrotising pneumonia. The incidence would thus depend on the burden of respiratory disease. This is in contrast to children at risk for lung abscesses, which would include children with impaired immunity (e.g., human immunodeficiency virus (HIV) or cystic fibrosis), an underlying anatomical abnormality (e.g., congenital cystic adenomatoid malformation or bronchopulmonary sequestration), or at risk for aspiration (e.g., neurodevelopmental anomalies or cerebral palsy).

Pathophysiology and Pathology

A pulmonary abscess develops when a localised infection within the parenchyma becomes necrotic, with subsequent cavitation. Several mechanisms exist for this process. The first is an unchecked infection secondary to impaired immunity, clearance of the organism, or virulence of the organism. Patients with impaired cellular or humoral immunity, which may be congenital or acquired, are unable to eradicate the infection, leading to breakdown. Nutritional deficiency can be a significant cofactor in Africa. Inadequate clearance may be secondary to a congenital cystic pulmonary lesion, an inhaled foreign body or bronchial narrowing. The latter, especially in the African setting, may occur secondary to tuberculosis (TB) lymphadenitis with a superadded infection. Cystic fibrosis also will lead to inadequate clearance, potentially leading to a lung abscess. Infection with a virulent organism, typically anaerobes, *Staphylococcus aureus*, streptococcal species, and *Klebsiella*, can cause a lung abscess. Delay in antimicrobial therapy in treating pneumonia is often causative in a lung abscess because the infection remains unchecked for a prolonged period. Unfortunately, in Africa, due to difficult health access, easily treated conditions may lead to significant morbidity, and mortality.

Second, pulmonary aspiration is a central contributing factor to lung abscess formation in many children. Aspiration usually occurs in children with a neurological deficit, particularly cerebral palsy. Any acquired depressed level of consciousness, such as trauma or postanaesthesia, would also place a child at risk. Children with incoordinate swallowing or muscle weakness are a second group of patients who frequently aspirate. Last are children with oesophageal abnormalities, including dysmotility, achalasia, and unrecognised trachea-oesophageal fistulas.

A final mechanism involves patients who develop a lung abscess secondary to septic emboli. This may be seen in children with right-sided endocarditis, long-term lines, or, rarely, in children with haematogenous spread from thrombophlebitis. *S. aureus* septicaemia may frequently result in this mechanism of lung abscess formation.

Clinical Presentation

The differentiation of pneumonia and lung abscess on purely clinical grounds is difficult. Fever and cough predominate but are not universal. Other findings include chest pain, anorexia, productive sputum, malaise, haemoptysis, chills, and halitosis. Signs of lung abscess are varied, but may include tachypnoea, dullness, bronchial breathing, amphoric breathing, and crepitations over the affected area.

Investigations

Radiology typically shows a cavity with an air fluid level; this needs to be differentiated from a pneumatocoele, complicated hydatid, or pyopneumothorax. Occasionally, to further delineate the anatomy, to exclude an underlying abnormality, or to facilitate percutaneous intervention, a computed tomography (CT) scan must be done. Ultrasound can be used if the abscess abuts the hemidiaphragm or chest wall, thus creating an acoustic window to enable visualisation.

Bacteriology, sputum, or pus, if intervention is performed, is invaluable in guiding antibiotic therapy. Ideally, this intervention should occur prior to commencement of antibiotic therapy. This may be done in the older child by using an induced sputum and in the younger child by bronchoscopy, if safe facilities exist.

Management

The mainstay of therapy involves prolonged antimicrobials. The exact duration and route of administration have not clearly been delineated in the literature. It would seem that it would be prudent to begin with intravenous antibiotics until signs and symptoms have settled, following which the remainder of the 4–6 week course may be given orally.

Drainage of the lesion can usually be achieved by using physiotherapy with postural drainage and percussion. In children unable to adequately expectorate, bronchoscopy can be a useful adjunct.

Antimicrobials should ideally be microbiologically directed, but empiric antibiotics with a B-lactam is usually adequate in the absence thereof. If there is consideration of coliforms, an aminoglycoside may be added, and if aspiration or anaerobes are considered to be causative, the addition of metronidazole or clindamycin is warranted. The latter makes an excellent single agent provided coliforms have been excluded. For primary abscesses, staph, strep, and coliforms should be considered; for secondary abscesses, it is important to cover anaerobes.

A significant morbidity is associated with surgery, such as empyema and air leaks, with mortalities of 5–10% having been reported. The need for surgery has further been minimised by percutaneous drains where interventional radiology is available. Thus, in most instances, surgical intervention should be reserved for underlying congenital anomalies and treatment failures. This would include large chronic abscesses, significant haemoptysis, bronchial stenosis, bronchiectasis, or massive necrosis.

Prognosis and Outcome

The outcome for lung abscesses is excellent, provided that appropriate antibiotics and postural drainage are instituted in a timely manner. Complications for surgery can be high; thus, surgery should be reserved for specific indications. Overall morbidity should be less than 5% and would occur predominantly in those with secondary abscesses, usually secondary to the comorbidity. Long-term follow-up of patients with primary abscesses shows no residual deterioration in lung function and a return to normal health.

Evidence-Based Research

Currently, there is a paucity of literature from Africa, and the literature from the developed world is limited to case reports. Further studies are needed, especially to look at the duration of antibiotic therapy.

CHAPTER 48
OESOPHAGEAL ATRESIA

Peter Beale
Kokila Lakhoo

Introduction

Little from Africa has been reported or written on the subject of oesophageal atresia (OA). The frequency of diagnosis and especially survival is widely variable, depending on available resources and expertise. In some areas, the incidence of diagnosis and survival is unlikely, whereas in a developing country such as South Africa, where facilities are good and a limited number of dedicated paediatric surgeons accumulate a large amount of experience, results are comparable to those of the developed world.

Demographics

The incidence of oesophageal atresia in Africa is unknown but would appear to be no different from that in other populations. Amongst South Africa's multicultural population, the incidence in the white population seems to be higher; however, this was very likely a spurious impression due to missed diagnoses.

In 2008, Nandi and colleagues reported equivalent incidences of oesophageal atresia/tracheo-oesophageal fistula (OA/TOF; 2.1% of all neonatal admissions) at two linked surgical departments in Europe and Africa: John Radcliffe, Oxford, United Kingdom; and Kilimanjaro Christian Medical Centre, Tanzania. Reports from Nigeria and Zimbabwe show an incidence comparable to that at Great Ormond Street Children's Hospital in London. The incidence in Africa probably corresponds to the 1 per 3,000–4,500 reported across the world in the literature.

Aetiology/Pathophysiology

The mechanisms of embryological development of OA/TOF occurs in the embryo at 3 weeks postfertilisation during the demarcation of the proximal foregut as the oesophagus with a gastric bubble caudally and a ventral lung bud cranially. During the subsequent phase of elongation of the oesophagus and lung bud, there is a further division of the tracheal primordium from the oesophagus.

The mechanism of development of tracheo-oesophageal fistula is the failure of apposition of longitudinal ridges, whereas the mechanism of the development of oesophageal atresia is apposition too posteriorly.

OA/TOF is classified into six types (see Figure 48.1):

A. Isolated oesophageal atresia (8%)

B. Upper pouch fistula with oesophageal atresia (1%)

C. Oesophageal atresia with tracheo-oesophageal fistula (86%)

D. Upper and lower pouch fistula (0.5%)

E. H-type fistula (4%)

F. Oesophagus with tracheal segment (0.5%)

Clinical Presentation

Prenatally, the condition may be suspected from maternal polyhydramnios and absence of a fetal stomach bubble at the 20-week anomaly scan. Prenatal scan diagnosis of OA/TOF is estimated to be less than 42% sensitive with a positive predicted value of 56%. Additional diagnostic clues are provided by associated anomalies, such as trisomy (13, 18, 21); VACTERAL (vertebral, anorectal, cardiac, tracheo-oesophageal, renal, limbs) sequence; and CHARGE (coloboma, heart defects, atresia choanae, retarded development, genital hypoplasia, ear abnormality) association. These associated anomalies are present in more than 50% of cases and worsen the prognosis; thus, prenatal karyotyping is essential. Duodenal atresia may coexist with OA/TOF. The risk of recurrence in subsequent pregnancies for isolated OA/TOF is less than 1%. Delivery is advised to be at a specialised centre with neonatal surgical input.

In the absence of prenatal diagnosis, the presentation may be respiratory distress, cyanotic spells, frothing around the mouth, and arrested passage of a nasogastric tube. Recurrent pneumonia or failure to feed are noted in delayed presentations. Presentation with gastric rupture, especially in low birth weight babies, is known to increase morbidity and mortality.

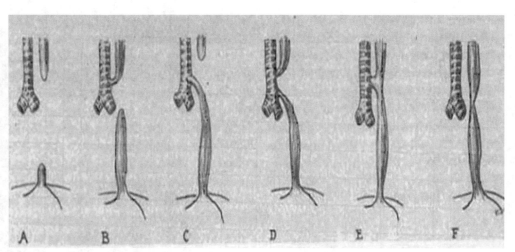

Figure 48.1: Types of oesophageal atresia and tracheo-oesophageal fistula.

Investigations

A babygram (Figure 48.2) with a radio-opaque nasogastric tube is the most informative imaging tool. This image helps with diagnosis, confirms OA+TOF or isolated OA, diagnoses the associated anomalies of VACTERL, and identifies associated duodenal atresia. Renal ultrasound is helpful in confirming renal anomalies, and a cardiac assessment may confirm the 30% associated cardiac anomalies. If dysmorhphic features are suspected, karyotyping may confirm chromosomal anomalies. However, if life-threatening chromosomal anomalies are suspected, the treatment may be delayed until karyotype results are obtained, which could be

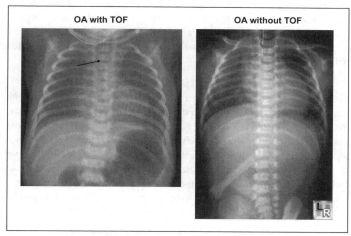

Figure 48.2: A babygram showing OA+TOF on the left and isolated OA on the right.

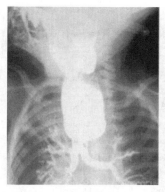 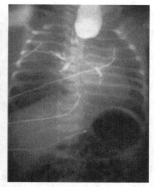

Figure 48.3: Examples of excessive volumes of contrast given to infants with oesophageal atresia, resulting in aspiration.

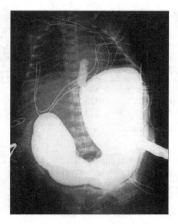

Figure 48.4: An on-table gastrogram in a baby with pure oesophageal atresia and duodenal atresia. A duodenoduodenostomy was performed, followed by oesophageal atresia repair after a 3-day interval.

within 48 hours. Contrast swallows are discouraged due to the risk of aspiration (Figure 48.3).

Cardiac echoes have proven unreliable in terms of identifying right aortic arch; however, this identification hasn't been particularly helpful because a right aortic arch has not been an impediment to repair via a right posterolateral extrapleural access. Routine preoperative bronchoscopy is advocated in some centres, but is not essential, and thus is not practiced by many centres.

In the event of a gasless abdomen and pure atresia, an initial gastrostomy may be required to establish the length of gap between proximal and distal segments of the oesophagus (Figure 48.4).

Management

Surgical intervention is urgent only in the event of abdominal distention causing ventilatory distress, gastric distention, or rupture. Otherwise, oesophageal atresia constitutes an urgent elective case to be repaired within 24 hours, preferably in the light of day, and after acquiring a cardiac echo and convening a suitable team of anaesthesiologist and operating room staff.

The patient is positioned in the left lateral position with a small strut under the left chest wall. Nasotracheal intubation is encouraged to ensure a stable endotracheal tube above the level of the carina. Surgery necessitates retraction of the right lung, so it is essential that the left lung is ventilated.

Depending on the size of the patient, a 16, 18, or 20 Wishard catheter is introduced into the proximal oesophageal pouch, replacing the Replogle tube, to be advanced by the anaesthetist when required.

An approximate 3-cm incision is made just below the angle of the right scapula, strictly in the skin lines to leave an optimal, almost imperceptible scar. Non–muscle-cutting access to the rib cage is established through the angle of auscultation between the latissimus and trapezius muscles.

The fourth intercostal space is opened on the superior margin of the fifth rib, maintaining an extrapleural plane. This is possible in most cases—a small breach of the pleura can be tied on a mosquito forcep at completion.

The azygos vein is tied and divided and the distal tracheo-oesophageal fistula is identified, isolated, and serially divided with a 1-mm cuff against the trachea, which is approximated with interrupted 6-0 proline or polydiaxonone sutures.

A feeding tube is passed down the distal oesophagus to ensure distal patency and to empty the stomach. The anaesthetist is then asked to advance the Wishard catheter, and the upper pouch is mobilised, if necessary, into the thoracic inlet and neck. This technique greatly facilitates mobilisation and separation in the plane of close adherence to the trachea.

The lower oesophagus is mobilised sufficiently to approximate the two segments. Where limited gap allows, the fistulous proximal end of the distal oesophagus is resected to achieve anastomosis to a better calibre, and to have mild distraction of the two ends.

A single transverse incision is made across the end of the upper pouch onto the Wishard catheter, and lateral and medial angle sutures are placed across the segments. The Wishard catheter is withdrawn, and the posterior anastomotic sutures are completed. The angle and posterior layer sutures are then tied. If necessary, the chest wall strut is removed to relieve tension. The anaesthetist is then asked to advance a Replogle or feeding tube, which is guided through the anastomosis. The anterior layer is completed.

The extent of proximal mobilisation overcomes most gaps. In the event of a 2.5cm+ vertical gap, options include the use of several techniques, including circular myotomies (Figure 48.5). If this is required, it is usually in the circumstance of a very high upper pouch, in which case the upper pouch needs to be mobilised out of the neck, myotomised, and placed back in the thoracic inlet. This is done with the Wishard catheter in the lumen prior to opening the apex of the pouch. Other options include an oesophageal flap (Figure 48.6).

Some recent controversy has arisen as to whether to drain the extrapleural para-anastomotic space when one is very confident of the

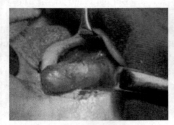
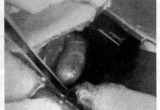

Circular Myotomy through the neck   Intrathoracic Circular Myotomy through the thoracotomy wound

Figure 48.5: Circular myotomy.

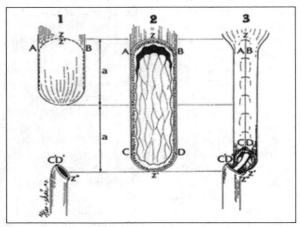

Figure 48.6: Flap technique: (1) the closed upper pouch; (2) the upper pouch is open and its lateral wall reaches the lower segment of the oesophagus; (3) the elongated upper pouch is anastomosed to the lower segment.

integrity of the anastomosis. A drain does no harm and can be removed in 2 or 3 days if one has confidence in the anastomosis. In cases anastomosed under tension, a para-anastomotic drain is retained for a week, and feeds are delayed until a contrast swallow confirms an intact oesophagus.

Gastrostomies are essentially used only for pure oesophagael atresia cases. The rest are fed via a transanastamotic tube initially, and subsequently are fed orally.

Minimally invasive endoscopic surgery has become the vogue in paediatric surgery, and has excellent application for a considerable range of procedures. Whether this is true for thoracoscopic repair of OA since the first report in 1999 is debatable. The foremost and most enthusiastic endoscopic surgeons promote this procedure and claim that their results and complication rates are at least comparable with open operative procedures. The technique may be used if equipment and expertise are available.

Postoperative Complications

An anastomotic leak may have dire consequences if a major intrapleural disruption occurs. Anastomotic leaks should be uncommon and, if extra-pleural and contained, can be treated expectantly by maintaining parenter-al nutrition and drainage until the leak seals and heals. A major intrapleural disruption can be life threatening and warrants early re-exploration. If total disruption occurs, the oesophagus may have to be abandoned and the upper pouch exteriorised as a cervical oesophagostomy.

A recurrent tracheo-oesophageal fistula requires operative interven-tion, closure, and tissue interposition, although endoscopic injection of glue has been described.

Another complication is stridor and cyanotic episodes related to tracheomalacia and a collapsing upper airway. The combination of gastro-oesophageal reflux and tracheomalacia may be particularly sinis-

ter and life threatening and require early intervention. Generally, gastro-oesophageal reflux is addressed first. Occasionally, infants cannot be fed at all without immediately refluxing and aspirating, and may be at risk of sudden infant death syndrome (SIDS).

Other postoperative complications include anastomotic stricture; gastro-oesophageal reflux; long-term Barrett's oesophagus due to chronic reflux; and chylothorax.

A well-recognised but uncommon pitfall in the operative management of OA, tracheo-oesophageal fistula occurs in the event of a carinal fistula with tracheal communication into the fork of the carina. In this situation, the relative position of the right main bronchus and distal oesophagus just below the fistula is reversed. The surgeon should always confirm that a structure isolated as the distal oesophagus is correctly identified by atraumatic occlusion and confirmation that the right lung still ventilates before dividing the structure.

Conclusion

In the Western world, current expectations of survival are that all patients with oesophageal atresia will survive unless there are major congenital malformations affecting other systems. There is no place for technical risk or error to compromise survival. In Africa, however, limiting fac-tors are delayed diagnosis and restricted access to a neonatal intensive care unit (NICU). Shortages of medical and nursing personnel demand techniques be selected that limit the NICU requirement, in-hospital stay, and complications. The potential to rescue patients with surgical compli-cations is probably not as good as it is in First World centres.

Evidence-Based Research

Table 48.1 presents a review of a 10-year personal experience with OA and TOF.

Table 48.1: Evidence-based research.

Title	Oesophageal atresia and tracheo-oesophageal fistula: review of a 10-year personal experience.
Authors	Adebo OA
Institution	Department of Surgery, University College Hospital and College of Medicine, University of Ibadan
Reference	West Afr J Med 1990; 9(3):164–169
Problem	Outcomes of TOF and OA repair in the African setting is poor.
Intervention	This study seeks predictors to improve outcome.
Comparison/ control (quality of evidence)	Eleven neonates with oesophageal atresia and distal fistula were managed between July 1977 and January 1987. The male-to-female ratio was 1.2:1. The patients were aged between 1 to 14 days (median of 7 days) and weighed 1.85 to 3.10 kg (mean of 2.6 kg) at presentation. Associated anomalies were present in 5, pneumonia in 4, and uraemia (mean serum urea of 88 mg%) in all patients. A primary repair and simultaneous gastrostomy (omitted in one) were performed for all cases. There were 5 operative deaths. Fifteen postoperative complications occurred in 10 patients, including septicaemia in 3, wound infection in 3, anastomotic leak in 1, and tracheal mucous plug in 1. Statistical analysis indicated no difference between survivors and nonsurvivors on the basis of age, weight, degree of uraemia, or presence of pneumonia. One of the 6 survivors (now 5 years after surgery) required bouginage after 26 months and has remained asymptomatic; the other 5 are well and without symptoms 3 to 11 months postoperative.
Outcome/ effect	High mortality and morbidity for this neonatal condition.
Historical significance/ comments	The most significant determinants of survival are the effectiveness of pre- and postoperative managements of patients.

Key Summary Points

1. The incidence of oesophageal atresia in Africa is comparable to that in the Western world.

2. Prenatal diagnosis of OA is rare.

3. Delayed presentation of OA with pneumonia, dehydration, and failure to feed is the norm in Africa.

4. Diagnosis of PA is confirmed with a nasogastric tube and high index of suspicion.

5. A babygram is the most useful image.

6. Outcomes depend on the availability of resources and technical skill.

Suggested Reading

Bar-Maor JA, Shoshany G, Sweed Y. Wide gap esophageal atresia: a new method to elongate the upper pouch. J Pediatr Surg 1989; 24(9):882–883.

Da Carvalho JL, Maynard J, Hadley GB. An improved technique for in situ esophageal myotomy and proximal pouch mobilization in patients with esophageal atresia. J Pediatr Surg 1989; 24(9):872–873.

Davies MRQ. Anatomy of the extrinsic motor nerve supply to mobilized segments of the oesophagus disrupted by dissection during repair of oesophageal atresia with distal fistula. Brit J Surg 1996; 83:1268–1270.

Goyal A, Jones MO, Couriel JM, Losty PD. Oesophageal atresia and tracheo-oesophageal fistula. Review. Arch Dis Child Fetal Neonatal Ed 2006; 91(5):F381–F384.

Holcomb GW, Rothenberg SS, Bax K, et al. Thoracoscopic repair of esophageal atresia and tracheoesophageal fistula: a multi-institutional analysis. Ann Surg 2005; 242(3):428–430.

Iliff PJ. Neonatal surgery in Harare Hospital. Cent Afr Jour Med 1990; 36(1):11–15.

Lugo B, et al. Thoracoscopic versus open repair of tracheoesophageal fistula and esophageal atresia. J Laperoendosc Adv Surg Tech 2008; 18(5):753–756.

Nandi B, Mungongo C, Lakhoo, K. A comparison of neonatal surgical admissions between two linked surgical departments in Africa and Europe. Pediatr Surg Int 2008; 24:939–942.

Puri P, Khurana S. Delayed primary esophageal anastomosis for pure esophageal atresias. Semin Pediatr Surg 1998; 7(2):126–129.

CHAPTER 49
GASTRO-OESOPHAGEAL REFLUX DISEASE

Merrill McHoney

Introduction

Gastro-oesophageal reflux (GOR) is defined as involuntary (passive) reflux of gastric contents into the oesophagus not caused by noxious stimuli. Gastro-oesophageal reflux disease (GORD) is defined as symptoms and complications arising from gastro-oesophageal reflux. GOR is present in many newborns, in whom it does not necessarily represent a clinical disease, but rather a somewhat delayed physiological development which occurs with time; some GOR can be considered "physiological" up to 3 months of age, and the reflux (without the disease) may also occur in many individuals during certain physiological processes and normal activities during the day. GORD, however, differs from this variant of normal physiological development, with complications and symptoms that lead to presentation and the need for medical or surgical intervention.

Demographics

As discussed further in the next section, GOR is common, but not necessarily pathological, in many newborns. GORD is not common in otherwise healthy children. There is no sex predilection. GORD itself has no age preponderance. The incidence in African countries and blacks is less than that seen in Westernised countries.[1-3] In one study, the prevalence was 4–7% of the population.[1]

GORD is more common in neurologically impaired children and those with neuromuscular disease. Congenital gastrointestinal anomalies associated with a high incidence are: oesophageal atresia, congenital diaphragmatic hernia, and abdominal wall defects. Populations in which the incidence or survival of premature neonates with neurological impairment is high may also have a higher incidence of GORD.

Aetiology/Pathophysiology

Several anatomical or physiological factors prevent GOR; they can be further broken down into oesophageal factors, diaphragmatic contribution, and stomach contribution.

Oesophageal clearance is thought to act as an antireflux mechanism. The presence of an oesophageal food bolus promotes lower (distal) oesophageal relaxation as a normal enteric reflex to allow swallowing. Therefore, a lack of oesophageal clearance can promote reflux by this effect. Also, if reflux does occur (which is an occasional event in most people; even those without GORD), oesophageal clearance rids the oesophagus of irritant acid (or alkali). Poor oesophageal clearance will increase contact time and promote oesophagitis and GORD.

One of the most important oesophageal contributions is the occurrence of a length of intraabdominal oesophagus. Intraabdominal pressure can reach 10 mm Hg. During times of increased intraabdominal pressure, and with changes during inspiration, there is a positive pressure gradient that can encourage reflux of stomach contents into the lower oesophagus. However, this positive pressure in the abdomen is transmitted to the entire length of intraabdominal oesophagus, which partially closes under this positive pressure and prevents reflux. If the length of oesophagus to which this pressure can be transmitted is decreased, the incidence of reflux is higher.

The importance of the presence of intraabdominal oesophagus is demonstrated by the fact that in patients who have a length of less than 1 cm, the incidence of reflux is high (85%). This is a common situation in the newborn period. This compares to the situation at 3 months of age, when the length of intraabdominal oesophagus reaches 3 cm and the incidence of reflux decreases. With an intraabdominal oesophagus length of 3–4.5 cm, reflux is mostly abolished. This development partially underlies the relatively common finding of reflux in young infants that abates with age.

Another important oesophageal factor is the presence of a high pressure zone (HPZ) in the lower oesophagus, also known as the physiological lower oesophageal sphincter (LOS). This mechanism is thought to contribute between 10 and 30 mm Hg pressure resistance to GOR. This HPZ is identifiable on manometry studies, but not anatomically. This HPZ relaxes in advance of a food bolus to allow swallowing to occur. One major contribution to GORD in children is thought to be inappropriate or excessive relaxation of this HPZ, called transient lower oesophageal sphincter relaxation (TLOSR).

These oesophageal mechanisms are reinforced by an important contribution from the crura of the diaphragm. The right crus of the diaphragm slings around the oesophagus, as the latter enters the abdomen. This provides a pinch-cock effect that contributes to the HPZ, and, more importantly, increases lower oesophageal pressure during inspiration, when thoracic pressure is most negative and would favour reflux.

A physiological mechanism contributed by the stomach is timely and efficient stomach emptying. Some studies have linked the presence of delayed gastric emptying (DGE) to reflux by demonstrating a higher incidence and recurrence rate of reflux in children who have DGE.[4] Some pharmacological treatments target DGE in an attempt to treat GORD.

Another anatomical contribution to reducing reflux is the presence of the acute angle of His between the oesophagus and the stomach. This acute angle allows a valve-like mechanism to occur. This arrangement is further supplemented by mucosal folds (rosettes) in the stomach. The contribution of this mucosal fold mechanism is minimal, and is thought by some not to contribute at all.

Some pathological causes and consequences of GORD with reference to these mechanisms are outlined in Table 49.1.

In addition to these pathophysiological changes, any process that leads to a significant increase in intraabdominal pressure sufficient enough to overcome these mechanisms may induce reflux and GORD. This may underlie the causation of GORD after tight abdominal closure (e.g., in gastroschisis and congenital diaphragmatic hernia).

Clinical Presentation

History

Infant

Vomiting is the most common symptom of GOR in an infant, and is usually nonbilious and effortless. The presence of bilious vomiting should prompt the search for another diagnosis. GOR should not be

Table 49.1: Possible pathological changes in GORD in relation to physiological factors preventing reflux.

Mechanism preventing reflux	Proposed contribution or pathology in GORD
Oesophageal clearance	Decreased in primary (e.g., oesophageal atresia/tracheo-oesophageal fistule (OA/TOF)) or secondary (e.g., severe oesophagitis) oesophageal motility disorders.
Length of intraabdominal oesophagus	Shortened in some congenital conditions including OA/TOF and sliding hiatus hernia.
Physiological lower oesophageal sphincter	Incriminated in transient lower oesophageal sphincter relaxation. Absent HPZ on manometry.
Diaphragmatic pinch-cock effect of crura	Abnormal anatomical configuration and/ or muscular weakness (e.g., in congenital diaphragmatic hernia, muscular dystrophies, scoliosis, and cerebral palsy) may contribute to reflux.
Angle of His	Altered in hiatus hernia and abdominal wall defects. May be altered by gastrostomy placement and other abnormalities of stomach anatomy.
Gastric emptying	Delayed gastric emptying in neurologically impaired and congenital gastrointestinal conditions contribute to, or worsen, reflux.
Mucosal folds (rosettes)	Possibly only a minor contribution.

assumed in these cases, although occasionally a bile vomit may be present in GOR.

Apnoeas and bradycardias are frequent presenting features in neonates and infants.[5] In some infants, these symptoms may progress to acute life-threatening events (ALTEs). ALTEs are acute respiratory events characterised by apnoeas, bradycardias, and acute respiratory distress, and sometimes respiratory arrest. They are thought to occur during aspiration episodes from GOR. They can lead to the need for ventilation or they can be present in neonates already ventilated on intensive care units.

Excessive vomiting can lead to failure to thrive, leading to presentation with poor or absent weight gain.

Older child
Vomiting and failure to thrive are the main presenting symptoms of GORD in older children. Haematemesis is an uncommon presenting feature, but may be present. Older children may be able to describe the typical heartburn associated with GORD. This retrosternal pain may be associated with a bitter taste in the mouth.

Respiratory symptoms of wheezing and recurrent pneumonias are uncommon but recognised features.[6] GORD should be suspected in children with these respiratory symptoms that are atypical and resistant to treatment. Patients who have resistant wheezing not typically responding to treatment should be investigated for GORD.

Physical Presentation
No physical findings are specific to GORD. Children who are failing to thrive may have evidence of weight loss and have a weight below the fifth centile or may be crossing down centiles. Children may have features of syndromes associated with GORD. Some children may have dental caries and poor general oral hygiene secondary to their reflux. Neurologically impaired children and those with other syndromes may exhibit features of abnormal posturing suggesting Sandifer's syndrome.

Late and atypical presentations and specific presenting syndromes
Sandifer's syndrome is constellation of abnormal posture (especially back arching) due to muscular spasm involving the back and neck muscles. It may also present as torticollis. The abnormal posturing may be related to feeding or occur soon after a feed, suggesting the associa-

tion. It is usually found in neurologically impaired children, in whom a differential diagnosis is often a neurological illness or fitting.

Regurgitation of undigested food is a sign of late disease with stricture formation. If food has not made it into the stomach, stricture formation should be suspected. This can also present as food bolus obstruction at the level of the stricture. Stricture formation is present at diagnosis in approximately 5% in Western countries. Where patients typically present late, the incidence may be higher. One South African study demonstrated an incidence of 12% in children presenting to the surgical unit.[7]

Iron deficiency anaemia may be a late presenting symptom. In one African study, GOR was present in 44% of patients investigated for refractory iron deficiency anaemia.[8]

Barrett's oesophagus is metaplasia in the lower oesophagus from squamous to specialised intestinal columnar mucosa with goblet cells. It is a precursor of dysplasia and progression to adenocarcinoma. It is present in approximately 5–10% of patients with GORD.[9] A prevalence of 2.5 per 1000 is quoted in one paediatric population-based study in the United States.[10] The incidence of Barrett's is lower in African compared to Western countries;[3] however, these patients tend to present later and have a higher rate of progression to adenocarcinoma.[2] There are no specific symptoms associated with Barrett's; it is discovered at endoscopy when biopsies are taken.

Differential diagnoses
The main differential diagnoses and the key features to differentiating them are:

• Malrotation and volvulus should be suspected if bilious vomiting is present. All patients with bilious vomiting should have an upper gastrointestinal (GI) contrast meal with follow through looking for malrotation.

• Urinary tract infection, meningitis and sepsis should be ruled out if there are signs of infection (urinary symptoms, fever, lethargy, and signs of meningism). It is important to rule out these out early or to start appropriate treatment if present. If diarrhoea is present, gastro-enteritis is the likely diagnosis.

• Intestinal obstruction usually presents with acute symptoms and is associated with distention and decreased passage of stool and flatus. Abdominal x-ray will reveal intestinal distention.

Investigations
The diagnosis of GORD is made by using a combination of three main investigative tools (pH study, contrast study, and upper GI endoscopy). The choice of first-line investigation is based on a combination of availability, expertise, and symptoms. Each has its advantages and disadvantages, and any one or all three may sometimes be necessary. Other extra investigations may be added as necessary.

A 24-hour pH study is considered by most as the gold standard investigation for the diagnosis of GORD. Originally described by Johnson and Demeester in 1974,[11] a pH probe placed in the distal oesophagus at the level of T10 is confirmed radiologically. The reflux index (percentage of total time that the oesophageal pH is less than 4) is the main assessment used for diagnosis. If pH is less than 4 for 5% or more of the total time, the study is positive. Twenty-four–hour pH studies have had up to 100% sensitivity and 94% specificity in some studies.[12] The apple juice pH study (using apple juice feeds instead of milk) has been shown to be more sensitive in babies on milk feed,[13] in whom milk may partially neutralise stomach acid and cause falsely high pH values in the presence of reflux.

An upper GI contrast study can also demonstrate reflux and is used to assess the anatomy of the oesophageal hiatus. It can reveal a sliding or rolling hiatus hernia if present. The contrast study is not mandatory, but it is useful in those not responding to treatment and should be done in those being considered for surgery. It can identify any stricture formation.

It is also useful for delineating the duodenojejugal (DJ) flexure to rule out malrotation.

Oesophagogastroduodenoscopy (OGD) is performed to assess the severity of oesophagitis, and biopsies are taken. Suspicious areas of Barrett's changes will also be assessed on histology.

Other investigations and their indications include:

- A multichannel impedance study can be combined with the pH study, and may become the "platinum standard" investigation.[6,14,15] It is thought to increase the sensitivity for reflux by allowing identification of nonacid reflux. Impedance detects changes in fluid contents in the oesophagus, and can determine the direction of flow to identify both acid and nonacid reflux. In patients in whom reflux is strongly suspected, and for whom all investigations have been normal, an impedance study may be warranted. Impedance can also be combined with manometry,[15] and together they can improve the understanding of pathophysiological mechanisms in paediatric GORD.

- A radioisotope gastric emptying scan (milk scan) can be used to assess gastric emptying and identify patients with significant DGE. However, there seems to be little correlation with surgical correction of DGE and outcome (see point 13 in section on Nissen fundoplication later).

- Bronchoscopy and broncho-alveolar lavage are sometimes used to detect lipid-laden macrophages as evidence of aspiration from reflux in those with respiratory symptoms. However more recent evidence has demonstrated a low sensitivity and specificity of this test.[16]

- Oesophageal manometry studies may be indicated in those cases of reflux stricture that cannot be distinguished from achalasia.

Management

Medical/Nonsurgical Management

Feed thickening

Feed thickening has been shown to reduce the clinical symptoms associated with GOR,[17;18] although this has not been proven to be the case in preterm infants in the neonatal intensive care unit (NICU).[19] Several thickening agents are available:

- Alginate (Gaviscon®) and pectin are gelling agents that can be added to milk feeds and result in a thickened feed that remains in the stomach easier than liquid feeds.

- Prethickened milk feeds (e.g., Enfamil® AR) contain an easy-to-digest rice starch that thickens in the stomach and is successful in helping reduce symptoms in some children. Carob-bean gum is another thickener that is added to prethickened feeds.

- Simple common household foods can be used as additives to reduce reflux in children. These can include cereals, breads, fruit purées, corn starch,[20;21] and other starches.

Overall, feed thickening offers moderate clinical improvement with less vomiting and improved weight gain in many infants and children.[22]

Postural changes

Changes in posturing immediately postprandial have been shown to decrease GORD both clinically and experimentally. The upright position is optimal in the postprandial period in infants and children at home or in general wards. Special nursing seats that maintain an upright position are used to reduce reflux. However upright positioning is not possible in all settings (e.g., in the NICU). Nursing infants in the prone position has been shown to reduce the instances of reflux, as demonstrated on dual pH and impedance monitors in the lower oesophagus in infants.[23] Others have shown that the ideal position is determined by the time after feeding, and changes from the right lateral in the early postprandial hour to left lateral later on.[24]

Feeding regimen

Changes in feeding pattern can be used to achieve a regimen that minimises symptoms. Smaller volumes and more frequent feeds can accomplish adequate calorific intake and achieve growth with minimal vomiting by reducing stomach distention with each feed. This may be especially useful in infants, most of whom will grow out of their reflux without major intervention.

All three of the above measures can be additive and should be tried together where possible.

Pharmacological treatment

Medical treatment of GORD usually involves therapy with an acid suppressant alongside a prokinetic agent in an attempt to reduce reflux and decrease complications.[25–28]

Gastrointestinal prokinetics are used to promote gastric emptying, reduce episodes of GOR, and improve symptoms. They may also act by increasing LOS tone. Common therapeutic agents are domperidone and erythromycin. Metoclopramide, an antidopaminergic and cholinomimetic drug, is a prokinetic agent that has also been used for medical management of GORD. However neurologic adverse effects (e.g., tardive dyskinesia) may occur. Cisapride is another very effective drug in this group, but has been taken off the market in most countries due to its cardiac side effects and is now available only in a limited-use protocol.

The H_2-recptor blockers (ranitidine, cimetidine) and proton pump inhibitors (omeprazole, lansoprazole) decrease acid output from the stomach and reduce both the symptoms and complications of GORD.[26] Oesophagitis has been shown to significantly improve on antacid therapy (particularly proton pump inhibitors). Proton pump inhibitors have become one of the main arms of maximal medical therapy in treating GORD and reversing the complications associated with the disease. Medical therapy with a thickener (such as Gaviscon), along with a prokinetic (domperidone) and a proton pump inhibitor have been used for 6 months as a maximal medical treatment to treat the disease. Patients who are not responsive to this treatment or need continuing therapy to control disease can be considered for step-up management (surgery).

Nasojejunal feeding is an alternative to operative intervention in those unfit for surgery or when surgery is not available. The incidence of complications and symptom resolution, however, may not be significantly different between operative intervention and jejunal feeding.[29] In appropriate clinical settings, the passage of a nasojejunal feeding tube (with radiological control or confirmation) may be enough to allow safe and effective feeding and sufficient time for growth, allowing the infant to "outgrow" GOR. Problems may arise with the presence of a long-term nasal tube (pressure effects, frequent dislodging, and difficulty with feeding regimen) and may push towards either a jejunostomy or definitive surgery.

Surgery

Surgery is usually contemplated only in those who do not improve on maximal medical management or need continuing medical treatment. The main (but not exclusive) indications for surgery include:

- ALTE;[30]

- presence of a hiatus hernia (GORD will not resolve with medical management);

- recurrent aspiration and pneumonias;[29]

- failure of, or need for, continued maximum medical management (decreases the need for long-term medical management,[31] particularly in neurologically normal children);

- stricture; and

- Barrett's oesophagus (relative indication).

Strictures are best treated initially by maximal medical treatment and dilatations. Dilatations may need to be repeated. Oesophageal dilatation can be performed either by bougie or balloon dilatation. There seems to be little difference in the incidence of complications (e.g., perforation) between the two approaches; however, balloon

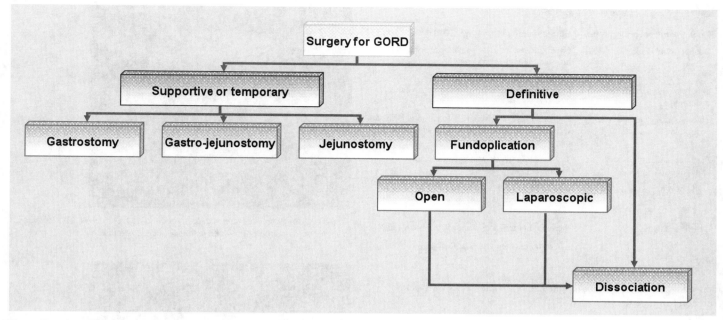

Figure 49.1: Operative intervention for GORD.

dilatation with radiological screening seems to be an inherently safer approach. Most patients then require surgery for their GORD. In one study in Cape Town, only 6 out of 31 patients with strictures secondary to GORD did not require antireflux surgery.[32] Overall, the approach of dilatation followed by antireflux surgery cures 75% of strictures. The remainder of patients may require further dilatations or resection of the strictured segment of oesophagus.

Barrett's oesophagus can also be considered a relative indication for antireflux surgery. There is a small incidence of adenocarcinoma secondary to Barrett's metaplasia. The evidence that surgical treatment is more effective than medical management in preventing progression to cancer has not been proven, however.[33] Laser ablation therapy has been shown in adult studies to be highly effective in curing Barrett's metaplasia[34;35] alongside medical or surgical management of the GORD. No data of its use in children have been published.

Surgery for GORD can be divided into either supportive/temporary or definitive (see Figure 49.1).

Supportive or Temporary Surgery

Gastrostomy for treatment of GORD is occasionally used as a means of establishing feeds and allowing the infant or child to thrive temporarily while maintaining minimal oral intake if possible. There is still some debate in the literature as to whether gastrostomy placement worsens reflux.[36] Some surgeons argue that a gastrostomy placed in the lesser curvature of the stomach is associated with less reflux, and may even improve symptoms.[37;38] Nevertheless, worsening of reflux is a possibility and should be taken into account; this possibility should be mentioned when obtaining consent for surgery. Gastrostomy placement may also be required in patients with severe strictures that need dilatation, both as a means of establishing feeds and a means of accessing the oesophagus for string-guided dilatations.[32]

Gastrojejunostomy is one step further along in the management of GORD in children. It offers advantages over gastrostomy in allowing feeding beyond the pylorus, thus significantly reducing reflux. It has the disadvantages of needing more time-consuming feeding regimens due to the inability to bolus feed. There are various methods of achieving gastrojejunostomy tube feeds. A feeding tube can be placed through an existing gastrostomy and confirmed by radiological imaging. Alternatively, custom-made devices, such as the percutaneous endoscopic gastrostomy–jejunostomy (PEG-J) tube, can be used.

This is placed endoscopically with the jejunostomy extension passed through the pylorus at the time of surgery and confirmed to be in the jejunum on x-ray. This tube also has the advantage of having access ports in the stomach to allow gastric feeding or decompression.

Placement of a jejunostomy tube directly into the jejunum is occasionally used. This is usually a tunnelled type (although a Roux-en-Y configuration is possible). Through a mini-laparotomy incision, a loop of jejunum, preferably 15 cm from the DJ flexure, is isolated as the insertion site. The silk jejunostomy tube is then tunnelled along the jejunum by imbricating the serosa around the tube by using sutures. The tube is then inserted into a stab incision in the jejunum and secured with a double purse string suture in a Stamm gastrostomy fashion. The jejunum, from the apex to the insertion site, is then sutured to the abdominal wall to complete the tunnel. The disadvantage of a jejunostomy is the difficulty in re-establishing the tube should it be pulled out. Displacement is possible, and caregivers should be aware of what should be done in the event of this occurrence. Jejunostomies are associated with higher complication rates compared to gastrojejunostomies (e.g., infections, leakage, feeding difficulties).

The options outlined above provide temporary treatment of GOR by allowing enteral intake and growth to be established before embarking on more major surgery. The infant/child can be tried on increasing oral intake while tube-feeding continues. Tube-feeding can then be stopped if full oral intake is achieved. These devices can then be removed on an outpatient basis without the need for surgery. Occasionally, a minor operation is needed if the stoma does not close.

Definitive Surgery

Definitive surgery (fundoplication) for GORD aims to address or augment the main contributing factors preventing reflux and to reverse any pathology present. Table 49.2 shows the key features of definitive surgery to correct GORD as it relates to the antireflux mechanism and pathology discussed earlier.

Nissen Fundoplication to Treat GORD

The operative details of Nissen fundoplication (360° wrap) are presented here because it is the author's operation of choice. Salient points on other operations are briefly presented in the next section.

1. A subcostal incision is appropriate in most cases. (Other options include rooftop, transverse supraumbilical or midline incisions,

Table 49.2: Surgical steps in treating GORD.

Mechanism preventing reflux	Surgical steps in treating GORD
Oesophageal clearance	Secondary effect from treating oesophagitis; however, a tight wrap can delay and cause dysphagia.
Length of intraabdominal oesophagus	Mobilisation of oesophagus and achieving an intraabdominal length of at least 2–3 cm.
Physiological lower oesophageal sphincter	Repairing hiatus hernia. Reinforcing the HPZ with a wrap of stomach around the abdominal oesophagus.
Diaphragmatic pinch-cock effect of crura	Tightening of hiatus with sutures. Repairing hiatus hernia.
Angle of His	Reinforcing acute angle between stomach and oesophagus (e.g., in Boix-Ochoa fundoplication).
Gastric emptying	Increased due to a decrease in stomach size. ± Pyloroplasty increases emptying

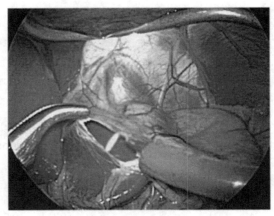

Figure 49.2: Incision in zona pellicuda over caudate lobe of liver. The incision is extended towards the crura, seen just superior to the incision.

depending on the body habitus and size of the patient as well as the surgeon's preference.)

2. The upper portion of the gastrohepatic ligament above the left gastric vessels over the caudate lobe of the liver (zona pellucida of the lesser omentum) is incised (Figure 49.2) and extended cranially and medially towards the oesophageal hiatus.

3. The crura of the diaphragm are then identified and dissected free while mobilising the oesophagus (incising the phreno-oesophageal ligament) to ensure an adequate intraabdominal length (usually 2–3 cm, depending on the size of the child).

4. If present, the sac of any hiatal hernia is excised, taking care not to enter the pleural cavity.

5. A window posterior to the oesophagus is created by dissection between it and the crura. The posterior vagus (and anterior, if possible) are identified during the dissection and kept with the oesophagus. The fundus of the stomach should be visible through this window.

6. The fundus of the stomach is freed from adhesions to the abdominal wall and spleen. Small peritoneal adhesions to the spleen are relatively common and need to be divided. Formal division of the short gastric vessels are not mandatory, but should be undertaken if needed to ensure a "floppy" wrap.

7. The oesophageal hiatus is then narrowed by using nonabsorbable sutures to approximate the crura posterior to the oesophagus (Figure 49.3). Usually, two sutures are needed, but this can vary. The crura are approximated enough to leave a small space between them and the oesophagus; this should be just enough for a fingertip.

8. The proximal oesophagus is sutured to the diaphragm by using a nonabsorbable suture to anchor it in place. This is optional, but adds stability to the oesophagus in the abdomen.

9. The fundus is then guided behind the oesophagus, ensuring that it is not under tension when wrapped around the lower oesophagus and that it is not twisted.

10. A floppy wrap is then constructed by using the fundus of the stomach, using three rows of nonabsorbable sutures placed widely on the fundus (Figure 49.4). These sutures can also be passed superficially through the oesophagus between the stomach ends (stomach-oesophagus-stomach).

11. The looseness of the wrap is tested by gently lifting the wrap off the oesophagus (or a gentle shoe-shining manoeuvre).

12. If required, a gastrostomy can be constructed in a Stamm fashion at the junction of the body and antrum.

13. A pyloroplasty is not routinely performed by this author, even in

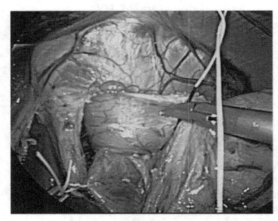

Figure 49.3: Second suture about to be placed to narrow the oesophageal hiatus. The anterior vagus is visible above the oesophagus.

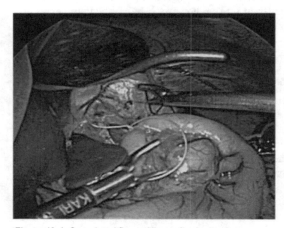

Figure 49.4: Completed floppy Nissen fundoplication.

those that have been shown to have delayed gastric emptying. Brown et al.[39] have demonstrated that a gastric outlet operation is not needed in most cases of fundoplication because almost 90% of patients have normalised gastric emptying after surgery. Also, Pacilli et al.[40] have demonstrated that gastric emptying, measured by using an isotope milk scan, increased following Nissen fundoplication without pyloroplasty. Therefore, a policy of fundoplication without pyloroplasty seems justifiable, leaving this option as a later addition in those that have continuing problems.

14. Pyloroplasty is performed by making a longitudinal incision along the pylorus through all layers. This is then closed transversely using interrupted sutures.

A laparoscopic approach to Nissen fundoplication is justifiable in surgeons with the expertise, with comparable outcomes compared to open surgery in randomised studies (in adults).[41] In a randomised trial, laparoscopic Nissen fundoplication in children was shown to preserve immune function in the postoperative period.[42] Laparoscopic antireflux surgery has now largely become the preferred approach in children where expertise exists (including our own institution). Day case laparoscopic Nissen fundoplication in South Africa has also been described,[43] and is a testament to the advances in recovery that can be achieved with the laparoscopic approach.

The other more common operations used to treat GORD include:

• Thal fundoplication (anterior 180° wrap).

• Toupet fundoplication (posterior 270° wrap).

• Boix-Ochoa fundoplication; additional steps after closing the hiatus involves stitching the fundus to the right crus of the diaphragm to restore the angle of His. The fundus is then plicated over the intraabdominal oesophagus as a partial anterior wrap up to the hiatus. The fundus of the stomach is then sutured to the undersurface of the diaphragm by using three sutures that suspend the fundus.

Many other versions and variations of antireflux surgery exist, with slight variations of the steps for Nissen fundoplication. There is little evidence that any one operation is superior to any other in terms of efficacy and outcome, and the choice of operation is usually up to the surgeon's choice and experience.

Total Oesophagograstric Dissociation

Total oesophagogastric dissociation (Roux-en-Y oesophagojejunal anastomosis and jejunojejunostomy with gastrostomy feeding tube) was initially proposed as a salvage operation for patients who have multiple failed fundoplications[44,45] (predominantly neurologically impaired children). It has now been proposed to include total oesophagogastric dissociation as a primary procedure in the severely neurologically impaired child or in difficult scenarios.[46,47] The author has no experience with this operation and further details are therefore not given here.

Complications

Bleeding from trauma to the liver or spleen can occur intraoperatively and should be anticipated with cross-matched blood. Rarely, splenectomy is required due to uncontrollable bleeding.

Perforation of the oesophagus during mobilisation is avoidable if careful dissection is performed. Occasionally, difficult dissection due to severe inflammation may make this complication more likely.

Respiratory complications, including pneumonia and atelectasis, occur mainly in the neurologically impaired or in those with neuromuscular disease. Pneumothorax may be caused during the dissection around the oesophageal hiatus if the pleura is accidentally incised. The consequence is usually mild, and the operation can be continued without intervention. Occasionally, a chest tube may be needed intraoperatively. If suspected and demonstrated on a postoperative x-ray, treatment should be on clinical grounds.

Gastrostomy-related complications include leakage, granuloma formation, infection, and tube dislodgement. Most gastrostomy

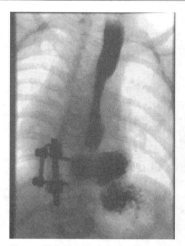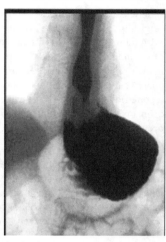

Figure 49.5: Contrast study after a Nissen fundoplication with recurrence of symptoms, demonstrating a sliding hernia. Note the indentation of the oesophagus, indicating the wrap is intact.

complications are treatable by conservative measures. Leakage from the stoma site is best addressed first by changing to a shorter button to achieve a better fit. Occasionally downsizing to a smaller gauge, to allow the stoma to shrink, then replacing with the original size is helpful. Granulomas can be treated with repeated silver nitrate cautery, which is effective in most cases. Occasionally, excision is required. Infections are treated with appropriate topical or systemic antibiotics, depending on prevalence and culture results. Parents and caregivers should always be warned of tubes falling out and advised of the action to take to maintain stoma patency. Occasionally, attempts at replacing the tube can lead to separation of the stomach from the abdominal wall, with peritonitis if feeds are then instilled into the abdominal cavity. This can be fatal if not recognised or if recognised too late.

Dysphagia is present in 5–10% of patients in the postoperative period. Most tend to resolve with time. A portion of patients continue to have significant problems and need dilatation; an even smaller portion need redo surgery.

Intestinal obstruction caused by adhesions can occur. This complication can be treated operatively or initially conservatively depending on clinical presentation. The incidence of adhesions may be lower after laparoscopic approach compared to open surgery.[48]

Retching after fundoplication occurs predominantly in the neurologically impaired group. This can resolve with changes in the feeding regimen and type of milk. In some patients, it persists, and a trial of alimemazine, an antihistaminic that has shown to improve this symptom, is sometimes effective.[49] Most patients with postoperative retching settle with conservative management. In the remainder, alimemazine has variable success. Gas bloat is also common due to the inability to burp up ingested air. Patients with gastrostomies can be vented regularly to avoid bloating.

Recurrence is seen in 5–25% of patients, depending on the series quoted.[27,31,50,51] The incidence is higher in patients with neurological impairment (20–40%) compared to neurologically normal children (5–10%).[31,51,52] The incidence is also higher in patients with congenital anomalies. If further surgical intervention is being considered, an upper gastrointestinal contrast study is performed to assess the integrity and position of the wrap. In most series, the cause of the recurrence is equally shared by wrap failure and wrap migration (into the chest). Figure 49.5 shows two contrast studies demonstrating intact wraps that have migrated into the chest. Recurrent herniations are best treated by redo surgery (redo of the wrap itself is not mandatory, however, if it appears sufficient at operation).

Barrett's oesophagus can occur despite surgical or medical treatment. In adults, it seems to be between 4 and 8 per 1,000 patient years, with no significant difference between those treated medically and those treated surgically.[33] The incidence in children is difficult to establish.

A mortality risk exists for children having Nissen fundoplication. Most of the mortality is late and due to associated conditions. Bradnock et al., in their series of 85 patients, found a late mortality of 7% in children who underwent laparoscopic fundoplication.[53] A similar rate of mortality was reported by Tovar et al[51] in their series of 252 children who had either open or laparoscopic fundoplication. In that series, 17 deaths (6.7%) occurred; 3 in the first postoperative month, with only 1 (0.4%) related to the operation.

Prognosis and Outcomes

In patients with mild disease that resolves on conservative management or with pharmacotherapy with no recurrence, the outcome is good. Resolution in infants usually takes 3 to 6 months.[54] Those with more severe symptoms may have ongoing disease even if improvement is noted.[55]

The main adverse determinants of outcome seem to be the presence of neurological impairment, the presence of associated congenital anomalies, and stricture.

Barrett's oesophagus is a precursor to malignant adenocarcinoma of the oesophagus. Endoscopic surveillance is advocated in older children into adulthood. The incidence of carcinoma in those diagnosed in childhood is not well established.

Prevention

There are no known preventive measures.

Evidence-Based Research

Tables 49.3 and 49.4 present trial studies on thickened-feed interventions in infants and a comparison of laparoscopic and open fundoplication in children, respectively.

Table 49.3: Evidence-based research.

Title	The effect of thickened-feed interventions on gastroesophageal reflux in infants: systematic review and meta-analysis of randomised, controlled trials
Authors	Horvath A, Dziechciarz P, Szajewska H
Institution	Department of Paediatrics, Medical University of Warsaw, Warsaw, Poland
Reference	Pediatrics 2008; 122:e1268–e1277
Problem	Currently, thickened feeds are increasingly being used to treat infants with gastro-oesophageal reflux, driven in large part by the baby food industry. Previous meta-analyses have shown that although thickened formulas do not seem to reduce measurable reflux, they may reduce vomiting. However, because data are limited, there is still uncertainty regarding the use of thickening agents.
Intervention	Meta-analysis of randomised controlled trials.
Comparison/ control (quality of evidence)	The Cochrane Library, Medline, Embase, and CINAHL databases and proceedings of the European and North American paediatric gastroenterology conferences (from 2000) were searched in May 2008; additional references were obtained from reviewed articles. Only randomised, controlled trials that evaluated thickened feeds used in infants for at least several days for the treatment of gastro-oesophageal reflux were considered for inclusion. Three reviewers independently performed data extraction by using standard data-extraction forms. Discrepancies between reviewers were resolved by discussion among all authors. Only the consensus data were entered.
Outcome effect	Fourteen randomised, controlled trials with a parallel or crossover design, some with methodologic limitations, were included. Use of thickened formulas compared with standard formula significantly increased the percentage of infants with no regurgitation, slightly reduced the number of episodes of regurgitation and vomiting per day (assessed jointly or separately), and increased weight gain per day. It had no effect on the reflux index, number of acid gastro-oesophageal reflux episodes per hour, or number of reflux episodes lasting >5 minutes, but significantly reduced the duration of the longest reflux episode of pH <4. No definitive data showed that one particular thickening agent is more effective than another. No serious adverse effects were noted.
Historical significance/ comments	Thickened food is moderately effective in treating gastro-oesophageal reflux in healthy infants.

Table 49.4: Evidence-based research.

Title	Clinical outcome after open and laparoscopic Nissen fundoplication in children: randomised controlled trial
Authors	McHoney M, Eaton S, Drake DP, Kiely EM, Curry J, Spitz L, Pierro A
Institution	Great Ormond Street Hospital for Children, London, UK
Reference	Abstract Canadian Association of Pediatric Surgery Conference, October 2004
Problem	There have been no randomised controlled studies comparing the outcome between open and laparoscopic fundoplication in children. The aim of this study was to compare the clinical outcome in children undergoing Nissen fundoplication who were randomised to open surgery or laparoscopy.
Intervention	Randomised to open and laparoscopic Nissen fundoplication.
Comparison/ control (quality of evidence)	Randomised control trial.
Outcome effect	Twenty patients in the open and 19 patients in the laparoscopic group. Median time to establish full feeds was 2 days in both groups. Median hospital stay was 4.5 days in the open group versus 5 days in the laparoscopic group, with no significant difference between groups. There was no significant difference in morphine requirements, although pain scores fell significantly faster in the laparoscopy group. Incidence of dysphagia, recurrence of reflux, and need for redo fundoplication were not significantly different between groups. At the time of follow-up, the incidence of retching was higher after open surgery (56%) versus laparoscopy (6%; p = 0.003).
Historical significance/ comments	This randomised trial demonstrated equal efficacy between laparoscopic and open fundoplication in children.

Key Summary Points

1. Gastro-oesophageal reflux is common in newborns and not necessarily related to disease pathology. Gastro-oesophageal reflux disease is more common in neurologically impaired children and those with congenital abnormalities of the upper GI tract.

2. Conservative and medical therapies are the mainstay of management, and surgery is reserved for those with complications and the need for ongoing maximal medical treatment.

3. Laparoscopic or open fundoplication is the operative procedure of choice, with a relatively good outcome, especially in neurologically normal children. There is a higher incidence of complications and recurrences in neurologically impaired children.

References

1. Sonnenberg A, El Serag HB. Clinical epidemiology and natural history of gastroesophageal reflux disease. Yale J Biol Med 1999; 72(2–3):81–92.

2. Mason RJ, Bremner CG. The columnar-lined (Barrett's) oesophagus in black patients. S Afr J Surg 1998; 36(2):61–62.

3. Segal I. The gastro-oesophageal reflux disease complex in sub-Saharan Africa. Eur J Cancer Prev 2001; 10(3):209–212.

4. Di Lorenzo C, Piepsz A, Ham H, Cadranel S. Gastric emptying with gastro-oesophageal reflux. Arch Dis Child 1987; 62(5):449–453.

5. Magista AM, Indrio F, Baldassarre M, et al. Multichannel intraluminal impedance to detect relationship between gastroesophageal reflux and apnoea of prematurity. Dig Liver Dis 2007; 39(3):216–221.

6. Rosen R, Nurko S. The importance of multichannel intraluminal impedance in the evaluation of children with persistent respiratory symptoms. Am J Gastroenterol 2004; 99(12):2452–2458.

7. Rode H, Millar AJ, Brown RA, Cywes S. Reflux strictures of the esophagus in children. J Pediatr Surg 1992; 27(4):462–465.

8. Fayed SB, Aref MI, Fathy HM, et al. Prevalence of celiac disease, *Helicobacter pylori* and gastroesophageal reflux in patients with refractory iron deficiency anemia. J Trop Pediatr 2008; 54(1):43–53.

9. Ahmed HH, Mudawi HM, Fedail SS. Gastro-oesophageal reflux disease in Sudan: a clinical endoscopic and histopathological study. Trop Gastroenterol 2004; 25(3):135–138.

10. El Serag HB, Gilger MA, Shub MD, Richardson P, Bancroft J. The prevalence of suspected Barrett's esophagus in children and adolescents: a multicenter endoscopic study. Gastrointest Endosc 2006; 64(5):671–675.

11. Johnson LF, Demeester TR. Twenty-four-hour pH monitoring of the distal esophagus. A quantitative measure of gastroesophageal reflux. Am J Gastroenterol 1974; 62(4):325–332.

12. Da Dalt L, Mazzoleni S, Montini G, Donzelli F, Zacchello F. Diagnostic accuracy of pH monitoring in gastro-oesophageal reflux. Arch Dis Child 1989; 64(10):1421–1426.

13. Tolia V, Kauffman RE. Comparison of evaluation of gastroesophageal reflux in infants using different feedings during intraesophageal pH monitoring. J Pediatr Gastroenterol Nutr 1990; 10(4):426–429.

14. Loots CM, Benninga MA, Davidson GP, Omari TI. Addition of pH-impedance monitoring to standard pH monitoring increases the yield of symptom association analysis in infants and children with gastroesophageal reflux. J Pediatr 2009; 154(2):248–252.

15. van Wijk MP, Benninga MA, Omari TI. Role of the multichannel intraluminal impedance technique in infants and children. J Pediatr Gastroenterol Nutr 2009; 48(1):2–12.

16. Rosen R, Fritz J, Nurko A, Simon D, Nurko S. Lipid-laden macrophage index is not an indicator of gastroesophageal reflux-related respiratory disease in children. Pediatrics 2008; 121(4):e879–e884.

17. Orenstein SR, Magill HL, Brooks P. Thickening of infant feedings for therapy of gastroesophageal reflux. J Pediatr 1987; 110(2):181–186.

18. Wenzl TG, Schneider S, Scheele F, et al. Effects of thickened feeding on gastroesophageal reflux in infants: a placebo-controlled crossover study using intraluminal impedance. Pediatrics 2003; 111(4 Pt 1):e355–e359.

19. Corvaglia L, Ferlini M, Rotatori R, et al. Starch thickening of human milk is ineffective in reducing the gastroesophageal reflux in preterm infants: a crossover study using intraluminal impedance. J Pediatr 2006; 148(2):265–268.

20. Chao HC, Vandenplas Y. Comparison of the effect of a cornstarch thickened formula and strengthened regular formula on regurgitation, gastric emptying and weight gain in infantile regurgitation. Dis Esophagus 2007; 20(2):155–160.

21. Chao HC, Vandenplas Y. Effect of cereal-thickened formula and upright positioning on regurgitation, gastric emptying, and weight gain in infants with regurgitation. Nutrition 2007; 23(1):23–28.

22. Horvath A, Dziechciarz P, Szajewska H. The effect of thickened-feed interventions on gastroesophageal reflux in infants: systematic review and meta-analysis of randomized, controlled trials. Pediatrics 2008; 122(6):e1268–e1277.

23. Corvaglia L, Rotatori R, Ferlini M, et al. The effect of body positioning on gastroesophageal reflux in premature infants: evaluation by combined impedance and pH monitoring. J Pediatr 2007; 151(6):591–596.

24. van Wijk MP, Benninga MA, Dent J, et al. Effect of body position changes on postprandial gastroesophageal reflux and gastric emptying in the healthy premature neonate. J Pediatr 2007; 151(6):585–590.

25. Cucchiara S, Minella R, Iervolino C, et al. Omeprazole and high dose ranitidine in the treatment of refractory reflux oesophagitis. Arch Dis Child 1993; 69(6):655–659.

26. Hassall E, Israel D, Shepherd R, et al. Omeprazole for treatment of chronic erosive esophagitis in children: a multicenter study of efficacy, safety, tolerability and dose requirements. International Pediatric Omeprazole Study Group. J Pediatr 2000; 137(6):800–807.

27. Cezard JP. Managing gastro-oesophageal reflux disease in children. Digestion 2004; 69 Suppl 1:3–8.

28. Pritchard DS, Baber N, Stephenson T. Should domperidone be used for the treatment of gastro-oesophageal reflux in children? Systematic review of randomized controlled trials in children aged 1 month to 11 years old. Br J Clin Pharmacol 2005; 59(6):725–729.

29. Srivastava R, Downey EC, O'Gorman M, et al. Impact of fundoplication versus gastrojejunal feeding tubes on mortality and in preventing aspiration pneumonia in young children with neurologic impairment who have gastroesophageal reflux disease. Pediatrics 2009; 123(1):338–345.

30. Valusek PA, St Peter SD, Tsao K, et al. The use of fundoplication for prevention of apparent life-threatening events. J Pediatr Surg 2007; 42(6):1022–1024.

31. Lee SL, Sydorak RM, Chiu VY, et al. Long-term antireflux medication use following pediatric Nissen fundoplication. Arch Surg 2008; 143(9):873–876.

32. Numanoglu A, Millar AJ, Brown RA, Rode H. Gastroesophageal reflux strictures in children, management and outcome. Pediatr Surg Int 2005; 21(8):631–634.

33. Corey KE, Schmitz SM, Shaheen NJ. Does a surgical antireflux procedure decrease the incidence of esophageal adenocarcinoma in Barrett's esophagus? A meta-analysis. Am J Gastroenterol 2003; 98(11):2390–2394.

34. Schulz H, Miehlke S, Antos D, et al. Ablation of Barrett's epithelium by endoscopic argon plasma coagulation in combination with high-dose omeprazole. Gastrointest Endosc 2000; 51(6):659–663.

35. Morino M, Rebecchi F, Giaccone C, et al. Endoscopic ablation of Barrett's esophagus using argon plasma coagulation (APC) following surgical laparoscopic fundoplication. Surg Endosc 2003; 17(4):539–542.

36. Razeghi S, Lang T, Behrens R. Influence of percutaneous endoscopic gastrostomy on gastroesophageal reflux: a prospective study in 68 children. J Pediatr Gastroenterol Nutr 2002; 35(1):27–30.

37. Plantin I, Arnbjornsson E, Larsson LT. No increase in gastroesophageal reflux after laparoscopic gastrostomy in children. Pediatr Surg Int 2006; 22(7):581–584.

38. Stringel G. Gastrostomy with antireflux properties. J Pediatr Surg 1990; 25(10):1019–1021.

39. Brown RA, Wynchank S, Rode H, Millar AJ, Mann MD. Is a gastric drainage procedure necessary at the time of antireflux surgery? J Pediatr Gastroenterol Nutr 1997; 25(4):377–380.

40. Pacilli M, Pierro A, Lindley KJ, Curry JI, Eaton S. Gastric emptying is accelerated following laparoscopic Nissen fundoplication. Eur J Pediatr Surg 2008; 18(6):395–397.

41. Catarci M, Gentileschi P, Papi C, et al. Evidence-based appraisal of antireflux fundoplication. Ann Surg 2004; 239(3):325–337.

42. McHoney M, Eaton S, Wade A, et al. Inflammatory response in children after laparoscopic vs open Nissen fundoplication: randomized controlled trial. J Pediatr Surg 2005; 40(6):908–913.

43. Banieghbal B, Beale P. Day-case laparoscopic Nissen fundoplication in children. J Laparoendosc Adv Surg Tech A 2007; 17(3):350–352.

44. Bianchi A. Total esophagogastric dissociation: an alternative approach. J Pediatr Surg 1997; 32(9):1291–1294.

45. Islam S, Teitelbaum DH, Buntain WL, Hirschl RB. Esophagogastric separation for failed fundoplication in neurologically impaired children. J Pediatr Surg 2004; 39(3):287–291.

46. Lall A, Morabito A, Bianchi A. «Total gastric dissociation (TGD)» in difficult clinical situations. Eur J Pediatr Surg 2006; 16(6):396–398.

47. Lall A, Morabito A, Dall'Oglio L, et al. Total oesophagogastric dissociation: experience in 2 centres. J Pediatr Surg 2006; 41(2):342–346.

48. Gutt CN, Oniu T, Schemmer P, Mehrabi A, Buchler MW. Fewer adhesions induced by laparoscopic surgery? Surg Endosc 2004; 18(6):898–906.

49. Antao B, Ooi K, Ade-Ajayi N, Stevens B, Spitz L. Effectiveness of alimemazine in controlling retching after Nissen fundoplication. J Pediatr Surg 2005; 40(11):1737–1740.

50. Mattioli G, Esposito C, Lima M, et al. Italian multicenter survey on laparoscopic treatment of gastro-esophageal reflux disease in children. Surg Endosc 2002; 16(12):1666–1668.

51. Tovar JA, Luis AL, Encinas JL, et al. Pediatric surgeons and gastroesophageal reflux. J Pediatr Surg 2007; 42(2):277–283.

52. Esposito C, Montupet P, van Der ZD, et al. Long-term outcome of laparoscopic Nissen, Toupet, and Thal antireflux procedures for neurologically normal children with gastroesophageal reflux disease. Surg Endosc 2006; 20(6):855–858.

53. Bradnock T, Hammond P, Haddock G, Sabharwal A. A roadmap for the establishment of pediatric laparoscopic fundoplication. J Laparoendosc Adv Surg Tech A 2009; 19(s1): s41-s45.

54. Tolia V, Wuerth A, Thomas R. Gastroesophageal reflux disease: review of presenting symptoms, evaluation, management, and outcome in infants. Dig Dis Sci 2003; 48(9):1723–1729.

55. Gold BD. Is gastroesophageal reflux disease really a life-long disease: do babies who regurgitate grow up to be adults with GERD complications? Am J Gastroenterol 2006; 101(3):641–644.

CHAPTER 50
ACHALASIA

George G. Youngson
Lohfa B. Chirdan

Introduction

Achalasia is an uncommon oesophageal problem in children and consequently can be slow to diagnose. It is a condition of unknown aetiology characterised by poor or absent motility of the body of the oesophagus and the failure of the lower oesophageal sphincter to relax. Infants may present with failure to thrive, pulmonary symptoms, vomiting, dysphagia, and growth retardation, but due to the rarity of the condition, many children present late with any of the above symptoms as well as with significant nutritional compromise. In the absence of an identifiable cause, treatment is directed at symptoms.

Demographics

The prevalence of this condition is unclear; a worldwide survey of paediatric surgeons with experience in achalasia in childhood, however, documented information concerning 175 children.[1] The condition appears to be more common in boys, and familial cases do exist but are rare. Regurgitation of food and dysphagia are common. Profound weight loss is a significant feature and is the most frequent symptom, with 18% of patients presenting in infancy but only 6% diagnosed during that time frame. Fewer than 5% of the cases are diagnosed in childhood. The mean age for diagnosis in adult life is 45 years, and the incidence is approximately five new cases per million population per year.

Aetiology/Pathophysiology

Achalasia is a motor disorder of unknown aetiology characterised by the failure of relaxation of the lower oesophageal sphincter along with poor peristalsis of the oesophagus. The three manometric requirements of the diagnosis of achalasia are: (1) hypertension of the lower oesophageal sphincter, (2) incomplete or absent relaxation of the lower oesophageal sphincter, and (3) weak or absent peristalsic contractions in the body of the oesophagus after swallowing. Transient achalasia can be due to corrosive ingestion and ganglion cell damage, as seen in *Trypanosoma cruzi*, or Chagas disease.[2]

Poor clearance of foodstuffs and saliva produces stagnation with a consequent structural change in the calibre of the oesophagus and a change in the mucosal integrity with resultant oesophagitis. Overflow and aspiration are responsible for the respiratory symptoms associated with this condition. The condition is associated with a late incidence of oesophageal carcinoma.[3]

History

Multiple, quite disparate presentations make achalasia a difficult diagnosis in some children. The diversity of symptomatology, ranging from foregut symptoms to advanced pulmonary sepsis as a consequence of aspiration, can distract from the diagnosis. The relative rarity of the condition compounds the situation. Nevertheless, typical features are pain on swallowing, dysphagia, vomiting, failure to thrive, and respiratory symptoms including chronic lung sepsis with wheezing. A family history of achalasia is present on rare occasions.

Physical Examination

Similarly, physical examination covers a range of findings from mild weight loss to an advanced pulmonary sepsis and severe malnutrition. Achalasia can be associated with adrenocorticotropic hormone (ACTH)-resistant adrenal insufficiency and alacrima (an absence of tears).[4] Hence, presentation may have the features of achalasia, addisonianism, and alacrima (triple A, or Allgrove syndrome). All other physical findings are nonspecific.

Investigations

Chest x-ray can demonstrate an air-fluid level in the oesophagus with a characteristic absence of the gastric air bubble on an erect film. In the absence of standard facilities (as is the case in most centres in Africa and other developing countries), a high index of suspicion as well as appropriate use and interpretation of a barium swallow are necessary for prompt diagnosis of achalasia. The barium swallow typically demonstrates a dilated oesophagus above a narrowing "rats tail" or "bird's beak" (see Figure 50.1).

Manometry is the confirmatory investigation with a resting lower oesophageal pressure in excess of 15 to 20 mm Hg and a failure of

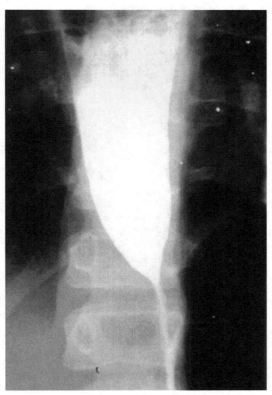

Figure 50.1: Typical barium swallow in an oesophageal achalasia patient.

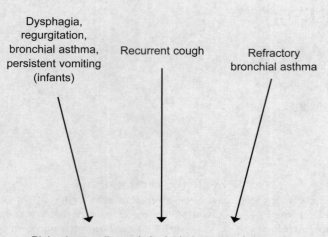

Dysphagia, regurgitation, bronchial asthma, persistent vomiting (infants)

Recurrent cough

Refractory bronchial asthma

Plain chest radiograph (to include upper abdomen)
• Widened mediastinum
• Fluid level in mediastinum
• Pneumonic changes in lung fields
• Absent air shadow in gastric fundus

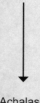

Barium oesophagogram
• Dilated proximal oesophagus
• Smooth tapering of distal oesophagus
• Ineffective peristalsis in proximal oesophagus

Achalasia

Source: Adapted from Chirdan LB, et al., Childhood achalasia in Zaria Nigeria. E Afr Med J 2001; 78:497–499.

Figure 50.2: Algorithm for the diagnosis of oesophageal achalasia in children in countries with limited diagnostic facilities.

the lower oesophageal sphincter to relax on swallowing, along with an absence of peristalsis being the confirmatory features. Endoscopy excludes other causes of organic obstruction or infection in the distal oesophagus.

An algorithm for the diagnosis of achalasia in children in the developing countries and countries with limited diagnostic facilities, seen in Figure 50.2, has been suggested by Chirdan et al.[5]

Management

The three therapeutic modalities of achalasia management are pharmacological treatment, pneumatic dilatation, and esophageal myotomy. An overriding consideration is the nutritional status of the child at outset, and due to the unpredictability of the efficacy of any of the procedures, restoration of good nutritional status is paramount. That can be effectively achieved with nasogastric feeding.

Pharmacological Treatment

Per-endoscopic four quadrant injection of botulinum toxin (100 unit) has been shown to substantially reduce the lower oesophageal sphincter pressures (preinjection, 44 mm Hg; postinjection, 16 mm Hg) with substantial sphincter relaxation. The clear disadvantage of this technique is the need for its repeated application.[6]

The calcium channel blocker nifedipine has been used with good effect in adults, but its use has been limited to those adults unfit for any other form of intervention.[7]

Pneumatic Dilatation in Children

The aim of pneumatic dilatation in children is to relieve obstruction by a gentle disruption of the lower oesophageal sphincter. This procedure is carried out under anaesthesia using radiological and manometric control. An upper gastrointestinal contrast study is performed following the procedure to exclude oesophageal perforation. The number and periodicity of repeat dilatations is patient-specific. It is the recommended initial therapeutic method of choice in older children, but if initial attempts fail to provide satisfactory relief, surgical treatment is then indicated. Only 25% of children show significant improvement with pneumatic dilatations alone, and few children under the age of 9 years have responded to this treatment.[8]

Oesophageal Myotomy

The operative approaches include an abdominal approach, an open thoracic approach, or—more recently—an endoscopic approach through the chest or abdomen.[9] These approaches share the same objective of performing a modified Heller's procedure, which includes a myotomy of the lower oesophagus, preserving the integrity of the oesophageal mucosa. (Heller initially performed his procedure on both sides of the oesophagus; that is, a double oesophagomyotomy.) This is often accompanied by a subsequent fundoplication to prevent gastro-oesophageal reflux frequently produced by the Heller's procedure, and some authorities restrict the myotomy to 0.5 cm on the cardia, thereby reducing the need for antireflux procedures. In those patients for whom transabdominal or a laparoscopic oesophagomyotomy has been performed, this is very frequently accompanied by an antireflux procedure,[9] although some recent authors evaluating the long-term results have suggested that symptomatic improvement in the longer term can be equally effectively obtained without an antireflux procedure.[10]

Surgical Procedure

Oesophageal myotomy through the abdominal route is described in detail in this section. An antireflux procedure is usually not necessary because reflux is rare among African children.

Position and Anaethesia

General anaesthetic with endotracheal intubation is used, with precaution taken to avoid aspiration of oesophageal contents, especially during induction.[11] The child is placed in the supine position. In centres where paediatric endoscopes are available, preoperative oesophagoscopy is used to ensure complete evacuation of retained food and secretions from the oesophagus. A nasogastric tube of appropriate size is passed into the stomach.

Incision and Exposure

An upper midline abdominal incision extending from the xiphisternum to the umbilicus is used. The incision could be extended to just below the umbilicus to give more access. Once the peritoneum is opened, adequate exposure of the abdominal oesophagus is gained by retracting the left lobe of the liver with a wide liver retractor anterosuperiorly. Alternatively, the left triangular ligament is divided in its avascular plane, and the left lobe of the liver is retracted towards the midline.

Mobilisation

The next stage of the operation is the exposure of the oesophageal hiatus and mobilisation of the distal oesophagus. For those who want to add a floppy Nissen fundoplication, the fundus of the stomach is freed by ligating and dividing the short gastric vessels in the gastrosplenic ligament. The phrenicoesophageal membrane is then stretched by applying downward traction on the stomach and retracting the diaphragm upwards. The avascular membrane is incised with a scissors, exposing the muscularis of the oesophagus, and the anterior vagus nerve is seen on the oesophagus. The exposed distal oesophagus is now encircled by using a combination of blunt and sharp dissection, taking care not to injure the posterior vagus nerve. A rubber sling or nylon tape is then placed around the distal oesophagus, and 5–8 cm of the oesophagus is exposed by using blunt dissection.

Myotomy

The myotomy is done on the anterior oesophagus extending to 1 cm of the fundus of the stomach. An incision is made in the distal oesophagus; the divided muscle is then parted with a blunt haemostat, exposing the mucosa. The muscle is separated from the underlying mucosa by pledget dissection. This is continued to about at least half the circumference, freeing the oesophagus from the constricting muscle. This is extended to 1 cm of the fundus. The stomach and oesophagus are then distended with air from the nasogastric tube, and the exposed mucosa is carefully inspected for perforation. In the event of a perforation, the mucosal defect is closed with polyglycolic acid sutures. Finally, the hiatus is narrowed posteriorly by placing deep sutures through the diaphragmatic crura, leaving sufficient space along the oesophagus that can admit the tip of the finger.

Wound Closure

The abdominal wound is closed in layers with nylon sutures. The skin is closed with subcuticular suturing.

Laparoscopic Approach

When a laparoscope is available, the pneumoperitoneum is established through standard procedure and a 5–10 mm camera port is placed through the infraumbilical skin crease. Three to four additional 5-mm ports are placed to permit retraction and dissection of the oesophageal hiatus. The same principles are adhered to as in the open operation, with mobilisation of the distal oesophagus under direct vision. Following circumferential encircling of the oesophagus with the umbilical tape and with caudal retraction on this tape, the distal oesophagus is dissected and

exposed for several centimetres. A myotomy is performed on the distal oesophagus vertically with extension just distal to the cardio-oesophageal junction. The muscle is elevated on either side of the myotomy with graspers anchoring the edge of the muscle and with the dissection of the muscle from the mucosa performed with endoscopic scissors.

Postoperative Care

Intravenous fluid is stopped after 3–4 days, and the nasogastric tube is removed by day 4.

The most worrying postoperative complication is leakage from an undetected perforation of the oesophageal mucosa, making a subsequent contrast study a requirement of the postoperative period.

Prognosis and Outcomes

The vast majority of patients have an immediate and lasting benefit from their surgery. Failure of the initial operation should be managed by an attempt at a second myotomy (on the contralateral side of the oesophagus), but more than 80% of patients have long-term relief of symptoms and resumption of appropriate growth following the first operation.

Evidence-Based Research

Due to the rarity of achalasia in children, no prospective studies exist that compare the various modalities of treatment and their long-term outcome in Africa. Guidance is derived mainly from retrospective experiences. Table 5.1 presents evidence-based research using Heller's procedure.

Table 50.1: Evidence-based research.

Title	Evaluating long term results of modified Heller limited esophagomyotomy in children with esophageal achalasia
Authors	Vaos G, Demetriou L, Velaoras C, et al.
Institution	Second Department of Pediatric Surgery, P and A Kyriakou Children's Hospital, Athens, Greece; First Department of Pediatric Surgery, P and A Kyriakou Children's Hospital, Athens, Greece; Department of Pediatric Surgery, Penteli General Children's Hospital, Athens, Greece
Reference	J Pediatr Surg 2008; 43:1262–1269
Problem	The role of modified transabdominal Heller's myotomy in the long-term outcome of children with achalasia.
Intervention	Heller's limited oesophagomyotomy.
Comparison	To evaluate long-term symptom relief after intervention using subjective outcome, Ba esophagogram, esophageal pH, and oesophageal manometry.
Outcome/effect	Excellent to good results observed in 93.3% of patients, late Ba oesophagogram showed a significant decrease in oesophageal diameter compared to preoperative values (p < 0.01), and the late oesophageal manometry showed a significant decrease of lower oesophageal sphincter pressure (p < 0.05).
Historical significance/ Comments	This report, although retrospective and in a small population of children, showed that the long-term outcome of children treated with modified Heller's myotomy can be quite satisfactory.

Key Summary Points

1. Achalasia is often diagnosed late in childhood.

2. An awareness of the condition as it affects children is key to diagnosis.

3. A combination of failure to thrive, respiratory symptoms, and food aversion should prompt investigation of upper gastrointestinal (GI) tract.

4. Heller's myotomy (open or laparoscopic) should follow correction of nutritional deficit, with good results being expected.

5. Strict attention must be paid to ensuring mucosal integrity.

References

1. Myers NA, Jolley SG, Taylor RI. Achalasia of the cardia in children: a worldwide survey. J Pediatr Surg 1994; 29:1375–1379.

2. Speiss AE, Kahriles PJ. Treating achalasia. JAMA 1998; 280:638–642.

3. Meijssen MA, Tilanus HW, Blankenstein M, Hop WC. Achalasia complicated by oesophageal squamous cell carcinoma: a prospective study in 195 patients. Gut 1992; 33:155–158.

4. Allgrove J, Clayden GS, Grant DB. Familial glucocorticoid deficiency with achalasia of the cardia and deficient tear production. Lancet 1978; 8077:1284–1286.

5. Chirdan LB, Ameh EA, Nmadu PT. Childhood achalasia in Zaria Nigeria. E Afr Med J 2001; 78:497–499.

6. Walton JM, Tougas G. Botulinum toxin use in pediatric esophageal achalasia: a case report. J Pediatr Surg 1997; 32(6):916–917.

7. Traube M, Dubovich S, Lange RC. The role of nifedipine therapy in achalasia: results of a randomised, double-blind, placebo-controlled trial stop. Am J Gastroenterology 1998; 84:1259–1262.

8. Azizkhan RG, Tapper D, Eraklis A. Achalasia in childhood: a 20-year experience. J Pediatr Surg 1980; 15(4):452–456.

9. Rothenberg SS, Partrick DA, Bealer JF, Chang JHT. Evaluation of minimally invasive approaches to achalasia in children. J Pediatr Surg 2001; 36(5):808–810.

10. Vaos G, Demetrou I, Velouras C, Skondras C. Evaluating long-term results of modified Hellers limited oesophagomyotomy in children with oesophageal achalasia. J Pediatr Surg 2008; 43:1262–1269.

11. Spitz L. Achalasia. In: Spitz L, Coran A, eds. Rob and Smith's Operative Surgery (Pediatric Surgery), 5th ed. Chapman and Hall, London: Pp 333–340.

CHAPTER 51
CORROSIVE INGESTION AND OESOPHAGEAL REPLACEMENT

Sameh Abdel Hay
Hesham Soliman El Safoury
Kokila Lakhoo

Introduction

Caustic ingestion can produce a progressive and devastating injury to the oesophagus and stomach. Caustic material ingestion is most frequently encountered in children who accidentally swallowed caustic materials or in adults who ingested caustic materials for suicidal purposes.[1,2] Alkaline caustics and acids are the commonest chemicals implicated in caustic burns. Stricture formation with inability to swallow food after the injury is inevitable in some cases. Many different therapies have been recommended. The literature regarding the treatment of these patients is quite controversial and inconclusive. Repeated dilatations to maintain an adequate lumen diameter were given in patients with chronic strictures. In more severe strictures, due to the complications and ineffectiveness of the dilatation, surgical replacement of the oesophagus may be required.

The causative caustic agent is either acid or alkali with different reactions and sequelae. The concentration and amount of the ingested material have an important impact on the injury. Lye is a broad term for a strong alkali used in cleansing agents.[3] For example, sodium and potassium hydroxides in granular, paste, and liquid forms are used in drain and oven cleansers as well as washing detergents. Also, button batteries, which contain high concentrations of sodium and potassium hydroxides, can cause severe injuries. Acids are commonly available in toilet bowel cleansers (sulfuric, hydrochloric); battery fluids (sulfuric); and swimming pool and slate cleansers (hydrochloric).[3] The majority of cases in Egypt are due to caustic potash, with three to five new cases every month and an overall ratio of eight alkali cases for every acid case.

Prevention

A public health drive is required to educate the population to the dangers of these corrosive products. Safe storage of corrosive liquids, out of reach from children, is needed. Also, corrosive products must be stored in containers with hazard labels rather than in soft drink bottles to reduce the accidental ingestion of corrosive material.

Directives to change the chemical composition of these products and institute safer preparation of button batteries should be given to commercial institutions.

Pathogenesis and Pathology

The extent of damage to the gastrointestinal tract depends on the agent, its concentration, amount, physical state, and the duration of exposure.[3,4] Acidic solutions usually cause immediate pain, and—unless ingestion is intentional—the agent is rapidly expelled. Alkali solutions, however, are often tasteless and odorless and are swallowed before protective reflexes can be evoked.[1]

Caustic agents in solid form and granules often adhere to the mucous membranes of the mouth, thereby preventing further movement of lye into the oesophagus. The most severe caustic injury generally occurs in the narrowest portion of the oesophagus, usually the midoesophagus in the region of the aortic arch.[5,6]

The primary difference between alkaline and acidic injury is rapid penetration into the tissue by alkali. Alkali has a potent solvent action on the lipoprotein lining, producing a liquefaction necrosis. Thrombosis of adjacent vessels results in further necrosis and bacterial colonisation. Granular agents often produce focal injury to the oropharyngeal and proximal oesophageal mucosa. Liquid alkaline solutions can cause extensive damage to the entire oesophagus and stomach.

Acidic agents produce a coagulation necrosis, resulting in a firm protective eschar that delays injury and limits penetration. The naturally alkaline environment, low viscosity, and rapid transit limit injury of the oropharynx and oesophagus by the acid compounds. Accordingly, acidic agents were thought to spare the oesophagus and injure the stomach. However, ingestion of highly concentrated sulfuric or hydrochloric acid penetrates the oesophageal mucosa and produces severe injury. When the stomach is empty, caustic acids will affect the gastric mucosa along the lesser curvature to the antrum, and when the stomach is full, the acidic agents cause diffuse injury.

Caustic injuries to the gastrointestinal tract are classified pathologically into three degrees according to the depth of injury,[1] as shown in Table 51.1.

Table 51.1: Degree of oesophageal burns

Degree of burn	Oesophageal depth
First-degree	Superficial, confined to mucosa, heal without stricture formation
Second-degree	Penetration into muscularis layer
Third-degree	Entire wall of gastrointestinal tract, with or without perforation

Clinical Features

The clinical picture on presentations depends mainly on the site and depth of injury caused by the caustic agent. Early manifestations include persistent salivation, dysphagia, hoarseness of voice and stridor, retrosternal chest pain, and hematemesis. Severe gastric injury may present as epigastric pain; retching; or emesis of tissue, blood, or coffee-ground material. Fever, shock, dyspnoea, and acute abdomen strongly indicate oesophageal or gastric perforation.[7]

Late complications of caustic injuries include dysphagia due to the establishment of oesophageal stricture within 1 to 2 months. Early satiety, weight loss, and progressive emesis suggest gastric outlet obstruction. Repeated chest infections may indicate acquired tracheo-oesophageal stricture.

Diagnosis

Due to the poor correlation between signs and symptoms and the degree of injury, endoscopic examination of the upper gastrointestinal tract is essential in most patients with a history of caustic ingestion. There is great controversy regarding the proper timing of the endoscopy. Many centres have performed the procedure in the first 24 to 48 hours after ingestion with excellent results, and have found the procedure to be safe and accurate. The endoscopic grading of the injury can predict the treatment and outcome, and unnecessary treatment is avoided when oesophageal injury is excluded by endoscopy. In the presence of stridor and respiratory problems, however, early endoscopy is hazardous because it may aggravate the airway obstruction.

Endoscopic grading of corrosive oesophageal and gastric burns is shown in Table 51.2. Grade I and grade IIA injuries do not result in strictures, whereas 70% to 100% of circumferential burns (grade IIB) and grade III lesions result in strictures.[5]

It has been suggested that most patients with severe injury have one or more clinical signs or symptoms (drooling, dysphagia, vomiting, and abdominal pain), and that 50% or more of patients who present with vomiting, stridor, and drooling have associated oesophageal injury. Furthermore, asymptomatic patients are deemed to be unlikely to have lesions that progress to stricture or perforation. Based on these data and on the absence of proven therapy to prevent stricture, the suggestion is that patients require endoscopy only if they are symptomatic.[3,7] Most authorities recommend performing upper endoscopy as soon as the patient is stable.[3,8]

The practice in Egypt is that endoscopy is not done in the acute stage but postponed for 6 weeks and performed only for symptomatic patients.

Table 51.2: Endoscopic grading of corrosive oesophageal burns.

Grade	Finding
Grade I	Oedema and erythema
Grade IIA	Haemorrhages, erosions, blisters, superficial ulcer, exudate (patchy or linear)
Grade IIB	Circumferential lesions
Grade III	Multiple deep brownish-black or gray ulcers
Grade IV	Perforation

Radiologic Studies

X-ray

Plain chest and abdominal x-rays should be performed in the acute phase of caustic injury. This may reveal evidence of perforation such as pneumothorax, pleural effusion, or air under the diaphragm. If perforation is still suspected despite negative plain films, a study with the use of water-soluble contrast material may reveal extra luminal contrast.[3–7]

Computed Tomography

Computed tomography (CT) of the oesophagus and stomach with orally administered contrast is the most sensitive method of detecting early perforation.[3] With this approach, life-threatening injuries can be identified and treated at an early stage.[9] In the chronic stages of the illness, maximal wall thickness of oesophageal stricture can be measured with a contrast-enhanced CT scan.[3]

Contrast studies (see Figures 51.1 and 51.2) are most useful in evaluating the inlet of the upper gastrointestinal tract, the oesophageal body, and the stomach outlet at approximately 3 weeks after injury.[3] Oesophageal body strictures can be of variable length, shape, and number. Most strictures are at the region of the aortic arch.[7] It is of utmost importance to study the inlet of the gastrointestinal tract before surgery to plan for the site of the proximal oesophagocolic anastomosis, and to study the outlet to detect any antral stenosis. Any missed strictures at the inlet or outlet after substitute organ replacement of the oesophagus may affect the success of the surgery.

Endoscopic Ultrasound

It is likely that endoscopic ultrasound (EUS) provides better determination of the depth of injury and may prove to be adjunctive or even superior to endoscopy in staging caustic oesophageal injury.[7]

Treatment Options

The goals of therapy are to prevent and treat perforation as early as possible, to avoid strictures of the oesophagus and stomach, and to replace or bypass the damaged organ to allow normal swallowing of food.

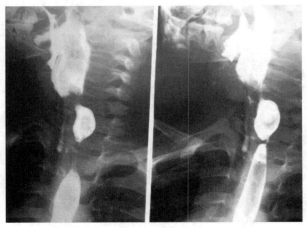

Figure 51.1: Multiple oesophageal strictures.

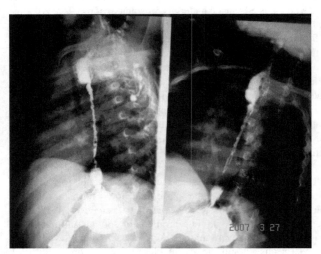

Figure 51.2: Long oesophageal strictures.

Surgery

Although emergency surgery is indicated in cases of perforation, it is difficult initially to predict which patients will develop this complication.[3] Early surgery is essential to improve the prognosis in cases of oesophageal or gastric perforation.[10] Although most investigators state that in selected cases, early surgery would be prudent, the criteria on which to base selection of surgical cases are not well defined.[3] The reduced mortality achieved through early detection of impending or actual perforations outweighs the morbidity and mortality rate associated with surgical exploration in patients with endoscopically diagnosed second-degree burns. However, many surgeons have condemned early surgery because the extent of the injury often cannot be delineated, leaks at anastomotic sites can occur, and surgery will not be needed in the majority of patients.

Neutralisation or Flushing

To be effective, neutralisation of caustics must be done within the first hour after ingestion of the caustic agent. Lye or other alkali can be neutralised with half-strength vinegar, lemon juice, or orange juice. Acids can be neutralised with milk, egg, or antacids.

Sodium bicarbonate is not used because it generates CO_2, which might increase the danger of perforation.[3–5] Water is used only to wash the mouth and not for dilution because it will take the remnant to the rest of the gastrointestinal tract (GIT). Emetics are contraindicated because vomiting renews the contact of the caustic substance with the oesophagus and can contribute to aspiration or perforation if it is too forceful.[3–5]

Collagen Synthesis Inhibitors

In experimental animals, collagen synthesis inhibitors, such as amino-proprionitrile, penicillamine, N-acetylcysteine, and colchicine, have been shown to prevent alkali-induced oesophageal strictures. These compounds impair synthesis of collagen by interfering with the covalent crosslink. However, no clinical studies have been performed with these agents.[3]

Nutrition

Intravenous (IV) nutrition is essential for patients in whom perforation has occurred or enteral feeding cannot be maintained. However, in some African institutions where IV nutrition is not available, patients may be started on oral alimentation or a nasogastric feeding tube. In many cases, a feeding gastrostomy or jejunostomy may provide the patient with the necessary nutritional requirement until surgical correction can be performed. A feeding gastrostomy can be used as a route for retrograde dilatation.[3]

Early Oesophageal Dilatation

Some investigators recommend eosophageal dilatation immediately after injury. Dilatation is performed at frequent intervals until healing occurs.[3] This approach, however, is controversial in that dilatations can traumatise the oesophagus, predisposing to bleeding and perforation, and same data indicate that excessive dilatations cause increased fibrosis.[5] Dilatation is recommended by some only when stricture formation develops. Others pass a string on the nasogastric tube as part of the initial therapy to maintain the oesophageal lumen.[3]

Corticosteroids

Studies by some investigators in animals have shown that corticosteroids given within 24 hours after alkali injury inhibits granulation and fibroblastic tissue reaction and decreases the incidence of oesophageal stricture.[3,11] Others, however, believe that corticosteroids may obscure evidence of peritonitis and mediastinitis and fail to reduce the incidence of stricture formation. Corticosteroid injections are used in localised strictures. Intralesional triamcinolone injections augment the effects of endoscopic dilatation.[12–14] Several studies have shown that local steroids improve and increase the intervals between dilatation but not the need for replacement.[15]

Oesophageal Stents

Some investigators have placed intraluminal silastic stents under endoscopic guidance in patients with deep circumferential burns. Unfortunately, the majority of these patients required oesophageal dilatation later.[3,16]

Endoscopic Dilatation

Treatment of strictures is endoscopic dilatation. Gradual dilatation is essential.[3] Dilatation can be done on a weekly or biweekly basis by using Savary-Gilliard® bougies, and is considered adequate if the oesophageal lumen could be dilated to 11 mm with complete relief of dysphagia. The Savary-Gilliard method is adequate for oesophageal dilatations in the paediatric population.[17,18,15] Balloon dilatation under endoscopic guidance and radiological screening of the oesophageal stricture is also successful (see Figure 51.3). The advantages of this method may be that its forces are exerted radially and the procedure may be performed under better control.[19] Perforation, bleeding, sepsis, and brain abscess may complicate dilatation, however.[3–20] Mitomycin C antibiotic has been recently used with promising results. After endoscopic dilatation, mitomycin can be applied onto the dilatation wound by using a rigid endoscopy.[21]

An adequate lumen should be reestablished within 6 months to 1 year, with progressively longer intervals between dilatations. If, during the course of treatment, an adequate lumen cannot be established or maintained, surgery should be considered. Surgical intervention is indicated in the following cases:

• Patients with failure to swallow solid food, which may lead to deformities of the mandible, temporomandibular joint, and teeth.

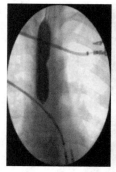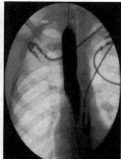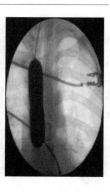

Figure 51.3: Balloon dilatation.

• Patients with complete stenosis, in which all attempts have failed to establish a lumen.

• Patients with multiple, tortuous, or very long (more than 5 cm) strictures.

• Patients with severe peri-oesophageal reaction or mediastinitis, and in the development of tracheo-oesophageal fistula.

• Patients who are unwilling or unable to undergo prolonged periods of dilatation.

Treatment Recommendations

During the acute phase, we give oral feeding as tolerated; otherwise, the patients are kept on IV fluid until oedema subsides; if dysphagia persists, we prefer to perform gastrostomy to keep the general condition of the patient maintained until an upper endoscopy is performed after 6 weeks. In Egypt, we are performing the gastrostomy by laparoscopy, with better results and fewer adhesions (see Figure 51.4). Our protocol for oesophageal dilatation starts after 6 weeks and is repeated every 2 weeks for 6 months by using the Savary-Gilliard dilator.

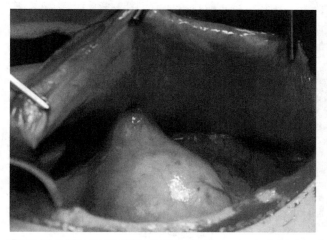

Figure 51.4: Appearance of the stomach after laparoscopic gastrostomy (no adhesions).

Surgical Interventions

The variety of abnormalities seen requires that creativity be used when considering oesophageal reconstruction. Skin tube oesophagoplasties are now used much less frequently and are mainly of historical interest. Currently, the stomach, jejunum, and colon are the organs used to replace the oesophagus through either the posterior mediastinum or the retrosternal route. A retrosternal route is chosen when there has been a previous oesophagectomy or if there is extensive fibrosis in the posterior mediastinum. When all factors are considered, the order of preference for oesophageal substitution depends on the experience of the surgeon and the practice in the institution.[5]

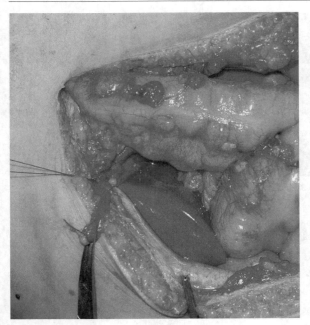

Figure 51.5: Fixing the round ligament to the sternum.

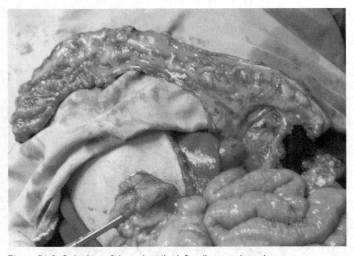

Figure 51.6: Colonic graft based on the left colic vessels and sigmoid vessels (double blood supply).

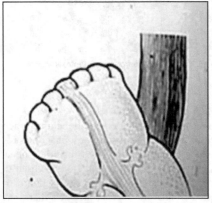

Figure 51.7: End-to-side oesophagocolic anastomosis.

Colon Substitution

The isoperistaltic left colon segment based on the left colic vessels is a very suitable substitute for the oesophagus in children. A sufficient length is available to replace the whole oesophagus and even the lower pharynx if needed. The blood supply from the left colic vessels is robust and rarely prone to anatomic variations. The close relation between the marginal vessels and the border of the viscus results in a straight conduit with little redundancy. The left colon seems to transmit food more easily than the right colon, and has proved to be relatively acid resistant.[22-24]

The transhiatal oesophagectomy with posterior mediastinal isoperistaltic left colon has been the most direct and shortest route for the oesophageal substitute between the neck and abdomen. It permits the removal of the scarred oesophagus, which has a definite increased risk of malignant changes, cyst formation, and empyema if left in place. [22-24]

The retrosternal route is still an ideal route for many surgeons. Retrosternal colon by-pass avoids any thoracic dissection and preserves the vagus nerves. It takes less operative time and avoids injuries to such intrathoracic structures as trachea and major vessels. The postoperative period is less stormy than the transhiatal route, and few patients require postoperative ventilations. Many modifications have been performed to make a straight route out of the anterior mediastinal/retrosternal route. Dividing the strap muscles in the neck and fixing the falciform ligament to the sternum (Figure 51.5) avoids the colon being stretched over the liver when the child is in an erect position. [22-24]

An equal number of each technique were performed at Ain Shams University in Cairo. We prefer using the transverse colon, based on a double blood supply from the left colic vessels (Figure 51.6) with comparable results for retrosternal and transhiatal techniques. Usually, we add an antireflux procedure while performing the cologastric anastomosis by wrapping the lower colon by stomach in the transhiatal approach and creating an angle between the lower colon and the anterior gastric wall. The length of tucking of the colon to the anterior gastric wall to create an antireflux mechanism should be 4–5 cm.

Leakage from the cervical oesophagocolic anastomosis has been reported to be 12–71% and is usually followed by varying degrees of stricture after the cessation of leakage. Performing an end-to-side anastomosis between the unequal diameters of the oesophagus and colon has decreased the incidence of leakage from the neck anastomosis (Figure 51.7). The use of a double blood supply to the colonic graft and the use of a vascularised omental flap to wrap the anastomosis have also reduced the leakage rate.[22-24]

Long-term follow-up for patients with colonic replacement of the oesophagus have shown excellent results. Late complications, such as strictures of the cervical end, may lead to varying degrees of dysphagia. Strictures may be dilated; however, the majority will need revision of the anastomosis. Redundancy of the interposed colonic graft in the chest may lead to stasis and dysphagia due to kinking of the graft (Figure 51.8). Proper measurement of the graft length and avoiding opening the pleura may decrease the incidence of redundancy of the colonic graft.[22-24]

Gastric Substitution

In gastric substitution, a cervico-abdominal approach is used. The neck incision may be right- or left-sided. The abdominal incision may be upper umbilical midline or transverse. The gastrostomy is carefully taken down and closed in two layers. The vessels on the greater curvature of the stomach are preserved for the gastric transposition or if a carefully constructed gastric tube is used. Where possible, a posterior mediastinal route is preferred to a retrosternal route. The fundal end of the stomach is anastamosed to the oesophageal stump in the neck, securing the neck anastomosis with sutures to the retro clavicular tissue. A wide bore nasogastric tube is introduced into the thoracic stomach to avoid acute gastric distention. Gastrohiatal sutures are applied to prevent herniation of abdominal contents. A pyloroplasty is performed and the pylorus is kept below the diaphragm (Figures 51.9

and 51.10) A feeding jejunostomy rarely is required for caustic injuries. Reported complications from Great Ormond Street Children's Hospital in London are as follows:[25] Mortality, 5.2%; anastamotic leaks, 12%; oesophageal strictures, 38%. All leaks but one closed spontaneously, and all strictures except three responded to dilatation. Transient dumping syndrome and delayed gastric emptying were also noted. Results were excellent in 90% of patients with minimal impact on growth, development, and respiratory function.

Jejunal Substitution

The jejunum is more commonly used in adults. It is used mainly as a free graft with microvascular anastamosis. Due to the popular use of the colon or stomach as replacement organs with good results, jejunal substitution is used less in the paediatric population.

Surgical Technique

The most critical point in the planning of the operation is the selection of the site for proximal anastomosis. The site of the upper anastomosis depends on the extent of the pharyngeal and cervical oesophageal damage. When the cervical oesophagus is destroyed and a pyriform sinus remains open, the anastomosis can be made to the hypopharynx. When the pyriform sinus is completely stenosed, a transglottic approach is used to perform an anastomosis to the posterior oropharyngeal wall.

Recovery is long and difficult and may require several endoscopic dilatations and, often, reoperations. Sleeve resections of short strictures are not successful because the extent of damage to the wall of the oesophagus can be greater than realised, and almost invariably the anastomosis is carried out in a diseased area. The management of a bypassed damaged oesophagus after injury is problematic. The extensive dissection necessary to remove the oesophagus, particularly in the presence of marked perioesophagitis, is associated with significant morbidity. Leaving the oesophagus in place preserves the function of the vagus nerves and, in turn, the function of the stomach. Leaving a damaged oesophagus in place, however, can result in multiple blind sacs and subsequent development of mediastinal abscesses years later. Most experienced surgeons recommend that the oesophagus be removed unless the operative risk is unduly high.[5]

Antral stenosis may develop rapidly 3 to 6 weeks after the injury, but in some cases it may appear only after several years.[26] Therefore, long-term follow-up is required even though the initial symptoms of the patients are minimal.[26] Some surgeons perform a Billroth I procedure for severely injured mucosa with complete pyloric obstruction, and pyloroplasty for moderate mucosa injury associated with partially obstructed but still viable pylorus.[27] However, distal gastric resection is usually recommended. Although many patients are initially achlorhydric, vagotomy is usually performed because acid production may return. With extensive injury, subtotal or total gastrectomy or partial oesophagectomy may be necessary.

A strong association exists between caustic injury and squamous cell carcinoma of the oesophagus. From 1% to 7% of patients with carcinoma of the oesophagus have a history of caustic ingestion. A 1000- to 3000-fold increase has been estimated in the expected incidence of oesophageal carcinoma after caustic ingestion.[3–7] Because of the markedly increased incidence of cancer in these patients, many authors have recommended yearly endoscopic surveillance beginning 20 years following caustic oesophageal injury.[7]

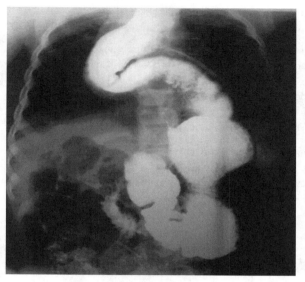

Figure 51.8: Retrosternal colonic graft.

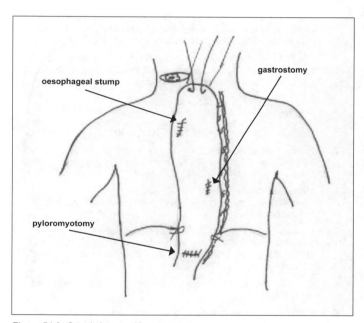

Figure 51.9: Gastric interposition.

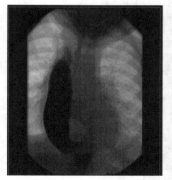
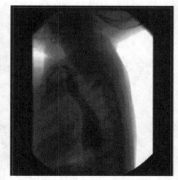

Figure 51.10: Contrast of gastric interposition.

Key Summary Points

1. A preventive scheme is essential to avoid the devastating accidental injuries due to corrosive ingestion.

2. Alkaline injury is more extensive than acid injury due to the delay in the protective reflexes in an acid injury and rapid penetration of alkali into the tissues.

3. The most severe caustic injury generally occurs in the narrowest portion of the oesophagus, usually the midoesophagus in the region of the aortic arch.

4. Early clinical manifestations include persistent salivation, dysphagia, hoarseness of voice and stridor, retrosternal chest pain, and hematemesis.

5. Fever, shock, dyspnoea, and acute abdomen strongly indicate oesophageal or gastric perforation.

6. Dysphagia is the late presentation due to stricture.

7. Diagnosis is by imaging and endoscopy.

8. The goals of therapy are to prevent and treat perforation as early as possible, to avoid strictures of the oesophagus and stomach, and to replace or bypass the damaged organ to allow normal swallowing of food.

9. Therapy is variable.

References

1. Havanond C. Clinical features of corrosive ingestion. J Med Assoc Thai 2003; 86:918–924.

2. Rodriguez MA, Meza Flores JL. Clinical-epidemiological characteristics in caustics ingestion patients in the Hipolito Unanue National Hospital. Rev Gastroenterol Peru 2003; 23:115–125.

3. Loeb-Abram PM, Eisenstein M. Caustic injury to the upper gastrointestinal tract. In Sleisenger and Fordtran's Gastrointestinal and Liver Disease, 6th ed. W. B. Saunders Company; 1998, Pp 335–342.

4. Gorman RL, Khin Maung Gyi MT, Klein Schwartz W, et al. Initial symptoms as predictors of esophageal injury in alkaline corrosive ingestion. Am J Emerg Med 1992; 10:189–194.

5. Peters JH, Demeester TR, Esophagus and diaphragmatic hernia. In: Schwartz ST, Shires GT, Spencer FC, et al., eds. Principles of Surgery, 7th ed. McGraw Hill, 1999, Pp 1158–1161.

6. Makela JT, Laitine S, Salo JA, Corrosion injury of the upper gastrointestinal tract after swallowing strong alkali. Eur J Surg. 1998; 164:575–580.

7. Douglas O, Fanigel M, Fennerty B. Miscellaneous disease of the esophagus. In: Yamada T, Alpers DH, et al., eds. Textbook of Gastroenterology, 3rd ed. Lippincott, Williams & Wilkins, 1999, Pp 1316–1318.

8. Gumaste VV, Dave PB. Ingestion of corrosive substances by adults. Am J Gastroenterol 1992; 87:1–5.

9. Guth AA, Pachter HL, Albanese C, Kim U. Combined duodenal and colonic necrosis. An unusual sequel of caustic ingestion. J Clin Gastroenterol 1994; 19:303–305.

10. Cotton P, Munoz-Bongrand-N, Berney T, Halimi B, Sarfati E, Celeriver M. Extensive abdominal surgery after caustic ingestion. Ann Surg 2000; 231:519–523.

11. Howell JM, Dalsey WC, Hartsell FW, Butzin CA. Steroids for the treatment of corrosive esophageal injury: a statistical analysis of past studies. Am J Emerg Med 1992; 10:421–425.

12. Gunnarsson M. Local corticosteroid treatment of caustic injuries of the esophagus. A preliminary report. Ann Otol Rhinol Laryngol 1999; 108:1088–1090.

13. Zarkovic S, Busic I, Volic A. Acute states in poisoning with corrosive substances. Med Arh 1997; 51:436–438.

14. Kochhar R, Ray JD, Sriram PV, et al. Intralesional steroids augment the effects of endoscopic dilation in corrosive esophageal strictures. Gastrointest Endosc 1999; 49:509–513.

15. Hamza A, Salam MAA, Naggar OA, Soliman HA. Endoscopic dilatation of caustic esophageal strictures in children. J Egypt Soc Surg 1998; 17:435–440.

16. Berkovits RN, Bos CE, Wijburg FA, Holzki J. Caustic injury of the esophagus. Sixteen years experience, and introduction of a new model esophageal stent. J Larynogol Otol 1996; 110:1041–1045.

17. Guitron A, Adalid R, Nares J, et al. Benign esophageal strictures in toddlers and pre school children, result of endoscopic dilation. Rev Gastroenterol Mex 1999; 64:5–12.

18. Asensio Llorente M, Broto Mangues J, Gil-Vernet Huguet JM, et al. Esophageal dilatation by Savary-Guillard bougies in children. Cir Pediatr 1999; 12:33–37.

19. Appignani A, Trizzino V. A case of brain abscess as complication of esophageal dilation for caustic stenosis. Eur J Pediatr Surg 1997; 7:42–43.

20. Sandgren K, Malmfors G, Balloon dilation of esophageal strictures in children. Eur J Pediatr Surg 1998; 8:9–11.

21. Uhlen S, Fayoux P, Vachin F, et al. Mitomycin C: an alternative conservative treatment for refractory esophageal strictures in children? Endoscopy 2006; 38(4):404–407.

22. Bahnassy AF, Bassiouny IE. Esophagocoloplasty for caustic strictures of the esophagus: changing concepts. Pediatr Surg Int 1993; 8:103.

23. Bassiouny IE, Bahnassy AF. Transhiatal esophagectomy and colonic interposition for caustic strictures. J Pediatr Surg 1992; 27:1091–1096.

24. Hamza AF, Abdelhay S, Sherif H, Hassan T, Soliman HA, Kabish A, Bassiouny I, Bahnassy AF. Caustic esophageal strictures in children: 30 years' experience. J Pediatr Surg 2003; 38:828–833.

25. Spitz L, Kiely E, Pierro A. Gastric transposition in children—a 21 year experience. J Pediatr Surg 2004; 39:276–281.

26. Wilasrusmec C, Sirikolchayanonta V, Tirapanitch W. Delayed sequelae of hydrochloric acid ingestion. J Med Assoc Thai 1999; 82:628–631.

27. Giftic AO, Senocak ME, Buyukpamukcu N, Hicsonmez A. Gastric outlet obstruction due to corrosive ingestion: incidence and outcome. Pediatr Surg Int 1999; 15:88–91.

CHAPTER 52
AERODIGESTIVE FOREIGN BODIES IN CHILDREN

Neetu Kumar

Ashish Minocha

With minor contributions by
David Msuya

Introduction

Aerodigestive foreign bodies are common causes of morbidity and mortality in infants and children worldwide. It is difficult to eradicate the problem, as children, by nature, are curious and exploratory. Possibly the only difference from one country to another is in the nature of foreign bodies commonly encountered. It is important to develop a comprehensive approach to the early recognition and timely management of aspirated and ingested foreign bodies, as complications from delayed diagnosis can have significant health implications. Serious complications from aspirated foreign bodies such as severe airway obstruction and death, tend to occur in infants and younger children due to the small size of their airways.

Chevalier Jackson's initial description of endoscopic removal of foreign bodies in 1936[1] revolutionised the treatment options for management of aerodigestive foreign bodies.[2] Associated developments in radiology have played an important role in the rationalised and safe management of these cases.

Epidemiology

Foreign body ingestion and aspiration are common childhood adverse events. They form the third leading cause of death in children under the age of 1 year and the fourth leading cause in the age group 1–6 years. The maximum prevalence is seen between the ages of 1 and 2 years; however, no age group is completely immune.[3–5]

Children younger than 5 years of age represent the highest risk group. This risk is increased if the child has neurological impairment.[6] Unfortunately, these children are often not viewed with a high index of suspicion when they present with nonspecific symptoms. Children known to have congenital anatomic or physiologic abnormalities of the oesophagus, such as diffuse oesophageal spasm, oesophageal atresia, and/or tracheo-oesophageal fistulas, or those who had previous bowel surgery are at increased risk of complications.

The commonly encountered foreign bodies vary geographically. Coin ingestion seems to be the commonest worldwide problem.[7] Other common nonfood items are school stationery, balloons, and toys. Pharyngeal fish bones are well reported from countries where fish forms a part of the staple diet. Over the years, there has been a rise in the incidence of disk-type battery ingestion in the paediatric population, which can lead to serious consequences.[8]

Seeds and nuts are frequent causes of tracheobronchial obstruction worldwide. Accidental aspiration of peanuts is commonly responsible for airway obstruction in children in Southeast Asia and Africa, and kola nuts, which are traditionally used in Africa, may be inhaled accidentally.

Clinical Presentation

Children present in myriad fashions, both with typical and not so typical or convincing stories. The problem is worse when no witness is available or parents are unsure of the sequence of events. In addition, older children may be reluctant to divulge the initial details for fear of punishment or due to embarrassment. Such enquiries should therefore be made discreetly and tactfully.

Tracheobronchial foreign bodies typically present with shortness of breath, wheezing, stridor, cough without associated illness, recurrent or migratory pneumonias, and even acute aphonia. When the diagnosis is initially missed, children often present with recurrent respiratory tract infections (pneumonia, empyema, and abscess formation).

Oesophageal foreign bodies typically present with odynophagia, drooling, spitting, vomiting, or even secondary airway compromise from foreign body impingement. Episodic vomiting may be the only presentation in some cases.[9]

Pathophysiology

Certain characteristics can predispose children to the likelihood of an aerodigestive mishap. Their underdeveloped posterior dentition, along with their immature swallowing mechanism, is no match for their oro-exploratory behaviour.

The process of aspiration or ingestion of foreign bodies can present in three different stages.[10] The first (or acute) stage characteristically involves a phase of coughing, choking, and gagging. This history is often easily elicited. Typically, an asymptomatic period follows the first phase. The diagnosis is potentially missed if the patient presents during this time. The third phase is a period of chronicity characterised by failure to thrive, recurrent lung infestations, wheeze, dysphagia, or even more severe manifestations such as intrathoracic abscesses and vascular catastrophes secondary to foreign body fistulation.[11]

Investigations

Nothing can substitute for a high index of clinical suspicion. However, clinicians must understand the role and limitations of emergency radiography. Plain radiographs should be assessed in two dimensions.[12,13] Radio-opaque foreign bodies are often easily seen, but more important is accurate anatomical localisation to assist retrieval. Follow-up radiographs are often essential if the preliminary studies have been negative. If a foreign body has not been visualised in the cervical or thoracic regions, it may well have passed into the small and large bowel; such relevant body parts may also need imaging. At times, there are indirect signs that assist in making a diagnosis. For example, air trapping on expiratory chest radiographs may be indicative of an obstructing foreign body not otherwise visible. In a considerable number of cases, plain radiography is unrevealing and secondary signs are not convincing enough to make a confirmed diagnosis. Some children may need urgent fluoroscopy to look for "filling defects" in the digestive tract.[14]

Bronchoscopy can be both diagnostic and therapeutic. Foreign bodies more distally located in the respiratory tree may warrant an urgent bronchogram. Computed tomography (CT) and even magnetic resonance imaging (MRI) may be employed to detect foreign bodies that are not found during endoscopic examination or if migration from the airway or oesophagus is suspected.[15]

Management

"Prevention is better than cure"—this proverb holds utmost conviction when it comes to aerodigestive foreign bodies in children. Public awareness and education are key elements to help foster a culture of preventive medicine.

In the emergent situation, paediatric life-support algorithms should be employed in a conscious child presenting with known foreign body airway obstruction. This involves voluntary coughing in older children and back blows between the shoulder blades in infants to dislodge the impacted foreign body. Crucial steps in acute management are the ABCs: optimisation of **A**irway, **B**reathing, and **C**irculation.

For both tracheobronchial and oesophageal foreign bodies, the definitive and safest treatment option is endoscopic retrieval under general anaesthesia. In a few cases, however, a more proximal foreign body may be removed under local anaesthesia. Risks and complications (aspiration) due to accidental dislodgement must be carefully considered before such an undertaking, though.

Some centres have reported success in the retrieval of smooth foreign bodies of the airway by using guide wire and angioplasty catheters.[16] The successful use of a Foley catheter with balloon inflation, with or without fluoroscopic guidance, to retrieve an oesophageal foreign body such as a coin, has been reported in older literature and is still practiced successfully with minimal morbidity in countries where endoscopic facilities may not be readily available.

Timing of an endoscopy is crucial. It may be required urgently in the following situations: (1) any suggestion of airway compromise, (2) a history of aspiration of dried peas or beans because they have a hygroscopic potential to swell up and block distal airways, (3) batteries impacted in the oesophagus because they can cause early caustic mucosal damage and even perforation, and (4) any suggestions of oesophageal perforation.[17,18]

The success of intervention depends on the experience and skill of the endoscopist and the local availability of the optimal instruments. The bronchoscope or oesophagoscope should be carefully sized to the predicted size of the child's airway/oesophagus and the foreign body.

Foreign bodies impacted in the pharynx/upper airway are usually visible during intubation and may be taken out by an anaesthetist using a Magill's forceps.

A rigid bronchoscope can be successfully used for removal of foreign bodies from the trachea or one of the main bronchi. Once the foreign body is localised, appropriate suction is introduced and grasping forceps help to engage the body. The endoscope is advanced to cover the object completely. The endoscope, forceps, and foreign body are then removed simultaneously. Good anaesthetic support is a must for success.[19] More distal foreign bodies need retrieval by flexible bronchoscopy.

Oesophageal foreign bodies are best retrieved by rigid oesophagoscopy. The same principles as for a flexible broncoscopy apply. Occasionally, if the retrieval looks challenging and the type of foreign body is definitely known to be inert, it may be pushed further into the stomach. This avoids the risks of aspiration and dislodgement. Nature can then be allowed to take its course. Disk batteries stuck in the oesophagus could cause serious harm and should be retrieved endoscopically as a matter of urgency.

Foreign bodies in the stomach and bowel usually do not need taking out unless they are harmful (e.g., sharp objects, batteries that have shown no progression beyond the stomach over a 48-hour period, or toxic foreign bodies). Long foreign bodies (>6 cm), such as tooth brushes and pens, and wide foreign bodies (> 2 cm), such as some toys, are also likely to remain stuck in the stomach. Ingestion of more than one magnet has been reported to cause necrosis of the intestine trapped

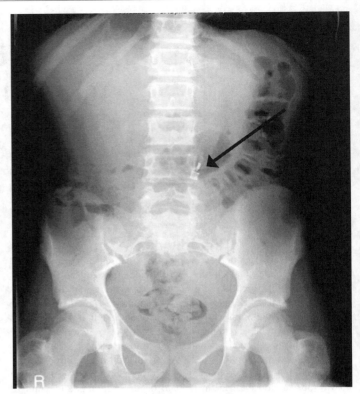

Figure 52.1: A retained pen in the stomach. There was no change in the position of the foreign body on a chest radiograph, 10 days after accidental ingestion.

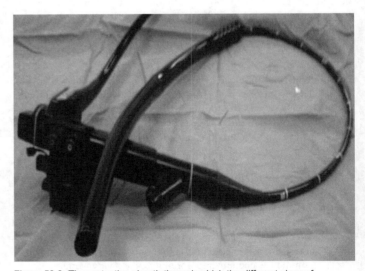

Figure 52.2: The protective sheath through which the different sizes of endoscopes can be easily guided. Preplacement of the protective sheath protects the oesophagus from accidental damage during retrieval of a sharp or pointed object.

between the two magnets;[20] therefore, it may be advisable to retrieve the magnets while they are still accessible in the oesophagus or stomach.

When the ingested foreign bodies are not retrieved, patients and parents are advised to look for foreign bodies in the stool. If not egested in a week to 10 days, repeat check x-rays are taken, and if no further distal movement of the foreign body is demonstrated beyond the stomach (see Figure 52.1), it is best retrieved endoscopically. Laparoscopic, or laparotomy-assisted, retrieval may be indicated very rarely, except for the situation of a secondary complication of obstruction or perforation. One reason to attempt a proactive laparoscopic or laparotomy retrieval is the risk of a secondary complication outweighing the chances of spontaneous passage of the foreign body.

Most of the endoscopic interventions are done as day procedures. Postinterventional care is straightforward and should be tailored to the specific need. Antibiotics are administered only if complications are suspected.

Practical Hints and Tips

The endoscopist must be aware of the following situations:

1. There may be more than one foreign body. This situation is more common and relevant with tracheobronchial foreign bodies such as aspirated food items, nuts, and seeds. Therefore, a thorough assessment of the airway is important.

2. The suction device "tip" should not be used to remove the object because it is not strong enough to hold the object during transit to the external world.

3. The dangerous end of sharp foreign bodies should be carefully covered by the scope (in case of a rigid scope) or a flexible endoscope protective sheath prior to removal (Figure 52.2).

4. Good haemostasis should be maintained.

5. Repeat inspection of the airway or digestive tract for any evidence of secondary or iatrogenic injury once the foreign body is retrieved.

Key Summary Points

1. Inhalation or ingestion of a foreign body by a child is a common accident that may cause significant morbidity or even mortality.

2. The situation worsens when the foreign bodies are initially missed and then later the patient presents with pneumonia, atelectasis, abscess, or bleeds.

3. Radiography, fluoroscopy, bronchogram, CT, and MRI have all been used to make a confirmatory diagnosis.

4. Of utmost importance are a good history and clinical suspicion.

5. The treatment of choice remains endoscopic retrieval under general anaesthesia.

6. Success is ensured by careful assessment of the airways or oesophagus as well as foreign body size and shape prior to skilled endoscopy retrieval.[21]

References

1. Jackson C, Jackson, CL. Diseases of the Air and Food Passages of Foreign Body Origin. Saunders, 1936.

2. Boyd AD. Chevalier Jackson: the father of American bronchoesophagoscopy. Ann Thorac Surg 1994; 57(2):502–505.

3. Steen KH, Zimmermann T. Tracheobronchial aspiration of foreign bodies in children: a study of 94 cases. Laryngoscope 1990; 100(5):525–530.

4. Mu L, He P, Sun D. Inhalations of foreign bodies in Chinese children: a review of 400 cases. Laryngoscope 1991; 101:657–660.

5. Diaz GA, Valledor L, Seda F. Foreign bodies from the upper-aerodigestive tract of children in Puerto Rico. Bol Asoc Med PR 2000; 92(9–12):124–129.

6. DeRowe A, Massick D, Beste DJ. Clinical characteristics of aero-digestive foreign bodies in neurologically impaired children. Int J Pediatr Otorhinolaryngol 2002; 62(3):243–238.

7. Mahafza TM. Extracting coins from the upper end of the esophagus using a Magill forceps technique. Int J Pediatr Otorhinolaryngol 2002; 62(1):37–39.

8. Higo R, Matsumoto Y, Ichimura K, Kaga K. Foreign bodies in the aerodigestive tract in pediatric patients. Auris Nasus Larynx 2003; 30(4):397–401.

9. Messner AH. Pitfalls in the diagnosis of aerodigestive tract foreign bodies. Clin Pediatr (Phila) 1998; 37(6):359–365.

10. Tan HKK, Brown K, McGill T, et al. Airway foreign bodies (FB): a 10-year review. Intl J Pediatr Otorhinolaryngol 2000; 56(2):91–99.

11. Remsen K, Lawson W, Biller HF, Som ML. Unusual presentations of penetrating foreign bodies of the upper aerodigestive tract. Ann Otol Rhinol Laryngol Suppl 1983; 105:32–44.

12. Herdman RC, Saeed SR, Hinton EA. The lateral soft tissue neck x-ray in accident and emergency medicine. Arch Emerg Med 1992; 9(2):149–156.

13. Lue AJ, Fang WD, Manolidis S. Use of plain radiography and computed tomography to identify fish bone foreign bodies. Otolaryngol Head Neck Surg 2000; 123(4):435–438.

14. Koempel JA, Hollinger LD. Foreign bodies of the upper aerodigestive tract. Ind J Pediatr 1997; 64(6):763–769.

15. Sethi DS, Stanley RF. Migrating foreign bodies in the upper digestive tract. Ann Acad Med Singapore 1992; 21(3):390–393.

16. Briggs G, Walker RWM. Retrieval of an endobronchial foreign body using a guide wire and angioplasty catheter. Anaesthesia and Intensive Care 2007; 35(3):433–436.

17. Ginsberg GG. Management of ingested foreign objects and food bolus impactions. Gastrointest Endosc 1995; 41:33–38.

18. Friedman EM. Tracheobronchial foreign bodies. Otolaryngol Clin North Am 2000; 33(1):179–185.

19. Swanson KL, Edell ES. Tracheobronchial foreign bodies. Chest Surg Clin N Am 2001; 11(4):861–872.

20. Vijaysadan V, Perez M, Kuo D. Revisiting swallowed troubles: intestinal complications caused by two magnets—a case report, review and proposed revision to the algorithm for the management of foreign body ingestion. J Am Board Fam Med 2006; 19(5):511–516.

21. Reilly JS, Walter MA, Beste D, et al. Size/shape analysis of aerodigestive foreign bodies in children: a multi-institutional study. Am J Otolaryngol 1995; 16(3):190–193.

CHAPTER 53
CHEST WALL DEFORMITIES

Michael Singh
Dakshesh Parikh
Brian Kenney

Pectus Carinatum

Introduction

Pectus carinatum (PC), or pigeon chest, is a spectrum of anterior chest wall anomalies characterised by protrusion of the sternum and adjoining costal cartilages (Figure 53.1). The sternal (gladiolus) protrusion can be associated with symmetrical or asymmetrical protrusion of the lower costal cartilages. The other uncommon variant is the chondromanubrial protrusion of the manubrium, sternum, and adjoining costal cartilages. There are varying degrees of asymmetry and tilting of the sternum with associated depression of the lower anteriolateral chest.

Aetiology

The underlying aetiology for PC is unknown and thought to be related to overgrowth of the costal cartilages. A familial incidence of PC is seen in up to 26% of patients. There is an association with connective tissue disorders, such as Marfan's syndrome, scoliosis (34%), and congenital heart disease (6%).[1,2]

Clinical Presentation

Most patients present after 10 years of age, when there is an increased prominence of the sternum during the adolescent growth spurt. PC is four times more common in males. Symptoms include exertional dyspnoea, decreased exercise tolerance, and precordial chest pain. The majority of patients, however, present because of the cosmetic deformity.

Investigation

Either a PA and lateral chest x-ray or a CT scan will allow good visualisation of the extent of the abnormality. Any spinal abnormality should also be evaluated. The respiratory and cardiac functions should be assessed.

Surgical Procedure

The most widely adopted surgical procedure was described by Ravitch. Either a transverse or chevron incision is made on the chest at a point that allows good access to the entire length of the deformity. In teenage girls, the incision can be hidden in the inframammary fold. The subcutaneous flaps are raised off the pectoralis major with diathermy superiorly to the manubrium and inferiorly to the rectus insertion. The medial attachments of the pectoralis major are incised and the muscle is reflected laterally. Inferiorly, the rectus abdominis is detached from its costal insertions. The costal cartilages of the lower offending ribs on both sides are resected subperichondrally. Care is taken not to damage the underlying pleura.

A transverse osteotomy is made in the anterior table of the sternum just proximal to the beginning of the sternal protrusion. By placing a wedge of resected cartilage into the osteotomy, the sternum can be tilted farther down. The pectoralis and rectus muscles are approximated in the midline with a continuous suture. Inferiorly, the rectus abdominis is sutured to the pectoralis muscle margin. This helps to keep the sternum depressed in its new position. A suction drain may be used. The subcutaneous tissues and skin are closed.

Postoperative analgesia is maintained by either an epidural or opioid infusion. The suction drains are removed once drainage has ceased.[1]

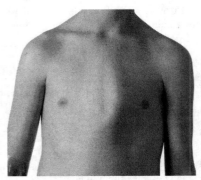

Figure 53.1: Pectus carinatum, chondrogladiolar deformity.

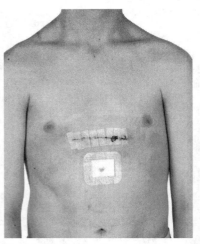

Figure 53.2: Postoperative result after correction of pectus carinatum.

Postoperative complications with the Ravitch technique are uncommon (11–22%). The reported complications following PC correction are seroma, pleural effusion, pneumothorax, and atelectasis. Hypertrophic scarring can occur in 15% of patients.[1,2]

Recently, external dynamic compression has been described as the nonoperative treatment of PC.[2] The dynamic compression system (DCS) consists of a compression plate on a brace and harness. The plate and brace applies external anterior posterior compression to the still compliant chest wall, allowing its gradual remodelling over time. Patients have to wear the brace overnight and for as long as possible during the day. Patients are required to wear the brace for a minimum of 7 months. Complications occur in 12% of patients, involving back pain, skin ulceration, and haematoma. Skin ulceration is managed by stopping the compression temporarily. Recurrence of PC has been reported in 15% during the rapid growth spurt. This can be treated with reuse of the DCS. Overall good to excellent correction has been reported in 88% of cases (Figure 53.2).[2]

Pectus Excavatum

Introduction

Pectus excavatum (PE), or funnel chest, describes a posterior depression of the lower sternum and costal cartilages into the thoracic cavity. Cosmetic appearance is the main presenting reason in asymptomatic patients. The asymmetrical depression is not unusual, and is associated with sternal torsion.

Demographics

Pectus excavatum is an uncommon abnormality with an incidence of 38 per 10,000 and 7 per 10,000 births in the Caucasian and African populations, respectively. It is four times more common in males than females. A family history of PE is reported in 43% of patients, and familial association is seen in 7% of patients with pectus carinatum .[3,4] The incidence of PC in our experience is equal to that of PE; however, the literature suggests that it is less common than PE.

Aetiology

The sternal depression is thought to result from asymmetrical growth of the costochondral cartilages. However, the exact aetiology is unknown. There is an association with connective tissue disorders such as Marfan's syndrome (21.5%) and Ehlers-Danlos syndrome (2%).[3]

Clinical Presentation

Thirty percent of PE patients present in early childhood, with the majority presenting during the pubertal growth spurt. Common symptoms attributed to PE include exercise intolerance, dyspnoea, chest pain with and without exercise, and palpitations. The majority of patients are healthy, and they present because of the cosmetic appearance (Figure 53.3). Patients often have a slouched posture, and young children have an associated protuberant abdomen. Almost a quarter of PE cases are associated with scoliosis, and hence the spine should be investigated in all cases.

Several variations in the sternal abnormality have been described. A cup-shaped appearance describes an abnormality with localised, steeply sloping walls. A saucer-shaped appearance is a diffuse and shallow sternal depression. A long asymmetrical trench-like deformity may also be found. Varying degrees of asymmetry of the chest wall may be present. Sternal torsion may be clinically obvious. A mixed carinatum/excavatum is an uncommon variation with the presence of a carinatum (protuberance) of the manubrium and excavatum of the sternum (Figure 53.4).[5]

Investigations

Cardiac

Cardiac abnormalities have been known to be associated with PE and should be investigated in all cases with electrocardiography and echocardiography. Compression of the right atrium and ventricle by the depressed sternum has been implicated to cause mitral or tricuspid valve prolapse in up to 17% of patients.[3] This has not been our experience in the United Kingdom; however, we have rarely found associated cardiac abnormalities in PE patients. Conduction abnormalities on electrocardiogram (ECG), such as right heart block, first-degree heart block, and Wolff-Parkinson-White syndrome, may be present in up to 16% of patients.[4]

Respiratory

Respiratory function should be assessed preoperatively at least with spirometry. Restrictive lung functions have been reported, with decreases in forced vital capacity (FVC) of 77%, forced expiratory volume in 1 second (FEV_1) of 83%, and forced expiratory flow during the middle portion of expiration ($FEF_{25-75\%}$) of 73%.[4] It is useful to identify any underlying respiratory abnormalities prior to surgery, both for anaesthesia and to see whether correction results in improvement.

Radiology

Chest x-rays, both anteroposterior (AP) and lateral, are routinely performed, which may help to define the severity of the deformity as well

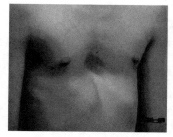

Figure 53.3: Pectus excavatum severe deformity.

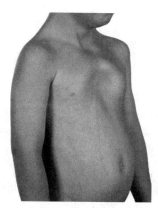

Figure 53.4: Mixed deformity with the presence of a carinatum (protuberance) of the manubrium and excavatum of the sternum.

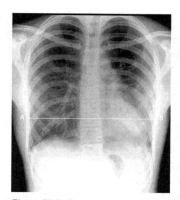

Figure 53.5: Chest x-ray AP view showing shift of heart towards left and a line across the chest (AB) that can be used to calculate the Haller index.

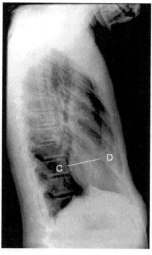

Figure 53.6: Lateral chest x-ray showing the depth of sternal depression (CD).

as help to evaluate the thoracic spine (Figures 53.5 and 53.6).[6] A computed tomography (CT) scan of the chest has been considered the gold standard investigation in PE (Figure 53.7). It allows the calculation of the Haller index, the ratio of the transverse to the AP diameter at the lowest point of the depression. Other information obtained includes the length of the depression, degree of sternal torsion, and presence of chest wall asymmetry.[5] Although recommended by some, we do not routinely carry out a CT scan of the chest or calculate the Haller index, as they do not influence the operative technique or outcome.

Indications for Surgery

Surgery for PE is carried out mainly to improve the appearance of the deformity. However, in some severe cases, two or more of the following are considered an indication for surgery:[7]

- a Haller index of greater than 3.25 plus the presence of cardiac or pulmonary compression.

- Demonstrable cardiac abnormalities.

- Decreased pulmonary function; and

- Previous failed repair by Ravitch or Nuss procedures.

The Nuss procedure is ideally performed between 10 and 12 years of age, taking advantage of the pliability of the chest wall. The child in this age group, however, is often immature and unable to make an educated decision on whether to undergo such a major procedure mainly for cosmetic reasons. The patient should be Gillick competent to give informed consent. A single bar achieves good correction at this age. Two bars are recommended for the postpubertal patient, long or extensive depressions, or the presence of connective tissue disorders.[7]

Surgical Procedure

The Ravitch procedure was the first widely accepted procedure for treatment of pectus excavatum. As has been described above for pectus carinatum, the cartilages are exposed and removed. The anterior table of the sternum is divided transversely to flatten the protrusion and the sternum is stabilized as described for the carinatum, but often with the addition of a transverse fixation bar, which is removed 6-12 months later.

In the past decade, the minimally invasive repair (MIR), or Nuss procedure, as described by Dr. Donald Nuss, has become the most accepted technique for the correction of PE in developed countries.[3,8]

The patient is positioned supine with both arms abducted to 70° to 80° at the shoulder. Prophylactic intravenous antibiotics (e.g., cefuroxime) are given. An extensive skin preparation with an alcohol-based antiseptic solution of the anterior and lateral chest wall is essential.

The distance is measured between the midaxillary points at the deepest part of the sternal depression. One inch is subtracted from this measurement to determine the length of the bar. The bar is then bent symmetrically into a semicircular shape. It is important to have a 2–4 cm flat segment at the centre of the bar to support the sternum. A slight overcorrection is advisable.[3]

The most elevated point in line with the deepest point of excavatum on the costal ridges is marked (Figure 53.8). Transverse incisions are made across the midaxillary line at the level of the lowest point of the depression bilaterally. A subcutaneous tunnel is dissected to the top of the ridges. A 5-mm thoracoscope is inserted into the interspace inferior to the proposed site of bar insertion on the right side. A pneumothorax is maintained at a pressure of 5 to 7 mm Hg with a flow rate of 1–2 l/min. The rest of the procedure is performed under thoracoscopic visualisation.

An introducer is then inserted from the midaxillary incision along the previously created subcutaneous tunnel, through the marked intercostal space (Figure 53.8). This introducer is used to carefully dissect the space between the sternum and pericardium under thoracoscopic vision. The introducer is brought out through the left symmetrically opposite, previously marked intercostal space. After passing the introducer through to the opposite midaxillary incision, both ends of the introducer are lifted

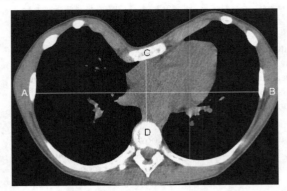

Figure 53.7: CT scan showing sternal torsion, asymmetrical chest, and a measure for the Haller index by calculating AB/CD.

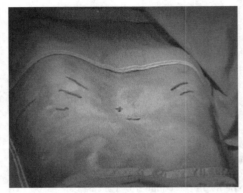

Figure 53.8: Markings on the chest wall: lateral transverse incisions perpendicular to midaxillary line, incision for the thoracoport, and the most elevated point in line with the deepest point of excavatum on the costal ridges.

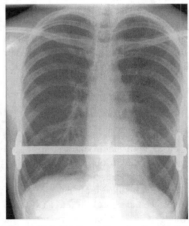

Figure 53.9: Postoperative chest x-ray showing bar in position.

while the costal margins and flared ribs are pushed down. This corrects the deformity and loosens up the connective tissue around the sternum.

An umbilical tape is attached to the end of the introducer and pulled across the retrosternal space by withdrawing the introducer. The bent bar is attached to the end of the tape and pulled into the chest, across the mediastinum, and out through the left with the convexity facing posteriorly. The bar is then flipped by using bar flippers so that the convex surface is facing the sternum. This produces an instant correction of the depression.

A single bar stabiliser is placed on the right side and sutured to the adjacent muscle with 1/0 polypropylene sutures. In addition, on the right side, the bar can be fixed to the adjacent rib with pericostal

1/0 polypropylene sutures guided by thoracoscopy. In the past, two stabilizers were used, one on either side. This practice has been abandoned by most because, as the chest wall grows, the patient can develop an hourglass deformity due to restriction in lateral growth, a problem that does not occur with the use of a stabilizer on only one side. The subcutaneous tissues and skin are closed. The lungs are expanded with positive pressures, and pneumothorax is relieved by putting a tube underwater through a thoracoscopy port site.[7]

A chest x-ray is obtained on day 1 postoperatively (Figure 53.9). Analgesia is maintained with epidural or a patient-controlled morphine infusion in combination with nonsteroidal anti-inflammatory drugs (NSAIDS). A graded programme of incentive spirometry and physiotherapy is commenced postoperatively. The epidural or morphine infusion is usually stopped after the third postoperative day. Oral NSAIDS and codeine may be required for up to 3 weeks postoperatively. Patients are advised to avoid sporting activity for 3 months postoperatively. This allows sufficient scar tissue to develop around the bar, thus fixing it in place and preventing displacement.

Complications

In experienced hands, surgical complications, summarised in Table 53.1, are uncommon. The majority of early postoperative complications can be managed conservatively.[7] Late postoperative complications also are uncommon (see Table 53.1). Bar displacement is caused by inadequate fixation of the bar. Hence, it is recommended that the bar be fixed by using a bar stabiliser and pericostal sutures. Persistent postoperative pain should be investigated for bar or stabiliser displacement, a tight or too long bar, sternal or rib erosion, infection, and bar allergy (i.e., allergy to nickel).[7]

Bar Removal

The bar is generally removed after 3 years. Under general anaesthesia, both lateral incisions containing the stabilizer bar is reopened. All visible sutures around the stabiliser are excised. The bar is straightened

Table 53.1: Early and late postoperative complications following bar insertion.[6]

Early postoperative complications	Pneumothorax small; most common, conservative treatment
	Pneumothorax large; chest drainage
	Horner's syndrome; transient, epidural related
	Stitch site or wound infection
	Pneumonia
	Haemothorax
	Pericarditis (postcardiomyotomy syndrome); oral indomethacin
	Pleural effusion; chest drainage
Late postoperative complications	Bar displacement. Major displacement revision required
	Overcorrection
	Bar allergy
	Recurrence
	Skin erosion

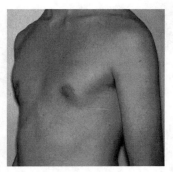

Figure 53.10: Long-term outcome after removal of pectus bar (Nuss bar).

by using the bar reverse bender. Once reasonably loose, it is pulled out from the right side of the chest. The bar should not be forcibly extracted. In the event of difficulty, any residual scar tissue impinging on the bar should be excised before removal. Bar removal is generally uncomplicated. A postoperative chest x-ray should be obtained to rule out pneumothorax. Pneumothorax following bar removal usually is self-limiting and does not require any intervention.[7]

Outcomes

The long-term cosmetic results from the Nuss procedure are as follows: excellent, 86%; good, 10.3%; fair, 2.4%; and failed, 1.3% (see Figure 53.10).[7]

Poland's Syndrome

Introduction

Poland's syndrome is a rare congenital malformation involving the chest wall and variable severity of other defects involving the areola, subcutaneous tissues, muscles, ribs, hand, and heart. The extent of these defects varies significantly from the absent sternocostal head of the pectoralis major and/or minor with normal breast and underlying ribs to complete absence of anterior portions of second to fifth ribs and cartilages. Breast involvement is frequent and is a disfiguring defect in girls. The hand deformity on the side of the defect is also associated in variable frequency from syndactyly to hypoplastic fingers.[6]

Demographics

The reported incidence of Poland's syndrome is low (1 in 30,000) and sporadic in nature. The exact aetiology of this defect is unknown. The proposed aetiology is a disruption in the subclavian arterial blood supply of the limb bud during the 6th foetal week.[9,10]

Clinical Features

The anatomical abnormalities of Poland's syndrome are usually unilateral. Clinically, these patients have an absent anterior axillary fold with the posterior axillary fold being easily visible from the front. The nipple and areola may be hypoplastic or absent with deficient subcutaneous tissues. The chest is depressed on the affected side due to hypoplasia or absence of the underlying 2–4 or 3–5 ribs and cartilages. Rarely, the lung may herniate through the defect in the chest wall, giving a flail segment. This may cause respiratory distress in the newborn period. Dextroposition of the heart is common in Poland's syndrome, rather than dextrocardia.

Surgical Options

The surgical reconstruction options depend on the age of the patient and the extent of the defect. In the neonate, a flail chest may require reconstruction in order to provide a rigid support to counteract the paradoxical movement. Split rib grafts harvested from the contralateral unaffected ribs are generally preferred for the replacement of the missing medial aplastic ribs. The grafts are then attached to the lateral border of the sternum. A mesh sheath can also be used to help bridge large defects. In older patients, a latissimus dorsi muscle flap can be used to correct the defect in muscle mass or anterior axillary fold. For girls with breast hypoplasia, myocutaneous flaps or silicone implants can be used for post pubertal breast reconstruction. Various combinations of procedures may have to be used to achieve a satisfactory cosmetic result.

Jeune's Syndrome

Introduction

Jeune's syndrome, also known as asphyxiating thoracic dystrophy, is a rare autosomal recessive disorder. It is characterised by dwarfism, foreshortened horizontally placed ribs, and short limbs. Thoracic cage abnormalities (osteochondro dystrophy) result in a markedly small chest with severe restriction of expansion, pulmonary hypoplasia, and severe respiratory distress. Its characteristic feature is a "bell-shaped" chest and a protuberant abdomen.

Surgical Procedure

The aim of surgery is to expand the chest wall and increase the thoracic volume, allowing lung expansion. Multiple surgical procedures have been described. Using a median sternotomy, the two halves of the sternum are stented apart by using rib drafts or methyl methacrylate. Another option is dividing the ribs laterally in a staggered arrangement. The divided ribs are then fixed by using titanium plates. This allows for gradual chest expansion. Recently, a form of expansion thoracoplasty by using a vertical expandable prosthetic titanium rib (VEPTR) has shown encouraging results. It allows for serial expansion of the thoracic wall. Despite these techniques, patients have only a modest improvement in respiratory function. The mortality from this condition still remains high.[11]

Sternal Cleft

Introduction

Sternal clefts result from failure of fusion of the mesenchymal plate during the eighth embryonic week. The defect can be partial (superior or inferior) or complete. These rare abnormalities represent 0.15% of all chest wall anomalies.[12]

The superior clefts consist of a U-shaped sternum with a bridge connecting both halves of the sternum inferiorly (Figure). There may be a scar on the overlying skin with varying degrees of herniation of the great vessels or heart. The inferior cleft consists of an inverted-V defect with a midline cord-like scar running inferiorly to the umbilicus (Figure 53.12). Inferior clefts may also form part of the pentalogy of Cantrell. Cardiac pulsation may be seen through the defect. The complete cleft consists of two separated sternal bars. There is an association with congenital heart disease and craniofacial haemangioma.

Preoperative investigations should include ECG, echocardiogram, and a three-dimensional (3D) CT scan for complex defects (Figure 53.13).

Surgical Procedure

The aim of surgery is to provide protection for the mediastinum by bridging the defect. This also stops the paradoxical mediastinal movement with respiration and improves cosmetic appearance. The surgical procedure employed depends on the age of the patient. Surgical correction in the neonatal period is now preferred, as the chest wall is more compliant, allowing for primary closure of the defect.[13] Access to the sternal bars is obtained by a midline incision and mobilisation of the skin and subcutaneous tissue flaps. The medial insertions of the pectoralis major and rectus abdominis are mobilised and reflected. The medial perichondrium or periosteum is mobilised and approximated.

For a neonatal repair of the superior sternal cleft, the inferior sternal bridge is excised converting it to a complete cleft. Multiple lengths of polydioxanone (PDS) sutures are then placed around both sternal bars. The sutures are then tied one at a time from inferior to superior. Collaboration with the anaesthetist is essential at this time, as respiratory compromise may occur. A retrosternal drain is inserted, the rectus and pectoralis muscles are reattached, and the subcutaneous tissues and skin are closed.[14]

Older patients, due to a less compliant chest wall, require bridging the defect with autologous bone or artificial mesh. The defect is bridged by using a cancellous bone graft from the iliac crest or split rib grafts.[12,13] For wider defects, a combination of transverse rib struts covered by synthetic mesh can be used.[12]

The long-term outcomes following sternal reconstruction are good. Some patients may develop mild pectus excavatum, however.[12]

Evidence-Based Research

Table 53.2 presents a large series (303 patients) by an expert in pectus excavatum repair.

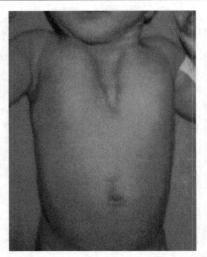

Figure 53.11: Superior sternal U cleft deformity in a neonate.

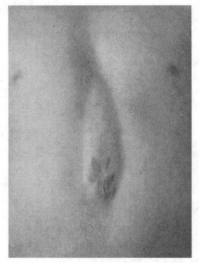

Figure 53.12: Inferior sternal cleft with diverification of recti and umbilical hernia.

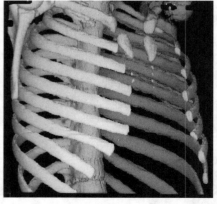

Figure 53.13: Three-dimensional CT scan of a 9-year-old girl with a complete sternal cleft repaired with a cancellous free bone graft from her iliac crest, with a very good result.[13]

Table 53.2: Evidence-based research.

Title	Experience and modification update for the minimally invasive Nuss technique for pectus excavatum repair in 303 patients
Authors	Croitoru DP, Kelly RE Jr, Goretsky MJ, Lawson ML, Swoveland B, Nuss D
Institution	Department of Surgery, Children's Hospital of the King's Daughters, Norfolk, Virginia, USA
Reference	J Pediatr Surg 2002; 37:437–445
Problem	Blind passage of bar across the anterior mediastinum was previously done. Significant incidence of bar displacement due to inadequate fixation.
Intervention	Introduction of thoracoscopy allows visualisation of introducer and bar during passage across the anterior mediastinum. Introduction of bar stabilisers and pericostal sutures.
Comparison/ control (quality of evidence)	No control group. A large series by an expert in the procedure.
Outcome/effect	Very good cosmetic repair with this minimally invasive technique. Safer passage of the bar across the mediastinum with the use of a thoracoscope, thus preventing cardiac injury. Reduced incidence of bar displacement by using bar stabilisers and pericostal sutures.
Historical significance/ comments	This represents significant refinement of the operative procedure by the inventor, which has improved safety and reduced complications.

Key Summary Points

1. Chest wall deformity is associated with cardiac and respiratory problems and connective tissue disorders.

2. Pectus excavatum is essentially a cosmetic problem.

3. The minimally invasive repair is safe, with low complication rates in experienced hands.

4. Thoracoscopy is strongly recommended while performing a Nuss repair of pectus excavatum.

5. Other chest wall anomalies are rare and are best managed in specialist centres for optimal results.

References

1. Fonkalsrud EW, Beanes S. Surgical management of pectus carinatum: 30 years' experience. World J Surg 2001; 25:898–903.

2. Martinez-Ferro M, Fraire C, Bernard S. Dynamic compression system for the correction of pectus carinatum. Seminars in Pediatric Surgery 2008; 17:194–200.

3. Croitoru DP, Kelly RE Jr, Goretsky MJ, Lawson ML, Swoveland B, Nuss D. Experience and modification update for the minimally invasive Nuss technique for pectus excavatum repair in 303 patients. J Pediatr Surg 2002; 37:437–445.

4. Kelly RE. Pectus excavatum: historical, clinical picture, preoperative evaluation and criteria for operation. Seminars in Pediatric Surgery 2008; 17:181–193.

5. Cartoski MJ, Nuss D, Goretsky MJ, Proud VK, Croitoru DP, Gustin T, et al. Classification of the dysmorphology of pectus excavatum. J Pediatr Surg 2006; 41:1573–1581.

6. Mueller C, Saint-Vil D, Bouchard S. Chest x-ray as a primary modality for preoperative imaging of pectus excavatum. J Pediatr Surg 2008; 43:71–73.

7. Nuss D. Minimally invasive surgical repair of pectus excavatum. Seminars in Pediatric Surgery 2008; 17:209–217.

8. Nuss D, Kelly RE Jr, Croitoru DP, Katz ME. A 10-year review of a minimally invasive technique for the correction of pectus excavatum. J Pediatr Surg 1998; 33:545–552.

9. Folkin AA, Robicsek F. Poland's syndrome revisited. Ann Thorac Surg 2002; 74:2218–2225.

10. Moir C, Johnson CH. Poland's syndrome. Seminars in Pediatric Surgery 2008; 17:161–166.

11. Duncan J, Van Aalst J. Jeune's syndrome (asphyxiating thoracic dystrophy): congenital and acquired. Seminars in Pediatric Surgery 2008; 17:167–172.

12. Acastello E, Majluf R, Garrido P, Barbosa LM, Peredo A. Sternal cleft: a surgical opportunity. J Pediatr Surg 2003; 38:178–183.

13. Abel RM, Robinson M, Gibbons P, Parikh DH. Cleft sternum: case report and literature review. Pediatr Pulmonol 2004; 37:375–377.

14. Daum R, Zachariou Z. Total and superior sternal clefts in newborns: a simple technique for surgical correction. J Pediatr Surg 1999; 34:408–411.

CHAPTER 54
MEDIASTINAL MASSES

Jonathan Karpelowsky
Kokila Lakhoo

Introduction

Mediastinal masses are a heterogeneous group of lesions that can provide significant diagnostic and management challenges to the paediatric surgeon. The lesions vary from slow-growing congenital cysts to aggressive neoplasms. The symptomatology can be quite varied, and a high index of suspicion needs be maintained to make the diagnosis.

Demographics

Due to the variety of mediastinal masses, it is not possible to determine the true prevalence of these lesions. Each type of lesion, barring mediastinal lymphadenopathy, is quite uncommon. The spectrum of lesions seen on the African continent would include lesions traditionally seen in the developed world, but with infectious causes playing a much larger role in any differential diagnosis. Furthermore, the human immunodeficiency virus (HIV) epidemic has presented myriad presentations not previously seen.

Pathology

Mediastinal masses can be practically classified by the lesion's location within the mediastinum, namely, anterior, middle, and posterior. The location of the mass usually gives a good indication as to the differential diagnosis of the lesion.

The anterior mediastinum extends from the inner aspect of the sternum to the anterior aspect of the trachea, pericardium, and great vessels. Its contents would include the thymus (Figure 54.1), ectopic thyroid or parathyroid, lymph nodes, and connective and adipose tissue. Thymic lesions would include hyperplasia (see Figure 54.1), cysts, thymoma, and thymic carcinoma. Disorders of the lymph nodes would be lymphoma (Figure 54.2), both Hodgkin's and non-Hodgkin's, and more recently an increasing number of patients with tuberculous adenopathy; germ cell tumours, both benign teratomas and malignant seminomas; and lymphatic anomalies, such as lymphatic malformations or lymphangiomas. Uncommon lesions include a retrosternal goitre or ectopic thyroid and malignancies of adipose tissue, a lipoblastoma. A Morgagni diaphragmatic hernia would come to lie in the inferior anterior mediastinum and would thus be considered in the differential of lesions in this location.

The middle mediastinum is situated from the pericardium anteriorly to the prevertebral fascia posteriorly. It contains the major mediastinal viscera, including the oesophagus, trachea, heart, and great vessels. Minor constituents would be the paratracheal spaces and lymphoid tissue. Lesions would thus arise from the aforementioned disorders of the lymphoid tissue (i.e., lymphoma and tuberculosis); congenital anomalies of foregut development (i.e., bronchogenic and enteric, or duplication, cysts); and uncommon lesions related to the heart and pericardium.

The posterior compartment contains the space between the trachea and the spine and the paravetebral sulcus on each side. The contents would include the thoracic spinal ganglia, the sympathetic chain, the proximal part of the intercostal vessels and nerves, lymphatics, and connective tissue. Consequently, lesions in this position are

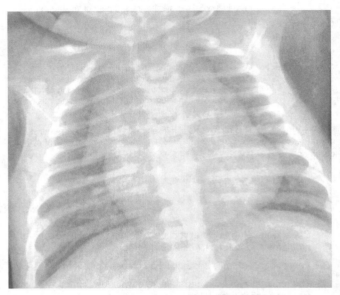
Figure 54.1: Normal thymus in the anterior mediastinum of a neonate.

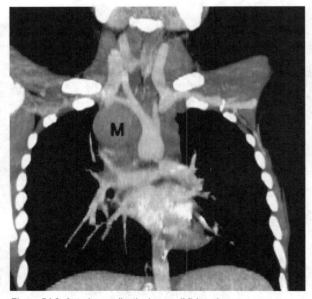
Figure 54.2: Anterior mediastinal mass (M) lymphoma.

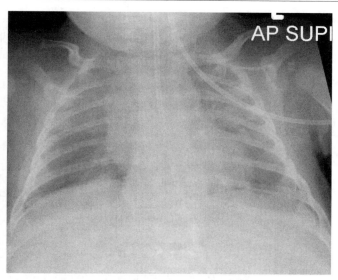

Figure 54.3: Posterior mediastinal mass (neuroblastoma).

typically neurogenic in origin—namely, neuroblastoma (Figure 54.3), ganglioneuroma, neurofibroma, neurilemoma, paeochromocyctoma, and neuroenteric cysts. Other, less common lesions would include a primitive neuroectodermal tumour (PNET) and hamartomas. Lastly, as for the mediastinal compartment, occasionally cystic lesions in the inferior posterior compartment may represent a sliding or paraoesophageal hiatus hernia.

A further mechanism for classifying mediastinal masses are as cystic and solid. Cysts are usually congenital in nature. Cystic lesions would include bronchogenic, duplications, neuro-enteric dermoids, lymphatic, and pericardial cysts. Solid masses are usually neoplasms, which may be benign or malignant and are well detailed in the preceding section.

Clinical Presentation

The location and the age of the patient are often the most useful factors in making a diagnosis. As discussed in the previous section, certain lesions have characteristic sites of occurrence.

Mediastinal lesions are often asymptomatic; many of them are found on routine chest radiology (see Figures 54.1 and 54.3). Symptoms usually occur secondary to a mass effect of the lesion on adjacent structures in the mediastinum. The symptoms, when present, are usually a cough, respiratory distress, wheeze, stridor, or dysphagia. In malignant mediastinal lesions, or occasionally in tuberculous lymphadenopathy, children can present with a superior vena caval syndrome, representing both vascular and airway compression. Depending on the rate of growth of the lesions, the presentation may be insidious; in malignant lesions, however, it may occur over a few weeks, or in lesions complicated by superadded infection or haemorrhage, it may present as a life-threatening emergency over days or even hours.

Posterior mediastinal lesions will usually present with pain secondary to bony erosions or neuralgia. Occasionally, with neurogenic tumours, patients may present with loss of power to the lower limbs and paraplegia secondary to a dumbbell lesion and cord compression. Neurological symptoms can be found with neuro-enteric cysts, but usually take the form of recurrent meningitis and only rarely paraplegia.

Systemic symptoms of loss of weight and night sweats are usually the initial symptoms for both tuberculosis (TB) and lymphoma. Differentiation between these two diseases in the African setting can often be difficult, especially in children coinfected with HIV. Both TB and lymphoma have an atypical and more aggressive course. In younger children, TB is the most common of the mediastinal lesions causing compressive symptoms of the airways. This is secondary to subcarinal and peribronchial nodes.

In the clinical examination, it is important to pay attention to a systemic examination. Features of weight loss, lympahedenopathy, visceromegaly, or skin lesions will all contribute to making the clinical diagnosis. A systematic approach to examination is important and can also provide a valuable alternative for a tissue diagnosis.

Investigations

Diagnostic studies will be directed by the type and severity of the symptoms and location of the mass.

Radiology

The initial radiological work-up will be the anteroposterior (AP) and lateral chest x-rays. An enormous amount of information can be gained from this affordable and widely available investigation (see Figures 54.1 and 54.3). Most important, one needs to assess the position of the mass, especially on the lateral film, which would place it in either the anterior, middle, or posterior compartments. The airways can be well assessed by looking for compression and deviation of the trachea and major bronchi.

In instances where dysphagia is a predominant symptom, a contrast swallow would be helpful to identify the location and extent of the oesophageal compression. In instances of foregut duplication, this will communicate with the normal oesophagus in 20% of the cases.

The mainstay of investigation will be the computed tomography (CT) scan, which provides an excellent outline of the mediastinum and major airways (see Figure 54.2). It gives a precise relationship of the mass to the airway, oesophagus, and major vascular structures. In instances where one suspects a foregut duplication, imaging should continue into the upper abdomen, as these lesions may extend below the diaphragm. CT scans should be kept to an absolute minimum amidst concerns of radiation-induced neoplasia.

In children who present with neurological symptoms, magnetic resonance imaging (MRI), where available, should strongly be considered, as—especially with dumbbell lesions—cord compression may be present.

Occasionally, radioisotope studies may be required, notably a metiodobenzylgaunidine (MIBG) scan, which is both specific and sensitive for neuroblastoma or phaechromocytoma.

The goal of the radiological work-up is to aid diagnosis and to help define the optimal surgical approach.

Laboratory Testing

Specific laboratory tests can aid in the diagnosis of mediastinal masses. Serum lactate dehdrogenase (LDH) is a sensitive but nonspecific marker of lymphoma and neuroblastoma. Homovanillic acid (HVA) or vanillulmandelic acid (VMA) are both markers of neurogenic tumours, and these tests should be done in posterior mediastinal lesions.

Finally, TB testing, either in the form of skin antigenicity (Mantoux or PPD—purified protein derivative) or white cell interferon-gamma testing (ELISpot or QuantiFERON®-TB Gold) should be performed. This testing must be correlated with the clinical picture—either induced sputum or gastric washings, depending on the age of the child. One note of caution: if TB is diagnosed, it can coexist with lymphoma, and hence failure to respond or progression on TB treatment should alert one to an alternative diagnosis.

Histology

Ultimately, treatment of solid mediastinal masses rests on the histological diagnosis. This is usually most pertinent to masses in the anterior mediastinum, where lymphoma is suspected. In these cases, peripheral nodes may provide the answer and avoid entrance of the thoracic cavity. In cases of smaller masses or cysts, excision biopsy can be done.

Treatment

The treatment for mediastinal masses ranges from curative excision to medical management, depending on the cause. In general, however, apart from lymphoma and TB, most lesions will require excision.

Airway Management

A compromised airway is often the reason for emergent presentation of these lesions. Airway compromise secondary to mediastinal lesions can be particularly difficult to manage, as the area of compression may often be at a carinal level and hence not alleviated by intubation or a tracheostomy. At presentation, patients may be unable to lie flat, and if given any sedation or anaesthetic will completely lose their airway.

The best form of management would be avoidance of any sedation. Obtaining tissue under local anaesthetic from other sites is preferable. If this is not possible, then careful liaison with anaesthetic services and use of a CT scan best identify the degree and location of the compression. A rigid bronchoscope is a necessity, as it may be the only option to re-establish an airway distal to the carina. Full intensive-care facilities must be available. Discussion with oncology services should be undertaken to balance the risk of biopsy, or empirical initial therapy to alleviate some of the airway compromise, with the disadvantage of losing valuable histological information.

Definitive Management

Surgical involvement is twofold: first, obtaining tissue for histology in unresectable lesions; and second, for excision of cysts and masses.

Careful attention needs to be paid to the access incision that is to be made. Anterior mediastinal lesions are best performed through a sternotomy, and middle and posterior lesions via a posterior lateral thoracotomy. Lesions that have a spinal component should either have a combined procedure, or alternatively have the spinal component done first, as failure to do so could result in paraplegia. In rare cases, thoracic foregut duplication cysts may transverse the diaphragm and end in the abdomen, requiring a combined abdominal and thoracic approach.

Occasionally, surgical intervention will be required for node decompression in cases of TB.

Thoracoscopic surgery offers an excellent diagnostic and therapeutic tool when available, but expertise and equipment may make this a limited option in most African settings.

Postoperative Complications

Postoperative complications are usually secondary to inadequate analgesia, resulting in pulmonary atelectasis. Incompletely excised lesions may recur, especially lymphatic malformations and malignant lesions.

Prognosis and Outcome

Generally, the prognosis for mediastinal masses is excellent. Mediastinal cysts that are excised offer complete cysts. Effective medical therapy for tuberculosis can prevent damage to the bronchi and lungs. Malignant lesions would depend on the histology, but most of the lesions found in the mediastinum are responsive to chemotherapy.

Evidence-Based Research

The wide spectrum of disorders that make up mediastinal masses do not lend themselves to comparative trials. Each of the neoplastic lesions (i.e., lymphoma, germ cell tumours, and neuroblastoma) has been extensively studied with respect to multimodal therapy, but these are not specific for mediastinal masses.

The largest case series is that of Grosfeld et al. (see Suggested Reading). Most subsequent series focus on thoracoscopic approaches to these lesions. Table 54.1 presents an analysis of mediastinal masses in 29 children. Table 54.2 discusses a study of airway obstruction and management in mediastinal tumours.

Table 54.1 Evidence-based research.

Title	When is a mediastinal mass critical in a child? An analysis of 29 patients
Authors	Lam JC, Chui CH, Jacobsen AS, Tan AM, Joseph VT
Institution	Department of Paediatric Surgery, KK Women's and Children's Hospital, Singapore
Reference	Pediatr Surg Int 2004; 20(3):180–184
Problem	The aims of this study were to determine the pattern of presentation of childhood mediastinal masses in our community and to identify factors associated with the development of acute airway compromise.
Intervention	The authors retrospectively reviewed the records of 29 consecutive patients with mediastinal masses managed at their institution between January 1995 and December 2001. Demographic data, mass characteristics, clinical presentation, and surgical procedures were recorded.
Comparison/ control (quality of evidence)	Seven patients (24.1%) were asymptomatic at presentation. Eight (27.6%) were classified as having acute airway compromise at presentation. Respiratory symptoms and signs were the most common mode of presentation (58.6% and 55.2%, respectively). The most common histological diagnosis was neurogenic mass (37.9%), followed by lymphoma (24.1%). Most masses were located in the superior mediastinum (41.1%). Factors associated with the development of acute airway compromise were (1) anterior location of the mediastinal mass (P=0.019); (2) histological diagnosis of lymphoma (P = 0.008); (3) symptoms and signs of superior vena cava syndrome (P = 0.015 and 0.003, respectively); (4) radiological evidence of vessel compression or displacement (P = 0.015); (5) pericardial effusion (P=0.015); and (6) pleural effusion (P = 0.033).
Outcome/ effect	Clinical presentation of childhood mediastinal masses is often nonspecific or incidental. Yet they have the propensity of developing acute airway compromise, which is closely associated with superior vena cava obstruction. Such patients should be managed as a complex cardiorespiratory syndrome, termed "critical mediastinal mass syndrome", by an experienced multidisciplinary team.

Table 54.2 Evidence-based research.

Title	Mediastinal tumors-airway obstruction and management
Authors	Robie DK, Gursov MH, Pokorny WJ
Institution	Cora and Webb Manning Department of Surgery, Baylor College of Medicine, Houston, Texas, USA
Reference	Semin Pediatr Surg 1994; 3(4):259–266
Historical significance/ comments	Large mediastinal masses can cause compression of surrounding mediastinal structures. Patients may have symptoms of airway obstruction or cardiovascular compromise. The additive effects of anaesthetics, paralysis, and positioning during biopsy can lead to acute airway obstruction and death. In some cases, tissue diagnosis can be achieved and treatment initiated without general anaesthesia. When general anaesthesia is necessary, specific measures should be taken to avoid disaster or immediately alleviate obstruction should it occur. Some patients at greatest risk will require pretreatment of the mass before tissue diagnosis. This article reviews these issues and provides a useful algorithm for managing patients with mediastinal masses.

Key Summary Points

1. Mediastinal masses are presented by their anatomical location into anterior, middle, and posterior mediastina.

2. The location usually indicates the differential diagnosis.

3. Chest x-ray and CT scan are the most useful imaging modalities for mediastinal masses.

4. Most lesions require excision (except infective causes and lymphoma).

5. Airway management is paramount.

Suggested Reading

Engum SA. Minimal access thoracic surgery in the pediatric population. Semin Pediatr Surg 2007; 16:14–26.

Grosfeld JL, Skinner MA, et al. Mediastinal tumors in children: experience with 196 cases. Ann Surg Oncol 1994; 1:121–127.

Hammer GB. Anaesthetic management for the child with a mediastinal mass. Paediatr Anaesth 2004; 14:95–97.

Jaggers J, Balsara K. Mediastinal masses in children. Semin Thorac Cardiovasc Surg 2004; 16:201–208.

Williams HJ, Alton HM. Imaging of paediatric mediastinal abnormalities. Paediatr Respir Rev 2003; 4: 55–66.

CHAPTER 55
CHYLOTHORAX

Jean-Martin Laberge
Kokila Lakhoo
Behrouz Banieghbal

Introduction

Chylothorax is a rare entity and is defined as an effusion of lymph in the pleural cavity. The chyle may have its origin in the thorax or in the abdomen or in both. Leakage usually occurs from the thoracic duct or one of its main tributaries.

Demographics

There are no known racial, gender, age, or geographical variations to chylothorax. This is due to its aetiology. However, it is known to occur in up to 4% of patients after cardiothoracic surgery.

Pathophysiology

The thoracic duct develops from outgrowths of the jugular lymphatic sacs and the cisterna chyli. During embryonic life, bilateral thoracic lymphatic channels are present, each attached in the neck to the corresponding jugular sac. As development progresses, the upper third of the right duct and the lower two-thirds of the left duct involute and close. The wide variation in the final anatomic structure of the main ductal system attests to the multiple communications of the small vessels comprising the lymphatic system. The thoracic duct originates in the abdomen at the cisterna chyli located over the second lumbar vertebra. The duct extends into the thorax through the aortic hiatus and then passes upward into the posterior mediastinum on the right before shifting toward the left at the level of the fifth thoracic vertebra. It then ascends posterior to the aortic arch and into the posterior neck to the junction of the subclavian and internal jugular veins.

The chyle contained in the thoracic duct conveys approximately three-fourths of the ingested fat from the intestine to the systemic circulation. The fat content of chyle varies from 0.4 to 4.0 g/dl. The large fat molecules absorbed from the intestinal lacteals flow through the cisterna chyli and superiorly through the thoracic duct. The total protein content of thoracic duct lymph is also high. The thoracic duct also carries white blood cells, primarily lymphocytes (T cells)—approximately 2,000 to 20,000 cells per milliliter. When chyle leaks through a thoracic duct fistula, considerable fat and lymphocytes may be lost. Eosinophils are also present in a higher proportion than in circulating blood. The chyle appears to have a bacteriostatic property, which accounts for the rare occurrence of infection complicating chylothorax.

Aetiology

Effusion of chylous fluid into the thorax may occur spontaneously in newborns and has usually been attributed to congenital abnormalities of the thoracic ducts or trauma from delivery. The occurrence of chylothorax in most cases cannot be related to the type of labor or delivery, and lymphatic effusions may be discovered prenatally.

Chylothorax in older children is rarely spontaneous and occurs almost invariably after trauma or cardiothoracic surgery; however, some patients with thoracic lymphangioma may present in this older age group. Operative injury may be in part a result of anatomic variations of the thoracic duct. Neoplasms, particularly lymphomas and neuroblastomas, have occasionally been noted to cause obstruction of

the thoracic duct. Lymphangiomatosis or diffuse lymphangiectasia may produce chylous effusion in the pleural space and peritoneal cavity. Extensive bouts of coughing have been reported to cause rupture of the thoracic duct, which is particularly vulnerable when full following a fatty meal. Other causes include mediastinal inflammation, subclavian vein or superior vena caval thrombosis, and misplaced central venous catheters (Table 55.1).

Table 55.1: Causes of chylothorax.

Lymphatic malformation (nontrauma)
Thoracic duct atresia/aplasia/hypoplasia/dysplasia
Lymphangioma
Lymphangiomatosis
Intestinal lymphangiectasia (protein-losing enteropathy)
Fontan procedure
Thoracic duct injury (trauma)
Cardiothoracic operations
Oesophageal atresia
Diaphragmatic hernia
Penetrating trauma (stab or gunshot injury)
Malignant
Lymphoma
Kaposi sarcoma
Mediastinal teratoma
Infectious
Tuberculosis
Filariasis
Pneumonia
Pleuritis and empyema
Idiopathic (associated with)
Down syndrome
Noonan syndrome
Gorham's disease
Hydrops foetalis
Turner syndrome
Lymphoedema
Transudative
Cirrhosis of the liver
Fontan procedure
Heart failure
Nephritic syndrome
Miscellaneous
Sarcoidosis
Amyloidosis

Clinical Presentation

The accumulation of chyle in the pleural space from a thoracic duct leak may occur rapidly and produce pressure on other structures in the chest, causing acute respiratory distress, dyspnea, and cyanosis with tachypnea. In the foetus, a pleural effusion may be secondary to generalised hydrops, but a primary lymphatic effusion (idiopathic, secondary to subpleural lymphangiectasia, pulmonary sequestration, or associated with syndromes such as Down, Turner, and Noonan) can cause mediastinal shift and result in hydrops or lead to pulmonary hypoplasia. Postnatally, the effects of chylothorax and the prolonged loss of chyle may include malnutrition, hypoproteinaemia, fluid and electrolyte imbalance, metabolic acidosis, and immunodeficiency.

In a neonate, symptoms of respiratory embarrassment observed in combination with a pleural effusion strongly suggest chylothorax. Similar findings are noted in the traumatic postoperative chylothorax. In the older child, nutritional deficiency is a late manifestation of chyle depletion and occurs when dietary intake is insufficient to replace the thoracic duct fluid loss. Fever is not common.

Diagnosis

Chest roentgenograms typically show massive fluid effusion in the ipsilateral chest with pulmonary compression and mediastinal shift. Bilateral effusions may also occur. Aspiration of the pleural effusion reveals a clear straw-colored fluid in the fasting patient, which becomes milky after feedings. Analysis of the chyle generally reveals a total fat content of more than 400 mg/dl and a protein content of more than 5 g/dl. In a foetus or a fasting neonate, the most useful and simple test is to perform a complete cell count and differential on the fluid; when lymphocytes exceed 80% or 90% of the white cells, a lymphatic effusion is confirmed. The differential can be compared to that obtained from the blood count, where lymphocytes rarely represent more than 70% of white blood cells.

Lymphangiography is useful for defining the site of chyle leakage or obstruction with penetrating trauma, spontaneous chylothorax, and lymphangiomatous malformation. However, in a nontraumatised patient, the site of lymphatic leakage is often difficult to localise. Lymphoscintigraphy may be an alternative to lymphangiography, as it is a faster and less traumatic procedure.

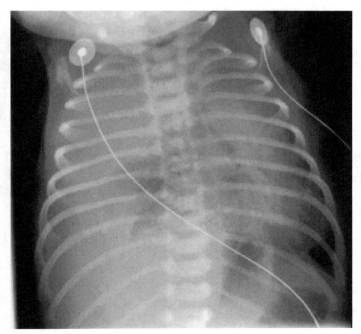

Figure 55.1: Right-sided congenital chylothorax in a newborn.

Management

Nonoperative Management

Thoracentesis may be sufficient to relieve spontaneous chylothorax in occasional infants; however, chest tube drainage will be necessary for the majority of patients. Further, tube drainage allows quantification of the daily chyle leak and promotes pulmonary re-expansion, which may enhance healing. Chylothorax in newborns usually ceases spontaneously. In some cases of congenital chylothorax, supportive mechanical ventilation may be necessary because of insufficient lung expansion, persistent foetal circulation, or lung hypoplasia. In cases of severe chylothorax leading to nonimmunologic hydrops foetalis, antenatal management by intrauterine thoracocentesis or pleuroperitoneal shunting should be considered in the absence of significant underlying malformations.

For postnatal chylothorax, since identifying the actual site of the fluid leak is difficult, surgery is often deferred for several weeks. Most cases of traumatic injury to the thoracic duct can be managed successfully by chest tube drainage and replacement of the protein and fat loss. Feeding restricted to medium- or short-chain triglycerides theoretically results in reduced lymph flow in the thoracic duct and may enhance spontaneous healing of a thoracic duct fistula. However, it has been shown that any enteral feeding, even with clear fluids, greatly increases thoracic duct flow. Therefore, the optimum management for chyle leak is chest tube drainage, withholding oral feedings, and providing total parenteral nutrition (TPN). Cultures of chylous fluid are rarely positive; therefore, providing long-term antibiotics during the full course of chest tube drainage is not considered necessary. In nonresolving chylothorax, subcutaneous injection of octeriotide, a somatostatin analogue, at 10 μg/kd/day in 3 divided doses is reported to have excellent results in a number of case reports and should be tried prior to surgical intervention.

Surgical Management

When chylothorax remains resistant despite prolonged chest tube drainage (2–3 weeks) and TPN, thoracotomy on the ipsilateral side may be necessary. The decision whether to continue with conservative management or to undertake surgical intervention should be based on the nature of the underlying disorder, the duration of the fistula, the daily volume of fluid drainage, and the severity of nutritional and/or immunologic depletion. Ingestion of cream before surgery may facilitate identification of the thoracic duct and the fistula. When identified, the draining lymphatic vessel should be suture ligated above and below the leak with reinforcement by a pleural or intercostal muscle flap. When a leak cannot be identified with certainty, or when multiple leaks originate from the mediastinum, ligation of all the tissues surrounding the aorta at the level of the hiatus provides the best results. Fibrin glue and argon-beam coagulation have also been used for ill-defined areas of leakage or incompletely resected lympangiomas.

Thoracoscopy may occasionally be used to avoid thoracotomy. The leak, if visualised, can be ligated, cauterised, or sealed with fibrin glue. If the leak cannot be identified, pleurodesis can be accomplished with talc or other sclerotic agents under direct vision through the thoracoscope, but this technique should probably be avoided in infancy due to the potential consequences on lung and chest wall growth. If there is concomitant chylopericardium, a pericardial window can be fashioned.

During any thoracotomy, if chyle leak is noted, the proximal and distal ends of the leaking duct should be ligated.

Pleuroperitoneal shunts have been reserved for refractory chylothorax. A Denver double-valve shunt system is the type most commonly employed; it is totally implanted and allows the patient or parent to pump the valve to achieve decompression of the pleural fluid into the abdominal cavity where it is reabsorbed.

Prognosis

Prognosis depends largely on the aetiology of the chylothorax. A mortality rate of 12.8% among paediatric patients with a nontraumatic chylothorax has been reported. This rate may be reduced by appropriate support with TPN and timely intervention.

Evidence-Based Research

Table 55.2 presents a systematic review of using someatostatin or octreotide as a treatment option for childhood chylothorax.

Table 55.2: Evidence-based research.

Title	Somatostatin or octreotide as treatment options for chylothorax in young children: a systematic review.
Authors	Roehr CC, Jung A, Proquitte H, Blankenstein O, Hammer H, Lakhoo K, Wauer RR.
Institution	Department of Neonatology, Charité Campus Mitte, Universitätsmedizin Berlin, Berlin, Germany; John Radcliffe Hospital, Department of Paediatric Surgery, Oxford, UK.
Reference	Intensive Care Med. 2006; 32(5):650–657. Epub 2006 Mar 11.
Problem	Chylothorax is a rare but life-threatening condition in children. To date, there is no commonly accepted treatment protocol. Somatostatin and octreotide have recently been used for treating chylothorax in children
Intervention	Summarisation of the evidence on the efficacy and safety of somatostatin and octreotide in treating young children with chylothorax
Comparison/ control (quality of evidence)	Design: Systematic review: literature search (Cochrane Library, EMBASE and PubMed databases) and literature hand search of peer reviewed articles on the use of somatostatin and octreotide in childhood chylothorax. Patients: Thirty-five children treated for primary or secondary chylothorax (10/somatostatin, 25/octreotide) were found.
Outcome/effect	Ten of the 35 children had been given somatostatin, as intravenous (IV) infusion at a median dose of 204 µg/kg per day, for a median duration of 9.5 days. The remaining 25 children had received octreotide, either as an IV infusion at a median dose of 68 µg/kg per day over a median 7 days, or subcutaneous injection at a median dose of 40 µg/kg per day and a median duration of 17 days. Side effects such as cutaneous flush, nausea, loose stools, transient hypothyroidism, elevated liver function tests and strangulation-ileus (in a child with asplenia syndrome) were reported for somatostatin; transient abdominal distention, temporary hyperglycaemia and necrotising enterocolitis (in a child with aortic coarctation) for octreotide.
Historical significance/ comments	A positive treatment effect was evident for both somatostatin and octreotide in the majority of reports. Minor side effects have been reported; however, caution should be exercised in patients with an increased risk of vascular compromise to avoid serious side effects. Systematic clinical research is needed to establish treatment efficacy and to develop a safe treatment protocol.

Key Summary Points

1. Chylothorax may be congenital or traumatic, most commonly postoperative.

2. Diagnosis is by means of pleural tap analysis showing more than 80% lymphocytes on the differential count.

3. Optimum treatment includes chest tube drainage, nothing by mouth and nutritional support with total parenteral nutrition (TPN). Feeding restricted to medium chain triglycerides may be tried in the absence of TPN, and is often used once the leak has subsided with the patient on TPN.

4. A somatostatin analogue may be tried before surgical intervention.

5. Surgery is reserved for the refractory chylothorax with either direct ligation of the leak where feasible, ligation of the duct and all periaortic tissues at the aortic hiatus, or utilisation of a pleuroperitoneal shunt.

References

1. Browse NL, Allen DR, Wilson NM. Management of chylothorax. Br J Surg 1997, 84:1711–1716.

2. Büttiker V, Fanconi S, Burger R. Chylothorax in children: guidelines for diagnosis and management. Chest 1999; 116:682–687.

3. Chan EH, Russell JL, William WG, et al. Postoperative chylothorax after cardiothoracic surgery in children. Ann Thorac Surg 2005; 80:1864–1870.

4. Cheung Y, Leung MP, Yip M. Octreotide for treatment of postoperative chylothorax. J Pediatr 2001; 139:157–159.

5. Christodoulou M, Ris HB, Pezzetta E. Video-assisted right supradiaphragmatic thoracic duct ligation for non-traumatic recurrent chylothorax. Eur J Cardiothorac Surg 2006; 29:810–814.

6. Horn KD, Penchansky L. Chylous pleural effusions simulating leukemic infiltrate associated with thoracoabdominal disease and surgery in infants. Am J Clin Pathol 1999; 111:99–104.

7. Levine C. Primary disorders of the lymphatic vessels—a unified concept. J Pediatr Surg 1989; 24:233–240.

8. Light RW. Pleural Diseases, 3rd ed. Baltimore: Williams and Wilkins, 1995, Pp 284–289.

9. Nygaard U, Sundberg K, Nielsen HS, et al. New treatment of early fetal chylothorax. Obstet Gynecol 2007; 109:1088–1092.

10. Podevin G, Levard G, Larroquet M, et al. Pleuroperitoneal shunt in the management of chylothorax caused by thoracic lymphatic dysplasia. J Pediatr Surg 1999; 34:1420–1422.

11. Pui MH, Yueh TC. Lymphoscintigraphy in chyluria, chyloperitoneum and chylothorax. J Nucl Med 1998; 39:1292–1296.

12. Robinson CLN: The management of chylothorax. Ann Thorac Surg 1985, 39:90–95.

13. Romero S. Nontraumatic chylothorax. Curr Opin Pulm Med 2000; 6:287–291.

14. Staats BA, Ellefson RD, Budahn LL, et al. The lipoprotein profile of chylous and nonchylous pleural effusion. Mayo Clin Proc 1980; 55:700–704.

15. van Straaten HL, Gerards LJ, Krediet TG. Chylothorax in the neonatal period. Eur J Pediatr 1993;152:2–5.

ABDOMINAL WALL

CHAPTER 56
CONGENITAL ANTERIOR ABDOMINAL WALL DEFECTS: EXOMPHALOS AND GASTROSCHISIS

Iyekeoretin Evbuomwan

Kokila Lakhoo

Introduction

Exomphalos and gastroschisis are the common forms of presentation of congenital abdominal wall defect.

Exomphalos (from the Greek *ex* = out; *omphalos* = umbilicus) refers to protrusion into the umbilicus. In its very mild form, a small loop of intestine protrudes into the base of the umbilicus; this is a hernia into the umbilical cord. In the more severe form, the defect allows protrusion of small intestine and other viscera, pushing the umbilical cord forward and distending its base into a cystic mass containing the viscera. This constitutes an omphalocele (from the Greek *omphalos*, *kele* = hernia, tumour). Omphalocele is more common, with a general incidence of 1:4,000 births. Omphalocele is a result of failure of formation and closing in of the anterior abdominal wall and could therefore be associated with other forms of impaired organ formation, which will determine the general prognosis.

Gastroschisis is a defect in the full anterior abdominal wall (from the Greek *gastro* = stomach—the term generally used for abdomen; *schisis* = fissure, tear, or gape) through which the abdominal content protrudes into the amniotic cavity.

Gastroschisis occurs in 1:10,000 births; although this is less common than exomphalos, in the Western world an increased incidence of tenfold is noted in young mothers with substance abuse. Gastroschisis is not due to or associated with impaired organ formation, but there could be complications from mass protrusion of viscera through a small defect, including vascular compromise, which in early foetal life could result in bowel atresia.

Demographics

The estimated birth prevalence of omphalocele in western countries is about 1 in 10, 000 births while that of gastroschisis is about 2.5 in 10, 000 births. The prevalence in sub Saharan Africa is not known as there are no population based studies. While the birth prevalence of omphalocele has remained generally stable over the years, reports from industrialized countries (Europe, United States, Japan) indicate that the rate for gastroschisis is on the increase. When omphalocele is associated with other abnormalities, the aetiology is multifactoral and incidence varies with age of the mother. These abnormalities occur more in younger mothers; omphalocele alone is more prevalent in older mothers, however.

Aetiology/Pathophysiology

The aetiology of these conditions is not known. For omphalocele, the pathogenesis is related to the formation of the anterior abdominal wall and return of the midgut into the abdominal cavity. At the third week of gestation, three primitive divisions of the gut are identifiable as foregut, midgut, and hindgut. By formation of the folds, intraembryonic coelom becomes gradually separated from extraembryonic coelom. The fold initially consists of ectoderm and endoderm. The mesoderm later forms in between, and the folds close in on the umbilical cord and thus complete the anterior abdominal wall. Failure of mesoderm development results in defects. At the cranial portion, the defect could affect the anterior wall of the chest (sternum, pericardium, and the heart, causing the classic features of the pentalogy of Cantrell). In the caudal aspect of the anterior abdominal wall, the defect may be associated with bladder exstrophy or varying degrees of anorectal anomalies. In the female, there may be a cloacal anomaly. Other anomalies that have been described as being associated include trisomy 13, 18, or 21 anomaly and the Beckwith-Weidemann syndrome.

The most common form is the central omphalocele, due to failure in the lateral folds. It may be classified in terms of shape, size, content, whether there are associated other anomalies, and whether the membrane coverage is intact or ruptured. More specifically:

1. Shape:
   - Conical: includes hernia of the umbilical cord; usually small with broad skin edge diameter
   - Globular: in which there is a large sac hanging on a relatively small diameter base and small abdominal cavity

2. Size of defect:
   - Small diameter up to 5 cm, described as minor
   - Diameter more than 5 cm, described as major

3. Content of the sac:
   - Bowel loops only, small and large intestine sometimes on part of the stomach, bladder, and occasionally the ovary
   - Bowel loops and liver

4. Associated with cardiac or other gross anomalies:
   - Syndromic
   - Nonsyndromic

5. Membrane coverage:
   - Intact
   - Ruptured membrane

For gastroschisis, a vascular accident of the right omphalomesenteric artery and abuse of vasoactive drugs have been implicated in the aetiology.

Clinical Presentation

Omphalocele (Figure 56.1) is an obvious abnormality in the newborn, presenting as a mass arising from a defect in the anterior abdominal wall covered by a membrane. The membrane is composed of an inner layer of peritoneum and an outer layer of amniotic membrane with Wharton's jelly between. It is attached by its base circumferentially to the skin of the anterior abdominal wall. The diameter of the base, the content of the sac, and the size relative to the size of the abdominal cavity will influence the decision for the method of management. Also important are whether the membrane is intact or not all around the circumference and whether the membrane or part of it is infected.

Other features to be examined are the possible associated congenital abnormalities. Such features as ectopia cordis, sternal defect, bladder exstrophy, and anorectal anomaly are suggestive of a syndromic omphalocele. When loops of bowel are eviscerated, it is important to evaluate whether it is an omphalocele in which the membrane has ruptured or the diagnosis should be a gastroschisis.

In gastroschisis (Figure 56.2), the eviscerate bowel segment is commonly loops of small intestine and colon, sometimes stomach. The umbilicus is attached to the normal site in an intact anterior abdominal wall and the defect through which the bowel has herniated is usually in the right side of the umbilicus, separated from it by a small bridge of skin. There is no membrane over the bowel. A large segment of bowel with oedematous and congested bowel wall is seen in cases presenting late after birth. A bowel segment wholly covered by fibrinous material—not an obvious membrane as in omphalocele— suggests the gastroschisis had occurred early in utero. The fibrinous cover is a result of reaction to amniotic fluid.

Investigations

A normal, generally healthy-looking baby in whom the only obvious anomaly is the omphalocele needs immediate urgent exclusion of hypo-glycaemia before routine investigation of haemoglobin and electrolyte checks are done. Other required investigations will be determined by evidence of associated anomalies. Abdominal ultrasound is used to ascertain the kidney, echocardiography is used if there are clinical signs of cardiac anomalies, and x-ray of the chest is used if there are signs relating to pulmonary anomalies. Chromosomal analysis may be required to rule out trisomy.

Gastroschisis requires a haemoglobin and electrolytes check as for preoperative preparation.

Treatment

Management of a baby with omphalocele or gastroschisis takes into consideration the following:

• treatment and care of the general state of the baby;

• specific treatment of the omphalocele; and

• management of associated anomalies.

General Care

The neonate should be well wrapped up in warm clothing to prevent hypothermia. Intravenous fluid should be commenced and the stomach should be kept decompressed with a nasogastric tube. The omphalo-cele, or the eviscerated bowel in the case of gastroschisis, should be well covered to reduce loss of heat and prevent injury. In intact ompha-locele, when there are no signs of intestinal obstruction or anorectal anomaly, the baby can be commenced on oral fluids and feed. The baby should be transferred to a neonatal unit for further care.

Nutrition in Omphalocele and Gastroschisis

Small lesions may be expected to have no problem with normal feeds. When the baby vomits frequently in the early days of life, intestinal obstruction should be suspected. Commonly, it is due to ileus and bowel oedema. Atresia or malrotation are indications for early exploration. Babies with gastroschisis have poor bowel motility due to the long exposure of the bowel loops to the amniotic fluid in utero; thus, delay in enteral feeding is frequently experienced. It is advisable to commence parenteral nutrition where available and continue until the baby estab-lishes normal gastrointestinal function.

Treatment of Omphalocele

The primary aim of treatment of omphalocele is to return the bowel into the abdominal cavity and close the anterior abdominal wall. The possibility to do so will depend on whether the viscera can be placed in the abdominal cavity without tension on the anterior abdominal wall, without intraabdominal compartment syndrome, and without pressure on the diaphragm, which would impair respiration.

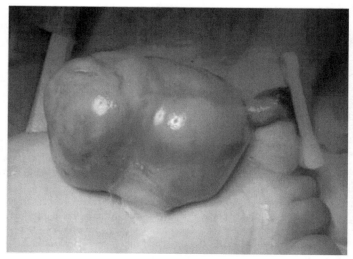

Figure 56.1: Exomphalos major.

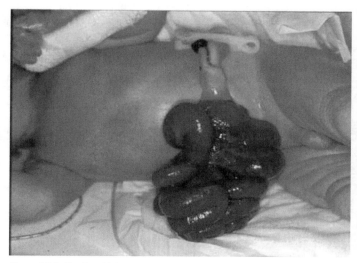

Figure 56.2: Gastroschisis.

Closure of Omphalocele Minor

Primary closure

Primary closure of the defect is possible in almost all cases of minor omphalocele. The membrane is cleaned and excised. The edges of the defect are determined and the fascial edges are closed, followed by skin closure.

Delayed primary closure

Primary closure may need to be delayed in minor omphalocele with an infected sac and oedematous abdominal wall. The sac is cleaned thoroughly, covered with Sofratulle® and gauze, and then wrapped with a soft crepe bandage. This is done daily, twice a day, morning and eve-ning. If there is slough on the sac, the slough should be excised gently without causing bleeding. After 6 or 7 days, the omphalocele may be closed by excising the sac and closing the fascia and the skin. When closing the skin, an attempt should be made to construct a navel.

Closure of Omphalocele Major

Primary closure

The abdominal cavity is closed with or without excision of the sac. During primary closure, it is important to exclude intraabdominal compartment syndrome, which is determined by poor urine output, tight abdominal cavity, respiratory compromise due to splinting of the diaphragm, and oedematous or dusky lower limbs due to poor venous return. The fascial layer and skin are closed separately, with possible constuction of an umbilicus. Muscle flaps are sometimes created by making a release incision on the sides of the peritoneal cavity and mobilising the muscle medially to obtain fascial closure.

Staged abdominal wall closure

If closure of the fasciomuscular layer is not possible due to undue pressure on the diaphragm, only the skin may be undermined, stretched, and closed. This will heal, leaving a ventral hernia that can be closed at a later age.

Postoperatively, the child is monitored for adequate respiration and urine output. Oral feeds are commenced as soon as the child can tolerate them.

Skin stretching may need to be attempted to increase the surface area of the abdominal skin wall. This is usually possible and reduces respiratory stress. Skin flaps are sometimes created by making release incisions on the sides of the abdomen and mobilising the skin medially without attempting to appose the fascia and muscles.

Secondary abdominal wall closure

Secondary abdominal wall closure is repair of the ventral hernia by achieving fascial closure with native body wall and, where not possible, the use of a prosthetic material (Gor-Tex®, Surgisis®, Permacol™) followed by skin closure.

The general condition of the child must be good, with good nutritional status and haemoglobin of at least 10 gm/dl. General anaesthesia is used. The scar of the healed omphalocele is excised. The skin is undermined, the fascial edge identified, and the fascia mobilised and muscle edge identified. Any adherent viscera are released. The peritoneum is closed without tension. The fascia is then closed longitudinally with monofilament-interrupted sutures. The effect of the closure on respiration should be monitored by the anaesthetist. If there is respiratory compromise, the sutures should be released and the use of a prosthetic material, such prolene mesh, Gor-Tex, Surgisis, or Permacol, should be considered, followed by skin closure.

Application of silo

Silo material is silicon or prolene or other nonirritant synthetic material that is nonporous and not adhesive. The mesh is constructed into a bag to fit firmly around the bowels and sutured tightly to the circumference of the fascia and subcutaneous tissues of the defect (Figure 56.3). Bogota bags or intravenous solution bags may be used as silos. Preformed silo bags are now available that can be placed on the omphalocele and applied firmly on the circumference; however, these are expensive. The baby is nursed in an incubator in supine position with the bag suspended from the roof of the incubator.

The baby is usually comfortable. Broad-spectrum antibodies are administered. The circumference suture area is firmly packed and monitored for soaking, infection, or evidence of detaching. Over the days that follow, the bowel content gradually reduces into the abdominal cavity. The bag can get loose on the omphalocele. Further sutures or bands are then applied on the bag to keep it firm on the bowels; this may be required every 2 days. By 7 to 10 days, the omphalocele can be reduced sufficiently to enable closure. The most serious difficulties with silos are infection and detachment at the suture line.

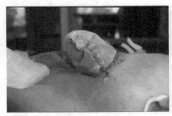 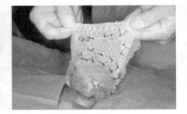

Figure 56.3: Traditional silo bag.

Conservative Treatment

Conservative treatment involves nonoperative measures aimed at escharisation of the sac, which progressively contracts the scar, and encouraging rapid epithelisation from the edge. Various materials have been used, including mercurochrome solution, dilute silver nitrate solution, and 70–90% alcohol. The effect and complications on the baby have caused these solutions to be used less frequently. A useful method of conservative treatment is the application of closed dressing, which is applicable only for an intact sac. When the sac is ruptured, the silo is preferable.

For the dressing, the whole abdomen is cleaned with a plain antiseptic lotion and dried. A layer of Sofratulle® is laid to cover the whole sac. Two or three layers of soft cotton gauze are placed to cover the whole lesion. A soft crepe bandage, 4 or 6 inches, is applied around the circumference of the abdomen, thus maintaining uniform pressure on the omphalocele (Figure 56.4). The dressing is kept on for 24–48 hours and repeated with fresh materials. If the sac appears moist, the dressing should be done once every day. If there is evidence of infection, the dressing should be done twice a day.

By this method, the baby can be kept in the hospital for a shorter time than for other methods, usually 7–10 days, and can be discharged to continue further dressing on an outpatient basis.

By the time the omphalocele heals, there is a ventral abdominal hernia (Figure 56.5). This is repaired at a later stage, as described above.

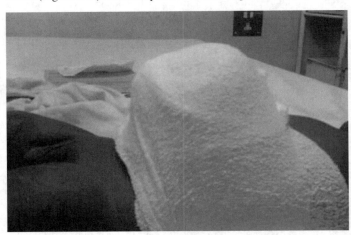

Figure 56.4: Conservative management of omphalocele.

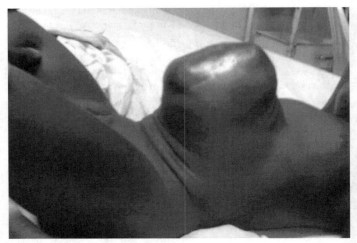

Figure 56.5: Ventral hernia formation.

Management of Gastroschisis

Gastroschisis has a better prognosis than omphalocele because the eviscerated bowel is usually a short loop of small intestine; the abdominal cavity would in most cases accommodate the herniated gut. There are usually no other serious associated congenital abnormalities.

Most gastroschisis can be repaired by primary closure. The small defect is extended, and exploration of the abdomen is done to exclude gut anomalies such as atresia or malrotation. The bowel is cleaned with warm saline and reduced into the abdominal cavity, and the wound is closed.

Gastroschisis is said to have occurred early in intrauterine life when the bowel has stayed out for long time before birth. The eviscerated loops are usually covered with fibrinous exudates due to amniotic fluid reaction. The abdominal cavity is usually small. Primary closure may not be possible. A silo is useful; the gut gradually reduces and the defect can then be closed.

Long delay before surgical intervention results in extrusion of more loops of bowel, which become oedematous and can be complicated by gangrene of the long segment of loop of gut. Resection of the gangrenous segment leaves a short length of small intestine.

Antenatal Diagnosis and Management

Omphalocele and gastroschisis can be detected early in pregnancy. Attempts to repair the defects intrauterine have not been successful. The main usefulness of antenatal detection is to transfer the baby in utero to a paediatric surgical centre and institute early treatment soon after birth. For large omphalocele, it may be preferred to deliver the baby by caesarean section to prevent rupture of the sac, which could occur during a normal vaginal delivery.

Key Summary Points

1. Omphalocele has a sac and has associated abnormalities that contribute to the mortality and morbidity of the condition.

2. Gastroschisis has no sac and has no associated abnormalities, except possible bowel atresia.

3. Primary repair has the best outcome; however, if this is not possible, consider other modalities to avoid intraabdominal compartment syndrome.

4. Hypoglycaemia must be excluded in omphalocele.

Suggested Reading

Bruch WS, Langer JC. Omphalocele and gastroschisis. In: Puri P, ed. Newborn Surgery. Hodder Arnold, 2003.

Patel G, Sadiq J, Shenker N, Impey L, Lakhoo K. Neonatal survival of prenatally diagnosed exomphalos. Pediatr Surg Int 2009; 25(5):413–416.

Sebakira J, Hadley GP. Gastroschisis: a third world perspective. Pediatr Surg Int 2009; 25:327–329.

CHAPTER 57
DISORDERS OF THE UMBILICUS

Jean Heuric Rakotomalala

Dan Poenaru

Ruth D. Mayforth

Introduction

Umbilical disorders are frequently encountered by paediatric surgeons. In the newborn, the umbilical cord typically desiccates and separates within three weeks, leaving a dry, "star-like" central abdominal scar that forms the umbilicus. Failure of the umbilical ring to completely close can result in an umbilical hernia, by far the most common umbilical disorder. Discharge or abnormal tissue from the umbilicus is most often due to an umbilical granuloma, but can result from incomplete involution of the urachus or omphalomesenteric duct. Any discharge, mass, or sinus tract is pathological and should be appropriately evaluated and treated. These and other umbilical disorders are discussed in further detail in this chapter.

Anatomy and Pathology

The umbilical cord is the main portal for entry and exit of blood from the placenta to the foetus during intrauterine life. In addition to the paired umbilical arteries and umbilical vein, the umbilical cord also contains the vitelline or omphalomesenteric duct (which connects the yolk sac to the midgut) and the allantois (the portion connecting the umbilicus to the bladder becomes the urachus). Usually, the vitelline duct obliterates by the 5th to 9th week of gestation, and the urachus obliterates to become the median umbilical ligament by the 4th to 5th month. After birth, the umbilical cord withers and separates, leaving no remnants. Umbilical abnormalities can arise, however, when embryological remnants persist or fail to completely involute.[1,2] Table 57.1 compares the embryological components of the umbilical cord with related disorders.

Like skin anywhere on the body, the umbilicus may also be affected by a variety of dermatological conditions, such as hemangiomas, dermoid cysts, or mechanical irritation. A number of syndromes, such as the Aarskog, Reiger, and Robinow syndromes, are associated with an abnormal umbilical appearance.[3] The umbilicus can also be found in an abnormal position or even absent, as in bladder exstrophy.

Classification of Umbilical Problems

Umbilical problems can be classified as follows, based on the aetiology of the abnormality:

- *acquired:* delayed umbilical separation, umbilical granuloma;

- *infectious:* omphalitis, umbilical vein phlebitis;

- *congenital:* omphalomesenteric duct remnant, umbilical polyp, patent urachus, umbilical hernia, dermoid cyst, umbilical dysmorphism; or

- *neoplastic:* rhabdomyosarcoma, teratoma.

Selected Umbilical Pathology

Delayed Umbilical Separation

The timing of umbilical cord separation may vary, depending on ethnic background, geographic location, and method of cord care. Cord separation usually occurs 1 week after birth; persistence beyond 3 weeks is generally considered delayed. Various umbilical cord antiseptics can prolong the separation time, however. For example, triple dye may

Table 57.1: Embryology and pathology of umbilical disorders.

Embryological element	Normal remnant	Pathological abnormality
Two arteries	Para-urachal lateral ligaments	Single umbilical artery*
One vein	Round ligament of liver	Phlebitis**
Allantois	Median umbilical ligament	Patent urachus, urachal cyst or sinus
Vitelline duct	None	Omphalomesenteric duct remnant, umbilical polyp, Meckel's diverticulum
Umbilical ring	Physiologic closure; fascia covering defect	Umbilical hernia Omphalocele

Source: Minkes R.K.. Disorders of the Umbilicus. EMedicine Specialities. Available at: emedicine.medscape.com/article/935618-overview; accessed 27 October 2008.

*Twenty-five percent of umbilical disorders with single umbilical arteries have associated congenital anomalies.

**A possible complication following umbilical vein catheterisation.

prolong separation of the cord for up to 8 weeks. Dry cord care has been found to be effective in developed countries;[4] however, in developing countries, antiseptic cord care continues to be recommended, and has been found to decrease the incidence of and mortality from omphalitis.[5] Agents that have been used include 70% alcohol, silver sulfadiazine, chlorhexidine, neomycin-bacitracin powder, and salicylic sugar powder.[6,7]

Aside from agents used in umbilical cord care, other factors that can delay umbilical cord separation include infection, underlying immune disorders (such as leukocyte adhesion deficiency), or an urachal abnormality.[7–10] On examination, the skin surrounding the umbilical cord remnant should be carefully examined for a urachal remnant or for any evidence of infection; omphalitis (see next section) can be rapidly progressive and life threatening in a neonate.

A complete blood count with a differential may be useful as an initial screen for leukocyte adhesion deficiency. Even in the absence of infection, leukocytosis and neutrophilia may be present in patients with leukocyte adhesion deficiency.[10] Rare neutrophil motility defects may require a more sophisticated immunologic work-up.

If a patient presents with delayed separation of the cord, it may be either gently removed manually or divided just distal to normal skin with scissors or a scalpel. After removal, the stump site should be cleansed with an antiseptic agent and exposed to air.

Omphalitis

Omphalitis is an infection of the cord stump or its surrounding tissues. It presents most commonly in the newborn; the mean age at onset is 5–9 days, or earlier in preterm infants. The risk of omphalitis is increased by a number of maternal factors (prolonged rupture of membranes, maternal infection, amnionitis), factors at delivery (nonsterile or home delivery, inappropriate cord care); and neonatal factors (low birth weight, delayed cord separation, leukocyte adhesion deficiency, neonatal alloimmune neutropaenia). The incidence of omphalitis in developing countries is significantly higher (as high as 6%) than in developed countries (0.7%).[7]

Proper umbilical cord care is important in decreasing the incidence of omphalitis as well as neonatal tetanus (which may or may not be associated with omphalitis). Public health interventions have proven effective in decreasing the incidence and death from these infections. In Nepal, for example, the use of chlorhexidine decreased the incidence of omphalitis by 75% and its mortality by 24% compared to dry cord care.[5]

More than a half million deaths occur yearly in newborn infants from neonatal tetanus. A high rate of neonatal tetanus was seen among the Maasai people in Kenya and Tanzania, who applied cow dung to the umbilical stumps of their infants. In one simple health programme among the Maasai people, the death rate from neonatal tetanus decreased from 82 per 1,000 in control groups to 0.75 per 1,000 in the intervention group.[11] Part of the success was in finding solutions that were culturally applicable and feasible (e.g., if clean water was unavailable, they advocated cleaning the stump with milk), obtaining support from within the community, and maintaining continued health promotion.

Patients with omphalitis present with erythema, oedema, and/or purulent drainage from the umbilical stump. Patients may also have systemic signs of sepsis, including lethargy, irritability, poor feeding, and fever or hypothermia. More extensive disease is seen with necrotising fasciitis or myonecrosis and may also include a rapidly progressive cellulitis, a peau d'orange appearance, violaceous discoloration, bullae, crepitus, and petechiae.

Patients with omphalitis should be admitted to the hospital and blood and wound cultures should be obtained. Omphalitis is usually polymicrobial; intravenous antibiotics covering gram-positive and gram-negative organisms should be initiated and the area of cellulitis marked and closely followed. Some authors also advocate anaerobic coverage, which certainly should be instituted if there is a concern of necrotising fasciitis. Newborns with sepsis should also have a lumbar puncture and supportive care instituted.

Patients with necrotising fasciitis or myonecrosis require emergent and complete surgical debridement of all affected tissue, including preperitoneal tissue, the umbilical vessels, and the urachal remnant. Necrotising fasciitis or myonecrosis can rapidly progress over a few hours; early and aggressive surgical treatment is critical to survival.

Complications of omphalitis include umbilical phlebitis, portal vein thrombosis (which may lead to portal hypertension), liver abscesses, peritonitis, and necrotising fasciitis or myonecrosis. The overall mortality of omphalitis is estimated at 7–15% and is significantly higher (37–87%) if complicated by necrotising fasciitis or myonecrosis.[12]

Umbilical Granuloma

Umbilical granuloma is the most frequent cause of "wet umbilicus." It presents as moist, raw, reddish-pink tissue arising from the base of the umbilicus after umbilical cord separation. An umbilical granuloma typically measures 0.1–1 cm in size and may be pedunculated. It is nontender (lacking innervation). Drainage may be clear or have the appearance of a fibrinous exudate. The tissue is friable and may bleed easily. Umbilical granuloma is due to the persistence of capillary and fibroblast cells, markers of an ongoing tissue growth. It may be difficult to distinguish from an umbilical polyp (discussed later in this chapter), which is usually brighter red, slightly larger, and represents remnant omphalomesenteric duct or urachal tissue.[7,8]

Management options for umbilical granuloma include repeated cauterisation with silver nitrate, ligation, use of alcoholic wipes, or, rarely, surgical excision. Care must be taken in applying silver nitrate, as contact with normal skin can cause a chemical burn. If the lesion fails to resolve with silver nitrate, the diagnosis should be questioned because umbilical polyps, which may look similar to umbilical granulomas, do not respond to silver nitrate. If the lesion is excised, histology should be

performed to rule out any retained omphalomesenteric duct or urachal remnants, which require further work-up.[1,7,13]

Dermoid Cyst of the Umbilicus

Dermoid cyst of the umbilicus is a rare umbilical mass caused by inclusion of skin epithelium below or within the normal skin of the umbilicus. On examination, the umbilicus appears wider and darker in color than normal, and shiny. No inflammation is noted unless the cyst is infected. The diagnosis is made at surgery on finding the characteristic toothpaste-like sebaceous material within the umbilical mass. Surgical excision is curative.

Omphalomesenteric or Vitelline Remnant

During early foetal development, the omphalomesenteric or vitelline duct serves as a conduit from the yolk sac to the midgut. It normally completely involutes by the 9th week of foetal life. However, a portion or all of the duct may fail to involute and present as one of the following:

• An umbilical polyp, as discussed in the next section.

• Meckel's diverticulum, in which only the diverticulum attached to the ileum has failed to involute. This is the most common vitelline remnant; it most often presents as a lower GI bleed caused by ectopic gastric mucosa, but rarely may present as diverticulitis, or it may function as the lead point for an intussusception.

• A persistent congenital band, which can act as a fixed point around which an intestinal volvulus may occur.

• A complete omphalomesenteric duct remnant with a patent conduit connecting the umbilicus to the ileum; this usually presents with pink mucosa protruding from the umbilicus (Figures 57.1 and 57.2) and usually minimal but persistent discharge of intestinal contents or stool.

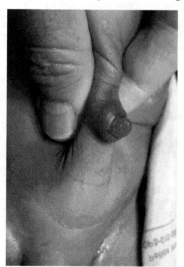

Figure 57.1: Omphalomesenteric fistula.

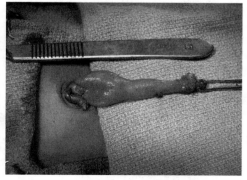

Figure 57.2: Omphalomesenteric fistula (intraoperative).

• An omphalomesenteric duct cyst, in which the proximal and distal ends have obliterated but a remnant persists in between; this may present with an infection or obstruction and is quite rare.

Diagnosis of an omphalomesenteric remnant is generally made on physical exam. An ultrasound may show a loop of bowel present under the umbilicus, but is not diagnostic and usually not necessary. A fistulogram may be helpful in clarifying the diagnosis.

All omphalomesenteric duct remnants should be surgically resected. A Meckel's diverticulum should be amputated at its base, the intestine closed transversely, and the vitelline artery ligated. A broad-based Meckel's diverticulum may require a formal resection with a primary anastomosis. Meckel's diverticula may contain ectopic gastric or pancreatic tissue on histology.[1,2,7]

Umbilical Polyp

An umbilical polyp (Figure 57.3) is a round, reddish mass at the base of the umbilicus that comprises embryologic remnants of the omphalomesenteric duct or, less commonly, the urachus. It is often brighter red and slightly larger than an umbilical granuloma. Unlike a granuloma, it does not respond to silver nitrate and must therefore be surgically excised and histologically evaluated to confirm the diagnosis. If an umbilical polyp is diagnosed, further work-up for an underlying omphalomesenteric duct or urachal remnant is warranted. One author reported a 30–60% chance of finding an underlying omphalomesenteric duct anomaly if an umbilical polyp was identified.[1,7,10,14]

Urachal Anomalies

In the foetus, the urachus is the embryonal duct connecting the dome of the urinary bladder to the umbilical ring. It is normally obliterated prior to birth, forming the median umbilical ligament. It forms in the pre-peritoneal space between the transversalis fascia and the peritoneum. Nonclosure of the entire tract leads to a patent urachus, whereas closure on the bladder side creates an umbilical sinus (Figure 57.4). Closure of both ends but patency of the tract in between may trap fluid in an urachal cyst (Figure 57.5), which is the most common urachal anomaly. A bladder diverticulum results when the distal tract involutes; it is the rarest urachal anomaly.

Both a patent urachus and a urachal sinus may present with clear drainage from the umbilicus, and careful examination demonstrates a sinus at the base of the umbilicus. A patent urachus drains urine and may predispose to cystitis or recurrent urinary tract infections. A urachal cyst most commonly presents once it has become infected. An affected patient will present with infraumbilical swelling, abdominal pain, and erythema. The symptoms may mimic appendicitis. Patients with delayed separation of the umbilical cord may have a urachal anomaly.[9]

Ultrasonography is often useful in diagnosing a urachal cyst, and will show a cystic hypoechogenic lesion in the preperitoneal space. The presence of a longitudinal double line from the bladder dome to the umbilicus is indicative of a urachal remnant. A sinogram may be used to identify the presence of a patent urachus or an urachal sinus. For a patent urachus, a voiding cystourethrogram (VCUG) should be obtained to exclude the presence of posterior urethral valves (back-up pressure from the distal obstruction may be keeping the urachus patent).

Treatment involves complete resection of any part of the tract that has failed to completely obliterate. It is important to remove a cuff of bladder when excising the urachus to prevent the risk of developing a urachal adenocarcinoma later in adulthood.[1,2,7]

Umbilical Hernia

An umbilical hernia is a full-thickness protrusion of the umbilicus with an associated fascial defect; it may contain peritoneal fluid, preperitoneal fat, intestine, or omentum.

In children, umbilical hernias often close spontaneously. Small defects (<1 cm) are much more likely to close than large defects (>2 cm). Meier et al. reported that umbilical hernias continue to close until the age of 14 years in African children.[16] The skin overlying an

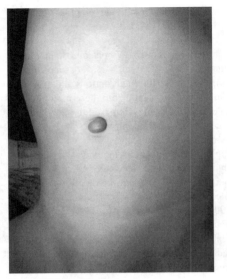

Figure 57.3: Umbilical polyp.

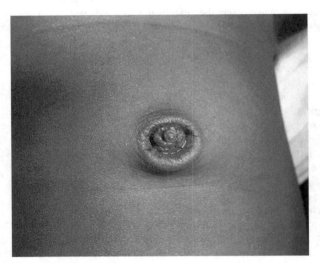

Figure 57.4: Urachal remnant.

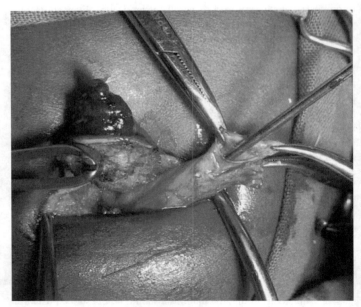

Figure 57.5: Urachal cyst (intraoperative).

umbilical hernia may continue to stretch and result in a proboscoid umbilical hernia. In Africa, most parents are very accepting of its appearance, in contrast to parents from developed countries. Once the umbilical defect has spontaneously closed, the nipple-like umbilical skin may continue to flatten, even during adolescence.

Aetiology

An umbilical hernia results when the umbilical ring fails to close. Umbilical hernias are more frequent in premature, low birth weight, and black infants. They also occur more often in children with ventriculoperitoneal shunts, ascites, obesity, and certain syndromes, including Beckwith-Wiedemann, Trisomy 21, and Marfan's syndromes.

Demographics

Umbilical hernias are common in Africa. In one study from Nigeria, umbilical hernias were found in 91% of under-6-year-olds; 64% of 6- to 9-year-olds, and 46% of 10- to 15-year-olds.[15] Meier found umbilical hernias with a fascial defect >1 cm in 23% of Nigerian children younger than 18 years old.[16] Surprisingly, when 6- to 9-year-old Nigerian children of high socioeconomic class were evaluated for an umbilical hernia, only 1.3% of 7,968 children had an umbilical hernia.[17] It is possible that nutrition may be a factor. Jelliffe found a higher incidence of umbilical hernias in malnourished versus well-nourished adults (27% versus 14%).[15]

Complications

Complications, including incarceration, strangulation, and rupture of umbilical hernias, may occur. In developed countries, the incidence of incarceration or strangulation is rare—one paper reported an incidence of 1 in 1,500 umbilical hernias.[18] Rupture of umbilical hernias with evisceration is even more rare, but has been reported in infants younger than 6 months of age.[19,20]

Even though the incidence of incarceration and strangulation in children with umbilical hernias in Africa is not known, it appears to be higher than in the West (although this may in part reflect the significantly higher prevalence of umbilical hernias in black children). For instance, at A. Le Dantec Hospital in Senegal, over a five-year period, 41 children had emergency operations for incarcerated or strangulated umbilical hernias.[21] At Jos University Teaching Hospital in Nigeria, over an eight-year period, 23 children underwent surgery for acute or recurrent incarceration.[16,19,22–24]

In contrast, Okada et al. reviewed the literature from 1957 to 1999 and found a total of only 38 cases reported in children *worldwide*.[25] In King's College Hospital in London, only 3 incarcerated umbilical hernias were treated in children over a 20-year period (and all 3 of these occurred in black children).[26] The fact that most umbilical hernias in the West are repaired by 4–5 years of age does not account for the apparent difference in the frequency of incarceration between the West and Africa. In both Senegal and Nigeria, most of the incarcerations reported occurred in patients younger than 5 years of age; in Senegal, the average age at incarceration was 14 months (range, 8 months–10 years); in Nigeria, the median was 4 years (range, 3 weeks–12 years). Most incarcerated hernias do not have an inciting factor; however, bezoars, digested vegetable matter, parasitic worms, or ascites have been implicated.[21,22,25]

Umbilical hernias can incarcerate regardless of the size of the fascial defect (Figure 57.6). In one report, a majority (52%) of the patients with incarcerated hernias had medium-sized (0.5–1.5 cm) fascial defects, whereas 24% occurred in small defects (<0.5 cm), and 24% in large defects (>1.5 cm).[25] Of the incarcerated hernias in which a measurement was documented in one study in Nigeria, all had defects greater than 1.5 cm in diameter (not all, however, were measured).[22]

Management

Factors that lead parents to seek medical care for their child in Africa include the age of the child, size of the defect, height of protruding

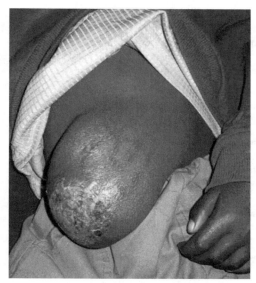

Figure 57.6: Giant ulcerated umbilical hernia.

umbilicus, and pain. On examination, a child with an umbilical hernia usually presents with a protrusion of the umbilicus with contents that are easily reducible. After reduction, the size of the fascial ring can be palpated; it can range from a few millimeters to more than 4 cm in diameter. No other investigations are required for diagnosis.

Umbilical hernia repair is one of the most frequent procedures performed by paediatric surgeons in developed countries.[1] In Africa, however, umbilical hernia repairs are more infrequent because the hernias are usually repaired only if symptomatic or complicated. Generally accepted indications for management in Africa compared to the West are highlighted next.

Due to the high rate of spontaneous closure and the fact that the appearance of a proboscoid umbilical hernia is well tolerated by parents in Africa, conservative management of asymptomatic, easily reducible umbilical hernias is recommended. In the West, conservative treatment is generally recommended for small asymptomatic umbilical hernias (<2 cm fascial defect) in children younger than 4–5 years of age.

In Africa, surgical repair is reserved for symptomatic umbilical hernias. Rarely, parents may request to have a proboscoid hernia repaired. (For further discussion, see the "Ethical Issues" section in this chapter.) In the West, surgical repair is generally recommended for hernias with large fascial defects (>1.5 cm), hernias that have failed to spontaneously close by 4 to 5 years of age, and umbilical hernias with significant proboscoid components.

A classic Mayo "vest-over-pants" procedure or simple approximation with long-lasting absorbable suture are both acceptable for conventional umbilical hernia repairs. For complicated umbilical hernia repairs, the use of mesh may be considered in the closure of a very large uninfected umbilical hernia to prevent excess tension on the fascia. The use of mesh also prevents the development of an abdominal compartment syndrome, which could result with significant fascial tension. Surgical complications are rare after umbilical hernia repairs. The outcome is excellent and the mortality approaches zero for elective repairs. Rare postoperative eviscerations can be prevented by meticulous surgical technique.

Other Umbilical Problems

Absent umbilicus

Malposition or absence of the umbilicus is encountered frequently in patients with bladder exstrophy. When the umbilicus is absent, an omphaloplasty may be performed, as many ethnic groups are culturally sensitive to the absence of the navel. Research has been performed to help the reconstructive surgeon locate the umbilicus in an aesthetically pleasing location.[27]

Stoma at umbilicus

Some paediatric surgeons in the West have advocated placing intestinal or urinary stomas in the umbilicus primarily for aesthetic considerations. Experience with this in Africa has been limited, and no papers adopting its use have been published in Africa to date.

Gastroschisis and omphalocele

These problems are discussed in Chapter 56.

Ethical Issues

As previously discussed, most African surgeons do not use the same indications for umbilical hernia repair as are used in developed countries. Instead, they recommend repairing only those umbilical hernias that are symptomatic in children. However, the incidence of incarceration or strangulation seems to be higher in Africa than in developed countries. Because of this, some African surgeons have recommended repairing all umbilical hernias in children.[21] Others, however, continue to recommend conservative treatment in spite of the risk of incarceration.[16,22] Part of the rationale given is the wide prevalence of umbilical hernias.

Even using selective criteria, Meier et al. have estimated that if all umbilical hernias >1.5 cm were repaired in young children in Africa, about 6–8% of children younger than 4 years of age would require repair;[16] the volume of cases would likely outstrip available surgical resources. The exact criteria for elective repair on which Meier et al. based their estimates were females older than 2 years of age and males older than 4 years of age with a fascial defect ≥1.5 cm in diameter; they estimated that 6% of 2-year-old females and 8% of 4-year-old males would need repair.[16]

If hernias with large (>1.5 cm) fascial defects are indeed the most likely to incarcerate in Africa, as reported by Chirdan et al.,[22] one could argue that they should be repaired, as they are the most likely to incarcerate and the least likely to spontaneously close. Consideration should also be given to closing umbilical hernias in patients who live more than one hour away from surgical resources. More research is necessary to determine the actual incidence of incarceration or strangulation, and to clearly define which umbilical hernias are at greatest risk.

Perhaps it is time to re-examine how current recommendations for umbilical hernia repair in Africa were developed or became generally accepted. Are the current recommendations truly the best for the patient, preventing many children with umbilical hernias from unnecessarily undergoing the risk of a surgical procedure and anaesthesia? Or did the current recommendations arise out of necessity, due to the wide prevalence of umbilical hernias, in an effort to strategically utilise surgical resources and time? If the latter is true, and umbilical hernias should be repaired by using the same criteria as those used in developed countries, there may be other creative solutions. For instance, just as health care workers have been specifically trained to suture lacerations or to perform caesarean sections, perhaps consideration should be given to specifically training them to perform simple, straightforward surgical procedures such as umbilical hernia repairs.

Evidence-Based Research

Table 57.2 presents the results of a trial involving application of chlorhexidine to the umbilical cord to prevent omphalitis and neonatal mortality.

Table 57.2: Evidence-based research.

Title	Topical applications of chlorhexidine to the umbilical cord for prevention of omphalitis and neonatal mortality in southern Nepal: a community-based, cluster-randomised trial
Authors	Mullany LC, Darmstadt GL, Khatry SK, et al.
Institution	DNepal Nutrition Intervention Project, Sarlahi, Kathmandu, Nepal; Institute of Medicine, Tribhuvan University, Kathmandu, Nepal; Department of International Health, Johns Hopkins Bloomberg School of Public Health, Baltimore, Maryland, USA
Reference	Lancet 2006; 365:910–918
Problem	Prevention of omphalitis and neonatal death related to umbilical cord care in southern Nepal.
Intervention	Topical application of chlorhexidine to the umbilical cord.
Comparison/ control (quality of evidence)	Prospective, community-based, cluster-randomised trial.
Outcome/effect	Compared to dry cord care, chlorhexidine reduced severe omphalitis by 75% and neonatal mortality by 24%.
Historical significance/ comments	Recent recommendations by the World Health Organization for dry umbilical cord care may be inappropriate in developing countries, where the risk of omphalitis and death related to umbilical cord care is higher than in developed countries.

Key Summary Points

1. Appropriate umbilical cord care is important in preventing omphalitis, which can be a life-threatening infection.

2. The presence of a remnant of the urachus or omphalomesenteric duct should be considered if there is an umbilical sinus, persistent drainage, or remnant tissue.

3. Ultrasonography can be useful in investigating umbilical disorders when the diagnosis is uncertain.

4. Any irreducible umbilical mass or persistent umbilical lesion needs surgical exploration and resection.

5. Umbilical hernias are more common in children in Africa than in the rest of the world, and the incidence of incarceration appears to be higher than in the West.

6. In Africa, proboscoid umbilical hernias are common, well-accepted, and treated conservatively.

7. Incarceration or strangulation of umbilical hernias is uncommon but has been reported more often in Africa than in developed countries. Complications remain the general indication for umbilical hernia repair in Africa.

8. An omphaloplasty may be indicated for cultural reasons.

9. After umbilical surgery, the prognosis is excellent and complications are rare.

References

1. Snyder CL. Current management of umbilical abnormalities and related anomalies. Semin Pediatr Surg 2007; 16:41–49.

2. O'Donnel KA, Glick PL, Caty MG. Pediatric umbilical problems. Pediatr Clin N Amer 1998; 45:791–799.

3. Friedman JM. Umbilical dysmorphology. The importance of contemplating the belly button. Clin Genet 1985; 28:343–347.

4. Zupan J, Garner P, Omari AA. Topical umbilical cord care at birth. Cochrane Database Syst Rev 2004; CD001075.

5. Mullany LC, Darmstadt GL, Khatry SK, et al. Topical applications of chlorhexidine to the umbilical cord for prevention of omphalitis and neonatal mortality in southern Nepal: a community-based, cluster-randomised trial. Lancet 2006; 365:910–918.

6. Pezzati M, Biagioli E, Martelli E, et al. Umbilical cord care: the effect of eight different cord care regimens on cord separation time and other outcomes. Biol Neonate 2002; 81:38–44.

7. Palazzi DL, Brandt, ML. Care of the umbilicus and management of umbilical disorders. Available at: www.uptodate.com; accessed 13 August 2008.

8. Minkes RK. Disorders of the umbilicus. EMedicine Specialities Available at: emedicine.medscape.com/article/935618-overview; accessed 13 August 2008.

9. Razvi S, Murphy R, Shalsko E, Cunningham-Rundles C. Delayed separation of the umbilical cord attributable to urachal anomalies. Pediatr 2001; 108:493–494.

10. Pomeranz A. Anomalies, abnormalities, and care of the umbilicus. Paediatr Clin N Amer 2004; 51:819–827.

11. Meegan ME, Conroy RM, Lengeny SO, et al. Effect on neonatal tetanus mortality after a culturally-based health promotion programme. Lancet 2001; 358:640–641.

12. Gallagher PG, Shah SS. Omphalitis. eMedicine Specialties. Available at: emedicine.medscape.com/article/975422; accessed 13 August 2008.

13. Daniels J, Craig F, Wajed R, Meates M. Umbilical granulomas: a randomised controlled trial. Arch Dis Child Fetal Neonatal Ed 2003; 88:F257.

14. Kutin ND, Allen JE, Jewett TC. The umbilical polyp. J Pediatr Surg 1979; 14:741–744.

15. Jelliffe DB. The origin, fate and significance of the umbilical hernia in Nigerian children (a review of 1,300 cases). Trans Royal Soc Trop Med Hyg 1952; 46:428–434.

16. Meier DE, OlaOlorun DA, Omodele RA, et al. Incidence of umbilical hernia in African children: redefinition of "normal" and reevaluation of indications for repair. World J Surg 2001; 25:645–648.

17. Uba AF, Igun GO, Kidmas AT, Chirdan LB. Prevalence of umbilical hernia in a private school admission-seeking Nigerian children. Niger Postgrad Med J 2004; 11:255–257.

18. Mestel AL, Burns H, Incarcerated and strangulated umbilical hernias in infants and children. Clin Pediatr 1963; 2:368–370.

19. Ameh EA, Chirdan LB, Nmadu PT, and Yusufu L. Complicated umbilical hernias in children. Pediatr Surg Int 2003; 19:280–282.

20. Weik J, Moores D. An unusual case of umbilical hernia rupture with evisceration. J Pediatr Surg 2005; 40:E33–E35.

21. Fall I, Sanou A, Ngom G, et al. Stangulated umbilical hernias in children. Pediatr Surg Int 2006; 22:233–235.

22. Chirdan LB, Uba AF, Kidmas AT. Incarcerated umbilical hernia in children. Eur J Pediatr Surg 2006; 16:45–48.

23. Mawera G, Muguti GI. Umbilical hernia in Bulawayo: some observations from a hospital based study. Cent Afr J Med 1994; 40:319–323.

24. Nmadu PT. Paediatric external abdominal hernias in Zaria, Nigeria. Ann Trop Paediatr 1995; 15:85–88.

25. Okada T, Yoshida H, Iwai J, et al. Strangulated umbilical hernia in a child: report of a case. Surg Today 2001; 31:546–549.

26. Papagrigoriadis S, Browse DJ, Howard ER. Incarceration of umbilical hernias in children: a rare but important complication. Pediatr Surg Int 1998; 14:231–232.

27. Abhyankar SV, Rajguru AG, Patil PA. Anatomical localization of the umbilicus: an Indian study. Plast Reconstr Surg 2006; 117:1153—1157.

CHAPTER 58
INGUINAL AND FEMORAL HERNIAS AND HYDROCELES

Francis A. Abantanga

Kokila Lakhoo

Introduction

In general, a hernia is defined as a protrusion of a portion of an organ or tissue through an abnormal opening (defect) in the cavity containing it. In children, the abnormal defect, which is congenital, is usually at the internal inguinal ring.

Groin hernias and hydroceles are extremely common conditions in infancy and childhood and form a large part of the general paediatric surgical practice. Inguinal hernias (IHs) and hydroceles in infants and children are overwhelmingly congenital, although a vast majority are noticed after the neonatal period. Most hydroceles in infants and children do not present any urgent problems.

Demographics

Groin hernias in children are mainly inguinal in nature (Figure 58.1). Inguinal hernias are indirect in nature in more than 99% of cases as a result of the presence of a patent processus vaginalis (PPV). In about 0.5–1% of cases, inguinal hernias in children may be direct and are said to be due to the weakness of the floor of the inguinal canal or occur after surgery to correct indirect inguinal hernias. The direct inguinal hernia bulges through the inguinal floor medial to the inferior epigastric vessels in the Hasselbach's triangle; the indirect hernia arises lateral to the inferior epigastric vessels. About 0.5% of groin hernias constitute femoral hernias (see Figure 58.1).

Incidence data with reference to groin hernias and hydroceles are not available in the literature from Africa; most reports are hospital-based retrospective studies. Such data from Africa on inguinal hernias show a male-to-female ratio ranging from 2.2:1 to 16.6:1. The reported incidence of clinically apparent inguinal hernias in term babies in the world literature ranges from 1% to 5% in large paediatric series, with males outnumbering females by 3–10:1. The incidence is considerably higher in premature babies, ranging from 7% to 35%. Inguinal hernias are found variously on the right side in about 60–70% of cases and on the left side in 25–30%. They are bilateral in about 5–10% of cases.

Inguinal Hernia

Embryology

The gonads develop along the urogenital ridge as retroperitoneal structures by the 6th week of gestation. The gonads are then differentiated into the testes or ovaries by the 7th to 8th week of intrauterine growth under hormonal influence. Retroperitoneal migration of the gonads, under the influence of hormones, results in their being at the internal inguinal ring around the 12th to 14th gestational week. A gubernaculum, which is attached to the lower poles of the testes, is a condensation of mesenchyme that contains cordlike structures within it. It appears to guide the testes into the scrotum. The testes remain quiescent at the internal inguinal ring until about 28 gestational weeks, when there is a rapid descent through the inguinal canal into the scrotum by the 36th to 40th week of intrauterine life.

An outpouching of peritoneum precedes the descent of the gonad (testis) through the inguinal canal at the level of the internal inguinal ring. This outgrowth of peritoneum is referred to as the processus

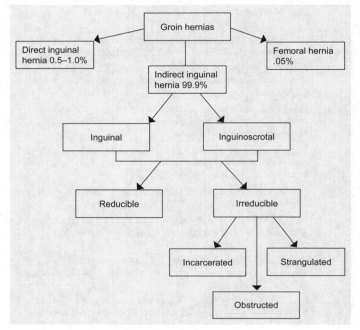

Figure 58.1: Classification of groin hernias.

vaginalis (PV) in the male or canal of Nuck in the female. As the testes descend, the PV is pushed ahead into the scrotum, and when descent is complete, the PV proximal to the testis obliterates either shortly before or just after birth, becoming a fibrous cord. This usually occurs later on the right side than the left, accounting for the greater frequency of hernias on the right. The portion of the PV adjacent to the testes remains patent and is referred to as the tunica vaginalis (which has a visceral and parietal layer) of the testes. In the female, the canal of Nuck ends in the labium majus and is also usually obliterated by the time of delivery of the baby.

As the testis descends into the scrotum, the layers of the anterior abdominal wall contribute to the formation of the layers of the spermatic cord. The transversalis fascia forms the internal spermatic fascia; the internal oblique and the transversus abdominis muscles form the cremasteric muscle; finally, the aponeurosis of the external oblique muscle contributes to the formation of the external spermatic fascia.

Pathophysiology

Failure of obliteration of the PV (or canal of Nuck) leads to the occurrence of hernias and hydroceles, the two most common problems of the region of the groin in children. The variety of degrees of patency of the PV account for the various pathologies seen in that region of the groin (Figure 58.2). Obliteration of the distal PV with the proximal portion still patent will lead to intestines herniating into it, resulting in the formation of an indirect inguinal hernia confined to the inguinal region (see Figure 58.2C). In the case of complete failure of obliteration of the

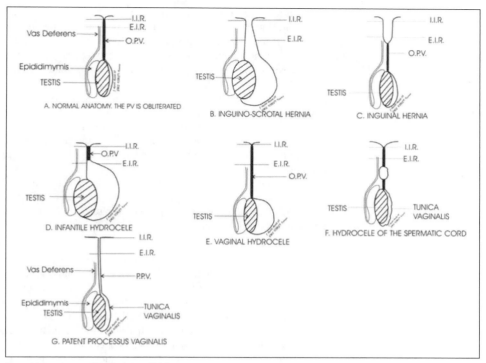

Note: I.I.R. = internal inguinal ring; E.I.R. = external inguinal ring; O.P.V. = obliterated processus vaginalis; P.P.V. = patent processus vaginalis.

Figure 58.2: Diagrammatic representation of different types of inguinal hernias and hydroceles in boys following the descent of the testes into the scrotum.

whole PV and in the presence of a wide neck, an inguinoscrotal (complete, scrotal) hernia will be the outcome (see Figure 58.2B).

Congenital hydroceles formed after the failure of fusion of the PV may be communicating or noncommunicating (see Figure 58.2D–G). Where the opening of the PV that has failed to obliterate completely is narrow and will not allow intestines to herniate but permits peritoneal fluid to trickle into it, a communicating hydrocele will result. Noncommunicating hydroceles can be of three types:

1. *vaginal or scrotal hydrocele,* formed when the proximal portion of the PV obliterates completely, leaving the distal tunica vaginalis to fill with fluid;

2. *infantile hydrocele,* formed when the proximal portion of the PV obliterates as far as the inguinal canal so that part of the PV is patent continuous with the tunica vaginalis; or

3. *encysted hydrocele of the spermatic cord*, or simply *hydrocele of the cord*, formed when there is complete involution of the proximal PV and the part above the tunica vaginalis, leaving an isolated cystic dilatation.

In the case of females in which the canal of Nuck is patent, a hydrocele or a hernia (usually containing intestine or ovary and fallopian tube) will form.

It is important to remember that the mere presence of a PPV does not automatically mean a hernia or a hydrocele necessarily occurs. The PPV may take about a year or two in some instances to obliterate completely, but not all children with a PPV will develop a hernia or a hydrocele.

Conditions associated with an increased risk of development of IH include positive family history, prematurity, low birth weight, undescended testes, hypospadias, epispadias, exstrophy of the bladder, ambiguous genitalia, ascites, gastroschisis, omphalocele, and male gender, among others (e.g., increased intraabdominal pressure).

Clinical Presentation

Inguinal hernias appear as intermittent, usually reducible, lumps in the groin (Figures 58.3 and 58.4) and are painless.

History

A careful and accurate history is taken, followed by meticulous examination of the child. There is usually a history (given by the mother or caregiver) of an asymptomatic bulge or mass in the groin or scrotum or labia, which is intermittent and originates from the internal inguinal ring. The mass appears on crying in the infant or younger child; in the older child, it may appear with coughing or walking or playing around (i.e., on increasing the intraabdominal pressure). Also of note in the history is that the bulge varies in size; it may periodically disappear spontaneously (when the contents completely return to the peritoneal cavity) or by application of gentle pressure by the parent. The mass usually does not cause pain or much discomfort to the child. Often the caregiver or the older child can point to the exact location of the bulge. Most hernias are seen in the first year of life, often when the parents are changing the diaper of a crying or straining child or bathing the child.

Physical examination

The history of a mass should be confirmed by examining the child in various positions, upright or supine. It is important to ascertain that the testes are in the scrotum because a retractile testis will mimic an inguinal hernia by causing a bulge at the external inguinal ring. One of the following procedures will increase the intraabdominal pressure in order to augment the demonstration of a groin mass.

1. Lie the infant supine with the hands held above the head and the lower limbs held straight down. This can be done by an assistant or the parent. This makes the child strain or cry, thus increasing the intraabdominal pressure and causing the bulge to appear if it is actually present. Standing the patient upright may help at times.

2. Ask the older child to jump or bounce up and down, which may allow the mass to appear in the inguinal region.

3. Ask the older child (>6 years of age) to cough or blow up a balloon. This will make the bulge appear. (Often, children <6 years of age just refuse to carry out instructions, even though they very well understand the request to do so.)

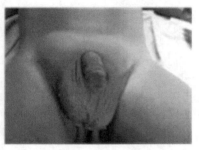

Figure 58.3: Bilateral reducible hernias. Both testes are in the scrotum.

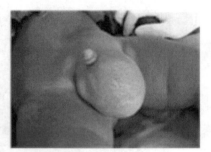

Figure 58.4: Reducible left inguinoscrotal hernia.

In the case where there is no bulge but there is the suspicion that a hernia sac may be present, gently but firmly palpate the cord structures in the male child or the round ligament of the ovary in the female child, sliding the structure over the pubic bone beneath the index finger medially and laterally. This will elicit a palpable thickening of the cord (or ligament of the ovary), usually referred to as the silk glove sign; this is suggestive of the presence of a hernia sac.

An inguinal hernia, if present, may be reducible or irreducible, complicated or uncomplicated. A reducible IH is one in which the contents of the sac return spontaneously to the peritoneal cavity or will do so with gentle manual pressure when the child is recumbent. In such situations, there is usually no pain associated with the mass. For an irreducible IH, the lump will not reduce spontaneously when the child lies supine, but may sometimes be reduced if some amount of pressure is exerted. The contents of the sac are trapped by a narrow neck. An irreducible hernia may or may not be tender.

In the case of an incarcerated IH, an example being the incarceration of the ovary with the fallopian tube in a hernia sac, the mass does not reduce spontaneously when the child lies down, and most often cannot be reduced by the physician examining the child. Note here that the mass is not tender and the contents (ovary and a portion of the fallopian tube) are usually a sliding component of the sac. In children, incarceration of inguinal hernias occurs at the external inguinal ring, whereas in adults, the hernia is normally obstructed at the internal inguinal ring.

The term "incarceration" does not imply obstruction, inflammation, or ischaemia of the herniated mass, although incarceration is necessary for obstruction or strangulation to arise. When an incarcerated hernia becomes painful and the examiner can elicit tenderness, then the IH is either obstructed or strangulated. When it is bowel that is trapped in the sac and the mass becomes tender and irreducible, then signs of intestinal obstruction will eventually occur. In such circumstances, there is usually no interference with the blood supply of the contents of the sac. Rectal examination in infants and small children may be diagnostic if the incarcerated bowel is palpated at the internal inguinal ring.

Strangulation is said to arise when the obstruction progresses to cause compromise to the blood supply of the contents (e.g., bowel or omentum); then bowel infarction leading to severe tenderness of the bulge will occur, and oedema and erythema of the overlying skin will appear. In such a case, the child may pass a bout of one or two bloody stools.

An obstructed or strangulated IH, especially where the contents of the sac are intestines, will lead to abdominal pain, vomiting, and constipation. If the obstruction is not relieved quickly, it may progress to bowel ischaemia, gangrene, perforation, and sepsis. There may also be compression of the spermatic cord, leading to ischaemia, necrosis, and secondary atrophy of the ipsilateral testis with the possibility of subfertility or infertility if, for one reason or another, the contralateral testis is abnormal. As such, incarceration of an IH should be taken seriously and steps initiated to exclude either an obstruction or strangulation. If an obstruction or strangulation is considered present, then the child should be admitted to hospital and managed appropriately to prevent complications.

The differential diagnoses of IH include: hydrocele, inguinal adenitis, femoral hernia, femoral adenitis, undescended testis, retractile testis, varicocele, torsion of the testis, testicular tumour, lipoma, and lymphangioma of the inguinal area.

Investigations

The diagnosis of IH in an overwhelming majority of cases is clinical (history and examination). In the few cases where the diagnosis cannot be made immediately, the child needs to be re-examined over a period of time to make a definitive diagnosis. Although imaging studies are generally not indicated for the diagnosis of IH, in the literature, ultrasonography has been used to confirm IH in selected patients; however, this is not the gold standard for diagnosing IH in children.

Other laboratory and radiographic investigations to determine the presence of IH in a child are usually not necessary or even indicated. In the African subregion, a full blood count with the determination of the sickling status of the child is usually all that is required to treat a child with a reducible, uncomplicated IH. If the hernia is complicated (obstructed or strangulated) and the child is being prepared for surgery, it is advisable to add blood urea, creatinine, and electrolytes determination to the investigations required before operation, especially if the obstruction or strangulation has been present for 24 hours or more (a frequent occurrence in the subregion).

Complications of an inguinal hernia include incarceration, intestinal obstruction, strangulation, gangrene of bowel, perforation of bowel, peritonitis, septicaemia, intraabdominal abscess formation, infarction of the testis, testicular atrophy, gangrene of the ovary and/or fallopian tube, and infertility.

Treatment

Inguinal hernias are not known to resolve spontaneously and must therefore be repaired surgically shortly after diagnosis on an elective basis; the definitive treatment for IH is early operation, a herniotomy. This will reduce the risks of incarceration with its attendant complications, such as obstruction and strangulation. A well-administered general anaesthesia is preferable and can be safely done by an anaesthesiologist experienced in the care of infants and children. Ketamine can also be used and is well tolerated by children.

The procedure (Figure 58.5) involves a herniotomy through a transverse or oblique incision made in the lowest inguinal skin crease (Figure 58.5A).

1. The incision is deepened through the Camper's fascia, subcutaneous fat, and Scarpa's fascia (in the process, one will encounter the superficial epigastric and the external pudendal vessels, which may be retracted aside, coagulated, or tied with a suture) until the aponeurosis of the external oblique abdominal muscle (Figure 58.5B) is reached. After clearing it of overlying fat, the external inguinal ring is identified.

At this stage, depending on the size of the hernia and the age of the child, a decision is made whether to open the aponeurosis. In neonates and infants, the external inguinal ring almost overlies the internal inguinal ring, so there may not be the need to open the aponeurosis of the external oblique muscle to get to the hernia. In large hernias, it is advisable to incise the aponeurosis of the external oblique to open into the inguinal canal before looking for the hernia sac. Here, too, one may decide to open the external oblique aponeurosis to include the external inguinal ring or not to include it in the incision.

2. The sac is normally found on the anteromedial aspect of the elements of the spermatic cord after bluntly spreading the fibres of the cremasteric muscle; it is picked up with haemostats (Figure 58.5C) and dissected free of the cord, using both blunt and sharp dissection.

3. Once the sac is dissected up to the internal inguinal ring, it is opened (Figure 58.5D), and its content(s) replaced into the peritoneal cavity to make sure it is empty. Figure 58.5E shows the vas deferens.

Where the sac is big and extends into the scrotum, no attempt should be made to dissect it completely into the scrotum. This will lead to unnecessary bleeding and haematoma formation postoperatively. Using sharp dissection and several haemostats (a minimum of 6), a large hernia sac can be circumferentially dissected, clamped, and amputated distally without having to follow it into the scrotum.

4. The dissection is then continued proximally towards the internal inguinal ring until the peritoneum (a white structure; see Figure 58.5F) or preperitoneal fat is visualised.

5. The sac is then twisted several times (Figure 58.5F) on itself to make sure the reduced content(s) stay in the peritoneal cavity out of harm's way, and the neck is then transfixed and ligated high up in the internal inguinal ring with Vicryl 3/0 or 2/0, and excess sac excised.

High ligation of the hernia sac is all that is required. Sometimes, an enlarged internal inguinal ring is narrowed at the medial margin by placing one or two sutures through the transversalis fascia.

6. Haemostasis is secured and, where the aponeurosis was opened, it is re-approximated with Vicryl and the skin closed with a suitable suture material. Usually, one Vicryl 2/0 or 3/0 suture of 90 cm in length is adequate enough to suture-ligate the sac, and close the aponeurosis and the skin, especially if one uses the subcuticular method of closure (Figure 58.5G).

For postoperative pain control, a local anaesthetic such as bupivacaine is injected into the wound during closure. The child can then be given either paracetamol, Tylenol® syrup, or a suppository for use in the house, as herniotomy is considered an outpatient procedure.

A controversial topic concerns the routine exploration of the contralateral side for an inguinal hernia. It is known that more than 50% of children younger than 2 years of age have a PPV, but only about 10% will eventually develop a clinical hernia; most PPV will spontaneously close and not develop into hernias. Many reports in the literature (including those from Africa) show that fewer than 7% of children who had a herniotomy done on one side will eventually develop a hernia on the contralateral side. This is a low incidence rate and does not, therefore, suggest or justify the need for routinely exploring the contralateral groin for a metachronous hernia.

Despite the above-stated argument, some paediatric surgeons will still routinely explore the opposite groin in children younger than 2 years of age, in older boys with a clinical hernia on the left, and in girls younger than 10 years of age because hernias on both sides for these groups are more common. Our experience, though, does not support this fact. Due to the high negative rate in exploration of the contralateral side and possible injury to the vas deferens and testicular vessels, it is strongly recommended to perform a unilateral repair of inguinal hernia if it is on only one side.

Herniotomy should be performed on premature babies before they are discharged home from hospital due to the frequent incarceration of IH in such children.

Findings in a hernia sac may include intestines, ovary with the fallopian tube, uterus (rare), ovotestis, omentum (in older children), appendix (Amyand's hernia; see Figure 58.6), Meckel's diverticulum (Littre's hernia), or Richter's hernia (entrapment of a portion of the antimesenteric wall of the bowel in the hernia sac).

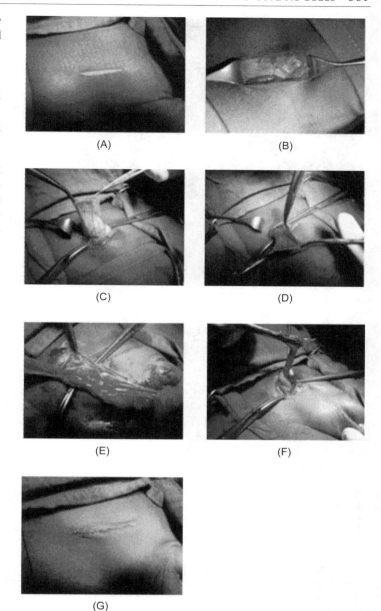

Figure 58.5A–G: The various steps of herniotomy of an inguinal hernia in a child.

The child with an irreducible (incarcerated) IH that is tender, making the child irritable, should be admitted to hospital and an attempt made to reduce the mass manually. Even in our subregion, where late presentation is the order of the day, an attempt should first be made to reduce all incarcerated hernias provided there are no signs and symptoms of peritonitis and toxicity. When this fails, surgery can then be performed. Most incarcerated hernias in children have not yet strangulated and can be manually reduced; this will prevent the need for an emergency surgery, with its attendant significantly increased risk to the constituents of the spermatic cord as a result of oedema of the tissues.

When manual reduction of a hernia is attempted on a child with an incarcerated hernia, the child should be given an analgesic (pethidine or tramadol at a dose of 2 mg/kg intramuscularly) and sedated with diazepam (2 mg intramuscularly or intravenously or even rectally), and the foot of the bed should be elevated slightly to allow the intraabdominal organs to fall back and to keep the intraabdominal pressure from being exerted on the inguinal area.

Manual reduction is then attempted as follows:

1. If the incarcerated hernia is on the right side, the thumb and index

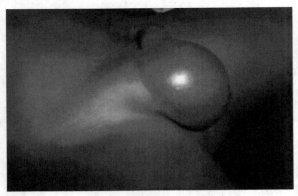

Source: By kind permission of the African Journal of Paediatric Surgery.

Figure 58.6: Amyand's hernia in a 5-year-old boy. Note the oedematous and shiny nature of the scrotum. Intraoperatively, an inflamed appendix was found.

finger of the left hand are placed on either side of the external inguinal ring (where the mass is usually obstructed) over the pubic tubercle. The fingers of the right hand compress the fundus of the hernia gently but firmly. The pressure should be gentle, firm, and sustained.

2. Meanwhile, the thumb and the index finger of the left hand attempt to disimpact the neck of the hernia from the narrow external inguinal ring and also prevent the contents of the sac from spreading to the sides and outwards.

3. When reduction is successful, the whole bowel is felt to return to the peritoneal cavity suddenly and with a gurgle or gush.

4. After successfully reducing an incarcerated hernia, the child is kept in hospital for at least 24 hours for observation, and herniotomy is planned for the next available elective list.

Other surgical methods available for repair of inguinal hernias in children consist of the different techniques of laparoscopic surgery. These include percutaneous internal ring suturing, laparoscopic flip-flap technique, and others.

Postoperative Complications

Complications of herniotomy can be immediate, early, or late. The immediate complications will include anaesthetic complications, such as nausea, vomiting, and laryngeal spasm or oedema. Other immediate complications are haemorrhage (which should be rare if haemostasis is meticulous) and haematoma formation in the wound.

If the vas deferens is transected intraoperatively and this is noticed, then it should be repaired by using fine monofilament sutures.

The early complications comprise

• haematoma formation in the wound or scrotum; such a haematoma will slowly resolve in 3–5 weeks if there is no superimposed infection;

• wound infection, which may occur as a result of anaemia and malnutrition in patients and especially after repair of incarcerated hernias;

• abscess formation in the wound or scrotal haematoma;

• intestinal obstruction; and

• faecal or urinary incontinence as a result of iatrogenic trauma to the bowel or urinary bladder.

Late complications comprise:

• stitch abscess, associated with the use of nonabsorbable sutures;

• undescended testis or high testis due to the fact that the surgeon did not make sure the testis was replaced in the scrotum when closing the inguinal incision;

• recurrence of the inguinal hernia (causes of recurrence include infection and missing the hernia sac during the first operation);

• hydrocele, which may resolve spontaneously or may require surgery;

• testicular atrophy as a result of transection of the vessels during the operation or, in the case of children presenting with incarcerated hernias, with evidence of infarction of the testis at operation;

• infarction of the ovary and fallopian tube (rare because there is usually no obstruction to the blood supply of these organs);

• subfertility or infertility if injury to the vas deferens is bilateral or is to the vas deferens of a solitary testis; and

• numbness of the inguinal region as a result of injury to the ileoinguinal nerve.

Femoral Hernia

Femoral hernia is an unusual hernia in the paediatric age group. A femoral hernia presents as a mass located lateral to and below the pubic tubercle, inferior and posterior to the inguinal ligament and medial to the femoral pulse. It occurs in about 0.5% of all groin hernias in children. The diagnosis of a femoral hernia is challenging, and the correct preoperative diagnosis is usually not made in many children. Most often, it is misdiagnosed, and only during surgery for a suspected inguinal hernia is the precise diagnosis made. Note that a diagnosis of a missed femoral hernia or a direct inguinal hernia should be considered if any child returns with an early recurrence of a groin bulge after an adequate herniotomy, as recurrent indirect inguinal hernias are rare. In the literature, some femoral hernias are reported to have occurred after an inguinal canal exploration or even as a result of iatrogenic disruption of the femoral canal. Most paediatric surgeons know of the existence of this entity but have not encountered it in their practice due to its rarity.

Aetiology

The aetiology of femoral hernias remains elusive. It is suggested that it may be due to either (1) a congenital narrow posterior inguinal wall attachment to Cooper's ligament with a resulting enlarged femoral ring (this is the anatomic aspect accepted by many paediatric surgeons); or (2) an acquired genesis related to increased intraabdominal pressure.

Anatomy

The anatomy of the femoral canal, which occupies the most medial compartment of the femoral sheath and extends from the femoral ring above to the saphenous opening below, has the medial border as the lacunar (Gimbernat's) ligament, posterior border as the pectineal (Cooper's) ligament, the lateral border as the femoral vein, and the anterior border as the inguinal ligament. It is usual to have a lymph node (Cloquet) within the canal.

In the available series of childhood femoral hernias, 60–65% are found on the right side, 25–30% on the left, and 10–15% are bilateral.

Presentation

The clinical signs and symptoms of a femoral hernia are a bulge below the inguinal ligament and lateral to the pubic tubercle; the mass appears on straining or coughing, and reduces in size or disappears when the patient lies supine; and there may be a cough impulse. A femoral hernia can remain unnoticed for a long period until it incarcerates, drawing the attention of the patient to the problem for the first time. Incarceration of paediatric femoral hernias is a very rare occurrence, however.

Diagnosis

The diagnosis of a femoral hernia is mainly clinical or at operation. For the diagnosis to be made preoperatively, the surgeon must consider it in the differentials of groin hernias. There are no known investigations to help confirm the diagnosis of a femoral hernia. The advent of laparoscopic surgery definitely helps with the diagnosis and repair of such hernias.

The differential diagnosis of a femoral hernia include inguinal hernia, ectopic testis, femoral aneurysm, sahpena varix, enlarged femoral lymph nodes, lymphadenitis, lipoma, psoas abscess, and lymphangioma.

Treatment

For uncomplicated femoral hernias, the treatment is surgical repair of the femoral defect as soon as the diagnosis is made. There are three methods of approaching the femoral canal for the repair of a femoral hernia:

1. a high or suprainguinal (transperitoneal or extraperitoneal) approach;

2. an inguinal approach; and

3. a low infrainguinal approach.

Irrespective of the method of approach used, the procedure is as follows:

1. The hernia sac is dissected free and opened to inspect the contents, which are then reduced back to the peritoneal cavity, if present.

2. The sac is then suture-ligated and the inguinal ligament is approximated to the pectineal ligament, thus effectively eliminating the defect.

Caution should be exercised not to strangulate the femoral vein, which will lead to compromised venous return, resulting in the swelling of the lower limb on the affected side. In an incarcerated femoral hernia, the transperitoneal approach may come in handy if there is the need to resect gangrenous bowel.

Femoral hernias can also be repaired laparoscopically.

Complications

Complications include recurrence of femoral hernia (mainly reported in patients who underwent simple herniotomy without any attempt to close the defect in the femoral canal), trauma to the femoral vessels, oedema of the lower limb, haemorrhage leading to haematoma formation, and wound infection.

Hydrocele

A hydrocele is an abnormal collection of fluid in the layers of the tunica vaginalis, the persistently patent processus vaginalis surrounding the testis. Hydroceles are common in infants. The PPV is found in about 90% of term babies at birth. This incidence rate will gradually decrease to about 40% at 2 years of age and then to about 10% in adulthood. A clinically apparent hydrocele is present in only 6% of term male children beyond the neonatal period.

Aetiology

In infants, hydroceles, which are mostly congenital, can be communicating or noncommunicating. A communicating hydrocele (Figure 58.7A) occurs when the proximal portion of the PV remains patent, allowing fluid from the abdominal cavity to trickle down its narrow neck into the scrotal sac, or tunica vaginalis. A communicating hydrocele fluctuates in size and is usually larger in ambulatory patients at the end of the day. It becomes small as the child lies down supine and the fluid trickles back into the peritoneal cavity (Figure 58.7B).

In the case of noncommunicating hydroceles (Figure 58.8), the PV is obliterated proximally with a collection of fluid distally in the tunica vaginalis alone or the tunica vaginalis and part of the PPV proximal to it. Thus, one can have (1) a vaginal (scrotal) hydrocele in which the whole PV is obliterated and there is fluid collection in the tunica vaginalis; (2) an infantile hydrocele, in which part of the PV proximal to the tunica vaginalis is still patent, and can sometimes extend into the inguinal canal as far as the internal inguinal ring; or (3) an encysted hydrocele of the spermatic cord (or, simply, hydrocele of the spermatic cord), in which there is a collection of fluid in a portion of PV somewhere along its length between the external inguinal ring and the testis. Most often, the cyst does not communicate with either the peritoneal cavity above or the tunica vaginalis below, and even may be considered as a third testis by the uninitiated (Figure 58.9). In the case of girls, the inguinal swelling filled with fluid is referred to as a hydrocele of the canal of Nuck.

Acquired hydroceles can be due to viral infection, trauma (called posttraumatic hydroceles), or testicular neoplasia.

Clinically, hydroceles are soft nontender masses within the hemiscrotum. The testis can usually be felt at the posterior aspect of

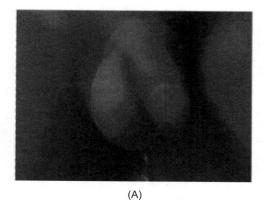

(A)

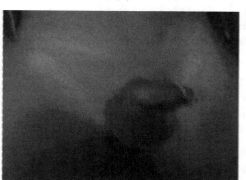

(B)

Figure 58.7: A communicating hydrocele in a 6-year-old boy: (A) in a standing position, fluid fills the tunica vaginalis and the hydrocele is apparent; (B) in a lying position, the fluid trickles back into the peritoneal cavity and the hydrocele empties.

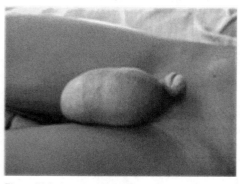

Figure 58.8: A vaginal (scrotal) hydrocele in a 10-year-old boy. The PV was completely obliterated above the hydrocele at operation.

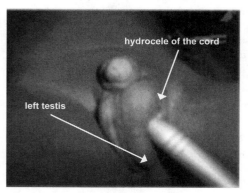

Figure 58.9: Encysted hydrocele of the left spermatic cord. Notice that the mass above the left testis transilluminates light brightly and is separate from the testis below it. Intraoperatively, the PV was found to be completely obliterated above and below the cyst.

fluid collection in the hemiscrotum. To diagnose a mass in the scrotum as a hydrocele, the following should be present:

1. One should be able to get above the mass. This is usually the case, except for the rare infantile hydrocele, which may extend into the internal inguinal ring.

2. The mass must be fluctuant. Always test for fluctuancy in two planes.

3. The mass must brilliantly transilluminate, especially when this test is done in a darkened environment. It must be remembered that hernias in infants can also transilluminate due to the thin walls of the bowel.

4. The mass cannot be emptied on applying pressure; this is very true for the noncommunicating hydroceles (Figure 58.8). For the communicating hydrocele (Figure 58.7A), on applying pressure, the mass empties very slowly; in the case of a reducible inguinoscrotal hernia, the emptying is relatively very fast and intestines are usually palpated in the scrotum.

Hydroceles in infants are often bilateral; like hernias, they are more common on the right than the left. Most hydroceles will resolve spontaneously by the age of 1 to 2 years, on the average by one and a half years of age. Therefore, hydroceles still in existence by this age should be electively repaired.

The diagnosis of a hydrocele in a child is usually clinical. There are no known imaging studies that are used routinely to diagnose the problem. However, ultrasonography may be used as a screening tool if a testicular tumour is considered as being a cause of the hydrocele.

The differential diagnosis of a hydrocele will include: an inguinal hernia, a testicular tumour, and epididymo-orchitis. The last two may have an associated hydrocele, which is usually reactive. For testicular tumours, such as malignant teratomas, measuring serum α-foetoprotein and human choriogonadotropin levels may help to establish the diagnosis. In the case of epididymitis and orchitis, urinalysis and urine culture and sensitivity may be of help in diagnosis and treatment.

Treatment

Hydroceles that are asymptomatic should be observed until the child is about 2 years old, at which time the PPV should close spontaneously. If a hydrocele does not resolve spontaneously by then, surgery is advised. The operation is performed through an inguinal approach, as in inguinal hernias, using one of the lowermost skin creases in the groin. Surgery involves, in the case of the communicating hydrocele, high ligation of the PPV within the internal inguinal ring. For encysted hydrocele of the spermatic cord, the hydrocele is usually easily dissected out without much of a problem. Care should be exercised, however, not to traumatise the vas deferens and its vessels. If the hydrocele is infantile or vaginal, then hydrocelectomy is carried out, also through a groin incision, with care not to traumatise the spermatic cord structures. In both cases, the PV proximal to the hydrocele is usually obliterated.

The child should be placed on analgesics after the surgery; Tylenol or a paracetamol suppository three times daily suffices in most cases. No antibiotics are required. Hydroceles in children should not be aspirated as a method of treatment because they have a natural history of resolution and will recollect after aspiration.

Postoperative Complications

The following complications are possible postoperatively:

• *Injury to the spermatic cord*. Careful surgery and avoidance of rough handling of the spermatic cord structures will prevent trauma to them.

• *Bleeding with possible scrotal haematoma formation*. This can be prevented if bleeding is meticulously controlled at every step during surgery. A diathermy machine (especially a bipolar diathermy), if available, is of great help, with careful avoidance of excessive burning of the tissues in order not to injure the vas deferens and its elements. Haematomas will resolve spontaneously in 3–5 weeks without surgery; if they persist beyond this period, surgical drainage may be necessary.

• *Wound infection*. Antibiotics may be necessary to treat the infection, depending on its severity.

• *Recurrence of the hydrocele*. Recurrence is rare.

Prognosis and Outcome

The prognosis is excellent for groin hernias and hydroceles if they are diagnosed and repaired early in childhood. Hernia surgery is safe and very effective in eliminating the problem; the outcome is usually good, and recurrence is rare (about 1%). Complications occur mostly in the difficult cases, such as in obstructed or strangulated hernias. An inguinal approach to the repair of hydroceles is extremely successful and should lead to less than a 1% recurrence rate.

Prevention

Groin hernias and hydroceles are congenital in nature, so prevention is geared towards preventing their complications and not towards preventing the occurence of these pathologies, per se. Complications of groin hernias can be prevented if they are treated timely, during childhood, on diagnosis. The risk of incarceration of inguinal hernias is high in children, and therefore elective repair is the treatment of choice. Premature babies with hernias should have an elective repair of the hernia done before discharge from hospital or as soon as practicable because their hernias are more prone to incarceration. A well-timed elective operation will prevent incarceration.

During laparoscopic repair of a groin hernia on one side, the contralateral side can be inspected for the presence of a metachronous hernia and a repair carried out as a preventive measure.

Evidence-Based Research

Table 58.1 presents a retrospective review of the incidence of complications following inguinal hemiotomy in newborns weighing 5 kg or less.

Table 58.1: Evidence-based research.

Title	The incidence of complications following primary inguinal herniotomy in babies weighing 5 kg or less
Authors	Nagraj S, Sinha S, Grant H, Lakhoo K, Hitchcock R, Johnson P
Institution	Department of Paediatric Surgery, Children's Hospital Oxford, John Radcliffe Hospital, Oxford, UK
Reference	Pediatr Surg Int 2006; 22(12):1033
Problem	Complications following inguinal hernia surgery in newborns.
Intervention	The aim of this study was to quantify the incidence of complications following inguinal herniotomy in small babies weighing 5 kg or less.
Comparison/ control (quality of evidence)	This was a retrospective review of inguinal herniotomies performed between December 1997 and March 2002 on babies weighing 5 kg or less. A total of 154 patients underwent hernia repair, of which 81% (125 patients; 221 hernias) were available for review. The median weight at surgery was 3.6 kg (range, 1.7–5 kg). Eighty-four patients (67%) were classified as premature (<36 weeks gestation). Thirty-three patients presented with an irreducible hernia, in whom all but one were successfully reduced prior to surgery. Patients were reassessed at a clinic following surgery, and follow-up data were obtained from the clinic notes after a median follow-up of three months (range, 1–60 months). Five cases (2.3%) of hernia recurrence occurred in 4 patients, and 6 patients (2.7%) experienced testicular atrophy. In the testicular atrophy group, 4 of the 6 patients presented with an incarcerated hernia, and of these, 3 were noted to have evidence of ischaemia at operation. There were 6 cases (2.7%) of high testes requiring subsequent orchidopexy.
Outcome/effect	Although neonatal inguinal herniotomy is a technically demanding procedure, this series has demonstrated a low complication rate. Testicular atrophy was associated with a history of preoperative incarceration in the majority of cases

Key Summary Points

1. Hernias and hydroceles in children are considered congenital and are diagnosed clinically (history and examination). Indirect inguinal hernias are overwhelmingly more common than other groin hernias.

2. Open herniotomy is the operation of choice for inguinal hernias in children in our subregion. These hernias can also be repaired laparoscopically.

3. Femoral hernias are very rare in children but should be kept in mind as a differential diagnosis for groin hernias. If there is recurrence after surgery for an indirect inguinal hernia in a child, it is important to exclude a direct inguinal hernia or a femoral hernia.

4. An attempt should be made to manually reduce all incarcerated hernias in children, especially in infants, under sedation and analgesia.

5. If manual reduction is successful, plan to operate on the child on the next available elective list, preferably within the next 72 hours because the oedema would have subsided by then.

6. If manual reduction fails, the child must be operated on immediately after the necessary preoperative preparations.

7. An encysted hydrocele of the spermatic cord may mimic an incarcerated hernia; therefore, careful examination of the child is important.

8. In the case of a dull transillumination of a groin mass, an attempt should be made to exclude an inguinal hernia, which in infants may transilluminate dimly.

Suggested Reading

Abantanga FA, Amaning EP. Paediatric elective surgical conditions as seen at a referral hospital in Kumasi, Ghana. ANZ J Surg (2002); 72:890–892.

Abantanga, FA. Groin and scrotal swellings in children aged 5 years and below: a review of 535 cases. Pediatr Surg Int 2003; 19:446–450.

Ameh, EA. Incarcerated and strangulated inguinal hernias in children in Zaria, Nigeria. East Afr Med J 1999; 76(9):499–501.

Calkins CM, St Peter SD, Balcom A, Murphy PJ. Late abscess formation following indirect hernia repair utilzing silk suture. Pediatr Surg Int 2007; 23:349–352.

Chen K-C, Chu C-C, Chou T-Y, Wu C-J. Ultrasonography for inguinal hernias in boys. J Pediatr Surg 1998; 33(12):1784–1787.

Collins, S. Hydrocele and hernia in children. Available at http://emedicine.medscape.com/article/1015147 (accessed 16 November 2008).

Davenport, M. ABC of general paediatric surgery: inguinal hernia, hydrocele, and the undescended testis. BMJ 1996; 312:564–567.

De Caluwe D, Chertin B, Puri P. Childhood femoral hernia: a commonly misdiagnosed condition. Pediatr Surg Int 2003; 19:608–609.

De Meulder F, Wojciechowski M, Hubens G, Ramet J. Female hydrocele of the canal of Nuck: a case report. Eur J Pediatr 2006; 165:193–194.

Fresno JCO, Alvarez M, Sanchez M, Rollan V. Femoral hernia in childhood: review of 38 cases. Pediatr Surg Int 1997; 12:520–521.

Hassan, ME. Laparoscopic flip flap technique versus conventional inguinal hernia repair in children. Ann Pediatr Surg 2005; 1(1):17–20.

Hebra, A. Pediatric hernias. Available at http://emedicine.medscape.com/article/932680 (accessed 14 December 2008).

Khanna PC, Ponsky T, Zagol B, Lukish JR, Markle BM. Sonographic appearance of canal of Nuck hydrocele. Pediatr Radiol 2007; 37:603–606.

Lau ST, Lee Y-H, Gaty MG. Current management of hernias and hydroceles. Sem Pediatr Surg 2007; 16:50–57.

Lee, S. Hydrocele. Available at http://emedicine.medscape.com/article/438724 (accessed 12 December 2008).

Lee SL, DuBois JJ. Laparoscopic diagnosis and repair of pediatric femoral hernia. Initial experience of four cases. Surg Endosc 2000; 14:1110–1113.

Lloyd, DA. Inguinal and femoral hernia. In Azizkhan RG, Weber TR Ziegler MM, eds. Operative Pediatric Surgery. McGraw-Hill Professional, 2003.

Luo C-C, Chan H-C. Prevention of unnecessary contralateral exploration using the silk glove sign (SGS) in pediatric patients with unilateral inguinal hernia. Eur J Pediatr 2007; 166:667–669.

Nmadu, PT. Paediatric external abdominal hernias in Zaria, Nigeria. Ann Trop Paediatr 1995; 15(1):85–88.

Nuss, D. The management of hernias, hydroceles and undescended testes. SA Med J, 1976; 548–549.

Osifo OD, Irowa OO. Indirect inguinal hernia in Nigerian older children and young adults: is herniorrhaphy necessary? Hernia 2008; 12:635–639.

Patkowski D, Czernik J, Chrzan R, Jaworski W, Apoznanski W. Percutaneous internal ring suturing: a simple minimally invasive technique for inguinal hernia repair in children. J Laparoendoscopic & Advanced Surg Techniques 2006; 16(5):513–518.

Rescorla, FJ. Hernias and umbilicus. In Colombani PM, Foglia RP, Skinner MA, Oldham KT, eds. Surgery of Infants and Children, Vol. 2. Lippincott Williams & Wilkins, 2005.

Shabbir J, Moore A, O'Sullivan JB, et al. Contralateral groin exploration is not justified in infants with a unilateral inguinal hernia. Irish J Med Sc 2003; 172(1):18–19.

Sklar C, Cameron BH. Achieving excellent outcomes and avoiding complications in pediatric inguinal hernia surgery. Available at: http://www.ptolemy.ca/members/archieves/2008/hernia.pdf (accessed 16 November 2008).

Stephens BJ, Rice WT, KouchyCJ, Gruenberg KC. Optimal timing of elective indirect inguinal hernia repair in healthy children: clinical consideration for improved outcome. World J Surg 1992; 16:952–957.

Usang UE, Sowande OA, Adejuyibe O, Bakare TIB, Ademuyiwa OA. Day case inguinal hernia surger in Nigerian children: prospective study. Afr J Paediatr Surg 2008; 5(2):76–78.

Woolley, MM. Inguinal hernia. In: Welch KJ, Benson CD, Aberdeen E, Randolph JG Ravitch MM. Pediatric surgery, Vol. 2. Year Book Medical Publishers, Inc, 1984.

Zamakhshary M, To T, Guan J, Langer JC. Risk of incarceration of inguinal hernia among infants and young children awaiting elective surgery. CMAJ 2008; 179(1):1001–1005.

ACRONYMS

3D	three-dimensional		BOO	bladder outlet obstruction
A&E	accident and emergency (department)		BP	blood pressure
AAS	Association for Academic Surgery		BPS	bronchopulmonary sequestration
ABL	allowable blood loss		BPSU	British Paediatric Surveillance Unit
ABR	auditory brainstem response		BRRI	Building and Roads Research Institute (Ghana)
ACE	antegrade continent enema			
ACS	American College of Surgeons		BSA	body surface area
ACTH	adrenocorticotropic hormone		BSO	bilateral salpingo-oophorectomy
ADA	adenosine deaminase		BWS	Beckwith-Weidemann syndrome
ADH	antidiuretic hormone		BXO	balanitis xerotica obliterans
ADL	African degenerative leiomyopathy		CA	condylomata acuminatum; choanal atresia
ADPKD	autosomal dominant polycystic kidney disease			
			CAEBV	chronic active Epstein-Barr virus
AER	air enema reduction		CAH	congenital adrenal hyperplasia
AF	anal fissure (fissure-in-ano)		CAIS	complete androgen insensitivity syndrome
AFB	acid-fast bacilli			
AFP	alpha-foetoprotein		CBF	cerebral blood flow
AFS	American Fertility Society		CCAM	congenital cystic adenomatous malformation (lung)
AGA	average for gestational age			
AIDS	acquired immune deficiency syndrome		CD	cluster of differentiation; Crohn's disease; compact disc
AIN	anterior interosseous nerve			
AIS	Abbreviated Injury Scale		CDH	congenital diaphragmatic hernia
AJOL	African Journals Online		CDLT	cadaveric donor liver transplantation
ALL	acute lymphocytic leukaemia		CECT	contrast-enhanced computed tomography
ALT	aspartate transaminase; akternative lengthening of telomeres			
			CESP	Confederation of European Specialists in Paediatrics
ALTE	acute life-threatening events			
AML	acute myelogenous leukaemia		CF	cystic fibrosis
AMREF	African Medical and Research Foundation		CFP 10	culture filtrate protein 10
AP	anteroposterior; Anatomical Profile		CFS	congenital fibrosarcoma
APC	adenomatous polyposis coli (gene)		CFTR	cystic fibrosis transmembrane (conductance) regulator
APSA	American Paediatric Surgical Association			
AR	androgen receptor; allergic rhinitis		CHARGE	Coloboma, Heart defect, Atresia choanae, Retarded growth and development, Genital hypoplasia, Ear anomalies/deafness (syndrome)
ARM	anorectal malformation			
ARPKD	autosomal recessive polycystic kidney disease			
			CHD	congenital heart disease
ART	antiretroviral treatment		CHEOPS	Children's Hospital of Eastern Ontario Pain Scale
ASA	American Society of Anesthesiologists			
ASCOT	A Severity Characterization Of Trauma		CHL	conductive hearing loss
ASSC	acute splenic sequestration crisis		CIC	clean intermittent catheterisation
AST	alanine transaminase		CIE	counterimmunoelectrophoresis
ATLS	Advanced Trauma Life Support		CIF	common intermediate format
ATRD	African Trauma Registry Database		CIIP	chronic idiopathic intestinal pseudo-obstruction
ATT	antitubercular treatment			
AVM	arteriovenous malformation		CIRM	International Radio Medical Centre
AVPU	alert, verbal, painful, unresponsive (method to assess level of consciousness)		CLD	chronic liver disease
			CLE	congenital lobar emphysema
AXR	abdominal x-ray; abdominal radiograph		CLO	congenital lobar overinflation
BA	biliary atresia		CMT	congenital muscular torticollis
BAC	bronchioloalveolar carcinoma		CMV	conventional mechanical ventilation; cytomegalovirus
BAHA	bone-anchored hearing aid			
BAPS	British Association of Paediatric Surgeons		CNI	calcineurin inhibitors
BCG	bacille Calmette-Guérin		CNS	central nervous system
b.d.	twice daily		CO	cardiac output
β-hCG	β-human chorionic gonadotropin		COPUM	congenital obstructive posterior urethral membrane
BMI	body mass index			

CORA	centre of rotational deformity	EIA	enzyme-linked immunosorbent assay
COSECSA	College of Surgeons of East, Central and Southern Africa	EIS	endoscopic injection sclerotherapy
		ELISA	enzyme-linked immunosorbent assay
CPA	conditioned play audiometry	EMG	electromyography
CPAM	cystic pulmonary adenomatous malformation (lung)	EMLA	eutectic mixture of local anaesthetics
		EMR	electronic medical record
CPAP	continuous positive airway pressure	ENT	ear, nose, and throat
CPC	cauterisation of the choroid plexus	ERCP	endoscopic retrograde cholangiopancreatography
CPP	cerebral perfusion pressure		
CPR	cardiopulmonary resuscitation	ERP	endorectal pull-through
CR	capillary refill	ESAT6	early secretory antigenic target-6
CRP	C-reactive protein	ESFT	Ewing's sarcoma family of tumours
CSF	cerebrospinal fluid	ESLD	end-stage liver disease
CT	computed tomography (scan)	ESPE	European Society for Paediatric Endocrinology
CTEV	congenital talipes equinovarus (CTEV)		
CVA	central venous access	ESR	erythrocyte sedimentation rate
CVP	central venous pressure	ESRD	end-stage renal disease
CXR	chest x-ray	ESRF	end-stage renal failure
DA	duodenal atresia	ESWL	extracorporeal shock-wave lithotripsy
DALYs	disability-adjusted life years	ET	empyema thoracis
DCS	dynamic compression system	ETF	enteral tube feeding
DDH	developmental dysplasia of the hip	ETRS	embryonic testicular regression syndrome
DEC	diethylcarbamazine	ETV	endoscopic third ventriculostomy
DES	diethylstilbesterol	EUS	endoscopic ultrasonography
DIC	disseminated intravascular coagulation	EUSOL	Edinburgh University solution of lime
DGE	delayed gastric emptying	EVD	external ventricular drainage
DHT	dihydrotestosterone	EWS/ETS	Ewing sarcoma breakpoint region/ erythroblastosis virus E26 oncogene transcription factor fusion gene
DJ	duodenojejunal		
DMSA	dimercaptosuccinic acid		
DNA	deoxyribonucleic acid	EXIT	ex-utero intrapartum treatment
DOA	dead on arrival	FAC	familial adenomatosis coli
DOT	directly observed therapy	FAO	foot-ankle orthosis
DPG	diphosphsglycerate	FAP	familial adenomatosis polyposis
DPL	diagnostic peritoneal lavage	FAST	focused abdominal sonography for trauma
DPPC	dipalmitoylphosphatidyl choline	FBC	full blood count
DRE	digital rectal examination	FDA	Food and Drug Administration (US)
DSA	digital substraction angiography	FEF	forced expiratory flow
DSD	disorders of sex differentiation; detrusor sphincter dyssynergia	FETO	fetal endoscopic tracheal occlusion
		FEV	forced expiratory volume
DSL	digital subscriber line	FFP	fresh frozen plasma
DTPA	diethylenetriamine penta-acetic acid	FGC	female genital cutting
DVD	digital video disc	FIA	fistula-in-ano
DYG	double-Y glanuloplasty	FLACS	Faces, Legs, Activity and Consolability Scale
EBV	Epstein-Barr virus		
ECG	electrocardiogram	fMRI	functional Magnetic Resonance Imaging
ECM	extracellular matrix	FNA	fine needle aspiration
ECMO	extracorporeal membrane oxygenation	FNAB	fine-needle aspiration biopsy
ECW	extracellular water	FNH	focal nodular hyperplasia
ED	Emergency Department (of a hospital)	FRC	functional residual capacity
EDNRB	endothelin B receptor gene	FSH	follicle-stimulating hormone
EF	examining finger	FVC	forced vital capacity
EFD	estimated (preoperative) fluid deficit	GA	general anaesthesia
EFR	estimated fluid requirement (maintenance fluids)	GABHS	group A beta-hemolytic streptococcal
		GCRG	giant cell reparative granuloma
EGD	oesophagogastroduodenoscopy	GCS	Glasgow Coma Scale
EGF	epidermal growth factor	GDNF	glial (cell line) derived neurotrophic factor
eGFR	estimated glomerular filtration rate	GDP	gross domestic product
EHBS	extra hepatic biliary system	GF	growth factor

GFR	glomerular filtration rate		ID	immunodiffusion
GGT	gamma-glutaml transpeptidase		IDA	iminodiacetic acid
GI	gastrointestinal		IF	intestinal failure
GID	gastrointestinal duplication		IFN-g	interferon gamma release protein
GIEESC	Global Initiative for Emergency and Essential Surgical Care		IgA, IgE, IgG, IgM	immunoglobulin A, E, G, M
GIT	gastrointestinal tract		IGF	insulin growth factor
GOR	gastro-oesophageal reflux		IH	inguinal hernia
GORD	gastro-oesophageal reflux disease		IHA	indirect haemogglutination antibody
GOS	Glasgow Outcome Scale		IHPS	infantile hypertrophic pyloric stenosis
GRWR	graft weight-to-recipient's body weight ratio (transplantation)		IJV	internal jugular vein
			IL	insensible losses (fluids)
GVHD	graft versus host disease		IM	intramuscular
GWD	guinea worm disease		INR	international normalization ratio
Gy	gray (radiation dose)		INSS	International Neuroblastoma Staging System
H&E	haematoxylin and eosin (staining)		IO	intraosseous
HAART	highly active antiretroviral therapy		IOM	Institute of Medicine
HAEC	Hirschsprung's-associated enterocolitis		IP	Internet protocol
HB	hepatoblastoma		IPAA	ileal-pouch anal anastomosis
HbAS	sickle cell trait		IQR	interquartile range
HbS/β thal	sickle cell thalassemia disease		IRA	ileorectal anastomosis
HbSC	sickle cell haemoglobin C disease		IRIS	immune reconstitution inflammatory syndrome
HbSS	homozygous sickle cell anaemia		IRS	Intergroup Rhabdomyosarcoma Study Group
HC	hydrocephalus			
HCC	hepatocellular carcinoma		INH	isoniazid
hCG	human chorionic gonadotropin		ISDN	Integrated Services Digital Networks
HCMV	human cytomegalovirus		ISfTeH	International Society for Telemedicine and ehealth
HCW	health care worker			
HD	Hirschsprung's disease		ISP	Internet service provider
HHML	hemihyperplasia-multiple lipomatosis syndrome		ISS	Injury Severity Score
			ITP	idiopathic thrombocytopaenic purpura
HIDA	hepato-iminodiacetic acid		ITU	International Telecommunication Union
HINARI	Health InterNetwork Access to Research Initiative		ITx	intestinal transplantation
			IV	intravenous
HIT	hydrodistention-implantation technique		IVA	ifosfamide, vincristine, and actinomycin D
HIV	human immunodeficiency virus			
HLA	human leukocyte antigen		IVC	inferior vena cavography; inferior vena cava
HMS	hyperactive malarial splenomegaly			
HO	hematogenous osteomyelitis		IVF	in vitro fertilisation
HPF	high-power fields		IVIG	intravenous immunoglobulin
HPN	home parenteral nutrition		IVU	intravenous urography
HPZ	high pressure zone		JCV	John Cunningham virus (but just say JC virus)
HR	heart rate			
HSCR	Hirschsprung's disease		JNA	juvenile nasopharyngeal angiofibroma
HSP	Henoch-Schönlein purpura		KS	Kaposi sarcoma
H-TOF	H-type tracheo-oesophageal fistula		KSHV	Kaposi sarcoma-associated herpes virus
HVA	homovallinic acid			
IBCA	isobutyl cyanoacrylate		KTS	Kampala Trauma Score
IBD	inflammatory bowel disease		LAD	leukocyte adhesion deficiency
IBI	intralesional bleomycin injection		LATS	long-acting thyroid stimulating (hormones)
ICCS	International Children's Continence Society			
			LB flap	lateral-based flap
ICP	intracranial pressure		LDH	lactate dehydrogenase
ICT	information and communication technologies		LDITx	living-donor intestinal transplantation
			LF	lymphatic filariasis
ICU	intensive care unit		LFT	liver function test
ICV	ileocaecal valve		LGA	large for gestational age
ICW	intracellular water			

LHR	lung-head ratio (foetal)		NEC	necrotizing enterocolitis
LLS	left lateral segment (liver)		NF	necrotising fasciitis
LMA	laryngeal mask airway		NGO	nongovernmental organisation
LMIC	low- and middle-income country		NGT	nasogastric tube
LOH	loss of heterozygosity		NHL	non-Hodgkin's lymphoma
LOS	length of (hospital) stay; lower oesophageal sphincter		NICU	neonatal intensive care unit
			NIO	neonatal intestinal obstruction
LPD	lymphoproliferative disorder		NJT	nasojejunal tube
LPP	leak point pressure		NK	natural killer (cell)
LPU	lower pole ureter		NMDA	N-methyl-d-aspartate
LRLT	living-related liver transplantation		NNBSD	nonneurogenic bladder sphincter dysfunction
L/S	lecithin/spingomyelin (ratio)			
LTB	laryngotracheobronchitis		NNIS	National Nosocomial Infection Surveillance (index)
LWAT	location without advanced technology			
LWPES	Lawson Wilkins Pediatric Endocrine Society		NOR	nonoperative reduction
			NPC	nasopharyngeal carcinoma
MACE	Malone antegrade continence enema		NPO	nothing by mouth, literally nil per os
MAG3	mercaptoacetyltriglycine		NPWT	negative pressure wound therapy
MAGPI	meatal advancement and glanuloplasty incorporated		NR	nephrogenic rests; nutritional rickets
			NRC	National Research Council (US)
MAP	mean airway pressure; mean arterial pressure; mutYH-associated-polyposis (gene)		NRSTS	nonrhabdomyosarcoma soft tissue sarcome
			NS	normal saline
MC&S	microscopy, culture, and sensitivities		NSAIDS	nonsteroidal anti-inflammatory drugs
MCDK	multicystic dysplastic kidney; multicystic diseased kidney		NSS	normal saline solution
			NTD	neural tube defect
MCUG	micturating cystourethrogram; micturating cystourethrography		NTSC	National Television Standards Committee
			NVB	neurovascular bundle
MD	Meckel's diverticulum		NWTSG	National Wilms' Tumour Study Group
MDGs	Millennium Development Goals		OA	oesophageal atresia
MDR	multidrug-resistant		OAE	otoacoustic emission
MEN2	multiple endocrine neoplasia type 2		OGD	oesophago-gastric-duodenoscopy
MFH	malignant fibrous histiocytoma		ONS	oral nutritional supplements
MIBG	metiodobenzylgaunidine (scan)		OPG	orthopantomogram
MIP	mega-meatus intact prepuce		OPSI	overwhelming postsplenectomy infection
MIR	minimally invasive repair		OR	operating room
MIS	Müllerian-inhibiting substance; minimally invasive surgery		ORIF	open reduction, internal fixation
			ORL	otorhinolaryngology
MMF	mycophenolate mofetil		ORS	ovarian remnant syndrome
MMP	matrix metalloproteinases		PA	pulmonary artery
MMR	measles-mumps-rubella (vaccine)		PAA	perianal abscess
MSP	manual separation with prophylaxis		PACU	postanaesthetic care unit
MRA	magnetic resonance angiography		PADUA	progressive augmentation by dilating the urethra anterior
MRCP	magnetic resonance cholangiopancreatography			
			PAIR	percutaneous aspiration, instillation, and reaspiration
MRI	magnetic resonance imaging			
MRKH	Mayer-Rokitansky-Kuster-Hauser (syndrome)		PAIS	partial androgen insensitivity syndrome
			PAL	phase alternating line
MSK	musculoskeletal		PAPSA	Pan African Paediatric Surgical Association
MSP	manual separation with prophylaxis			
MTC	medullary thyroid carcinoma		PAS	para-aminosalicylic acid; pyriform aperture stenosis
mTOR	mammalian target of rapamycin			
MTOS	Major Trauma Outcome Study		PAX/FKHR	Paxillin [Drosophila melanogaster])/ (forkhead box O1 [Homo sapiens]) fusion gene
NASA	National Aeronautics and Space Administration (USA)			
			PBM	pancreaticobiliary malunion
NBCA	n-butyl cyanoacrylate		PC	phosphatidyl choline (lecithin)
Nd:YAG	neodymium:yttrium aluminium garnet (laser)		PCA	patient-controlled analgesia

PCEA	patient-controlled epidural analgesia		RBC	red blood cells; red blood count
PCR	polymerase chain reaction		RBF	renal blood flow
PDS	polydioxanone		RCT	randomised controlled trial
PE	pleural effusion; pectus excavatum		rDNA	ribosomal DNA
PEB	cisplatin, etoposide, and bleomycin		RDS	respiratory distress syndrome
PEEP	positive end expiratory pressure		REAL	Revised Euro-American Lymphoma
PEG	percutaneous endoscopic gastrostomy		RET	REarranged during Transfection (gene)
PELD	Pediatric End-stage Liver Disease		RL	Ringer's lactate
PEP	post exposure prophylaxis		RMS	rhabdomyosarcoma
PEPFAR	President's Emergency Plan for AIDS Relief		RPC	recurrent parotitis in children
			RPL	recurrent pregnancy loss
PET	positron emission tomography (scan)		RR	respiratory rate
PFC	persistent foetal circulation		RRP	recurrent respiratory papillamatosis
PFIC	progressive familial intrahepatic cholestasis		RSV	respiratory syncytial virus
			RTS	Revised Trauma Score
PHT	portal hypertension		RUT	rapid urease test
PIC	percutaneously(or peripherally) inserted central (venous)		RVF	rectovaginal fistulae
			SARS	sacral anterior root stimulation
PICU	paediatric intensive care unit		SB	spina bifida; small bowel
PLP	pathological lead point		SBO	small bowel obstruction
PN	parenteral nutrition		SBP	systolic blood pressure
PNET	primitive neuroectodermal tumour		SC	sickle cell hemoglobin in sickle cell disease
PO	per os (by mouth, orally)			
PPD	purified protein derivative		SCD	sickle cell disease
PPF	periportal fibrosis		SCF	supracondylar fracture
PPHN	persistent pulmonary hypertension of the newborn		SCIWORA	spinal cord injury without radiographic abnormality
PPI	proton pump nhibitor		SCT	sacrococcygeal teratoma
PPS	post-polio syndrome		SCV	subclavian vein
PPV	patent processus vaginalis		SEER	Surveillance, Epidemiology and End Results (U.S. program)
P(s)	probability of survival			
PSARP	posterior sagittal anorectoplasty		SENIC	Study on the Efficacy of Nosocomial Infection Control (CDC)
PSE	passive stretching exercise			
PSI	pleural space infection		SGA	small for gestational age
PSS	postsplenectomy sepsis		SHML	sinus histiocytosis with massive lymphadenopathy
PSTN	public switched telephone network			
PSVT	Paroxysmal supraventricular tachycardia		SIDS	sudden infant death syndrome
PT	prothrombin time		SIOP	Société Internationale d'Oncologie Pédiatrique (International Society of Pediatric Oncology)
PTEN	phosphatase/tensin			
PTFE	polytetrafluoroethylene			
PTH	parathormone		SIRS	systemic inflammatory response syndrome
PTLD	posttransplant lymphoproliferative disorder		SIS	small intestinal submucosa
PTS	Paediatric Trauma Score		SLE	systemic lupus erythematosus
PTSD	posttraumatic stress disorder		SM	streptomycin
PTT	partial thromboplastin time		SMA	superior mesenteric artery
PUD	peptic ulcer disease		SMT	sternomastoid tumour
PUJ	pelviuretic junction. (see also UPJ)		SMV	superior mesenteric vein
PUV	posterior urethral valve		SNHL	sensorineural hearing loss
PV	processus vaginalis		SNS	sympathetic nervous system
PVO	portal vein occlusion		SOMI	sterno-occipito-mandibular immobilization
PVR	post-void residual		SPE	streptococcal pyrogenic exotoxins
PVT	portal vein thrombosis		SS	sickle cell hemoglobin in sickle cell disease
PZA	pyrazinamide			
QOL	quality of life		SSI	surgical site infection
RA	regional anaesthesia		STD	sexually transmitted disease
RAFT	Réseau en Afrique Francophone pour la Télémédecine		StAR	steroidogenic acute regulatory (protein function)
Rb	retinoblastoma (gene)		STEP	serial transverse enteroplasty procedure

STING	subureteric Teflon injection	UC	ulcerative colitis
StrepTSS	streptococcal NF associated with toxic shock syndrome	UDT	undescended testis
		UGI	upper gastrointestinal
STS	soft tissue sarcoma	ULE	unilateral limb enlargement
SVT	supraventricular tachycardia	UNFPA	United Nations Population Fund
TAP	tunica albuginea plication	UNICEF	United Nations Children's Fund
TB	tuberculosis	UPJ	ureteropelvic junction (see also PUJ)
TBA	traditional birth attendants	UPU	upper pole ureter
TCA	total colonic aganglionosis	URTI	upper respiratory tract infection
TEV	talipes equinovarus	US	United States; ultrasound, ultrasonography
TFL	tensor fascia lata	UVJ	ureterovesical junction; see also VUJ
TGD	total gastric dissociation	UTI	urinary tract infection
TGF	transforming growth factor	VAC	vacuum-assisted closure; vincristin, actinomycin D, and cyclophosphamide
TIP	typhoid intestinal perforation; tubularised incised plate		
		VACTERL	Vertebral and spinal cord, Anorectal, Cardiac, TracheoEsophageal, Renal and other urinary tract, Limb
TIPSS	transjugular intrahepatic portosystemic stent shunt		
TLOSR	transient lower oesophageal sphincter relaxation	VAPP	vaccine-associated paralytic poliomyelitis
		VATER	Vertebrae, Anus, Trachea, Esophagus, and Renal (association)
TMJ	temporomandibular joint		
TNF	tumour necrosis factor	VATS	video-assisted thoracic surgery
TNM	tumour, nodes, metastases (staging system)	VCUG	voiding cystourethrogram
		VDRL	Venereal Disease Research Laboratory
TOF	tracheo-oesophageal fistula; tetralogy of Fallot	VEPTR	vertical expandable prosthetic titanium rib
		VCUG	voiding cystourethogram
TORCH	Toxoplasmosis, Rubella, Cytomegalovirus, Herpes	VLBW	very low birth weight
		VMA	vanillylmandelic acid
TPA	tissue plasminogen activator	VP	ventriculoperitoneal (shunt)
TPPPS	Toddler-Preschooler Postoperative Pain Scale	VPI	velopharyngeal incompetence
		VSD	ventricular septal defect
TPN	total parenteral nutrition	VUJ	vesicoureteric junction; see also UVJ
TR	trauma registry	VUR	vesicoureteric reflux; vesicouretal reflux
TRH	thyrotropin-releasing hormone	WAGR	an acronym for WT, Aniridia, Genito-urinary malformations, mental Retardation
TRISS	Trauma and Injury Severity Score		
T-RTS	Triage RTS	WBC	white blood cells
TS	Trauma Score	WHO	World Health Organisation
TSH	thyroid-stimulating hormone	WT	Wilms' tumour
TSPY	testis-specific protein Y-encoded	WWW	worldwide web
TSS	toxic shock syndrome	XRT	x-ray therapy
TST	tuberculin skin test	YTP	inverted-Y tubularised plate
TV	tunica vaginalis		

INDEX